Free Student Aid.

Log on.

Explore.

Succeed.

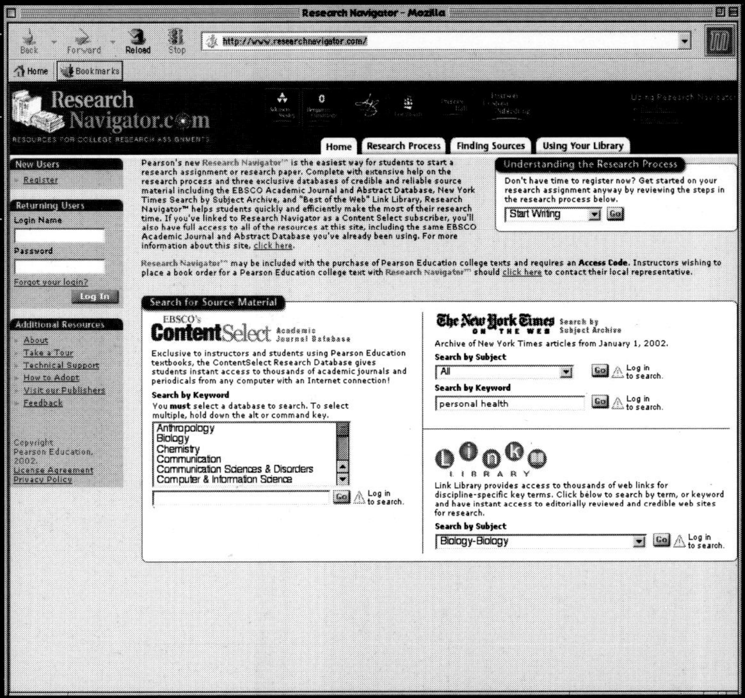

Research Navigator™ is a great media resource that can help you succeed in your personal health course. Offering three exclusive online databases of credible and reliable source material, Research Navigator™ includes EBSCO's Content Select Academic Journal Database, The New York Times Search by Subject Archive, and "Best of the Web" Link Library. Research Navigator™ can help you make the most of your research time.

What your computer system needs to use these media resources:

WINDOWS™

- 266 MHz minimum CPU
- Windows 98/NT4/2000/ME/XP
- 64 MB minimum RAM
- 800 x 600 screen resolution
- Thousands of colors
- 56K Internet connection
- Browsers: Internet Explorer 5.0 and higher; Netscape 4.7, 7.0
- Plug-ins: Adobe Acrobat Reader

MACINTOSH™

- 266 MHz minimum CPU
- OS 9.2 or higher
- 64 MB minimum RAM
- 800 x 600 screen resolution
- Thousands of colors
- 56K Internet connection
- Browsers: Internet Explorer 5.0 and higher; Netscape 4.7
- Plug-ins: Adobe Acrobat Reader

Got technical questions?

For technical support, please visit www.aw.com/techsupport. You can also call our tech support hotline at 800-6-Pro-Desk (800-677-6337) Monday-Friday, 8 a.m. to 5 p.m. CST.

Here's your personal ticket to success:

How to log on to Research Navigator™

1. Go to www.aw.com/pruitt
2. Click the Research Navigator™ link located on the left side of the web-site.
3. Click on the "Register" button located under the "New User" section on the left side of the Research Navigator™ homepage.
4. Scratch off foil below to reveal your pre-assigned access code.
5. Enter your access code exactly as it appears below.
6. Complete the online registration form to create your own personal Log In Name and Password.
7. Once your personal Log In Name and Password are confirmed by email, you can either go back to www.aw.com/pruitt and click Research Navigator™ or go to www.researchnavigator.com and type in your new Log In Name and Password under "Returning Users" and click "Log In."

Your Access Code is:

Record your new login name and password on the back of this card.

Cut out this card and keep it handy. It's your ticket to valuable information.

Important: Please read the License Agreement located on the launch screen before using Research Navigator™. By using the website, you indicate that you have read, understood and accepted the terms of this agreement.

0-321-10671-7

Decisions for Healthy Living

Decisions for Healthy Living

B.E. Pruitt
Texas A & M University

Jane J. Stein
The Stein Group

PEARSON
Benjamin Cummings

San Francisco Boston New York
Cape Town Hong Kong London Madrid Mexico City
Montreal Munich Paris Singapore Sydney Tokyo Toronto

Publisher: Daryl Fox
Acquisitions Editor: Deirdre McGill
Project Editor: Ellen Keohane
Associate Editor: Michelle Cadden
Development Manager: Claire Brassert
Managing Editor: Diane Southworth
Production Editor: Steven Anderson
Photo Researcher: Cypress Integrated, Brian Donnelly
Cover Design: Yvo Riezebos
Production Coordination & Composition: Elm Street Publishing Services, Inc.
Manufacturing Buyer: Stacey Weinberger
Marketing Manager: Sandra Lindelof
Cover Photo: DigitalVision/Getty Images

Photography and illustration credits appear on pp. 325–326

Library of Congress Cataloging-in-Publication Data
Pruitt, B. E.
Decisions for healthy living / B.E. Pruitt, Jane J. Stein.
p. cm.
Includes bibliographical references and index.
ISBN 0-321-10671-7
1. College students—Health and hygiene. 2. Health—Decision making. I. Stein, Jane. II. Title.
RA777.3.P778 2004
613'.0434—dc21

2003043606

PEARSON
Benjamin Cummings

www.aw.com/bc

1 2 3 4 5 6 7—VHP—07 06 05 04 03

To Katy and Bob, and our children and grandchildren; and to our readers as they make good decisions for healthy living.

Brief Contents

Contents

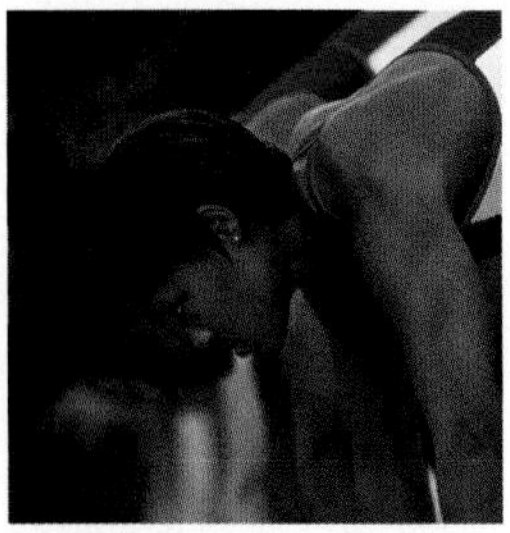

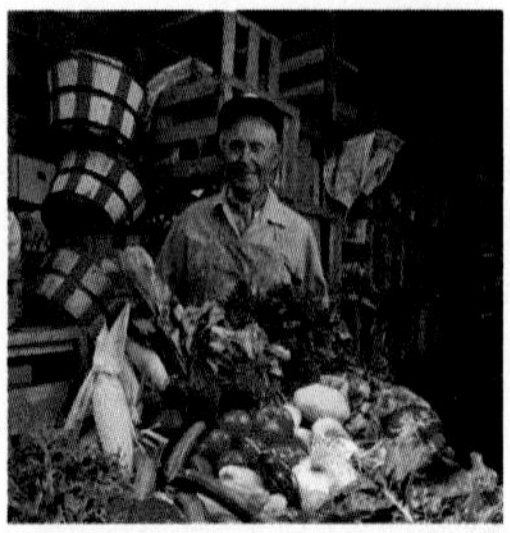

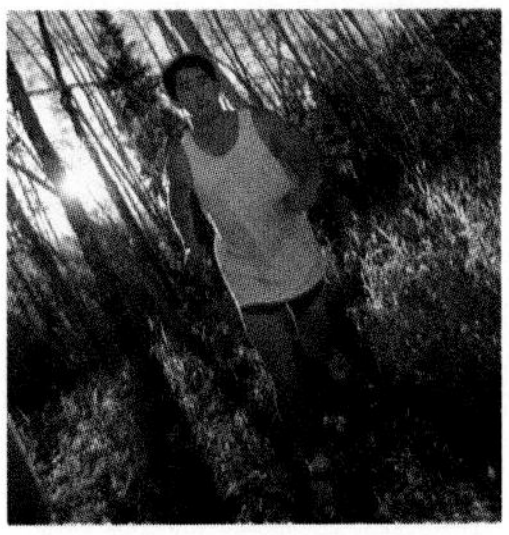

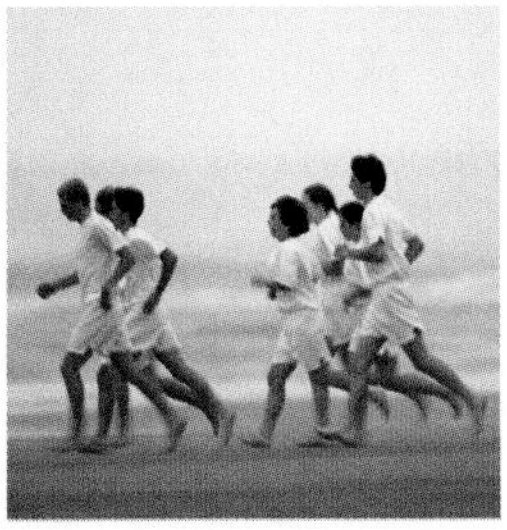

Part Three
Controllable Health Risks 95

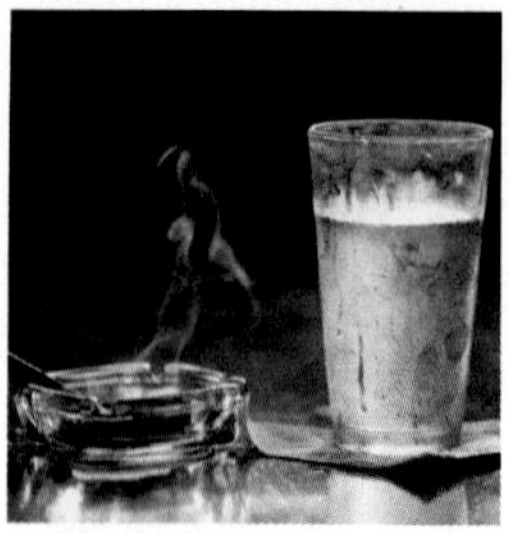

Chapter 7

The Health Effects of Smoking and Drinking 95

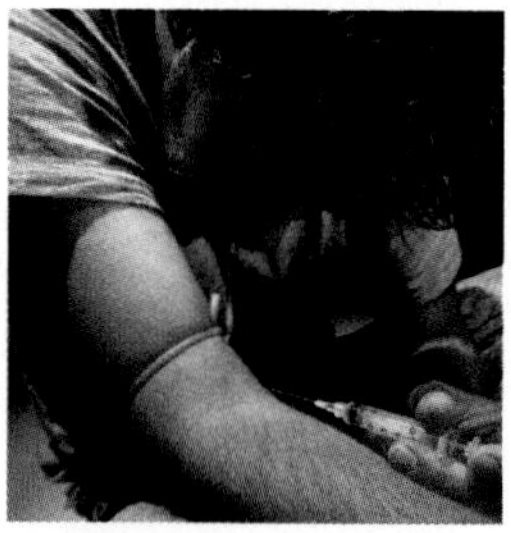

Chapter 8

Understanding the Dangers of Drug Use 114

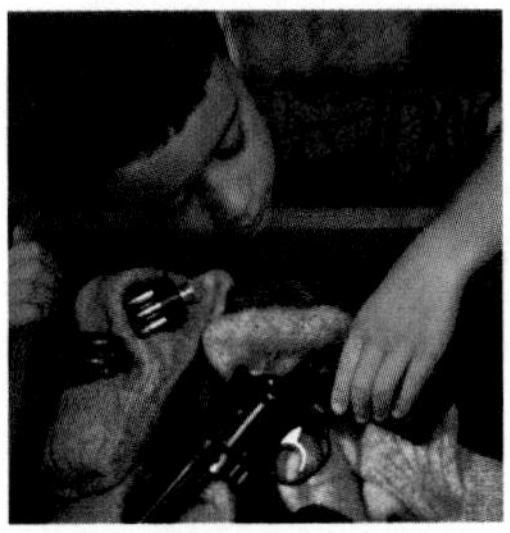

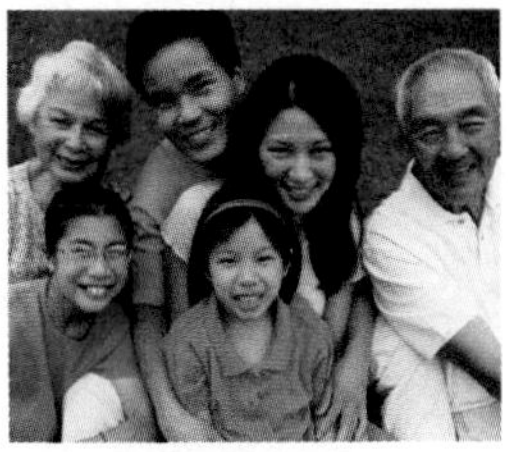

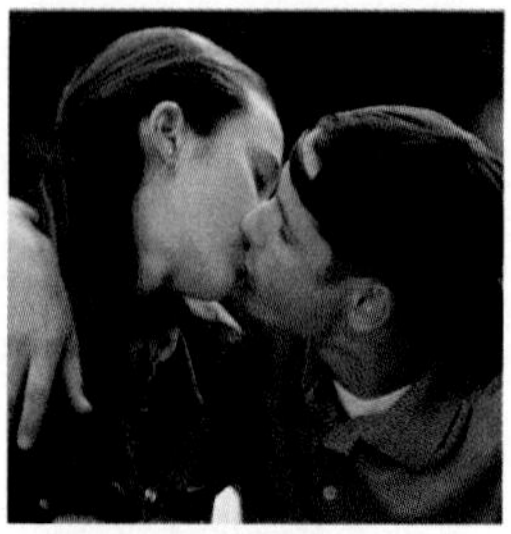

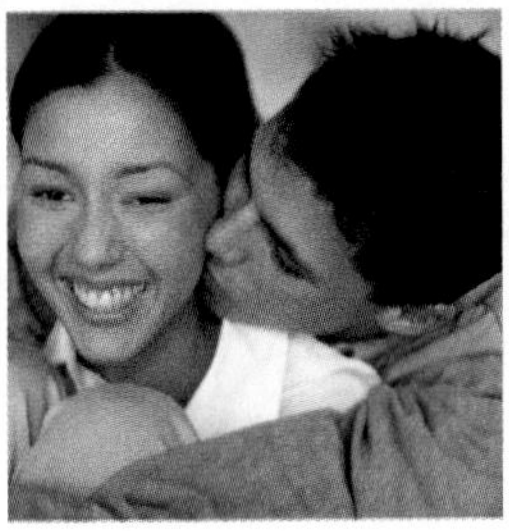

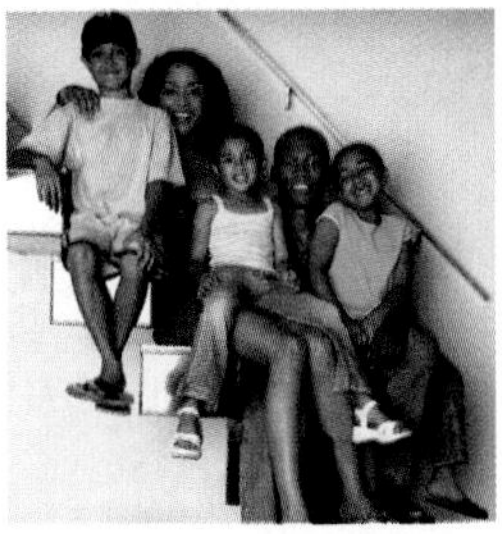

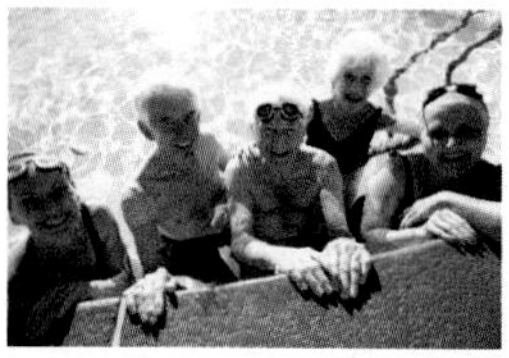

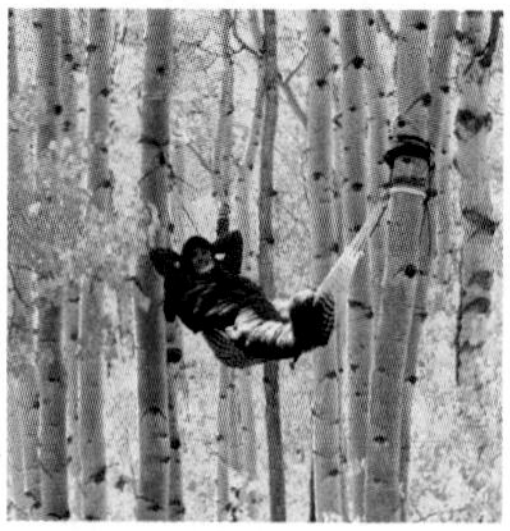

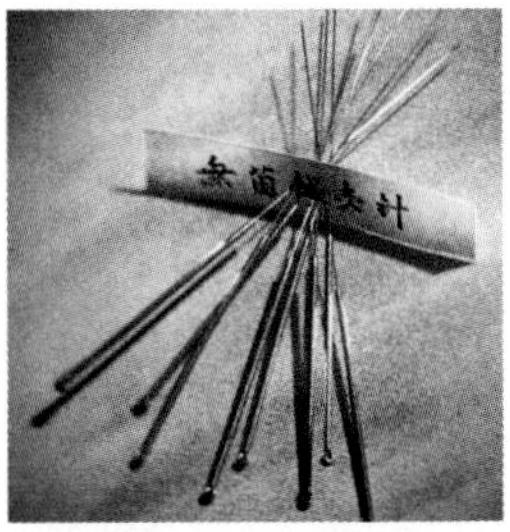

Feature Boxes

Cultural View

Developing Health Skills

Assess Your Health

Preface

Every day, college students make decisions that affect their own health, the health of their family and friends, and the health of their community. Some of these decisions seem simple—for example, what to eat for breakfast—while others could be a matter of life and death—such as whether or not to drink and drive. We strongly believe that with high-quality health information and a sound perspective on health and health behaviors, students can develop the necessary skills to evaluate their behavior and make healthy decisions. We wrote *Decisions for Healthy Living* to give students the basic building blocks for making those decisions. After completing a course of study using this textbook, students will be better prepared to face the varied decisions they'll encounter related to their personal health. They will become increasingly skilled as they put into practice what they have learned.

The approach of *Decisions for Healthy Living* is conceptual. We focus on big ideas rather than the specific details in each chapter. A clear, concise, and friendly writing style keeps students engaged in the material without bogging them down with technical details and without making judgments about their choices.

The organizational and topical approach to *Decisions for Healthy Living* was chosen after a thorough examination of the public health threats currently facing people in the United States. A commitment to comprehensive health education, as defined by leading professional health education organizations, accounts for the inclusion of the traditional topics. A recognition of the importance of *Healthy People 2010: National Health Promotion and Disease Prevention Objectives* accounts for the addition of nontraditional topics such as the health threats of violent behavior and the added emphasis on weight management. Also in keeping with *Healthy People 2010,* this textbook recognizes the importance of personal health assessment. Without an accurate measure of personal health—particularly benchmarks such as weight, pulse rate, and cholesterol levels—health improvement is difficult to attain. The importance of health assessment is evident in Chapter 1, *Health: Your Personal Responsibility,* and also in many of the pedagogical tools included throughout the book.

Much of what students will learn in *Decisions for Healthy Living* does not require a full understanding of how the human body functions biologically. One exception relates to sexuality. In this case, we recognize the importance of students knowing human anatomy and physiology. Accordingly, we have prepared a special appendix, *Your Sexual Body: A Primer on Reproductive Anatomy and Physiology.* This primer explains the biological functions of the male and female reproductive systems and includes high-quality, accurate art by Benjamin Cummings' renowned medical illustrators. It is intended to enhance students' understanding of material presented in other parts of the text relating to sex and sexuality. The appendix is designed for flexible use in the course.

Organization

Decisions for Healthy Living is organized into six parts—each part building on the information presented in earlier sections of the book.

Part One, Introductory Concepts, presents the basic definitions and concepts of health and well being that are the foundation of the book. It introduces students to the importance of taking responsibility for their own health, for minimizing risks through prevention, and for developing a plan for informed health decision making.

Part Two, The Basics of Good Health, teaches students many of the most basic components of a healthy lifestyle, including positive mental health, stress management skills, diet and weight control, and physical fitness.

Part Three, Controllable Health Risks, deals with some of the risk factors that account for health problems—those we can control. An understanding of the health threats of smoking, alcohol and drug use, accidents, and violent behavior are central to students taking control of these risks.

Part Four, Understanding the Disease Process, addresses chronic and infectious diseases and sexually transmitted infections including HIV/AIDS. Prevention and risk reduction of these diseases is a critical component of a healthy lifestyle.

Part Five, Sexuality and Relationships: A Life Span Approach, presents a social health perspective with a focus on the major stages of life from birth through to the end of life. It covers the importance of developing healthy relationships with other people (including healthy sexual relationships) and planning a family. It also covers end-of-life issues such as the aging process, dying, and death.

Part Six, Participating in a Healthy Community, deals with environmental health and consumer decisions related to health. These two concerns go beyond personal health to address the health of the community now and for generations to come.

Special Features and Learning Aids

The study of health is not a passive encounter with health facts. Therefore, *Decisions for Healthy Living* actively involves the reader in several ways.

Each chapter opens with a list of **Learning Objectives** as well as five **Test Your Knowledge** questions. The Learning Objectives provide the reader with an idea of the content of the chapter as well as a tool for evaluating understanding once the chapter has been completed. The Test Your Knowledge feature is a collection of true/false questions meant to challenge students' misconceptions or false impressions about particular health topics covered in each chapter. These questions motivate students to read on and learn the facts about topics they may have assumed they already understood. The answers to these questions are found at the end of each chapter. There are three special boxes that appear in many or all of the chapters to highlight, personalize, and otherwise bring special attention to critical, relevant health information.

Assess Your Health self-assessment boxes ask students to analyze their behavior, health skills, and personal choices. Such assessments provide the student with a reality check to make sure their attempts at health enhancement are based on objectively derived observations of health status—and not on misconceptions or misimpressions.

Developing Health Skills boxes stress behavior changes by providing information related to environmental, consumer, and general health education topics. This information helps students develop the abilities they need to achieve good health.

Cultural View boxes explore interesting health issues and concepts from a cross-cultural perspective. Many health decisions are influenced by cultural factors and these boxes acknowledge and promote respect for these cultural differences.

All boldfaced terms in the text are defined in the **Running Glossary,** which appears at the bottom of each page. There is also a complete glossary at the end of the book.

The following additional learning aids appear at the end of each chapter and are an integral part of *Decisions for Healthy Living:*

Case Studies provide realistic scenarios of how individuals face health-related decisions. Most of the cases involve two college students. One individual makes a positive health decision while the other does not. A series of "In Your Opinion" questions prompt students to analyze the scenarios in search of further understanding on the complexity of health-related behavior.

Several **Critical Thinking Questions** highlighted in each chapter prompt in-depth thinking and exploration of the dilemmas that often occur when studying health. In each chapter, at least two Critical Thinking Questions are based on the *Healthy People 2010* initiatives to further bolster the students' understanding of this important guide to public health.

A list of **Key Concepts** is provided at the end of each chapter for review as well as a list of **Review Questions** based on the contents of each chapter.

Health Hotlines provide a listing of toll-free telephone numbers for students to call to get health information that could directly affect them, their family, friends, and community.

HealthLinks give students access to current health information on the Internet, with websites specifically selected to include trends and data from credible sources.

A **Selected Bibliography** for each chapter is included for further exploration of the topics discussed.

A complete **Glossary** at the end of the book defines terms found in the text.

Instructor Supplements

Instructor's Resource Manual 0-8053-5371-2
This comprehensive resource features chapter-by-chapter learning objectives, lecture outlines, and key terms and concepts. Healthy Activities and Questions for Discussion sections provide engaging lecture ideas. Information about video resources is also listed.

Instructor's Resource Binder 0-8053-5567-7
Available as a separate item, this 2 1/2-inch ring binder will fit all print supplements that accompany *Decisions for Healthy Living.* All supplements are available separately.

PowerPoint® Presentation CD-ROM 0-8053-5375-5
With more than 320 pre-made PowerPoint® slides to choose from, this cross-platform CD-ROM makes preparing lectures easy. Each chapter presentation features lecture outlines, illustrations, and tables from the text.

Transparency Acetates 0-8053-5374-7
Full-color acetates include all illustrations and tables from the text.

Printed Test Bank 0-8053-5372-0

Computerized Test Bank 0-8053-5373-9
Including 60 multiple-choice, 10 fill-in-the-blank, 15 true/false, 10 matching, and 5 essay questions for each chapter, the test bank is available in print, on a cross-platform CD-ROM, and in the instructor section of MyHealthClass™ and Blackboard.

Instructor's Guide for StudentBody101.com 0-205-35084-4
This booklet offers a road map to the StudentBody101.com website. With teaching tips and collaborative learning exercises, this booklet shows you how to make the most of the materials on the site.

Blackboard
http://cms.aw.com/blackboard

MyHealthClass™
www.myhealthclass.com
In addition to Blackboard, we offer MyHealthClass™—an online standard course management system powered by CourseCompass™ that is loaded with valuable free resources for your students. MyHealthClass™ features preloaded content including the Behavior Change Log Book and Wellness Journal, Take Charge of Your Health! Worksheets, and links to the StudentBody101.com website and the *Decisions for Healthy Living* website. Also includes Research Navigator™, TestGen, PowerPoint® Slides, and Instructor's Resource Manual material. MyHealthClass™ can be packaged free with the text.

Discovery Health Channel Health & Wellness Lecture Launcher Videos

Volume I 0-8053-5369-0
Volume II 0-8053-6001-8

Created in partnership between Discovery Health Channel and Benjamin Cummings, these VHS tapes feature a series of quick lecture-launcher clips on topics from nutrition and stress management to substance abuse. There are 24 clips in all, each 5 to 10 minutes in length, and they are an excellent way to engage your students and enliven your lectures.

Benjamin Cummings Video Series

In addition to the Discovery Health Channel and Wellness Lecture Launcher videos, the following 15 videos are available free for adopters:

Promoting Healthy Behavior 0-205-29194-5
Coping with Stress 0-205-29196-1
Understanding Healthy Relationships & Sexuality 0-205-29197-X
Considering Birth Control, Pregnancy & Childbirth Options 0-205-29198-8
Eating for Optimal Health 0-205-29199-6
Managing Your Weight 0-205-29200-3
Keeping Fit 0-205-29201-1
Understanding the Risks of Tobacco and Caffeine 0-205-29204-6
Preventing Drug Abuse 0-205-29205-4
Reducing the Risk of Cardiovascular Disease 0-205-29230-5
Avoiding Infectious & Sexual Transmitted Diseases 0-205-29232-1
Living with Modern Maladies 0-205-29233-X
Accepting Life's Transitions 0-205-29234-8
Stemming Violence & Abuse 0-205-29235-6
Thinking Globally, Acting Locally 0-205-29236-4

Films for the Humanities

More than 80 videos from recognized sources are available for qualified adopters. Contact your local Benjamin Cummings sales representatives for more information.

Student Supplements

Decisions for Healthy Living Website

www.aw.com/pruitt

This powerful study tool offers a wide range of activities, including practice quizzes, critical thinking questions, self-assessments, weblinks, and audio and video clips to help students earn better grades. Online flashcards help students quiz themselves on key terms from the text, and an "Ask Buzz and Jane" section allows students to e-mail questions to the book authors. eThemes of the Times—containing 30 *New York Times* articles reporting on the latest health news and research—is also included.

StudentBody101.com
www.studentbody101.com
This dynamic website contains current articles, self-assessments, online discussions, and behavior-change tips. Accredited by Health on the Net, it can be packaged free with each new copy of the text.

Student Study Guide for StudentBody101.com 0-8053-4793-3
Guiding students through the material on the StudentBody101.com website, this valuable resource also contains new exercises, additional weblinks, and interviews with experts on health polls, surveys, and other topics. It can be packaged free with each new copy of the book.

Behavior Change Log Book and Wellness Journal 0-8053-5548-0
This assessment tool helps students track daily exercise and nutritional intake and create a long-term nutritional and fitness prescription plan. It also includes a Behavior Change Contract and topics for journal-based activities. This tool can be packaged free with each new copy of the book.

Take Charge of Your Health! Worksheets 0-8053-5573-1
Approximately 48 self-assessment activities that help students make positive behavioral changes in their lives. These worksheets can be packaged free with each new copy of the text.

Health on the Net 0-205-34669-3
This catalogue of Internet resources provides useful tips for online research, links to relevant websites, and MLA and American Psychological Association (APA) guidelines. It can be packaged free with each new copy of the text.

NutriFit CD-ROM 0-321-11218-0
Using this nutrition and fitness management software, students can track and analyze their daily food intake and exercise. A variety of assessment activities can be assigned to students for evaluation of nutrient balance and calorie expenditure. Various reports analyze their eating and exercise habits.

Research Navigator™ 0-321-18607-9
Complete with extensive help on the research process and three databases of credible and reliable source material—including EBSCO's Content Select™ Academic Journal Database, *New York Times* Search by Subject Archive, and "Best of the Web" Link Library—Research Navigator™ helps students quickly and efficiently make the most of their research time. A six-month subscription is included with all new copies of the text.

Stand-alone Blackboard Premium Access Code Card 0-321-19567-1

Stand-alone MyHealthClass™ Access Code Card 0-8053-5546-4
This access code card is for students who purchase used books. It includes all content from the *Decisions for Healthy Living* website.

A Word of Thanks

Dozens of health education experts have contributed to this book through their thoughtful reviews and suggestions. These reviewers teach health education in colleges and universities and work in the field of health education across the country. They are at the cutting edge of their profession and have ensured that the contents of *Decisions for Healthy Living* are on the cutting edge as well. We are deeply appreciative of the time they took to comment on our book.

Robert Alman II
Indiana University of Pennsylvania

Robert B. Beavers
Benedict College

Roger Bounds
Sam Houston State University

Liz Brown
Rose State College

Laura J. Burger
Grossmont College

Jean Dunlap
Rose State College

Mandi Dupain
Millersville University

Richard Mark Ellington
University of North Carolina–Wilmington

Rosemary Ferguson
University of North Carolina–Wilmington

Julie Sammarco Henderson
University of Utah

Loretta R. Herrin
Benedict College

J. David Holland
Springfield College, Illinois

Gwendolyn Holmes
Norfolk State University

Holli Hudson
Berea College

Loeen Irons
Baylor University

Karl Kleinkopf
College of Idaho

Robert Kostelnik
Indiana University of Pennsylvania

Ellen Lee
California State University–Fullerton

Greg Lonning
Luther College

Linda Ludovico
Tyler Junior College

Bonnie Luft
Baylor University

Danyte Mockus
San Diego State University

Helene Monthley
Pennsylvania State University

Valorie Nybo
Western Carolina University

Roseanne Poole
Tallahassee Community College

José E. Rivera
Indiana University of Pennsylvania

George Rosales
Ventura College

Jiri Stelzer
Valdosta State University

Robert Walker
John Brown University

Words on paper do not make a book. So we are especially grateful to the team at Benjamin Cummings for their creative input during the editorial and production process of *Decisions for Healthy Living*. Thanks to Deirdre McGill, Ellen Keohane, Sandra Lindelof, Michelle Cadden, Steven Anderson, Diane Southworth, Cheryl Cechvala, Erin Joyce, and Kari Dickenson. We'd also like to thank Heather Johnson at Elm Street Publishing Services, Inc.

Why Read *Decisions for Healthy Living*?

The knowledge and skills acquired through the use of this book are personal, relevant, and hold the potential to positively influence a student's quality of life both now and in the future. *Decisions for Healthy Living* is a textbook for the study of health and health behaviors. But it is much more than that. Welcome to a study of the most interesting and personally relevant subject in the college catalog.

Buzz Pruitt
College Station, TX

Jane Stein
Washington, DC

About the Authors

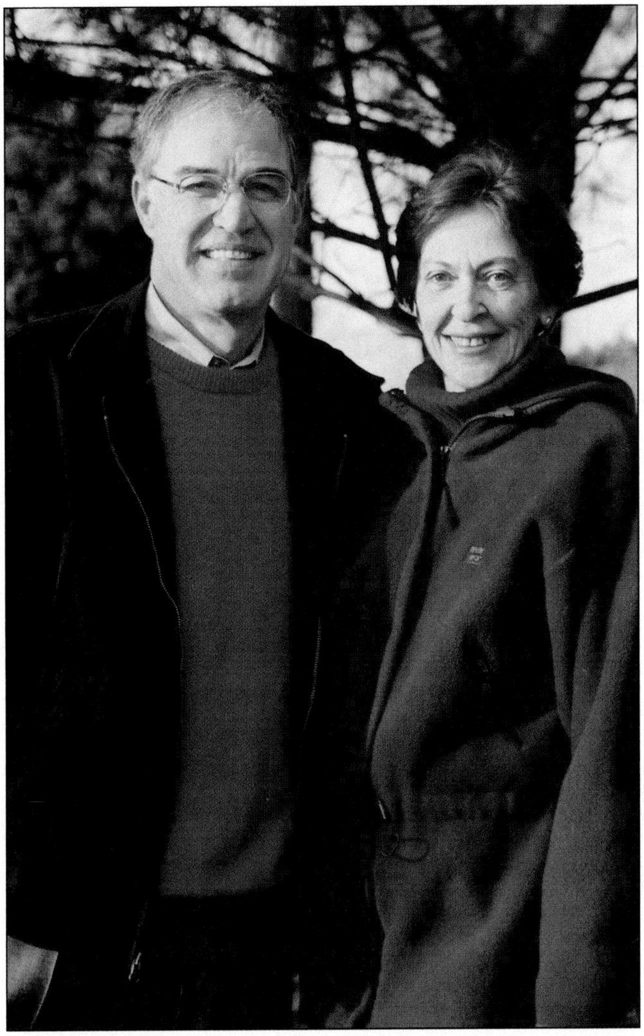

B.E. (Buzz) Pruitt
Buzz Pruitt has been a health educator for more than 30 years. He has directed major curriculum development projects related to drug-use prevention, sex education, and comprehensive health education. He presently conducts research and is a Professor of Health Education at Texas A & M University. *Decisions for Healthy Living* incorporates Pruitt's own philosophy of well-being. His approach is neutral and non-judgmental, particularly in the field of human sexuality, in which he specializes.

Buzz recently won the "2002 AAHE Professional Service Award" from the American Association for Health Education. He has also received honors from the Texas Association for Health, Physical Education, Recreation, and Dance (TAHPERD); the University of North Texas; the Association of Former Students of Texas A & M University; the Texas Association of School Administrators; Eric Clearinghouse on Teacher Education; Southwest Texas State University; the Association for the Advancement of Health Education; the U.S. Department of Health and Human Services; and the Danforth Foundation. He is an active member of the American Alliance for Health, Physical Education, Recreation, and Dance (AAHPERD) and the American School Health Association. He is also the founder and president of the Health Education Foundation of Texas.

Jane J. Stein
Jane Stein has spent more than 40 years writing about health care for the general public, translating often complex medical information into understandable terms for the lay reader. Her philosophy about how to communicate health issues is reflected in *Decisions for Healthy Living*. She is the author of *Making Medical Choices* and hundreds of articles in the popular press, and she has served as editor and publisher of national health publications. She is president of The Stein Group, a publications development and management firm specializing in health and health policy issues including women's health, mental health, substance abuse, and access to and quality of care.

Jane was a founder and former board member of Washington Independent Writers, is a lifetime member of the National Association of Science Writers, and has taught nonfiction writing at the American University in Washington, D.C.

CHAPTER

1

Health: Your Personal Responsibility

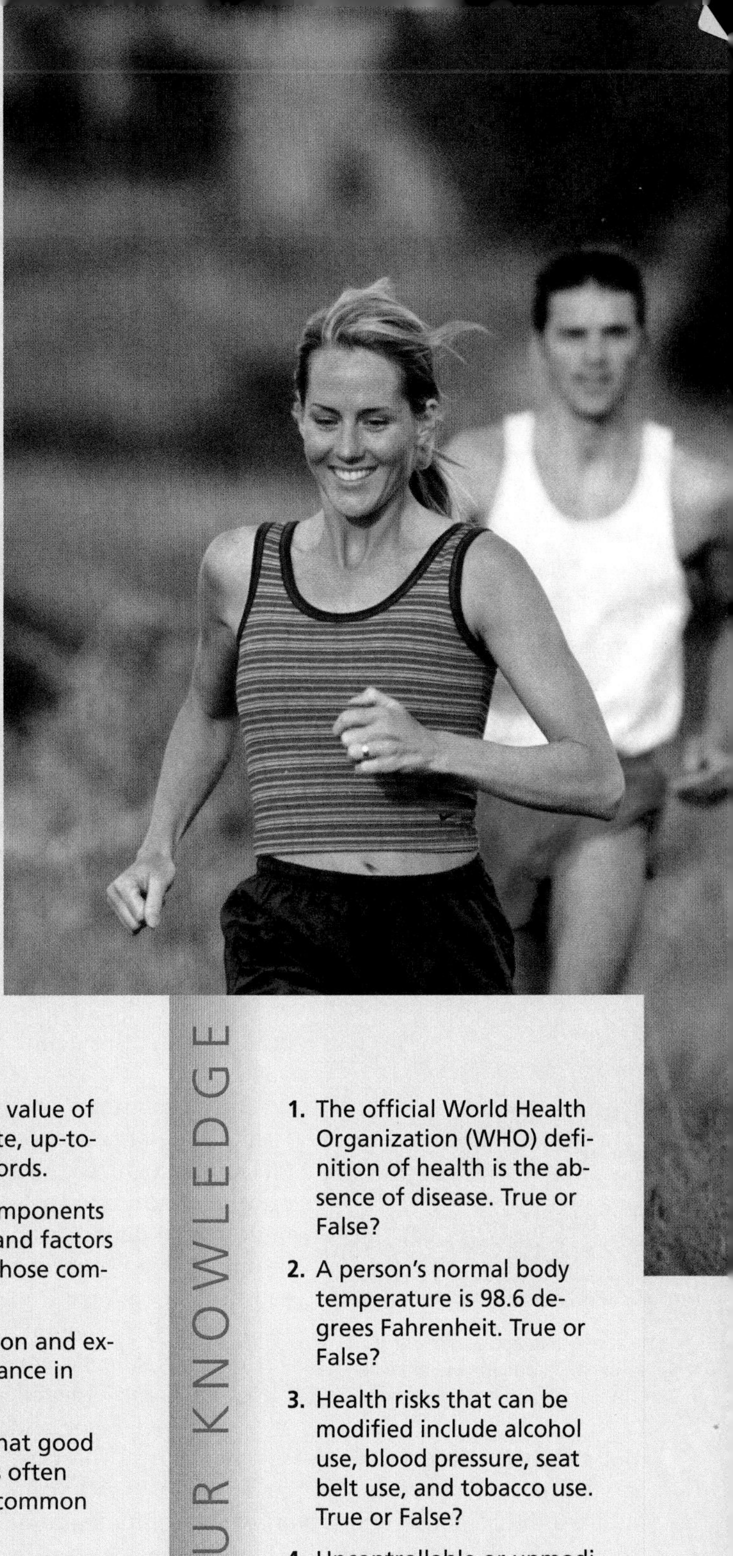

OBJECTIVES

When you finish reading this chapter, you will be able to:

1. Define health and describe a healthy person.
2. Describe the nature of becoming healthy.
3. Explain the importance of health knowledge and health skills to your overall well-being.
4. Differentiate among behaviors related to health.
5. Become familiar with different means of health assessment and ways to draw accurate conclusions about your health status from your observations.
6. List several healthy behaviors that may lead to health risk reduction.
7. Understand the value of keeping accurate, up-to-date health records.
8. Describe the components of health style and factors that influence those components.
9. Define prevention and explain its importance in your life.
10. Acknowledge that good health practices often come down to common sense.

TEST YOUR KNOWLEDGE

1. The official World Health Organization (WHO) definition of health is the absence of disease. True or False?
2. A person's normal body temperature is 98.6 degrees Fahrenheit. True or False?
3. Health risks that can be modified include alcohol use, blood pressure, seat belt use, and tobacco use. True or False?
4. Uncontrollable or unmodifiable risk factors include having a relative die of heart disease and witnessing a violent argument. True or False?
5. Healthy living is a matter of personal choice not influenced by friends or family. True or False?

Answers found at end of chapter.

Before you came to class today, did you have breakfast? Did you smoke a cigarette? Did you get seven to eight hours of sleep and wake up feeling alert? Did you work out in the gym or go for a swim or jog? The answers to these health-related questions are highly personal. That is why this book and this course of study focus on personal health. During the semester, you will learn that you can significantly influence how healthy you are by what you do and how you relate to the people around you.

This textbook is a guide to good health—a guide to things you can do to reduce your risks for disease and increase your overall well-being. *Decisions for Healthy Living* focuses on you and your abilities as well as on your interaction with the environment and with your community, society, and culture.

Defining Health

Health is an abstract idea for which there are many definitions. Once, it may have been appropriate to define it simply as the absence of disease. This definition is fraught with problems. Given our modern understanding of the nature of disease, it is highly unlikely that anyone would qualify as healthy under this definition.

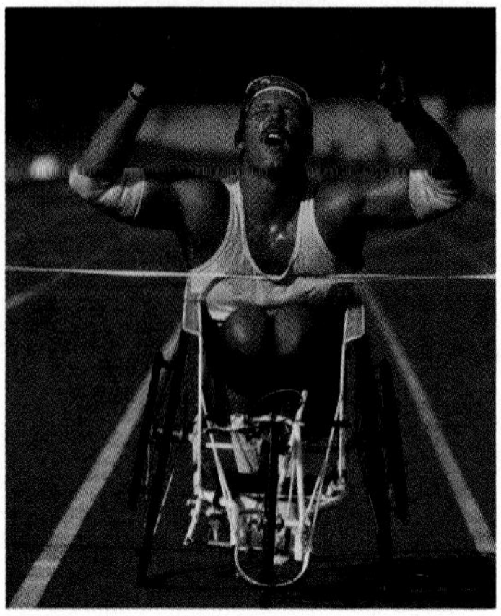

Personal health and wellness are measured individually and ultimately mean reaching your personal best.

Fortunately, the World Health Organization (WHO) recognized this difficulty and provided a multifaceted definition of health. In its founding constitution, adopted in 1946, WHO defined health as "a state of complete physical, mental, and social well-being and not merely the absence of disease or infirmity." This classic definition has become the guidepost for health care and health-promotion efforts worldwide (see the Cultural View box). By recognizing that health is a measure of well-being, the WHO definition has broadened our understanding of health so that it represents not only an end in itself, but also a means toward that end.

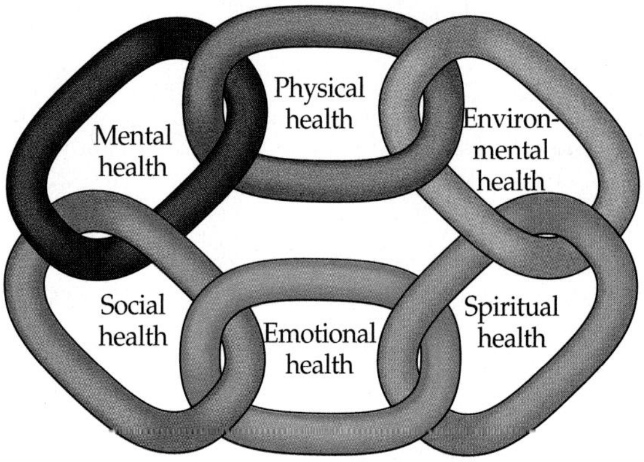

Figure 1.1 Holistic Health
Holistic health encompasses many aspects of a person's life—physiological, emotional, spiritual, and more. By taking a holistic approach to your health, you show that you understand that the whole is greater than the individual parts.

The WHO definition of health is contained in the concept of **holistic health.** In this broad concept, health encompasses physical, mental, emotional, social, spiritual, and environmental aspects of an individual as well as of the community in which he or she lives. The word *holistic* is based on the concept that the whole is greater than the sum of its parts (see Figure 1.1).

Even such expansive definitions of health, however, do not take into account the full nature of health and well-being. Most notably missing from the WHO definition or the holistic health concept is the idea of human potential. If health is viewed in terms of potential, everyone can be healthy—and the extent of health is determined not by an externally established standard but by personal potential. This line of thinking has led to the concept of wellness.

Wellness emphasizes your potential and responsibility for health. Physician Halbert Dunn, who coined the term *high-level wellness,* described it as follows: "You

health A state of complete physical, mental, and social well-being; not merely the absence of disease or infirmity.

holistic health The concept of health involving physical, mental, emotional, social, spiritual, and environmental aspects of an individual as well as of the community in which he or she lives.

wellness A description of health that includes the human potential for a high level of well-being while taking into consideration environmental and personal limitations.

Cultural View

A Multifaceted Definition of Health

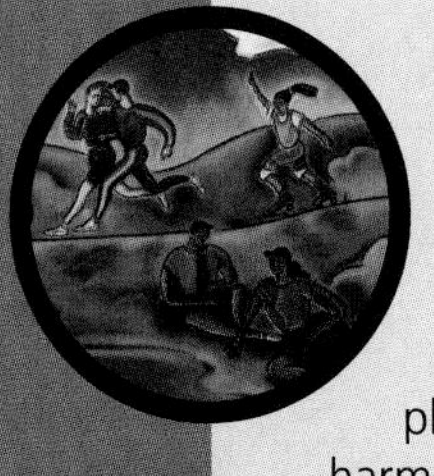

How broadly can health be defined? Very broadly, the World Health Organization (WHO) decided. According to WHO, the following principles relating to health are basic to the happiness, harmonious relations, and security of all peoples in all countries:

- Health is a state of complete physical, mental, and social well-being and not merely the absence of disease or infirmity.
- The enjoyment of the highest attainable standard of health is one of the fundamental rights of every human being without distinction of race, religion, political belief, or economic or social condition.
- The health of all peoples is fundamental to the attainment of peace and security and depends upon the fullest cooperation of individuals and states.
- The achievement of any state in the promotion and protection of health is of value to all.
- Unequal development in different countries in the promotion of health and control of disease, especially communicable disease, is a common danger.
- Healthy development of the child is of basic importance; the ability to live harmoniously in a changing total environment is essential to such development.
- The extension to all peoples of the benefits of medical, psychological, and related knowledge is essential to the fullest attainment of health.
- Informed opinion and active cooperation on the part of the public are of the utmost importance in the improvement of the health of the people.
- Governments have a responsibility for the health of their peoples, which can be fulfilled only by the provision of adequate health and social measures.

Source: Constitution of the World Health Organization

have energy to burn. You tingle with vitality. At times like these, the world is a glorious place." His concept was later portrayed in the form of a continuum. Think of health as a long line of events having premature death at one end and a high level of wellness at the other. An illness/wellness continuum, based on Dunn's original ideas, has been used for decades to illustrate the nature of health, including the potential for a high level of well-being (see Figure 1.2).

Wellness is an ongoing process in which you are always moving either toward or away from the most favorable level of health. According to the wellness model, a person with a physical disability who has good mental health, eats a nutritious diet, and participates competitively in wheelchair tennis tournaments may be healthier—and farther along the illness/wellness continuum—than a person who does not have physical disabilities but who is not as emotionally and physically fit.

Becoming Healthy

The concept of health is complex, regardless of the definition. So, too, is the process of attaining health—of becoming healthy. There are two ways to view the process of becoming healthy:

1. *You become healthy through developing healthy behaviors.* This assumes that you are healthy and that you move to a stronger position of health by taking health-promoting actions.
2. *You become healthy through behavior change.* You may have developed unhealthy behaviors, but you undergo a change in lifestyle or take specific actions that result in a healthier state.

In either case, personal involvement plays a critical role. You will be making decisions that affect your health throughout your life. By now, you have probably developed some good—and some bad—health habits. This book will help you expand your decision-making capabilities to enhance your health.

The process of becoming healthy is influenced by many factors, but significant among them are health knowledge (often expressed in terms of health literacy), health skills, and health behavior. Together, these components help you make decisions that result in healthy living.

Health Knowledge

Becoming healthy begins with health knowledge. **Health knowledge** is the accumulation of factual information that influences health decision making. High-quality health knowledge leads to high-quality health decision

health knowledge The accumulation of factual information that influences health decision making.

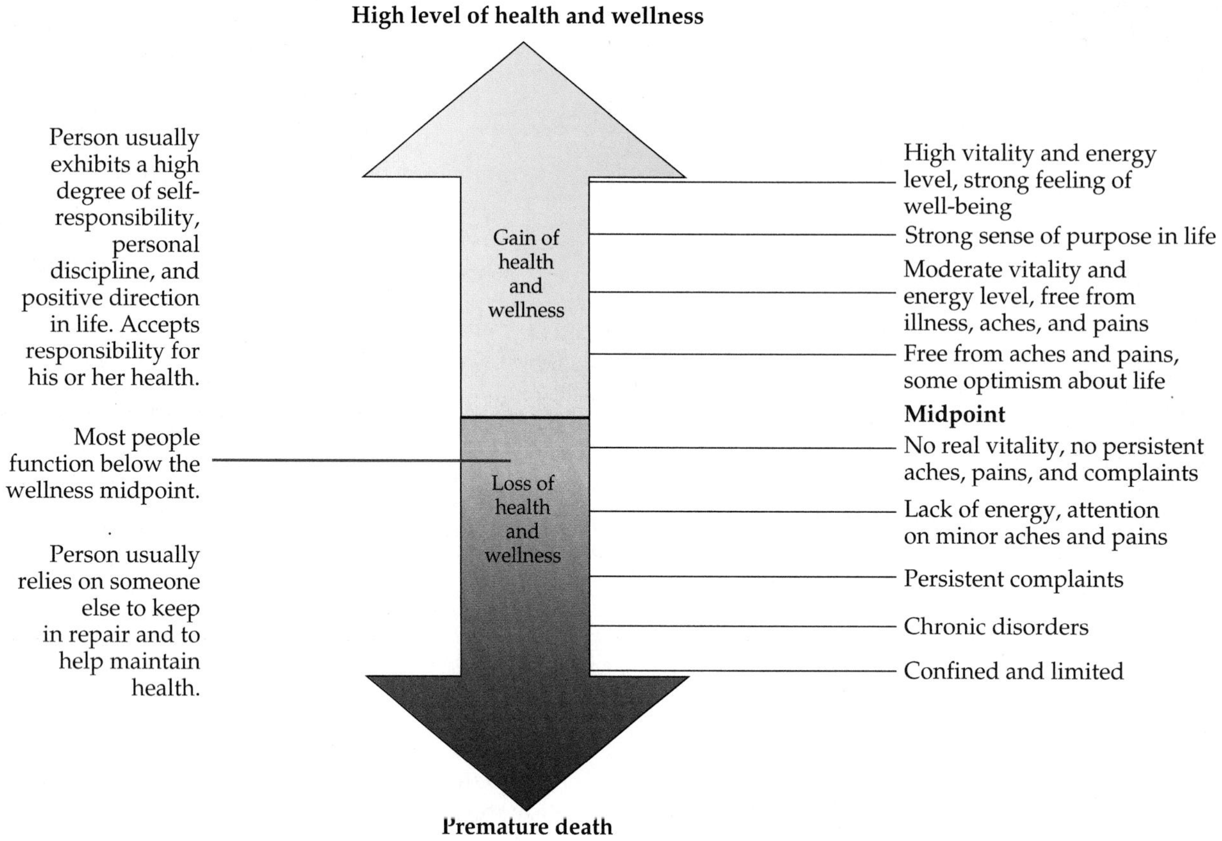

Figure 1.2 The Health and Wellness Continuum
Wellness is an ongoing process in which you are always moving toward an optimal level of health.

making. Low-quality health knowledge, alternatively, creates the potential for health-compromising decisions.

Where do you get your health information? From an advertisement in a fashion or sports magazine? A newspaper story? A television program? Your family physician? Or from family myths handed down from generation to generation ("You'll get a cold from wearing wet shoes.")? Do you think your sources of health information are adequate? To make good health decisions, you need accurate and unbiased information.

Health knowledge alone is not enough. You need to be able to use that knowledge—you need to be health literate as well. According to the National Health Education Standards, **health literacy** means being able to get, interpret, and understand basic health information and to use that information in ways that enhance your health—and the health of others.

health literacy The capacity of an individual to get, interpret, and understand basic health information and services and the competence to use such information and services in ways that are health enhancing.

There are four major components of health literacy:

1. *Self-directed learning.* Using a variety of sources to get current, credible, and applicable information can help you make sound health-related decisions.
2. *Critical thinking and problem solving.* Critical thinking skills can help you gather, analyze, and apply health information to meet your personal needs.
3. *Effective communicating.* There is a wide range of communication approaches—from listening to sharing information on the Internet—that you can use to learn about health issues. With effective communication skills, you can create a climate of understanding and support for others to learn about health.
4. *Being a responsible citizen.* Given your health knowledge, you are in a strong position to help keep yourself, your family and friends, and your community healthy (see the Developing Health Skills box).

Developing Health Skills

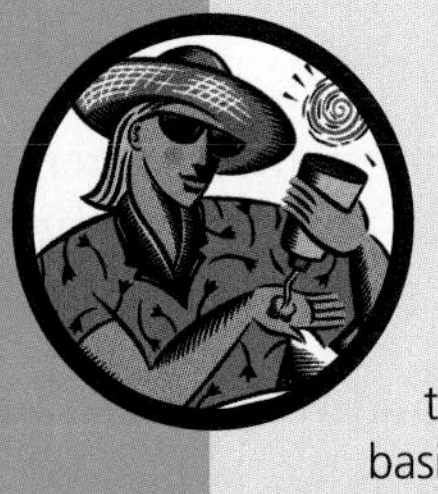

Healthy People 2010

Healthy People 2010 is a national initiative to assess the health of the nation. It continues a process begun in the 1980s to objectively measure the American population's health and to track disease and disease risk on a population-wide basis. The *Healthy People* initiative is an important means of understanding the health status of our population, of assessing progress toward health as a nation, and for planning effective prevention programs.

Healthy People 2010, which presents 467 objectives to improve the health of Americans, is designed to achieve two overarching goals: to help individuals of all ages increase life expectancy *and* improve their quality of life; and to eliminate health disparities among different segments of the population. Throughout *Decisions for Healthy Living,* you will find critical thinking questions based on *Healthy People 2010* objectives for the nation.

HEALTHY PEOPLE 2010

This document/article was neither reviewed nor approved by the U.S. Department of Health and Human Services. The views expressed herein are solely those of the issuing organization and do not necessarily reflect the official positions or policies of the U.S. Department of Health and Human Services. Healthy People 2010 documents are online at the Healthy People Web site at www.healthypeople.gov.

Health Skills

Skills are abilities that can help you achieve tasks. A skill is something you know how to do and feel comfortable doing. Once learned, a skill may become automatic. This is the case when you learn to drive a car safely. When you first start to drive, you have to think about when to signal before making a turn. With practice, however, signaling becomes a task that is done with little thought—it becomes automatic.

Health skills are abilities that can help you achieve good health. They are specific to healthy development or healthy behavior change. As with other skills, they evolve over time and with practice. The better you perform a health skill, the more likely you are to use it.

There are different ways to categorize health skills:

- *Motor skills* involve some physical movement, as in exercising or in brushing and flossing your teeth.
- *Intellectual skills* include gathering information, decision making, and using good judgment.
- *Emotional skills* involve managing stress, dealing with feelings, and using self-control.
- *Social skills* include listening, helping others, and asking for help.

The ability to assess blood pressure provides an example of how these skills interact. It requires (1) the motor skill of using a blood pressure measuring device properly; (2) the intellectual skills of knowing why it is important to know your blood pressure and what you can do if it is too high; (3) the emotional skill of practicing stress reduction as a way to control high blood pressure; and (4) the social skill of asking how to do any of the previous skills. You use health skills more often than you think you do. In fact, you use them as part of your daily living, learning, working, and playing activities.

Health Behavior

Health behavior is a complex, interlocked set of actions and reactions to a variety of stimuli. These actions and reactions may lead either to enhancement and protection of your health status or to its decline. There are three basic kinds of health behavior: preventive behavior, illness behavior, and sick-role behavior.

Preventive behavior helps you stay healthy. Examples of preventive behaviors are managing your weight, exercising at least three times a week, not smoking, and keeping your immunizations up to date. Preventive behaviors enhance health by reducing your risk for diseases or unintentional injuries.

health skills Abilities that influence health development, health status, and health maintenance.

health behavior Actions and habits that may lead either to enhancement and protection of a person's health status or to its decline.

preventive behavior Action taken by a person who is essentially healthy in order to remain healthy.

Illness behavior is what you do when you are not feeling well or have reason to believe you are not well. You respond to bodily signs and symptoms, for example, by taking your temperature or seeking the opinion of someone who has health expertise. Your health is enhanced when you engage health professionals in the diagnosis and treatment of an illness or disease. Failure to do so can delay your recovery and, in the case of an infectious disease, inadvertently spread illness.

Sick-role behavior is what you do after you have been diagnosed as sick. These are specific behaviors intended to address the acute nature of the diagnosed illness. An example is taking a drug prescribed by your physician to alleviate symptoms or cure a condition. By following the instructions of your physician, you contribute to your own recovery. By ignoring the instructions—such as by not taking prescription drugs as directed—you may jeopardize your health.

Assessing Your Personal Health

Becoming healthy is a lifelong process. But how will you know if you achieve that illusive goal? How do you know if you are healthy now? How do you know if you are not healthy? There are several ways to assess your personal health. Health assessment skills are critical to achieving health competence and, ultimately, to maintaining good health. The assessment of your own health begins with your skills of observation and data collection. Equally important, however, may be your knowledge about when to seek and how to respond to a health assessment expert—a physician, nurse practitioner, or health-promotion specialist.

Your health can change from one day to another, even from one second to another. You can be healthy today and suffer from a cold, influenza, or another communicable disease tomorrow. You can be active and able the second before you dive into shallow water and a quadriplegic the next second. Given the range of changes that might occur, it is not possible to know absolutely how healthy you will be at any moment. By conducting periodic assessments and by keeping good health records, you can determine what is normal for you so you can better notice when a change occurs.

A **self-assessment** occurs when an individual collects and interprets his or her own health-related baseline data. Obviously, this is a highly subjective means of health assessment and is often inaccurate. A **medical assessment** is conducted by a medical professional, such as a physician, and focuses on diagnosing whether you have a certain disease or medical condition. You can learn a lot about your personal health with each kind of assessment.

Observing Yourself

One of the most important ways to know if you are healthy is to observe yourself—conduct a self-assessment. This begins by asking simple questions such as "How do I feel?" and "Do I look healthy?" If you feel healthy, the likelihood is that you are relatively healthy. At the same time, if you feel ill, the chances are good that you are suffering from some form of health threat. Although there are many ways to observe yourself, three specific self-assessments are crucial to your lifelong well-being: assessment of body temperature, pulse rate, and body weight.

An easily observed marker of illness is body temperature. Most people have a thermometer and also have experienced a change in temperature. Body temperature is best measured by placing the thermometer under the tongue or in the armpit or anus. Normal body temperature has long been thought to be 98.6 degrees Fahrenheit, but recent studies indicate that it is 98.2 for adults and between 97.1 and 100 for infants and young children. Even so, some people have a slightly lower body temperature as their norm; others have a slightly higher normal body temperature. In general, women have a higher normal temperature (98.4) than men (98.1). And for everyone, temperature is highest between 4 P.M. and 6 P.M. and lowest at about 6 A.M.

A rise in temperature from your norm is an important sign that you may be sick. Such a rise is commonly called a **fever** and results when internal heat is formed faster than the body can get rid of it. No one fully understands the role of fever, but it is considered to be one way that the body fights illness. According to one theory, the increased heat weakens or kills pathogens. According to another, an infection causes the formation of chemicals in the body called **pyrogens,** a term that means "fire makers." In any case, there is no doubt that fever usually means that something may be wrong. There is one exception: Your temperature can rise as a result of exercise—a healthy rea-

illness behavior Action taken by a person who has reason to believe that he or she is not well.

sick-role behavior Action taken by a person who has been diagnosed as sick.

self-assessment An evaluation of health status based on data collected on oneself by oneself.

medical assessment An evaluation conducted by a medical professional that focuses on identification of the presence or absence of a disease.

fever Above-normal body temperature.

pyrogen A chemical that signals the brain to raise body temperature.

son for increased body temperature. After a cooling-down period, it should return to normal.

A drop in body temperature can be a sign of trouble. You can develop **hypothermia,** or a sudden drop in body temperature, from overexposure to cold (as in falling into freezing water) or from overexertion (as in running a marathon).

Your **pulse,** the regular beat in your arteries caused by the contraction of the heart, is another important measure of health that you can observe. The pulse can be felt on the inside of the wrist, in the neck, or over the heart itself. The normal pulse rate, which ranges between sixty and eighty beats per minute (women's rates are at the higher end of this range while men's are at the lower end), has a regular rhythm. An irregular pulse or heart rate may be serious. In adults, a pulse rate greater than 120 beats per minute, taken while resting, is cause to check with a physician.

Changes in body weight are frequently important measures of a change in health. Weight gain that results from poor eating and little or no exercise can lead to greater risk for a variety of diseases, including heart disease. An unexplained weight gain is reason to consult a physician. An unexplained weight loss could indicate the presence of a persistent infection or serious illness. Nearly everyone owns or has access to a scale. It is to your advantage to know your normal weight range and to take notice if it changes, by how much, and over what period of time. This does not mean you should weigh yourself every day or otherwise become obsessed with your weight. A few pounds up or down is normal for most people.

Other parts of your body to observe are your breasts (for females) and testes (for males) for suspicious lumps, your skin for color changes, and your legs or feet for swelling. Not all changes are worrisome or signs of serious illness. Aches, pains, and a slight rise in temperature may be best treated by taking two aspirin or acetaminophen (non-aspirin pain reliever) and resting in bed. Persistently elevated body temperature, severe discomfort, or dramatic changes from the norm such as blood in your urine or feces should lead you to contact your physician immediately.

A Medical Assessment

There are times when it is important to involve a medical professional in your health assessment. A physician will perform a health assessment in much greater detail and will look for the presence not only of disease risk but also of disease itself. When a physician examines you and assesses your health, he or she looks at three different measures:

- Your health history
- A personal examination
- Laboratory tests

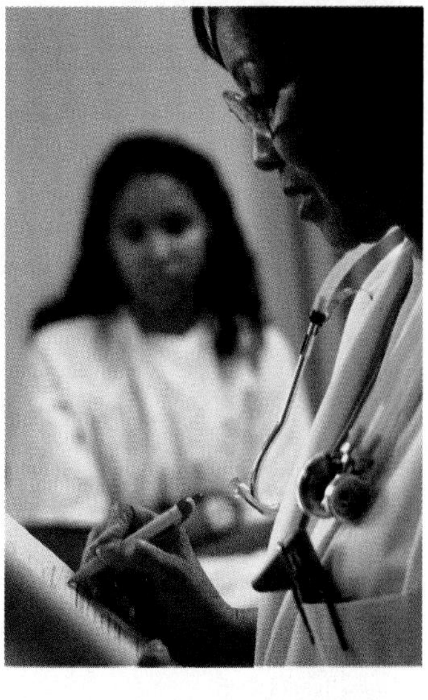

Have you talked with your physician about nutrition, safer sex, and other health-related issues that many college students think about? You can look to your physician for health counseling.

An assessment of your **health history** can often provide clues to disease or discomfort. Your physician needs to know what diseases, injuries, and other health-related experiences you have had. If you have an allergy to penicillin, for example, your physician needs to know that so he or she can choose a different antibiotic when one is needed. Similarly, if you show up at the emergency room with a deep cut on your foot as a result of stepping on a rusty nail, the physician needs to know when you had your last tetanus vaccination and whether you need a booster shot to avoid getting tetanus.

A history of your health should also include a history of your family's health. Has anyone in your immediate family died of heart disease or cancer? Is there a family history of diabetes, obesity, alcoholism, or mental illness? Because some diseases have a genetic link, this information can provide insights into your health as well as into your family's health (see the Assess Your Health box). For example, an ophthalmologist will ask if your parents have had glaucoma, an eye disease that can result in blindness. If so, you have a higher than usual chance of getting it, so your eyes should be checked regularly. Glaucoma can usually be controlled if it is caught in the early stages.

The **physical examination** involves inspection, **auscultation** (listening), and **palpation** (touching). By in-

hypothermia A drop in body temperature to subnormal levels; can result in mental confusion, unconsciousness, and death.

pulse The palpable flow of blood in the arteries caused by the regular contraction of the heart.

health history A history of the patient's health as well as of the health of his or her family.

physical examination An examination by a physician that involves inspection, auscultation, and palpation of the body.

auscultation Listening to the sounds made by various body structures.

palpation Touching body parts with the hands.

The Relative Risks in Your Family Tree

For early warning signs of health problems that may lie ahead, most doctors say, study the details of your family's medical past. No wonder. More than 3,000 ailments are now known to be inherited, including heart disease, cancer, diabetes, arthritis, Alzheimer's, and even alcoholism, depression, thyroid disease, and schizophrenia. New ones are added to the list every day.

If your own family's health history has gone largely unrecorded, there's no better time than now to get the crucial details down in writing. Here's how to do it:

Getting Started

Using the sample shown here as a guide, create your own "genogram," or health family tree. Starting with your grandparents, fill in their full names and their dates of birth and death.

Next, add as much as you can about the health of all your close relatives; include chronic ailments, such as ulcers or allergies, as well as major surgeries and causes of death. The more specific the information, the better. Some genetically linked cancers, for example, can be remarkably specific—right down to whether, say, a tumor first appears on the right or left side of the colon.

Dialing for Details

Where memories fail, official records may be useful. Death certificates, for example, typically contain information about the medical cause of death. To locate them, call or write the Division of Vital Records or Division of Statistics in the state where the relative died.

Some hospitals and doctors also keep permanent archives of medical records on microfilm. To get health records for your late Uncle Harvey or Grandma Rose, you'll need a letter of consent from the closest living relative, as well as a copy of the death certificate.

Looking for Patterns

When your genogram is complete, sit down with your family doctor and talk about any obvious patterns that show up. An illness or health condition that appears more than once—especially if it showed up in relatives before age fifty-five—should get special attention. Knowing your predisposition toward a disease makes preventing it easier, either by changing high-risk behaviors or simply by detecting the ailment early.

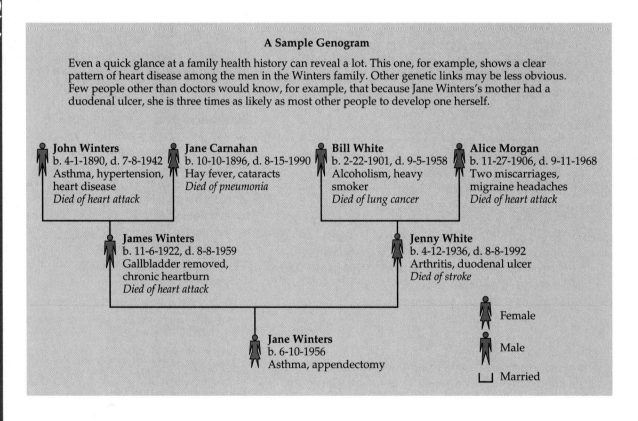

A Sample Genogram

Even a quick glance at a family health history can reveal a lot. This one, for example, shows a clear pattern of heart disease among the men in the Winters family. Other genetic links may be less obvious. Few people other than doctors would know, for example, that because Jane Winters's mother had a duodenal ulcer, she is three times as likely as most other people to develop one herself.

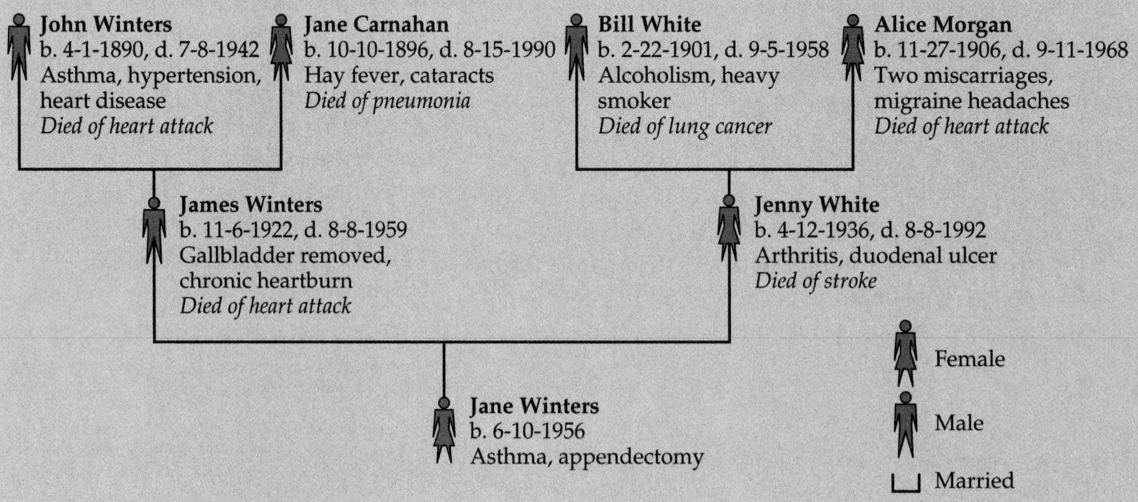

Source: "The Relative Risks in Your Family Tree," *Health,* January–February 1997. Reprinted by permission of Time Inc. Health

specting, or looking at, your body, the physician can find indications of disease by noting such signs as jaundiced (yellow) skin or extreme overweight. Through his or her trained sense of hearing, a physician listens for abnormalities in the sound of the heart or lungs. Finally, the physician's trained sense of touch permits the examination of body parts for growths and other abnormalities. To aid the physician in this examination, there are tools ranging from the simple flashlight, used to examine the ear canal, to ultrasound machines, used to visually examine a fetus at various stages of pregnancy.

When needed, physicians are assisted in their medical assessment by **laboratory tests,** which involve examining materials taken from the body, such as blood or urine. An automated blood test can analyze up to forty different blood chemicals at once, including cholesterol and glucose. A complete blood count, in addition, can detect disorders such as anemia or chemical or poison reactions. Urinalysis is useful in diagnosing urinary disorders and kidney and liver diseases. Other laboratory tests include throat cultures, used to see whether a bacterial organism such as streptococcus is causing a sore throat; electrocardiograms, used to evaluate heart rate and to reveal the presence and location of heart damage; and chest X-rays, used to detect abnormalities in patients who have chest symptoms.

These procedures are necessary to make an accurate diagnosis, but how many of them are needed and how often they should be performed is widely debated. The so-called annual physical examination may be a thing of the past. Much depends on your age and health history, but the best advice today is to have a physical examination to provide baseline data (for example, to record your normal blood pressure, pulse, and cholesterol level) and to have additional examinations only in specific circumstances. Children under age six and adults over age sixty are more likely to get sick, so they should have checkups about once a year even if they do not have any clinical symptoms or other signs of health problems. Adults whose parents, grandparents, or siblings have had heart disease, diabetes, or other conditions also may want to have checkups every year or two. Most people do not need an annual physical. But when you do have one, you may find that your physician is able to spend time counseling you on the dangers of smoking and alcohol, unsafe sex, and poor eating habits (see the Developing Health Skills box).

Defining Health Risks

Your personal health assessment involves not only self-assessment and medical assessment, but assessment of health risks as well. A **health risk** refers to the likelihood of having a certain health condition. It is usually defined in terms of behaviors and environment. A person working in a coal mine, for example, is at risk for contracting anthracosis, or black lung disease. This risk is significantly increased if that person smokes cigarettes. In contrast, another person of the same age, sex, and income level who lives and works in a relatively unpolluted community and who does not smoke is not at risk for black lung disease.

The situations that contribute to the risk a person faces are called **risk factors.** Some risk factors are disease-specific. For example, sexually active people who do not use condoms and injecting drug users are at risk for becoming infected with HIV, which causes AIDS. The risk factors are unprotected sex and/or use of unclean needles.

Risks are not the same for everyone, and not all risks need to be avoided all the time. If you generally

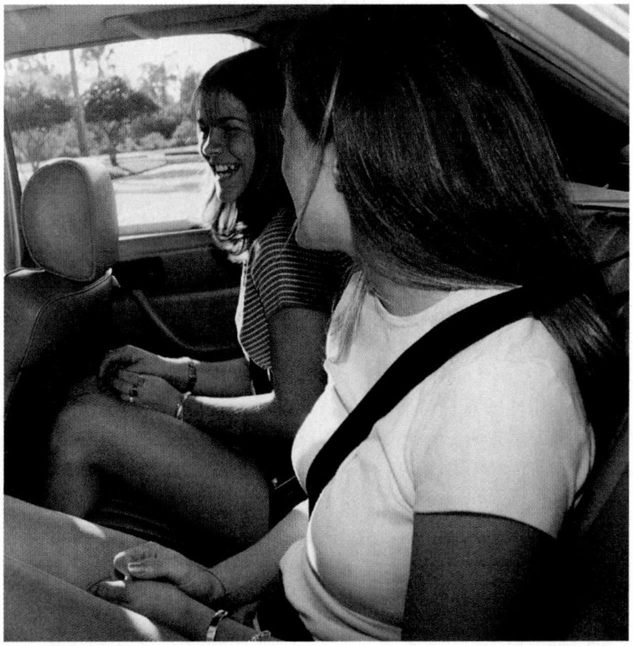

People face numerous risk factors every day, some more obvious than others. Knowing how to manage risk factors can help reduce your personal risk of injury.

laboratory tests Procedures that involve the examination of blood, tissue, and other biologic materials for the diagnosis, prevention, or treatment of disease.

health risk The likelihood of developing a certain disease or health condition.

risk factor A condition or habit that puts a person in danger of negative health occurrences.

Developing Health Skills

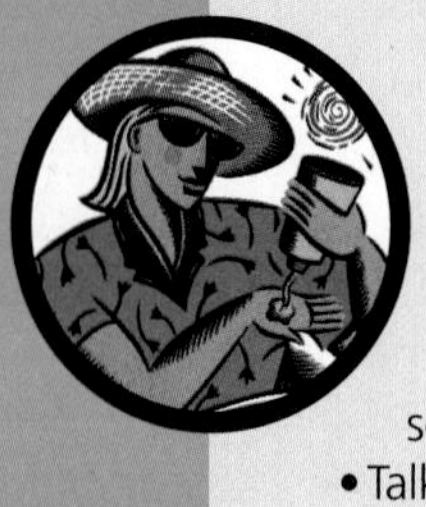

Knowing What to Expect from a Physical Exam

We seldom think of having a physical examination as requiring health skills. But to get the most from a physical examination, you need to apply some basic communication skills.

- Talk clearly and effectively about your wants and needs concerning the examination. Ask questions, expect answers, and probe for information.
- Provide accurate information to your physician. Just because you may have done something embarrassing—for example, having unsafe sex—is no reason to place yourself at greater risk by withholding information from the physician.
- When you go for a checkup, be sure your physician gives you the following preventive services, which are recommended for men and women ages nineteen to thirty-nine by the U.S. Preventive Services Task Force.

History and Counseling
Dietary intake
Physical activity
Tobacco/alcohol/drug use
Sexual practices

Physical Exam
Height and weight
Blood pressure
Complete oral cavity exam (for people who smoke or chew tobacco)
Clinical breast exam (for females)
Clinical testicular exam (for males)
Complete skin exam (for people with a family history of skin cancer)

Laboratory and Diagnostic Procedures
Blood cholesterol
Urinalysis
Pap smear (for sexually active females)
Testing for HIV and other STDs (for persons seeking treatment for STDs and those with multiple sexual partners)
Mammogram (for women with a family history of breast cancer)

Source: Adapted from the U.S. Preventive Services Task Force

follow a healthy diet, there is nothing wrong with occasionally having a one-inch steak smothered with onions sautéed in butter. Although this is an unhealthy load of cholesterol, it will not send you into cardiac arrest if you do it once in a while.

Daily exposure to unavoidable health risks is another matter. Return to the example of the coal miner: Merely going to work and breathing puts him or her at risk for black lung disease. Other risk factors over which you may have little control are a family history of heart disease, breast cancer, or diabetes; extreme stress due to a death in the family or job loss; and exposure to violence. Fortunately, many risk factors can be either controlled or modified.

Risk factors considered controllable or modifiable include:

- Alcohol use
- Blood pressure
- Drug abuse
- Hours of sleep
- Life satisfaction level
- Miles driven
- Physical activity level
- Seat belt use
- Strength of social ties
- Tobacco use

Risk factors considered uncontrollable or unmodifiable include:

- Exposure to environmental pollution
- Family history of breast cancer
- Family history of diabetes
- Family history of heart disease
- Having had a hysterectomy
- Abnormal Pap smear result
- Serious loss or misfortune in the past year
- Witnessing or involvement in a violent or potentially violent argument

Keeping Good Health Records

Health records are important because they are a way to keep track of your health history and a means of monitoring change in health status. Do you know when you had your last vaccination to protect you from getting tetanus? What would you tell the physician if you were to step on a rusty nail? Parents tend to keep health records for their children, but college students are less careful about keeping their own records current.

You should keep your health records easily retrievable in one place. For example, you could keep a copy on a computer and bring it up to date with each new event. Make a note of each diagnosis, the name and telephone number of the physician making the diagnosis, and the treatment taken. Pharmacies keep a record of prescriptions that you have ordered, but most people use more than one pharmacy, so the record in each place is not complete. You should develop your own complete prescription record. This can help in avoiding drug interactions—when two drugs or a drug and food taken at the same time produce a bad effect in the body. Your prescription record is also useful when you want to give an accurate health history to a new physician. Finally, if you travel internationally, it could be important for you to have a complete health history with you in case you get sick. For some countries, you will need evidence of certain vaccinations.

Your health records should include records of your health-promoting activities as well. A record of how much you exercise and how often, a record of your dietary fat intake, and a record of your sleep patterns can be important information when assessing your health status. For women, a record of menstrual cycles can provide critical information when the decision to become pregnant is made. Health records provide far more than a medical history. They provide documented evidence of positive, and negative, health behavior.

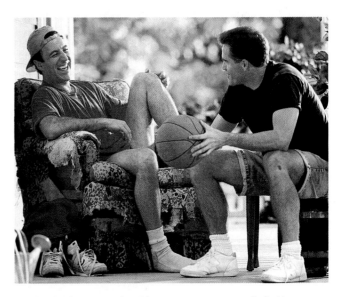

People who have a good social support system generally feel better than those who don't have close friends.

Establishing a Personal Health Style

The term **health style** is a shortened version of the two words *healthy* and *lifestyle.* A healthy lifestyle is one type of health style. An unhealthy lifestyle is another type of health style.

Health style is best described as the sum of your health values, beliefs, and actions. Each time you make a choice concerning your health, whether positive or negative, you are contributing to your health style.

Your health style is personal and, at the same time, interpersonal. It is an element of your life over which you can assert much control. It is influenced by (1) the factors that are involved in becoming healthy—health knowledge, health skills, and health behavior; (2) your health-related values; (3) your health-related attitudes and beliefs; (4) your social and cultural environment; and (5) the momentum developed by your health-related decisions and actions.

A value is something that is important to you. A **health value** is something related to health that is important. How prominent is health on your list of personal values? Many college students do not even think about health as a value. Good health is something that most of us are born with, and we think this state of good health will continue for a long time. This thought is at best wishful. People who value good health are more likely to make decisions that promote their health—decisions such as getting the right amount of sleep and eating a healthy diet—than are people who do not think of health as a value.

A **health attitude** is your behavioral intention concerning health. If you intend to exercise, then you are more inclined to do so than if you have no such intention. Likewise, if you intend to drink and then drive, the potential of your having a car crash is greater than if you have no such intention. Health attitudes are usually expressed as either positive or negative—positive if they contribute to good health, negative if they do not contribute to good health.

Just as your attitudes toward health influence your health style, so do your health beliefs. When you believe something to be true, whether it is true or not, that belief influences your behavior. A **health belief** is something you believe to be true about health. Health beliefs concerning disease prevention are especially important. For example, beliefs about your ability to practice good

health style The sum of health knowledge, health skills, and health behavior. Health style is most easily observed in personal health decisions.

health value Something of importance that is related to health.

health attitude A behavioral intention concerning health, usually expressed in positive or negative terms.

health belief A health-related concept thought to be true whether supported by evidence or not.

Table 1.1 One Bad Habit Can Lead to Another

A survey of people, twenty years or older, showed that smokers are more likely than nonsmokers to have other unhealthy habits.

	Smoking Habit		
Health Practice	**Never Smoked**	**Former Smoker**	**Current Smoker**
Never eats breakfast	18.3%	19.0%	37.6%
Heavy drinker*	7.2	11.9	20.1
Sleeps six hours or less	20.9	20.0	25.3
Less physically active	17.3	18.1	21.8

*At least five drinks on ten days or more in the past year

Source: National Center for Health Statistics

health behavior effectively ("I can stop smoking") or about what stands in your way ("I can't stop smoking because my roommate smokes") can influence your health style.

Your social and cultural environment also affects your health style. For example, people who have good social support systems report that they feel better than do those who don't have close friends to talk with. This seems to hold true for people of all ages and especially for those with life-threatening illnesses such as AIDS and breast cancer.

Even though your health style is very personal, it can affect others around you just as their health styles can affect you. For example, nearly half of all motor vehicle accidents involve a driver who had been drinking. So if you drink and drive, this health style can affect someone else. For another example, a motorcycle rider not wearing a helmet is more susceptible to serious injury if an accident occurs than one wearing a helmet. Serious injury results in extended medical care, which in turn results in increased medical costs passed on to you by hospitals and other health care providers and is reflected in your insurance premium.

A final factor that influences your personal health style is the **health momentum** established by your health-related decisions and behavior. Each time you take an action concerning your health, you influence the next action you take related to your health. For example, if you always wear a seat belt when you are in a car, you are more likely to wear a helmet when you bike. This is because you have established a momentum for safe health habits on the road. If you have established a momentum for an exercise program, it is likely that you will not smoke because smoking will compromise your aerobic capacity and other aspects of your fitness.

health momentum A perception of movement toward or away from good health that results from decisions and health behaviors of the past.

The opposite is also true: One bad habit can lead to another. According to a 2001 report from the National Center for Health Statistics, smokers tend to have other bad health habits. A nationwide survey of adults showed that heavy smokers were more likely to skip breakfast, to snack more during the day, to drink more alcohol, and to remain physically less active than nonsmokers. According to a health researcher analyzing the survey data, two possible factors are at work here. One is that this cluster of bad health habits is associated with a consumption-oriented lifestyle—smoking, drinking, and overeating. The second is that smokers are more prone to risk-taking behaviors and give less attention to healthier practices (see Table 1.1).

Prevention: The Best Alternative

At the turn of the twentieth century, the leading causes of death were infectious diseases. It was a time of great hope, and for most of these diseases, a vaccination or a cure was on the horizon. Today, just after the turn of the twenty-first century, however, most of the leading causes of illness and death are not infectious diseases but health-compromising behaviors. According to the National Center for Health Statistics, the leading causes of death in the United States in the year 2000 were heart disease, cancer, and stroke (see Table 1.2). These diseases may be the "official" causes of death, but the actual

Table 1.2 Nine Leading Causes of Death in the United States

All Ages

1. Heart disease
2. Cancer
3. Stroke
4. Chronic lower respiratory disease
5. Unintentional injuries
6. Diabetes
7. Influenza and pneumonia
8. Alzheimer's disease
9. Kidney disease

Ages Fifteen Through Twenty-Four

1. Unintentional injuries
2. Homicide
3. Suicide
4. Cancer
5. Heart disease
6. Congenital malformations
7. Chronic lower respiratory disease
8. HIV
9. Stroke

Source: National Center for Health Statistics

Table 1.3 Nine Leading Behavioral Causes of Death

1. Tobacco
2. Diet and activity patterns
3. Alcohol
4. Microbial agents
5. Toxic agents
6. Sexual behavior
7. Firearms
8. Motor vehicles
9. Drug use

Source: Adapted from McGinnis, J. M., and W. H. Foege. "Actual Causes of Death in the United States." *Journal of the American Medical Association* 270, no. 18 (1993): 2207–2212

causes are more likely poor health behaviors (see Table 1.3). For example, heart disease is the leading cause of death for people of all ages. For many people with heart disease, however, smoking is the actual cause of disease. Diets rich in cholesterol and fats are another actual cause of heart disease. Given that behaviors are often the actual causes of death, the best hope for reducing the number of deaths caused by many diseases lies not in finding cures for them but in changing the behaviors that lead to them in the first place.

Prevention means taking health-promoting action to reduce the risk of disease and injury. Prevention is the best strategy for achieving a healthy future. By following this strategy, you can make health-promoting decisions that reduce your risk of acquiring a disease or sustaining an injury. Prevention can be carried out on the personal as well as on the community level.

On the personal level, for example, you can make a decision not to smoke cigarettes and thereby to reduce your risk for a range of illnesses, including cancer, heart disease, stroke, and lung disease. Much can also be done on the community level. Many localities are passing laws that prohibit smoking in an increasing number of public places, including hospitals, office buildings, and bars. State and local taxes on cigarettes are rising in some places, and part of these revenues are used to educate the public—particularly young people—about the

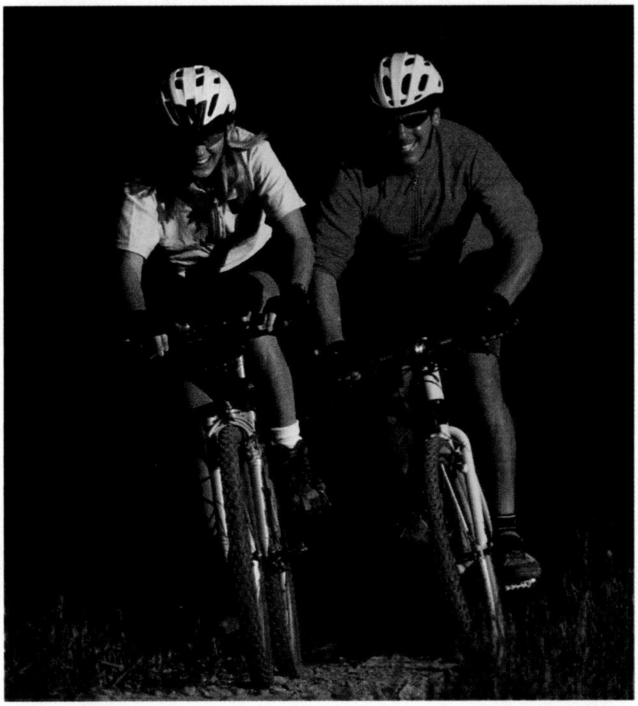

Prevention is the best strategy for achieving a healthy future. For bicyclists, this means wearing a helmet.

prevention Taking health-promoting action to reduce the risk of disease or injury.

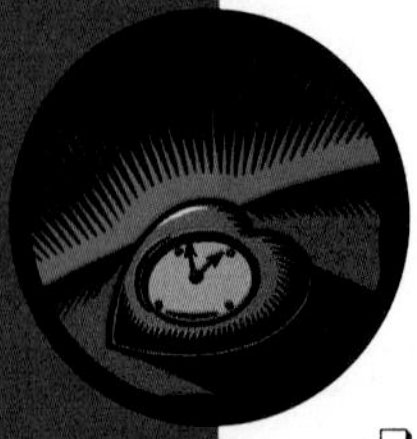

A Wellness Inventory

Put a check beside each statement that applies to you.

1. Alcohol Use

- ❑ I drink fewer than two drinks a day.
- ❑ In the past year, I have not driven an automobile after having more than two drinks.
- ❑ When I'm under stress, I do not drink more.
- ❑ I do not do things when I'm drinking that I later regret.
- ❑ I have not experienced any problem because of my drinking in the past.

2. Tobacco Use

- ❑ I have never smoked cigarettes.
- ❑ I haven't smoked cigarettes in the past year.
- ❑ I do not use any form of tobacco (pipes, cigars, chewing tobacco).
- ❑ I smoke only low-tar and low-nicotine cigarettes.
- ❑ I smoke less than one pack of cigarettes a day.

3. Blood Pressure

- ❑ I have had my blood pressure checked within the last six months.
- ❑ I have never had high blood pressure.
- ❑ I do not currently have high blood pressure.
- ❑ I make a conscious effort to avoid salt in my diet.
- ❑ There is no history of high blood pressure in my family.

4. Weight/Body Fat

- ❑ According to height and weight charts, I am in the average range.
- ❑ I have not been on a weight reduction diet in the past year.
- ❑ There is no place on my body that I can pinch an inch of fat.
- ❑ I am satisfied with the way my body looks.
- ❑ None of my family, friends, or health care professionals has ever urged me to lose weight.

5. Physical Fitness

- ❑ I do some form of vigorous exercise for at least thirty minutes three times a week or more.
- ❑ My resting pulse is eighty beats a minute or less.
- ❑ I don't get fatigued easily while doing physical work.
- ❑ I engage in some recreational sport such as tennis or swimming on a weekly basis.
- ❑ I would say that my level of physical fitness is higher than most of the people in my age group.

6. Stress/Anxiety Level

- ❑ I find it easy to relax.
- ❑ I am able to cope with stressful events as well as or better than most people.
- ❑ I do not have trouble falling asleep or waking up.
- ❑ I rarely feel tense or anxious.
- ❑ I have no trouble completing tasks I have started.

7. Car Safety

- ❑ I always use seat belts when I drive.
- ❑ I always use seat belts when I am a passenger.
- ❑ I have not had an automobile accident in the past three years.
- ❑ I have not had a speeding ticket or other moving violation for the past three years.
- ❑ I never ride with a driver who has had more than two drinks.

8. Relationships

- ❑ I am married and living with my spouse.
- ❑ I have a lot of close friends.
- ❑ I am able to share my feelings with my spouse and/or other family members.
- ❑ When I have a problem, I have other people with whom I can talk it over.
- ❑ Given a choice between doing things by myself or with others, I usually choose to do things with others.

9. Rest/Sleep

- ❑ I almost always get between seven and nine hours of sleep a night.
- ❑ I wake up few, if any, times during the night.
- ❑ I feel rested and ready to go when I get up in the morning.
- ❑ Most days, I have a lot of energy.
- ❑ Even though I sometimes have a chance, I never take naps during the day.

10. Life Satisfaction

- ❑ If I had my life to live over, I wouldn't make all that many changes.
- ❑ I've accomplished most of the things that I've set out to do in my life.
- ❑ I can't think of an area in my life that really disappoints me.
- ❑ I am a happy person.
- ❑ Compared with the people with whom I grew up, I feel I've done as well as or better than most of them with my life.

Scoring:

Record the number of checks (from zero to five) for each area. Then add up the numbers to determine your score.

Area	*Subscore*
Alcohol use	________
Tobacco use	________
Blood pressure	________

Area	Subscore
Weight/body fat	________
Physical fitness	________
Stress/anxiety level	________
Car safety	________
Relationships	________
Rest/sleep	________
Life satisfaction	________

Interpreting Your Score:

A score of 40–50	Healthier than average lifestyle
A score of 25–39	Average lifestyle
A score of 0–25	Below average: need for improvement
Scores of less than 3 in any of the 10 areas	Need for improvement in that area

health hazards of smoking. And health insurers are taking measures to reward nonsmokers by charging smokers higher premiums. See the Assess Your Health box to determine whether you have a healthy lifestyle.

Preventive Behaviors

Prevention usually comes down to a handful of actions that research has consistently found to be very positive contributors to a healthier and longer life. Here is a list of eight good health behaviors—prevention behaviors. The reason these are so positive is that each serves to reduce risk for a large number of health threats yet involves a small behavioral change.

- Avoid the use of tobacco.
- Get exercise on a routine basis.
- Maintain normal body weight.
- Drink alcohol in moderation, if at all.
- Practice safer sex.
- Wear a seat belt.

These prevention behaviors are much like the advice you've heard from your parents—just common sense. They are also the result of extensive research by some of the most respected health researchers. A good way to reduce risk is by increasing prevention behaviors. The following are some common-sense suggestions for healthy living. In subsequent chapters, you will find a more detailed discussion of each.

- Smoking has been identified as the most avoidable cause of death in our society. There is no question that it is dangerous to your health and to the health of those around you. Because of the impact of sidestream smoke that originates from the end of cigarettes, smoking is never simply a personal health decision: What a smoker does can affect the health of others as well. ***Common sense suggests that you do not smoke.***
- Researchers have found that regular physical activity is related to a reduction of risk for many health threats, including heart disease and hypertension. It is a valuable stress management tool and an important element of weight control and good sleep habits. ***Common sense suggests that you exercise on a regular basis.***
- Dietary factors have been linked to several health threats, particularly heart disease and cancer of the colon. There is consensus among health professionals that limiting fat consumption reduces health risk. ***Common sense suggests that you limit the fat in your diet.***
- Alcohol and other drugs have been found to relate to many threats to health, including violent actions, accidents, and some chronic diseases. If alcohol is consumed, it should be taken in moderation and under controlled circumstances that ensure safety. It should not be a means of stress management. ***Common sense suggests that if you drink alcohol, drink wisely.***
- Because of sexually transmitted infections, safer sexual practices have become an important part of healthy living. Although use of a condom is considered a highly effective preventive measure, abstinence and monogamy offer the best protection from the health threats of sexual encounters. ***Common sense suggests that you practice safer sex.***
- One of the leading causes of death and injury to college-aged students is automobile accidents, and the evidence is clear that wearing a seat belt greatly reduces the chances of injury or death in such an event. ***Common sense suggests that you wear your seat belt.***

By following common sense and good health practices, you can lead a healthy life—and still have fun. The best strategy for a healthy future is prevention—making health-promoting decisions that reduce your risk for acquiring a disease or sustaining an injury. Using common sense and practicing prevention are both elements of being personally responsible for your own health (see the Assess Your Health box).

Being Responsible

Despite all the advances in medical science—new surgical procedures, wonder drugs, diagnostics that picture the inner workings of your body—your health remains your responsibility. The good news is that acting on this

Assess Your Health

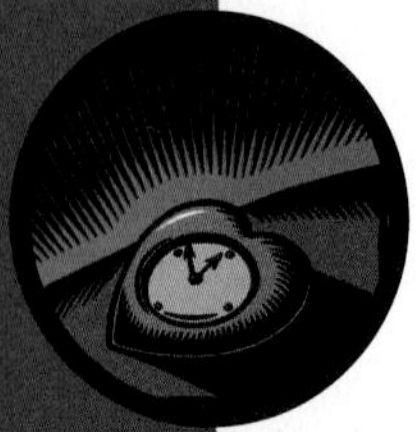

Your Health Habits

1. List four or five health habits you would like to develop (more sensible eating, regular exercise, coping with stress, etc.).
   a. ____________________
   b. ____________________
   c. ____________________
   d. ____________________
2. Now, go back and circle the habit you would most like to develop.
3. Turn your wish into a goal. Set target dates for starting toward and reaching that goal.
   ____
   ____
   ____
   ____
4. Helps and hindrances

   What will help you reach your goal? What will stand in the way?

   Helps
   ____
   ____

   Hindrances
   ____
   ____
5. Action plan:

Who? (name)	*Will do what?*	*Starting when? (date)*

6. Write down the names of a few people who will help you reach your goal.

   Wellness support system *Signatures (of support people)*

   Name ____________________

   Name ____________________

   Name ____________________
7. Evaluation of progress:

   Did I reach my goal? ____________________

   Did my support system help? ____________________

   Is it a permanent change? ____________________

   Do I feel better? ____________________

responsibility is not very difficult. As you have just read, for the most part it involves:

- Common-sense decisions made by a health-literate person.
- The use of health skills that develop with practice, particularly skills related to health assessment and health record keeping.
- Health behaviors, particularly prevention behaviors, that enhance rather than compromise health.

With few exceptions, positive health behaviors are a matter of voluntary action. You choose them; they cannot be forced on you. As you become more knowledgeable about your own health and about the health of others, and more competent in the application of that health knowledge, you will realize that healthy living offers the best prospect for a healthy, long, happy, and productive life.

CASE STUDY 1: Responsibility for Health

Although taking classes and working part-time keep Maria very busy, she still finds time to look after her health. In fact, leading a healthy life is an important priority for her, and she has planned her schedule to make time for a workout in the gym three times a week. She usually eats a balanced diet even though she often has to grab food on the run, and she gets the amount of sleep her body needs.

One reason Maria places such a high value on her health is that she knows the consequences of not doing so, including being at greater risk for sickness, feeling fatigued, and not being attentive in class. Maria carries her personal interest in health activities over to the community by volunteering to teach sports to children with disabilities. During the last election season, she worked for a candidate who supported increasing tobacco taxes to help pay for expanded access to health care.

Phil also goes to school and works part-time, but his health style is completely different—by choice. He feels stressed out by the end of the day, and instead of working off tensions with a brisk walk or a game of racquetball, he has a few beers at a local bar. He nibbles on chips and nuts before returning to the computer to finish his work. The idea of leading a healthier life seems never to occur to him.

How does Phil fare on the community level? Once a year, he joins a group of students to clean up bottles, cans, and other trash on the highway, but he views it more as a party than as something that can affect the health of the community. He votes in almost every election, but so far, he has not taken notice of the increasing number of health-related issues on the ballot or on candidates' agendas.

In Your Opinion

Both Maria and Phil are well-educated and well-read students, but only Maria has made a conscious decision to have a positive health style.

- Why isn't Phil maintaining a positive health style? Could he be afraid of not being able to change well-established habits?
- Could Phil's lack of health skills be a factor in his negative health style?
- Look ahead ten years. What kind of health style will Maria be leading? What about Phil?
- What steps would you suggest that Phil take to alter his way of living so that he has a healthier lifestyle?

KEY CONCEPTS

1. According to the World Health Organization, health is "a state of complete physical, mental, and social well-being and not merely the absence of disease or infirmity."
2. Health skills are abilities that can help you achieve good health. They include motor skills, intellectual skills, emotional skills, and social skills.
3. Health behaviors are actions related to the promotion or maintenance of good health. They include preventive behavior, illness behavior, and sick-role behavior.
4. Health literacy means being able to get, interpret, and understand basic health information and to use that information in ways to enhance your health—and the health of others.
5. Four categories of health skills are: motor skills, involving physical movement; intellectual skills, involving decision making and good judgment; emotional skills, involving stress management and self-control; and social skills, involving listening, helping others, and asking for help.
6. A health assessment is an analysis of a broad range of measures affecting an individual's health. Because a health assessment is a measure taken at only one point in time, it is necessary to assess your health and your health risks continually throughout your life.
7. The physical examination done by a physician involves inspection, auscultation, and palpation. Most people do not need an annual physical examination.
8. By keeping good health records, you can determine what is normal for you so you can better notice when a change occurs.
9. Your health style is best described as the sum of your personal health decisions, both those that affect you and those that affect others and your community.

10. The best strategy for a healthy future is prevention—making health-promoting decisions that reduce your risk for acquiring a disease or sustaining an injury.

REVIEW QUESTIONS

1. Explain why the absence of disease is an inadequate definition of health.
2. Differentiate between holistic health and wellness.
3. Give examples of healthy development and healthy behavior change.
4. List the three elements of health style.
5. Name three types of health behaviors and provide an example of each.
6. Explain how health beliefs and health attitudes influence health style.
7. Give three reasons for keeping good health records.
8. Explain the saying "an ounce of prevention is worth a pound of cure."
9. List eight health behaviors that research has proved to be health enhancing.
10. Explain how common sense can provide a clue to good health.

CRITICAL THINKING QUESTIONS

1. *Healthy People 2010* involves a large-scale assessment designed to get a picture of the health of the United States (see the Developing Health Skills Box, page 5). Do you believe the public has a right to know of the incidence and prevalence of diseases even when some diseases such as HIV/AIDS are very personal, and reporting them might invade someone's right to privacy?
2. Physical activity is recognized as important to the effort to reduce risk for heart disease as well as for other diseases. *Healthy People 2010* establishes a goal of increasing "the proportion of adults who engage regularly, preferably daily, in moderate physical activity for at least 30 minutes per day." What difficulties are apparent in any attempt to assess physical activity levels according to this standard?
3. Motorcyclists who wear helmets are less likely to be seriously injured in an accident than those not wearing helmets. Yet many motorcyclists are opposed to state laws requiring helmets, claiming that these laws are an infringement on their privacy. Can you justify helmet laws in terms of public health? How do you resolve the infringement question?
4. A familiar saying goes, "An ounce of prevention is worth a pound of cure." This is especially true when most chronic diseases result from chosen behaviors such as smoking cigarettes or eating high-fat foods. What are some of the diseases for which a cure is of no concern and prevention is the only option?

JOURNAL ACTIVITIES

1. Do you know if there are any health risks in your family's history? Make a list of causes of death of close family members. Do any of these suggest that you should change your health behaviors? Which ones, and why?
2. Starting now and for the remainder of this course, keep a record of health assessments that you make. This can include a record of your weight, medications that you take—even a record of your exercise.
3. Identify the three leading causes of death in your community. The community can be your college or university or your local city or county.
4. Conduct your own epidemiological study. Epidemiology is the study of epidemics—the occurrence of disease in a given population. Go to the student union or a local shopping mall and systematically observe 100 randomly selected individuals. Note their disease risk—their smoking behavior, your perception of their body weight and other health-risk indicators. From your observations, project the risk of disease among your research subjects.

SELECTED BIBLIOGRAPHY

Healthy People 2000 Review, 1998–1999. Hyattsville, MD: HHS, 1999.

Healthy People 2010: National Health Promotion and Disease Prevention Objectives. Washington, DC: U.S. Department of Health and Human Services, Public Health Service, 1999.

Institute of Medicine. *Improving Health in the Community.* Washington, DC: National Academy Press, 1997.

McGinnis, J. M. and W. H. Foege. "Actual causes of death in the United States." *Journal of the American Medical Association* 270: 2207–2212, 1993.

Morbidity and Mortality Weekly Report. Centers for Disease Control and Prevention (published weekly).

National Center for Health Statistics (NCHS). *Health, United States.* With urban and rural health chartbook. Hyattsville, MD: HHS. (Updated Annually)

Prevention Report. Washington, DC: U.S. Department of Health and Human Services, Office of Disease Prevention and Health Promotion (published quarterly).

University of California at Berkeley Wellness Letter (published monthly).

HEALTHLINKS

Websites for Better Health

You can access better health as it relates to this chapter by checking out some of the following sites on the Internet. These sites can be accessed directly from the *Decisions for Healthy Living* Website located at www.aw.com/pruitt.

Health Resources and Services Administration
Provides a link to news releases and general information on health issues, as well as a listing of employment opportunities and grant funding in the health sciences.

HealthGate
Online source for health, wellness, and biomedical information. Explores health issues from a holistic health perspective.

Healthy People 2010
Provides the latest facts on the nation's health initiatives.

International Healthy Cities Foundation
Network of interrelated groups dedicated to improving communities and cities and improving the health of the world's population.

Med/Access
An all-encompassing site with information and material on a broad spectrum of topics, all related to healthy living. It also offers a database of hospitals, specialty treatment centers, physicians, and HMOs, to name just a few, as well as overviews of the U.S. health care system.

National Center for Health Statistics
Definitive reference for vast array of national health statistics.

Office of Disease Prevention and Health Promotion
A division of the U.S. Department of Health and Human Services, the Office of Disease Prevention and Health Promotion provides fact sheets and information on areas of health promotion and disease prevention ranging from nutrition to consumer health.

HEALTH HOTLINES

Your Personal Responsibility

Health Resources and Services Administration, Office of Health Facilities
(800) 492-0359 (within Maryland)
(800) 638-0742 (outside Maryland)
5600 Fishers Lane
Rockville, MD 20857

National Institutes of Health, Division of Public Information
(800) 633-3425
9000 Rockville Pike, Building 1, Room 344
Bethesda, MD 20892-0188

TEST YOUR KNOWLEDGE ANSWERS

1. False. The World Health Organization (WHO) defines health broadly as "a state of complete physical, mental, and social well-being and not merely the absence of disease or infirmity."
2. False. Normal body temperature ranges from 97.1 to 100 degrees Fahrenheit, depending on age, sex, and time of day. The average for adults is approximately 98.2.
3. True. Health risks are not the same for everyone. You can modify or reduce some health risks by taking positive actions for healthy living.
4. True. Some health risks are unavoidable due to genetics or the environment in which you live.
5. False. Healthy living is positively influenced by a good social support system.

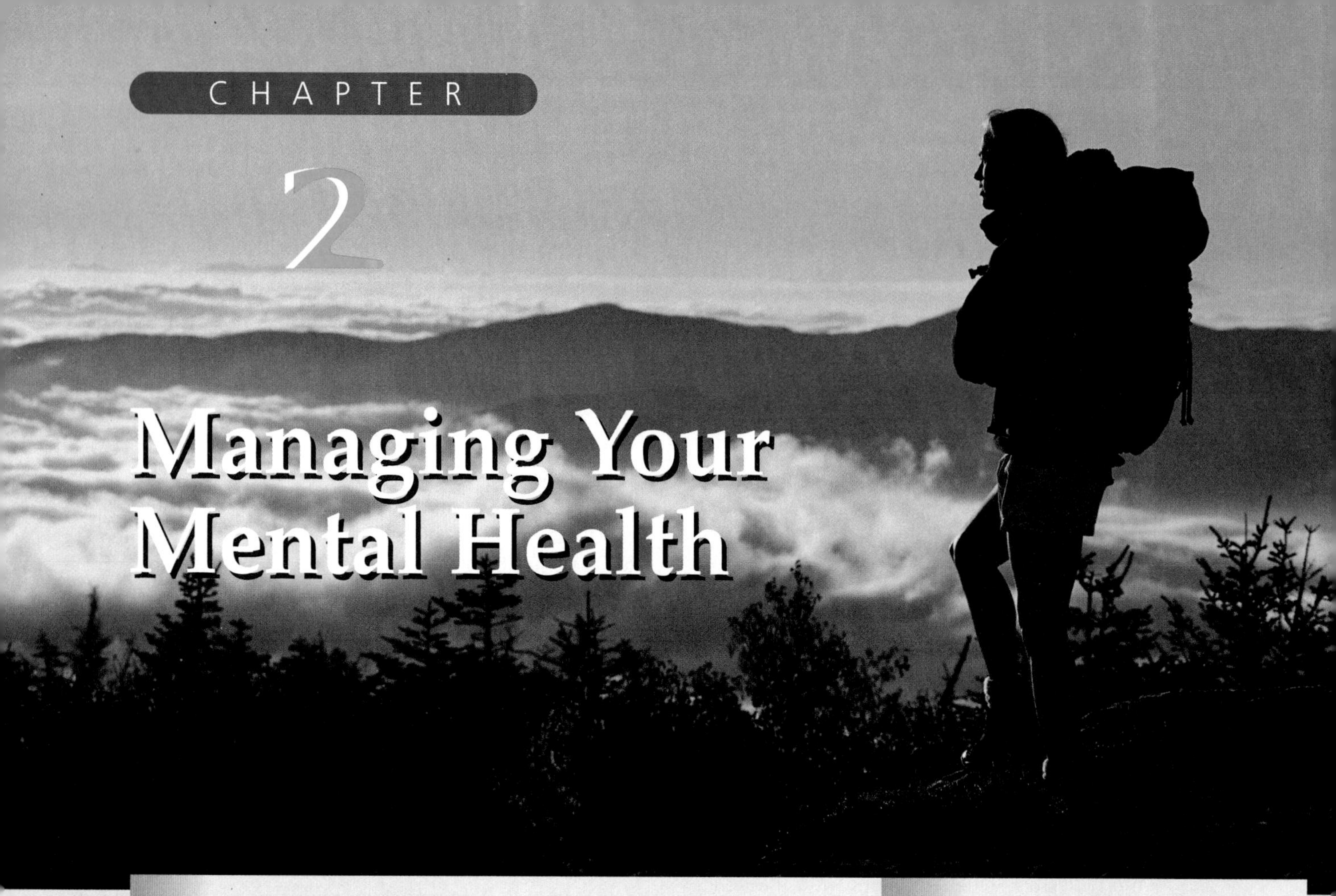

CHAPTER 2

Managing Your Mental Health

OBJECTIVES

When you finish reading this chapter, you will be able to:

1. Differentiate between a mentally well and a mentally ill person.
2. Explain what is meant by emotional and social wellbeing.
3. Identify the role of emotions in a healthy lifestyle and list several normal emotions along with positive and negative ways to express them.
4. Recognize the mental health benefits of sleep.
5. Understand the meanings of the terms *self-concept, self-esteem, self-efficacy,* and *self-actualization.*
6. Recognize a variety of mental illnesses, including anxiety, depression, and schizophrenia.
7. Differentiate between minor depression and major depression.
8. Recognize the characteristics of an individual contemplating suicide.
9. Name a variety of mental health professionals and understand how each addresses emotional problems.
10. Know when to call for help if you suspect that you are experiencing a mental health problem.

TEST YOUR KNOWLEDGE

1. A mentally healthy person is one who is happy with his or her life regardless of the circumstances within which he or she lives. True of False?
2. The American Psychiatric Association recognizes homosexuality as a "sexual orientation" and not a psychiatric condition subject to treatment. True or False?
3. During the REM period of sleep, repair work, including the regeneration of cells, is accomplished. True or False?
4. Suicide is the third leading cause of death among people aged fifteen to twenty-four, after unintentional injuries and homicide. True or False?
5. Although 60 percent of men and 50 percent of women experience traumatic events in their lifetime, most do not develop post-traumatic stress disorder. True or False?

Answers found at end of chapter.

When people ask, "How do you feel?" most often they mean, "How do you feel physically?" How you feel mentally is just as important and is a good indication of your mental health. **Mental health,** an abstract concept, is usually defined according to normal behavior. What defines normal, as you might expect, remains controversial.

As a healthy college student, you experience a range of emotions. Sometimes you are happy; sometimes you are sad. Sometimes you feel self-confident; sometimes you feel you can't do anything right. Knowing how to deal with your emotions and gaining personal insight and growth from these experiences are two important aspects of good mental health.

Mental health is the ability to negotiate the daily challenges and social interactions of life without experiencing undue emotional or behavioral incapacity. To understand mental health in general—and your mental health in particular—think of yourself as fitting into three systems: a biological system, a psychological system, and a social system. The psychological system is most important when considering mental health. But the relationships among the three systems are so close that the state of your psychological system directly affects the other systems. In other words, how you feel and how you interpret the events around you affect your biological and social well-being. Understanding mental health, therefore, is critical to maintaining an overall healthy life.

A Continuum of Well-Being

Mental health refers to your emotional and social well-being. Like so many terms in the mental health field, well-being suggests an abstract state. In a state of well-being, an individual is capable of (1) healthy interaction with his or her environment and (2) enduring the hard times of life with resilience. The absence of mental well-being is indicated by an inability to interact with the environment and/or a lack of resilience.

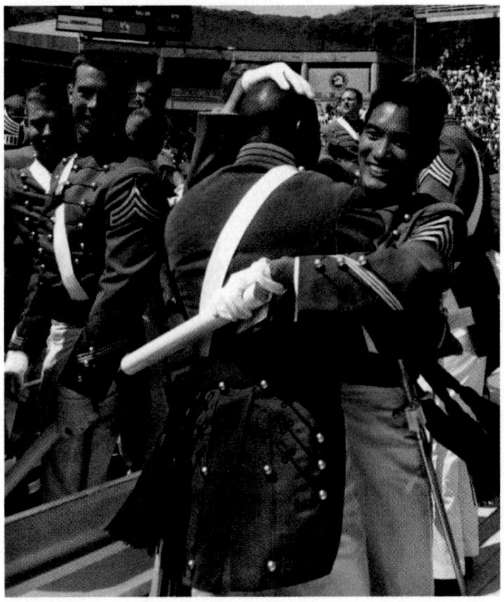

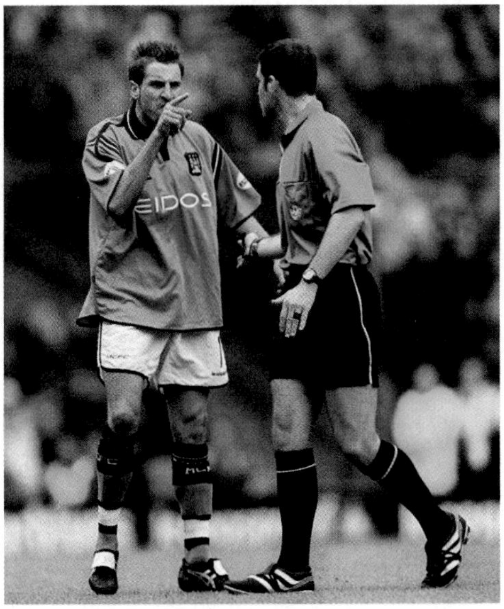

There are countless emotions, such as anger and joy. It is mentally healthy to express emotions, but there are more healthy and less healthy ways of doing so.

Imagine a continuum of mental well-being from mental health to **mental illness.** Most people do not have serious mental or emotional problems and therefore tend to identify with the mentally healthy side of the continuum. This does not mean that, as a mentally well person, you are free from life's stressors. Everyone experiences stress, but those who are mentally healthy are more capable of handling stress with a

mental health A state of emotional and social well-being; a state in which an individual is capable of healthy interaction with his or her environment and of enduring the hard times of life, with resilience.

mental illness A disorder or problem of the mind that prevents a person from being productive, adjusting to life, or getting along with other people.

minimum of difficulty. Everyone experiences important life transitions—going to college, starting a career, getting married or divorced, the death of a loved one. Stressful events present a significant challenge to your mental health. These transitions and the emotions they engender, however, are a part of normal life and are not a cause of pathological disease (see Chapter 3).

The mental illness side of the continuum represents a disorder or problem of the mind that prevents a person from being productive, adjusting to life, or getting along with other people. While most people weather at least one period of minor depression, extreme depression can lead to total incapacitation. Mental health and mental disorders can be affected by numerous factors including (1) genetics; (2) physical abilities, disabilities, or vulnerabilities; and (3) social and environmental conditions and stressors. The details of mental illness are addressed later in the chapter. But first, let us consider the mentally healthy person.

What Makes a Person Mentally Well?

The mentally well person is often referred to as well-adjusted. Note that the word *adjusted* connotes change. A well-adjusted person is not tied to one way of thinking about or doing things or even to maintaining so-called normal behavior. This is because norms change. What is normal today may be abnormal in the near future or may have been abnormal in the past. For example, until 1974, the American Psychiatric Association listed homosexuality among its mental disorders, diseases, and abnormalities. Now homosexuality is recognized as a sexual orientation, not a psychiatric condition subject to treatment.

What characterizes a mentally well-adjusted person? Numerous efforts have been made to define such a person. The following seven qualities might be found on many lists.

A well-adjusted or mentally well person is one who

1. has a positive self-image and good self-esteem;
2. experiences appropriate and stable moods;
3. maintains control of emotions and has the ability to love, feel guilt, and accept remorse;
4. demonstrates flexibility and adaptability in social situations;
5. acknowledges personal strengths and accepts personal limitations;
6. tolerates ambiguity and understands that conflict is normal and that final solutions to problems may not exist; and
7. does not distort reality, consciously or unconsciously.

None of us exhibits these qualities perfectly. We maintain a positive self-image and good self-esteem most of the time. We experience appropriate and stable moods most of the time. We tolerate ambiguity and understand that conflict is normal and that final solutions to problems may not exist most of the time. In other words, we do not live in a continuous state of psychological perfection. Variations and fluctuations of these qualities occur. In fact, it would be highly unusual to find someone who did not experience the natural highs and lows of daily living.

The Role of Your Emotions

There are countless emotions, just as there are countless combinations of pigment to form colors of skin. Anger, love, fear, sorrow, and joy are among the most easily identified and expressed emotions. Other emotions that are more difficult to recognize and deal with are guilt and hate. Guilt, for example, is one way for your conscience to distinguish between right and wrong. You can feel guilty over cheating on a test, not helping your roommate clean up the room, or putting off a visit to your grandmother in the nursing home. These are all so-called normal feelings of guilt, but if they build up and are not handled appropriately, they can stifle your enjoyment of living and can cause fears and anxieties that result in debilitating health problems.

It is mentally healthy to express emotions, but there are more healthy and less healthy ways of doing so. Consider the emotion of anger. Blowing up at your lab partner because his or her part of the experiment was not completed will not necessarily dissipate your anger. In fact, expressing rage might make you even angrier. Studies conducted at the University of Michigan show that the healthiest people use a reflective style of coping with anger. They put off venting it until they have cooled down. That way, they control their anger rather than letting the emotion control them (see the Assess Your Health box).

The Benefits of a Good Night's Sleep

College students are well-known for "all nighters," during which they stay up through the night to study for an exam or to finish—or even to start—a paper due in the morning. Lack of sleep is nothing to brag or laugh about. Sleep is vital to your life and can help you function at optimal levels both physically and mentally.

On the physical side, sleep helps regulate your metabolism and your body's state of equilibrium. On the mental side, it helps restore your ability to be optimistic and to have a high level of energy and self-confidence. To keep your body in balance, more sleep is needed when you are under stress, experiencing emotional fatigue, or undertaking an intense intellectual activity such as learning.

Assess Your Health

How Do You Respond to Normal Emotions?

The following are examples of normal emotions that everyone experiences from time to time. In most cases, these emotions do not threaten your health, but the way in which you respond to them may. Responses to emotions can be both positive and negative.

Anger: Anger is a strong feeling of being mad or unhappy. It is usually the result of an event or series of events that did not go as expected or desired.

\+ A positive response to anger is to go for a walk, count to ten, or just take some time to cool down.

– A negative response is to punch the wall, break something, drive fast, or drink a great deal of alcohol.

Frustration: Frustration is a feeling of disappointment, usually resulting when a goal has not been or cannot be met.

\+ A positive response to frustration is to talk with a friend, take some time to think about the problem, and plan a different approach to dealing with it.

– A negative response is to quit, yell at a good friend, or blame someone else.

Hostility: Hostility is a feeling of intense anger and anxiety, often an aggressive unfriendly attitude.

\+ A positive response to hostility is to take time to cool down, to talk with a friend or counselor, or simply to walk away from the problem.

– A negative response is to fight, say abusive words to the source of hostility, or undermine someone's reputation by talking behind his or her back in an angry manner.

Fear: Fear is a feeling of being frightened and of not knowing what to expect.

\+ A positive response to fear is to investigate exactly what causes the fear, name the source of the fear, and restructure your environment to eliminate the source.

– A negative response is to hide from the fear by staying at home, sleeping excessively, or taking drugs.

Love: Love is a strong feeling of affection and/or deep concern for another person. It may involve intimacy and/or commitment.

\+ A positive response to love is to feel pleasure at being loved.

– A negative response to love is denial, fear, or extreme emotional anxiety over the possibility of being rejected.

As you encounter these and other emotions in your daily life, think about how you can respond positively to them.

During sleep, most people experience periods of what is called rapid eye movement (REM). These movements can be observed beneath closed eyelids. In **REM sleep,** the body is quiet but the mind is active, even hyperactive. Some researchers believe that REM sleep helps you form permanent memories; others believe that this period of active brain waves serves to rid your brain of overstimulation and useless information acquired during the day. REM sleep is the time not only for dreams but also for acceleration of the heart rate and blood flow to the brain. Erections in males and engorgement of the clitoris in females are common. At the same time, skeletal muscles rarely move.

During **non-REM sleep,** in contrast, the body may be active—some people sleepwalk during this period—but the mind is not. In spite of this activity, non-REM sleep is the time when the body does its repair and maintenance work, including cell regeneration.

Although much still needs to be learned about sleep and its functions, few would disagree that sleep

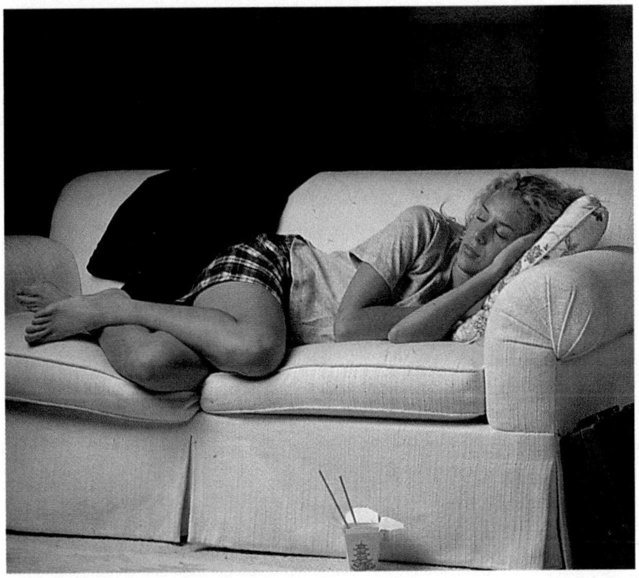

Getting enough sleep is important for your mental health. A catnap in the afternoon can make you feel more alert afterward, but it is not a substitute for a good night's sleep.

REM (rapid eye movement) sleep Sleep during which the eyes flicker back and forth behind closed eyelids; the period of sleep associated with dreaming.

non-REM sleep Sleep during which the eyes are relaxed and not moving; the period of sleep associated with cell regeneration.

Developing Health Skills

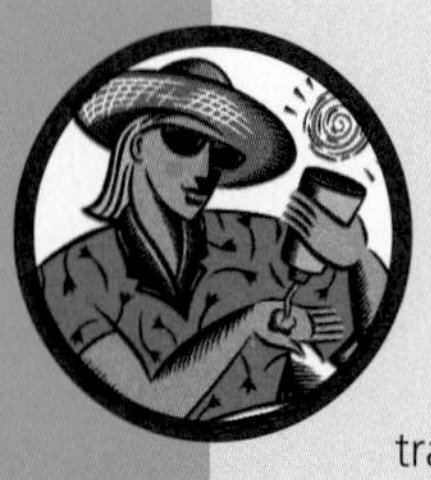

Gaining Strength from Solitude

One way to get to know yourself is through solitude. Being alone gives you a chance to think about yourself and your problems in a concentrated fashion.

Researchers have found that when people are put in isolated environments for even short periods, they are suddenly able to overcome difficulties that have been plaguing them for some time, such as overeating or smoking. Psychologists working on isolation studies conclude that these people mastered their problems because they had the time to sit and think about them.

Most people think of time spent alone as an obstacle to overcome—a void to fill. To gain strength from solitude, think of it instead as an opportunity for self-exploration. Here is some "alone time" advice from experts:

- Keep a journal. Think about yourself and put your thoughts on paper.
- Take on a major project. Instead of buying a bookcase, build one. Instead of reading a poem, write one.
- Develop an interest in something rewarding and intellectually stimulating that you can do by yourself—for example, bird-watching or playing the piano.
- Do something that will give you an immediate sense of accomplishment, such as going on a three-mile run or walk, painting the bathroom, or weeding the garden.

The trick to using your solitude effectively is to think of time alone as a luxury instead of a problem.

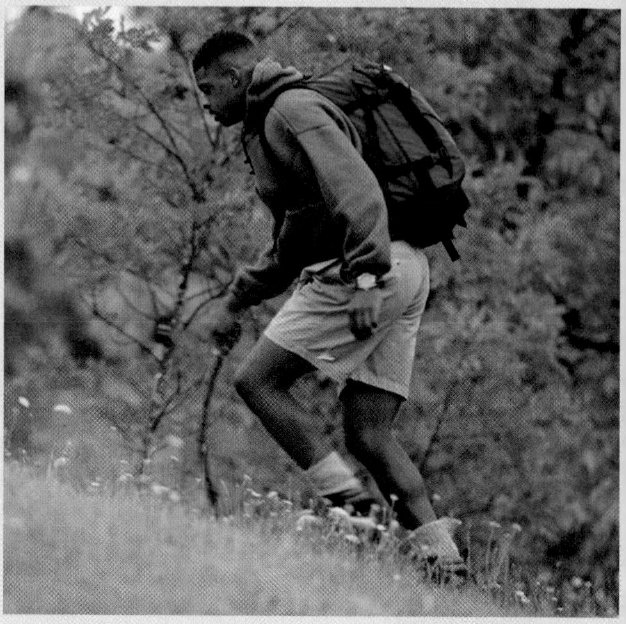

Sometimes it is important to be by yourself. Being alone doesn't necessarily mean being lonely. Solitude can give you time for self-exploration and personal growth.

plays a role in the maintenance of good mental health. Here is some advice from sleep researchers on how to get a better night's sleep:

- Go to bed every night and wake up every morning at about the same time.
- Exercise regularly, but not just before you go to bed.
- Avoid eating heavy meals for at least two hours before bedtime. Keep nighttime snacks light and easy to digest.
- Stay away from stimulants—coffee, cola drinks, tea, hot cocoa, and chocolate—before you go to bed.
- If you have trouble falling asleep, don't just lie there and become anxious. After thirty minutes, get out of bed, read a book, or do some other restful but productive activity. Then try to go to sleep again.
- Don't rely on over-the-counter sleeping aids to help you sleep. They don't always work, and they can have side effects. If you feel you need a sleeping aid more than four days a week or for more than two weeks, consult your physician.

A final point about sleep: Be aware that everyone has sleepless nights on occasion. It is a normal way for the body to adjust to certain situations.

self-concept A person's view of himself or herself gained through an assessment of strengths and weaknesses.

self-esteem How a person values himself or herself.

self-efficacy A person's belief that he or she is capable of accomplishing a task or series of tasks under certain conditions.

self-actualization The ability to seek the highest and most idealistic state that can lead to a person's fullest possible development.

Who Am I? The Importance of Knowing Yourself

Have you ever taken a good look at yourself in the mirror and asked, "Who am I?" The answer is important because who you think you are and what you think of yourself are key indicators of your mental health (see the Developing Health Skills box). Mentally healthy people have an accurate **self-concept** as well as a positive sense of **self-esteem**. They also have a good sense of what they can accomplish (**self-efficacy**) and the ability to fulfill their potential (**self-actualization**).

Self-Concept

Self-concept is how you see yourself. It includes a self-assessment of your strengths and weaknesses. Oliver Cromwell once commissioned a portrait of himself. When he noticed that the artist was painting the most flattering replica possible, even to the point of leaving out several blemishes, Cromwell said, "Paint me as I am, artist, warts and all!" What Cromwell was seeking was an honest assessment of his physical reality—warts and all.

Acknowledging your less attractive side—for example, a tendency to procrastinate—does not mean that you have to denigrate yourself. A person with an accurate self-concept fully acknowledges who he or she is—warts and all.

Self-Esteem

Self-esteem is how you value yourself. High self-esteem means that you respect yourself and consider yourself worthy. People with high self-esteem recognize their limitations, and they expect to grow and improve themselves. Having a positive sense of self-esteem can contribute to feelings of competence, worth, and acceptance. It can enhance the formation of meaningful relationships.

Health researchers often link low self-esteem to apathy, anxiety, alcoholism, drug dependence, poor physical health, and lack of accomplishment. In fact, almost every negative health behavior has been linked to some extent to low self-esteem. Without a good sense of self-esteem, you may find it difficult to overcome the fear of rejection or to accept your own limitations or those of others. People who don't have good self-esteem may be especially vulnerable to peer pressures, especially those concerning drug abuse or sexual promiscuity. Low self-esteem is also one of the personality traits of people with eating disorders (see Chapter 5).

Self-Efficacy

If you believe that you can get a job done in an appropriate and timely manner, you have a good sense of self-efficacy. Self-efficacy is more than knowing what to do. It also involves integrating that knowledge into your sense of who you are.

Self-efficacy is one indicator of how you are likely to perform in a specific setting. This sense of self-efficacy is critical to both your mental and physical health. If you believe you can lose weight or stop smoking, you are likely to do so. If you believe you cannot lose weight or stop smoking, your efforts are likely doomed.

Self-Actualization

According to the theory of self-actualization formulated by psychologist Abraham Maslow, people strive to

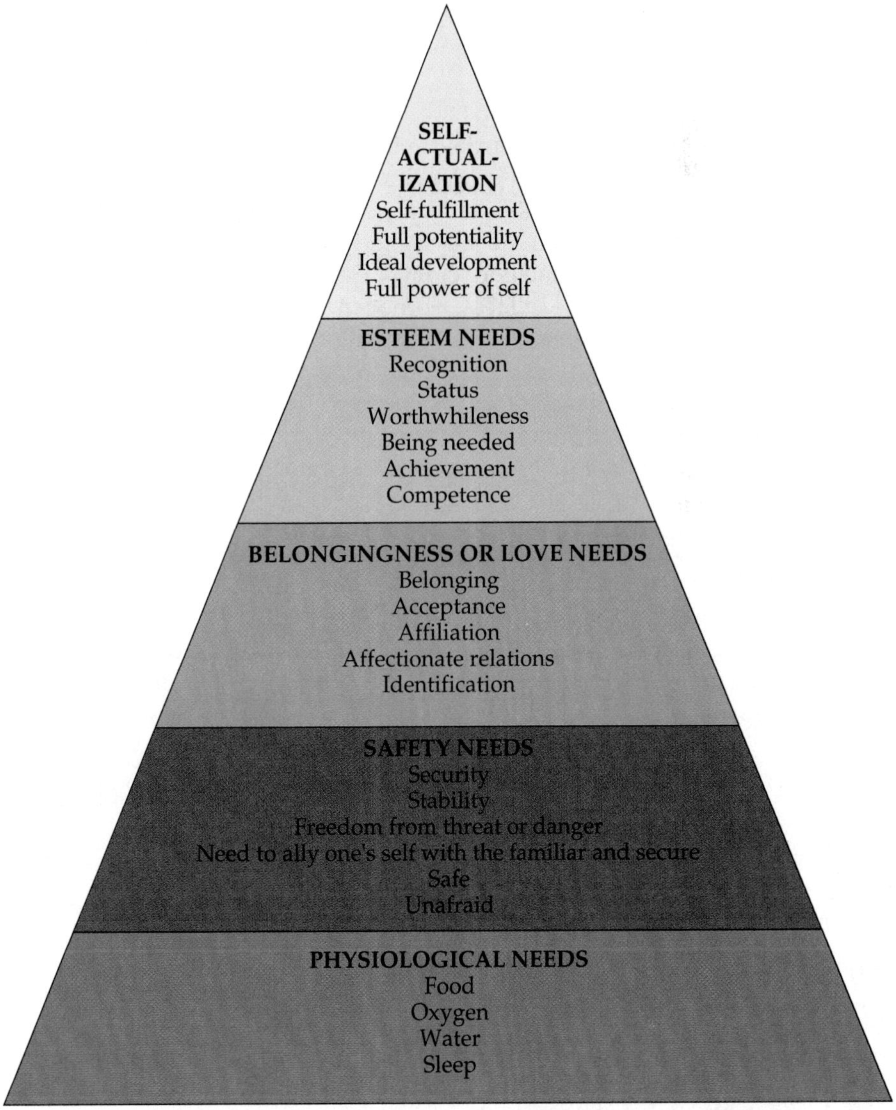

Figure 2.1 Maslow's Hierarchy of Human Needs
The theory of self-actualization holds that people tend to seek the highest and most idealistic aims that lead to their fullest possible development.

reach the highest and most idealistic levels of their capabilities. Maslow has proposed a hierarchy of human needs in which basic physiological needs are at the bottom and self-actualization is at the top (see Figure 2.1). Once physiological needs have been satisfied, human beings are free to proceed to the next level where they will pursue safety needs, followed by love needs, esteem needs, and, finally, self-actualization.

Self-actualization and good mental health are believed to go hand in hand. However, Maslow's theory does not lend itself to experimental proof or disproof, so psychologists must take it largely on faith.

A Continuum of Mental Dysorganization

Unfortunately, many people do not live up to their potential because they suffer from mental illness. According to *Healthy People 2010*, approximately 20 percent of the U.S. population is affected by mental illness during any given year. This in no way suggests that 20 percent of the country is "mad" or "crazy." Such terms, once associated with mental illness, do not fit in with today's concept of mental health and mental illness.

Psychiatrist Karl Menninger coined the word **dysorganization** to describe the difficult and painful experiences someone undergoes in trying to cope with difficult situations in life. According to Menninger, the degree of mental illness a person suffers is in direct proportion to the amount of **dysfunction** present (see Figure 2.2). A person at the first level of dysfunction is what is commonly called nervous; at the second level, neurotic; at the third level, openly aggressive; at the fourth level, psychotic; and at the fifth level, self-destructive. (*Dysorganization* is not the same as *disorganization*. *Dys-* means painful or difficult. In dysorganization, the process of organization or living is painful or difficult. Disorganization connotes a lack of organization, a state of disarray.)

Anxiety Disorders

Americans experience **anxiety** more than any other mental health problem (see Figure 2.3). Although anxiety disorders can cause emotional suffering, those affected usually can carry out day-to-day activities. Anxiety disorders are generally viewed as cognitive distortions or unsatisfactory ways of reacting to life situations.

Anxiety is often brought on by an imagined fear of impending danger. Most anxiety is normal and may play an important role in anticipating situations. For example, the fear of being attacked on a deserted street at night may cause a person to take appropriate actions to avoid such a possibility. You have probably experienced anxiety before taking a final exam. Some of the symptoms you may have had are sweating, dry mouth, heavy breathing, and trouble sleeping. This type of anxiety is in response to a realistic situation.

However, some people suffer anxiety over a long period of time and without any apparent cause. A person who has a **phobia,** for example, has an unreasonable fear of some object or situation. Simple phobias include fear of heights or fear of bees and usually do not interfere with daily activities. Some phobias, however, are more severe and can cause people to lead constricted lives. Because of their irrational fears, some people do not leave the house. Anxiety becomes a serious mental health problem when individuals suffering from it are so emotionally disabled that they cannot continue at school, hold a job, or otherwise lead a satisfying and productive life. Nearly half of the people with **post-traumatic stress disorder,** a condition that can result in persistent psychological and biological changes, also suffer from anxiety and social phobias (see the Developing Health Skills box).

Mood Disorders

Like anxiety, depression is a common disorder experienced by mentally healthy people from time to time. **Minor depression** is a mental state in which feelings of sadness, guilt, and hopelessness are exaggerated. Feeling depressed is so common an emotional state that it would be considered abnormal if you did not, on occasion, feel depressed or sad ("I have the blues today."). The breakup of a significant relationship or other traumatic changes involving personal relationships can bring on a brief period of sorrow. Most people rebound from temporary setbacks once the initial sense of loss wears off. If the depression continues, treatment with a mental health professional is recommended (see the Cultural View box).

Major depression is when a person experiences the feelings of sadness and hopelessness with such inten-

dysorganization Pain or difficulty in the process of organization or living.

dysfunction The inability to function properly.

anxiety A state of apprehension or tension, often accompanied by physiological signs.

phobia An unreasonable fear of some object or situation.

post-traumatic stress disorder A psychological condition affecting rape victims, combat veterans, and other trauma survivors.

minor depression An emotional state in which a person's normal feelings of sadness, guilt, and hopelessness are exaggerated.

major depression Depression that is extreme, more intense, and longer lasting than minor depression and that usually interferes with daily life; often characterized as a mood or affective disorder.

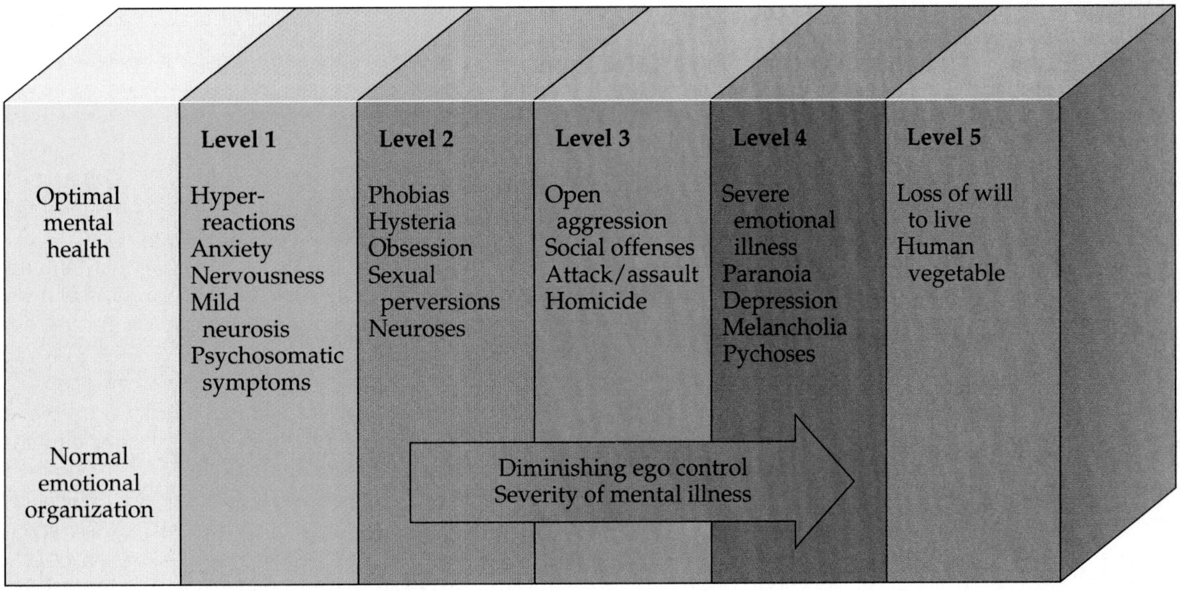

Figure 2.2 A Spectrum of Mental State
There is a wide range of mental dysfunction. At one end is mild nervousness, which most people experience at one time or another. At the other end is the self-destructive loss of the will to live. Dysorganization is the term that mental health professionals use to describe the difficult and painful experiences someone undergoes in trying to cope with difficult life situations.

sity or over such a long period of time that those feelings interfere with normal day-to-day activities. Some people have only one episode of depression in their lifetimes; others slip into depression from time to time. Severe depression takes many forms. Collectively, they are called mood or **affective disorders.**

Premenstrual dysphoric disorder (PMDD) is an example of a depressive disorder characterized by feelings of hopelessness, fatigue, mood swings, and other physical symptoms such as bloating, swollen hands or feet, headaches, and tender breasts. This is different from **premenstrual syndrome** (PMS), which has many of the same symptoms but to a much lesser degree. Although as many as 70 percent of menstruating women have some symptoms of PMS, only between 3 percent to 5 percent of women have the most severe form of PMDD. Both are examples of a disorder that involves the biological, as well as the psychological, system.

A form of severe depression, which is characterized by cycles of manic highs and depressive lows, is **bipolar disorder.** It is also called manic-depressive illness. Researchers have found that depression—particularly bipolar disorder—runs in families. Another form of depression is **seasonal affective disorder,** which is one reason some people get more depressed in the winter. It is believed that the absence of bright daylight causes chemical changes in the brain, which bring on depression.

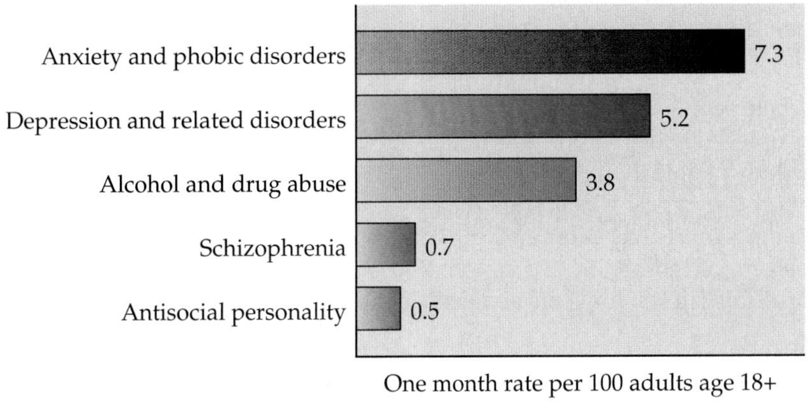

Figure 2.3 The Most Common Mental Health Disorders
More people experience anxiety than any other mental health problem. Anxiety often stems from an imagined fear of impending danger. (*Source:* National Institute of Mental Health)

affective disorder A condition in which moods or emotions become extreme and interfere with daily life.

premenstrual dysphoric disorder A form of depression occurring just prior to menstruation and characterized by fatigue, irritability, mood swings, and physical symptoms such as abdominal bloating, swollen hands or feet, headaches, and tender breasts; a severe form of premenstrual syndrome.

premenstrual syndrome A combination of emotional and physical features which occur before menstruation; characterized by mood changes, discomfort, swelling and tenderness in the breasts, a bloated feeling, headache, and fatigue.

bipolar disorder A form of depression characterized by cycles of manic highs and depressive lows; also called manic-depressive illness.

seasonal affective disorder A form of depression brought on by lack of sufficient daylight.

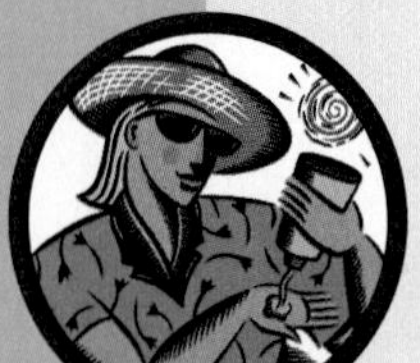

Developing Health Skills

Your Environment

The Psychological Wounds of Terror

The trauma of witnessing—and in some cases even thinking about—the collapse of the World Trade Center on September 11, 2001, stressed many Americans. Some people had stress symptoms such as dizziness, heart palpitations, nightmares, and pervasive fears that persisted for months after the event and were severe enough to interfere with their normal life. These people suffered from post-traumatic stress disorder (PTSD), a condition that also can affect rape victims, combat veterans, and survivors of traumatic experiences such as automobile accidents, aborted airplane takeoffs, earthquakes, floods, and other natural disasters.

About 60 percent of men and 50 percent of women experience a traumatic event in their lifetime, but most do not develop PTSD. Among those traumatized, more women (20 percent) than men (8 percent) develop the disorder. This difference may be explained because a higher proportion of people who are raped develop PTSD than those who suffer other traumatic events, and women are much more likely to be raped than men (see Chapter 9).

People with PTSD are more likely than others to abuse alcohol and drugs, and to have mental problems, especially depression, anxiety, and social phobias. After September 11, for example, PTSD symptoms included being afraid of crowded places and loud noises and being reluctant to leave the "safety" of home. In addition, people with PTSD have an increased risk of medical illness including heart attack.

Treatment can help ease the symptoms, but many people suffering from PTSD do not seek help. This is because some of the traumatic events are associated with shame—for example, rape or incest—which can make the victim feel helpless. Another reason is that after events such as natural disasters, people are so busy cleaning up that they do not think about tending to their mental health.

Treatment options for PTSD include individual and group therapy and antidepressants. Relaxation therapy and a method called exposure—which involves repeated recounting of the traumatic event—also are used. In some cases, a combination of treatments may be required. The goal is to calm the body and mind. The good news, according to PTSD experts, is that most people do get better.

Depression can emerge in early childhood and adolescence, but it usually first appears in young adults—when people are in their early twenties. Although most people with depression are under age forty-five, many elderly people thought to suffer from Alzheimer's disease and other types of **dementia** may instead have treatable depression. Medication and therapy can help about 80 percent of those with depression. Without treatment, depression can last for years and even lead to suicide.

Psychotic Disorders

Psychoses are mental disorders so serious that they result in loss of touch with reality and often require hospitalization. The most common and disabling psychosis is **schizophrenia,** a complex mental illness in which the person has his or her own view of reality. This view of the world is often very different from the view of normal people. For example, a schizophrenic might see things that do not exist, such as a dead mother, or live in a world without time, dimension, or color. Because of its complexity, few generalizations hold true for all people who are diagnosed as schizophrenic.

Schizophrenia takes two basic forms: acute and chronic. With the onset of delusional symptoms, a person is said to be experiencing acute schizophrenia. Some people may have only one episode in their lives; others have repeated acute episodes and lead relatively normal lives in between. The first symptoms of

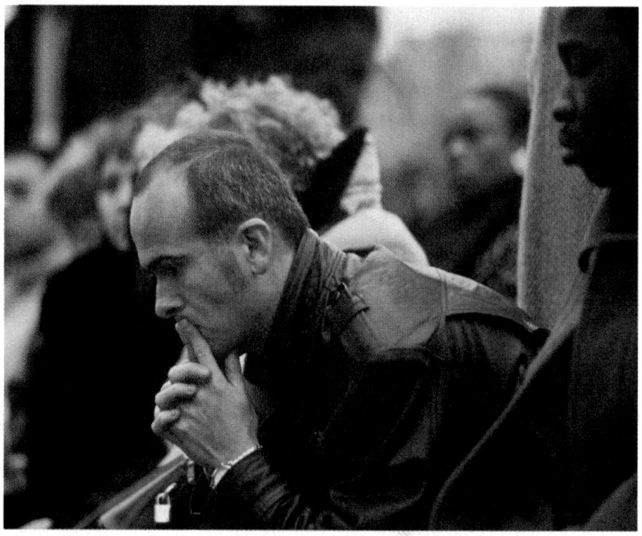

It is normal to be sad and depressed for a brief period of time, especially when you experience a significant loss. But depression can be a serious mental illness when it is accompanied by feelings of helplessness over a long period of time.

dementia Mental confusion and loss of brain function that can be caused by disease or old age.

psychosis A mental disorder that can result in losing touch with reality.

schizophrenia A complex mental illness in which an individual has a distorted view of reality.

Cultural View

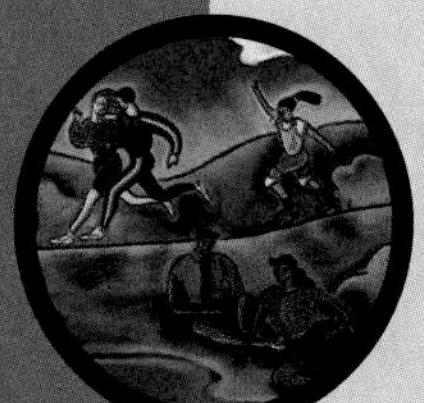

The Importance of Spirituality in Treating Depression among African Americans

In a small study of patients in an urban, university-based primary care clinic, African Americans were three times more likely than whites to rate spirituality as an extremely important dimension of depression care.

This finding comes from a survey of 49 whites and 27 African Americans. Survey respondents were asked to rate the importance of 126 aspects of depression care.

Thirty of the aspects rated most important by both groups came from the following nine categories: health professionals' interpersonal skills, primary care provider recognition of depression, treatment effectiveness, treatment problems, patient understanding about treatment, intrinsic spirituality, financial access, life experiences, and social support. Most aspects of depression care were rated similarly by both ethnic groups, with the exception of items that concern spirituality.

African Americans cited personal issues of spirituality—faith in God, belief in God's forgiveness, and prayer—as being among the 10 most important aspects of depression care. White participants rated these same aspects below the top 24 in importance. Less personal displays of faith, such as church attendance, rated below the top 30 across the entire sample.

Researchers note that disparities in mental health care usage, quality, and outcomes between whites and African Americans are long-standing and well documented. Along with cost issues, the fear of social stigma, mistrust toward mental health professionals, and fear of antidepressant or psychotropic drugs may prevent some African Americans from seeking depression care. Further, studies find that, when compared with whites, African Americans are more likely to drop out of psychotherapy, less likely to take their medications routinely, and less likely to be referred to mental health specialists, even though they report favoring counseling over medication to treat depression.

Even though African Americans are using more general medical services for mental health problems, studies show that they are not adequately treated for depression. Researchers believe the illness is poorly recognized by patients and providers.

The investigators say findings from their survey and previous studies indicate that patients with strong beliefs want physicians to discuss faith and spirituality during treatment. Yet physicians say they lack the time and training to do so. The researchers suggest that physicians could make referrals to pastoral counselors, with patients' consent. They say this exploratory study suggests that acknowledgement of spirituality within the context of care for depression may be particularly important for African Americans.

Source: Adapted from Cooper L., et al. "How Important Is Intrinsic Spirituality in Depression Care?" *Journal of General Internal Medicine* 16 (2001): 634–638. From *Advances*, The Robert Wood Johnson Foundation quarterly newsletter.

schizophrenia are often seen in the teens or twenties in men, and in the thirties and early forties in women. These symptoms include **hallucinations** (seeing or hearing things that are not present), **delusions** (false beliefs despite obvious proof to the contrary), **disordered thinking** (disconnected or incoherent thought processes and speech), and **inappropriate affect** (showing emotions that are inconsistent with the person's thoughts). Chronic schizophrenics never fully recover normal functioning.

Schizophrenia has no single cause, but it is likely brought on by a combination of factors. Schizophrenia has long been known to run in families, and the gene for at least one kind of schizophrenia has been identified. Close relatives of a schizophrenic are more likely to develop the disorder than are persons who do not have a schizophrenic relative. Twin studies provide another indication of a family tie. The development of schizophrenia in both members of a twin pair is more likely among identical twins than among fraternal twins. Researchers are studying other factors as well. For example, brain scans have disclosed that schizophrenics are more likely to have structural brain abnormalities than are normal persons of the same age.

Currently, no single cure exists for schizophrenia, although a review of 2,000 patients' records from first breakdown to old age suggests that 25 percent achieve full recovery, 50 percent recover partially, and 25 percent require lifelong care. Schizophrenia treatments include antipsychotic drugs, shock treatment, psychosocial and behavioral therapy, and skills training. Most patients are treated in halfway houses and group homes, although some chronic schizophrenics require prolonged hospitalization or residential care.

hallucination The sensation of seeing or hearing something that is not present.

delusion A false belief despite obvious truth to the contrary.

disordered thinking Disconnected or incoherent thought processes and speech.

inappropriate affect Showing emotions that are inconsistent with a person's thoughts.

Suicide: A Symptom of Mental Illness

Every year, there are more than 200,000 reported suicide attempts (an unsuccessful attempt to end one's life) and 30,000 completed suicides. In reality, there are countless more suicides. Suicide is heavily underreported as a result of the social stigma attached to it and the often uncertain circumstances in which it happens. For example, many single-car crashes may be suicides.

The reasons people commit suicide are complex, highly interrelated, and only partially understood. The major causes are psychological, biological, and sociological. Collectively, they contribute to the profile of a suicide.

Suicidologists, specialists who study suicide, report that a cluster of psychological symptoms can be warning signs of depression and possible suicidal behavior. These include a change in behavior, loss of interest in usual activities, weight loss or gain, withdrawal from friends and family, and feelings of hopelessness or guilt. Self-destructive behaviors such as excessive drinking or drug use also indicate an increased risk. According to the National Institute of Mental Health, 15 percent of depressed individuals die by suicide (see the Developing Health Skills box).

Suicide among Teens and Elders

It has never been easy being a teenager, but spurred by changing social patterns, suicide is increasingly becoming a way out of problems for young people. Suicide is the third leading cause of death among people aged fifteen to twenty-four, after unintentional injuries and homicide. As just one example, more than 60 percent of a group of 380 students attending an academically select public high school in New York City reported having thoughts about killing themselves. Nearly 10 percent reported that they had made at least one actual attempt to kill themselves.

What causes such feelings? According to one psychologist, suicidal teenagers talk about a recurring theme: hopelessness. In growing numbers, adolescents don't just "feel" hopeless; they say, "I am" hopeless. Compounding the problem, as many as 90 percent of suicidal teenagers believe that their parents do not understand them. The teens feel isolated and anonymous.

While adolescent suicide is a focus of media attention, the elderly are quietly taking their lives, too. The elderly comprise only 12 percent of the population but account for about 20 percent of all reported suicides. The most common reason for suicide among the elderly is depression associated with chronic physical ailments. A significant number of elderly suicides are probably unreported. Not eating or taking medications correctly are common ways in which an older person can slip into a nonreported suicide.

Getting Help for Mental Health Problems

Mild anxiety and depression can be treated over a relatively short period of time through professional counseling and/or stress management techniques (see Chapter 3). College and the years beyond it are among the most unsettling times of life, and people aged twenty-five to forty-five make nearly half of all visits to psychiatrists. There are several forms of therapy and types of therapists that you may find helpful at various points in your life.

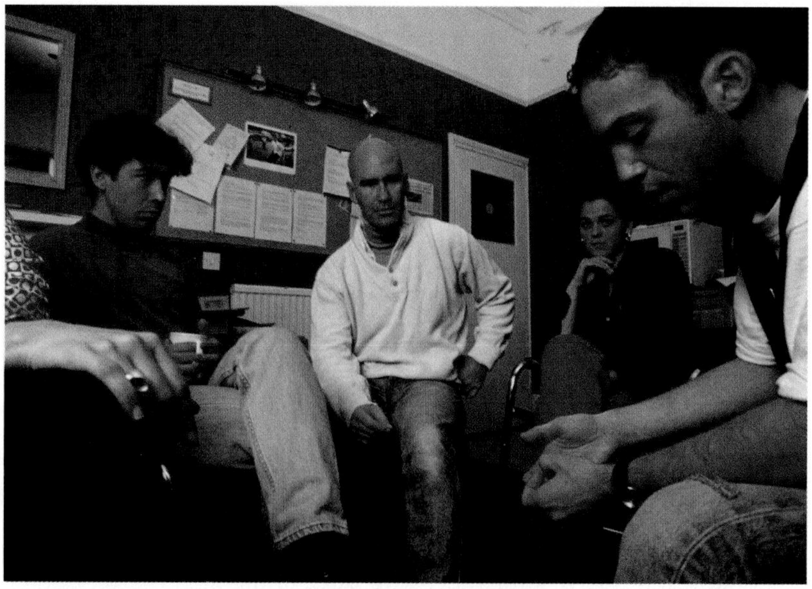

Group therapy has become increasingly popular as members with like issues, guided by the therapist, help each other with problems.

suicidologist A person who studies suicide.

The following is a list of some of the professionals who are trained specifically to assist with mental health problems:

Psychiatrists. A psychiatrist is a physician who has several years of specialty training in the diagnosis and treatment of mental problems. Psychiatrists understand both the physical and emotional aspects of their patients. Their broad training allows them to use many treatment approaches. Of the mental health professionals, only psychiatrists can prescribe antianxiety drugs, antidepressants, and other drugs. Child psychiatrists specialize in working with children; geriatric psychiatrists specialize in helping the elderly.

Psychologists. The field of psychology covers many specialties, including clinical treatment, testing, and research. Psychologists who conduct individual and group psychotherapy are generally called clinical or counseling psychologists. They work in many settings, including private practice, hospitals, mental health centers, and schools. In most states, a licensed psychologist has a doctoral degree in psychology.

Social workers. Some of the tasks that social workers are trained to perform involve individual and group therapy, diagnosis, and referral and consultation for mental health problems. Psychiatric social workers have master's degrees in social work and have completed field-placement programs in therapy and consultation.

Mental health counselors. A mental health counselor is trained to help with decision making. Counselors work with individuals and groups in private practice, business, schools, and mental health and other community agencies. A certified clinical mental health counselor has a master's degree and clinical training.

The following are examples of situations in which you may want to contact a mental health professional for help:

- If you have a problem accepting a new environment
- If a close family member or friend dies
- If you experience financial difficulty
- If you are fired from a job
- If you experience a personal injury or illness

Developing Health Skills

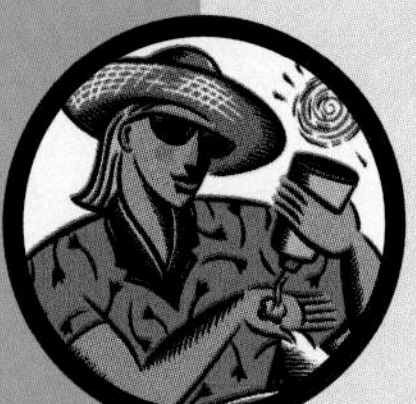

Suicide Warning Signs

Many suicides are preventable—if the clues are seen by others. There are many warning signals that you can watch for in classmates whom you think may be suicidal. Here are seven of them:

1. Depression
2. Drop in grades
3. Excessive worrying, especially over grades
4. Social isolation or withdrawal
5. Extreme pessimism
6. Substance abuse
7. Change in normal habits

What can you do if you believe a friend or classmate is suicidal? Here are some tips from psychologists who work with suicidal people.

- Confront the individual with your concerns in this matter. Don't mince words; speak honestly and directly. Ask the person: "Are you thinking about killing yourself?"
- Be a friend. Offer support and a listening ear. Suggest concrete alternative actions.
- Break confidentiality and tell someone else—a close relative, the dorm counselor or resident assistant, or a mental health professional.
- If you are really worried, remove all potentially lethal weapons from that person's house or room. Don't leave him or her alone.

In some situations help is absolutely necessary. Some examples are:

- If you lose control of your emotions
- If you lose the will to live
- If you can't sleep over a period of time
- If you have a constant feeling of hopelessness
- If you become dependent on alcohol or drugs
- If you develop an eating disorder
- If you think about suicide

Other situations may occur in which help is absolutely necessary. A brief period during which you lose control of your emotions does not necessarily mean you are having a breakdown or a serious mental upset. But in conjunction with not sleeping well and feeling hopeless, it is an indication of depression. In such a case, professional help is needed.

Calling for help is not a demonstration of weakness. In fact, it may be an important expression of inner strength—of good mental health.

CASE STUDY 2: Managing Mental Health

The more she thought about it, the more depressed Elaine became. Her grades began to drop and she was losing sleep over it.

What was happening? Her parents were expecting her to come home from college for the Christmas holiday and she didn't want to go. The holiday season always made her feel blue. Christmas Day was depressing. New Year's Eve was even worse.

Elaine decided to talk about it with Marie, her dorm counselor. Marie had helped Elaine work out some other problems. Marie told Elaine that she, too, sometimes felt blue when others were happy. Her solution in that situation was to treat herself to something special to perk herself up. Elaine promised to do the same, and she bought something special for herself. Her trip home turned out far better than she had anticipated. The holidays still weren't fun, but at least she wasn't insufferably sad.

Charles was pleased with how well he did during his first semester at school. His grades were good—A's and B's—and he had made some good friends. But all of a sudden—now that he was ready to go home for the holidays—he came crashing down. He was listless and had no energy or desire to do anything. Charles started cutting classes and not completing his schoolwork.

What had happened? Was there something going on in his life that had upset him? Were the demands he placed on himself realistic? Was he worried about going home and having a fight with his parents?

Charles didn't know the answers to these questions, but, more to the point, he didn't care. He was so depressed when he went home that he didn't return to school. He spoke to his family physician and got a psychiatric referral. Charles stayed in treatment for the next several months, and by the end of the summer, he was ready to go back to school. Charles was in good spirits, but he promised himself that if he got too far down in the dumps again, he would not wait until his depression was out of control before he sought help.

In Your Opinion

Elaine and Charles both faced the pre-holiday blues, but they handled their problems very differently. Elaine sought answers to her sadness; Charles avoided his problems, at least initially.

- What are the positive steps that both Elaine and Charles took?
- How could Charles have handled his situation differently so that he didn't have to take time off from school?
- With regard to their self-concept, self-esteem, self-efficacy and self-actualization, how do Elaine and Charles perceive themselves?
- Think about a recent situation in which you were depressed. What was going on in your life? Did you seek help? Did you work it out yourself? How might you do it differently today?

KEY CONCEPTS

1. Mental health refers to an individual's emotional and social well-being.
2. There are countless emotions, such as anger, love, fear, and joy. These emotions occur at different levels of intensity.
3. It is mentally healthy to express emotions, but there are more healthy and less healthy ways of doing so.
4. Self-concept, self-esteem, and self-efficacy are all elements of knowing oneself—self-assessment.
5. Mental illness is recognized in degrees. The degree of mental illness a person suffers is in direct proportion to the amount of dysfunction (pain or difficulty) present.
6. Some anxiety is normal and may play an important role in anticipating situations. Anxiety sustained over a long period of time, however, may result in physical symptoms such as muscle tension and back and neck pain.
7. It is common to feel sad and depressed from time to time, but depression becomes a mental illness when it is experienced with such intensity and over such a long period of time that it interferes with normal day-to-day activities.
8. Psychoses are mental disorders that are so serious as to result in loss of touch with reality. Schizophrenia is the most common and disabling psychosis.
9. Every year, there are more than 200,000 reported suicide attempts, and 30,000 are completed. Suicide is

the third leading cause of death among people aged fifteen to twenty-four years old.

10. Many types of professionals are trained specifically to assist with mental health problems, including psychologists, psychiatrists, and social workers.

REVIEW QUESTIONS

1. Differentiate between mental health and mental illness.

2. Explain the concept of "normal" as it is used to define both mental health and mental illness.

3. List seven characteristics of a mentally healthy (well-adjusted) individual.

4. Explain the difference between REM sleep and non-REM sleep and describe the benefits to be gained by each.

5. Describe the similarities and differences between the following elements of knowing yourself: self-concept, self-esteem, self-efficacy, self-actualization.

6. Rearrange the following mental states in order from least dysfunctional to most dysfunctional: psychotic, nervous, phobic, self-destructive, aggressive.

7. Explain how depression is both normal and abnormal, and differentiate between simply feeling sad and being clinically depressed.

8. Describe the symptoms of schizophrenia.

9. List the warning signs that suggest that an individual is contemplating suicide.

10. Differentiate between each of the following mental health professionals: psychiatrist, psychologist, social worker, mental health counselor.

CRITICAL THINKING QUESTIONS

1. We often hear that how we feel about our self is an indication of the state of our well-being or health. Is it possible to be healthy and still maintain a poor "self" component—either poor self-concept, poor self-esteem, or poor self-efficacy?

2. In *Healthy People 2010,* the following goal is stated: "Increase the proportion of people with mental disorders who receive treatment." Baseline data suggest that only 47 percent of such people currently obtain treatment. These data are based on self-reports. How accurate do you think self-reports are as a means of quantifying people who obtain treatment? What is another way to collect this information?

3. *Healthy People 2010* established a goal to "increase the proportion of adults with recognized depression who receive treatment." Baseline data from 1997 indicate that only 23 percent of adults diagnosed with depression received treatment. What strategies would you suggest for achieving this goal by the year 2010?

4. How accessible are mental health services in your community or on your campus? When considering this question, be sure to differentiate between accessibility and availability. Availability suggests that a service exists in your community or on your campus. Accessibility means that you can get to it. What barriers, both physical and psychological, prevent people from taking advantage of mental health services?

JOURNAL ACTIVITIES

1. Chart your emotions for a period of one week. Indicate when you are happy, sad, anxious, or distressed and when you experience other emotional states. What are the reasons for these emotional responses?

2. Identify a place where you can go by yourself to be alone with your thoughts. Make yourself stay for one full hour without reading, watching television, or experiencing any other diversions. Then write a paragraph describing how you feel about that experience.

3. Interview a dorm counselor and ask what are the most common problems that college students on your campus face.

4. Make a list of mental health resources available on campus or in the community where you can go for help if you or one of your friends needs it. Be sure to include the address and telephone number of each resource.

SELECTED BIBLIOGRAPHY

Chambless, D. L., et al. "An Update on Empirically Validated Therapies." *Clinical Psychologist* 49 (1996): 5–18.

Diagnostic and Statistical Manual of Mental Disorders (4th ed., rev.). Washington, DC: American Psychiatric Association, 2000.

Gorman, Jack M. *The Essential Guide to Mental Health*. New York: St. Martin's Press, 1996.

Jones, A. H. "Mental Illness Made Public: Ending the Stigma?" *Lancet 352* (1998): 1060.

Kessler, R. C., G. Borges, and E. E. Walters. "Prevalence of and Risk Factors for Lifetime Suicide Attempts in the National Comorbidity Survey." *Archives of General Psychiatry 56*, no. 7 (1999): 617–626.

Maslow, A. H. *Motivation and Personality* (3rd ed.). New York: Harper & Row, 1987.

Mental Health: A Report of the Surgeon General. Rockville, MD: U.S. Department of Health and Human

Services, Substance Abuse and Mental Health Administration, 1999.

National Center for Injury Prevention and Control. *Fact Book for the Year 2000: Suicide and Suicide Behavior.* http://www.cdc.gov/ncipc/pub-res/FactBook/suicide.htm.

Secker, J. "Current Conceptualizations of Mental Health and Mental Health Promotion." *Health Education Research 13* (1998): 57–66.

HEALTHLINKS

Websites for Information on Mental Health Issues

You can access better health as it relates to this chapter by checking out some of the following sites on the Internet. These sites can be accessed directly from the *Decisions for Healthy Living* Website located at www.aw.com/pruitt.

American Psychological Association

Includes APA newsletters, information on books, journals, and public practical and educational materials.

Center for Mental Health Services

The government agency that focuses on efforts to treat mental illness by promoting mental health and preventing the development or worsening of mental illness when possible.

National Institute of Mental Health

General information on mental disorders, diagnosis, and treatment, as well as the latest research in the field.

National Mental Health Association

The nation's only citizen volunteer advocacy organization dedicated to improving mental health of all individuals and achieving victory over mental illness.

American Foundation for Suicide Prevention

A voluntary organization dedicated to advancing our knowledge of suicide and our ability to prevent it.

HEALTH HOTLINES

Managing Your Mental Health

National Alliance for the Mentally Ill
(800) 950-6264
2107 Wilson Boulevard, Suite 300
Arlington, VA 22201

National Mental Health Association Information Center
(800) 969-6642
2001 N. Beauregard Street, 12th Floor
Alexandria, VA 22311

National Mental Health Consumer, Self-Help Clearinghouse
(800) 553-4539
1211 Chestnut Street, Suite 1207
Philadelphia, PA 19107

TEST YOUR KNOWLEDGE ANSWERS

1. False. Mental health is the ability to negotiate the daily challenges and social interactions of life without experiencing undue emotional or behavioral incapacity. A mentally healthy person experiences a wide range of emotions, including sadness, fear, and disappointment as well as joy and happiness.
2. True. In 1974, the American Psychiatric Association removed homosexuality from its list of mental disorders.
3. False. During REM sleep the body is quiet but the mind is active. During non-REM sleep, in contrast, the body may be active but the mind is not. It is during non-REM sleep that the body does its repair and maintenance work.
4. True. Every year, there are more than 200,000 reported suicide attempts and 30,000 completed suicides. The suicide rate is especially high among teenagers and people in their early twenties.
5. True. Of all individuals experiencing traumatic events, 20 percent of women and 8 percent of men will develop post-traumatic stress disorder.

CHAPTER

3

Coping with Stress

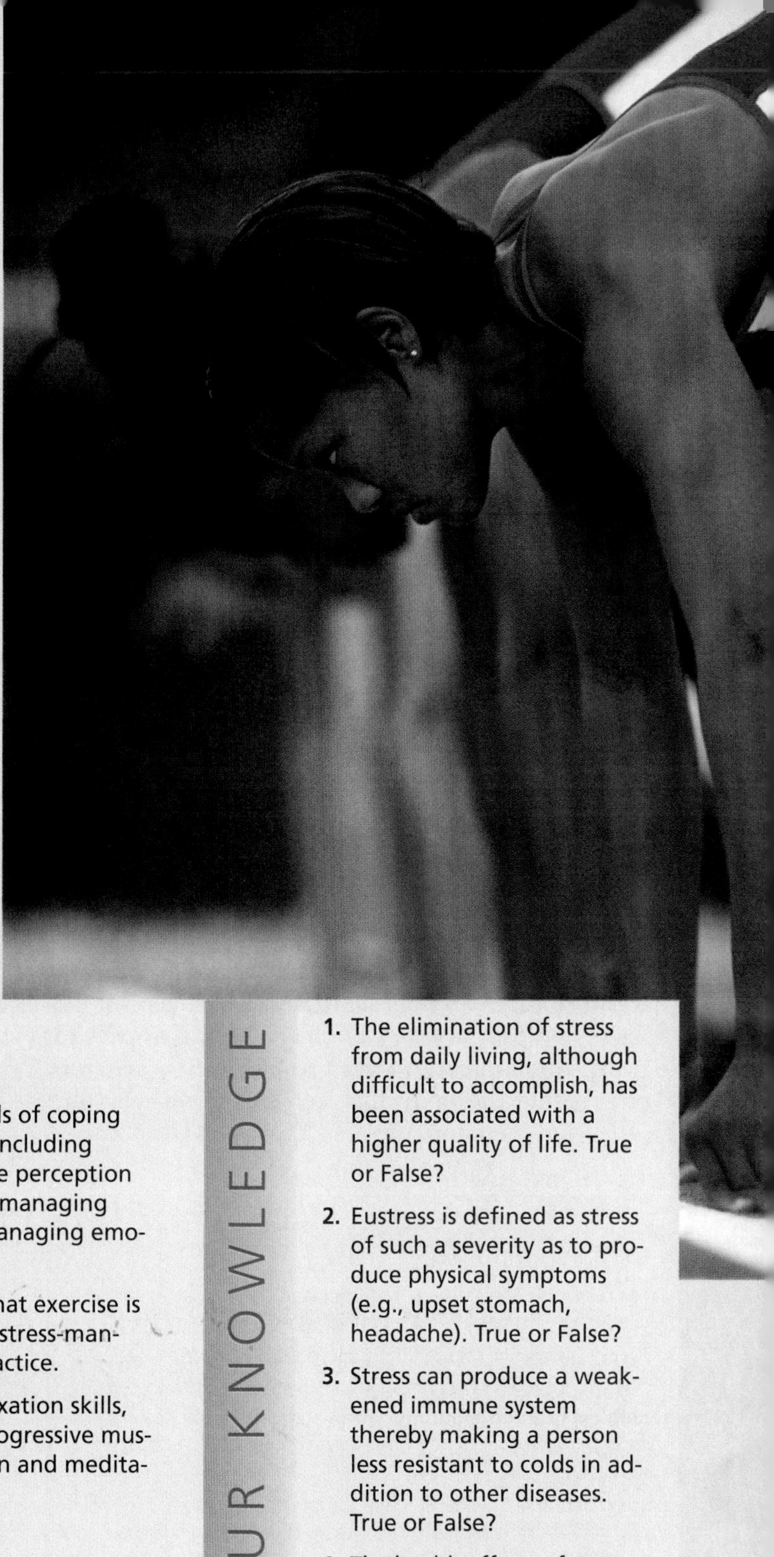

OBJECTIVES

When you finish reading this chapter, you will be able to:

1. Define stress and recognize it as a part of your daily life.
2. List several common stressors and the source of each.
3. Differentiate between primary stressors and secondary stressors, and explain the effect of each.
4. Understand that stress results from a reaction to events, not from the events themselves.
5. Differentiate between distress and eustress.
6. Recognize the scientific connection between too much stress and the incidence of disease.
7. Describe sources of stress in college life and in the work environment.
8. Develop skills of coping with stress, including changing the perception of stressors, managing time, and managing emotions.
9. Recognize that exercise is an effective stress-management practice.
10. Practice relaxation skills, including progressive muscle relaxation and meditation.

TEST YOUR KNOWLEDGE

1. The elimination of stress from daily living, although difficult to accomplish, has been associated with a higher quality of life. True or False?
2. Eustress is defined as stress of such a severity as to produce physical symptoms (e.g., upset stomach, headache). True or False?
3. Stress can produce a weakened immune system thereby making a person less resistant to colds in addition to other diseases. True or False?
4. The health effects of stress include asthma, amenorrhea, back pains, chest pains, and diarrhea. True or False?
5. Stress in the workplace has been found to be lower among workers who are not engaged in the decision-making process and who have little control over their work—for example, receptionists or junior assistants. True or False?

Answers found at end of chapter.

Imagine life without stress. It might sound like a good thing to you, especially when you are facing the pressures of exams, conflicts at home or at work, and daily hassles such as running to catch a bus or looking for a parking space.

In reality, there is no such thing as a stress-free life. However, there are positive and negative stressors and positive and negative ways of coping with them. Low levels of stress can act as motivators. For example, the stress caused by having done poorly on a test can prompt you to study and do well on the final exam. But too much stress and poor coping strategies can be harmful to your health and can lead to a wide range of conditions, including migraine headaches, rashes, ulcers, anxiety, depression, and heart disease.

Some stressors can be avoided or the impact of them made less taxing. You can drop a course that is too difficult or find a tutor to help you keep up with the class. Other stressors, such as the sickness or death of a loved one, are totally unavoidable. Whether avoidable or unavoidable, stress and how you deal with it can have a significant impact on your health.

Defining Stress

Stress is a perception of an external situation or event that can result in an internal response such as nervous tension, an upset stomach, or other physical or psychological symptoms. The **stress response** is a series of events within the body that involves chemicals, hormones, and neural impulses. The stress response is caused by **stressors,** specific events that disrupt equilibrium and initiate this complex biochemical response. Stress is highly individualized, and what one person perceives as stressful may be thought of as highly stimulating and not at all stressful by another. This is why the scientist Hans Selye described stress as the "nonspecific response of the body to any demand."

stress A reaction of the body and mind to the mental and emotional strain placed on them.

stress response A series of events, caused by stressors, within the body that involve chemicals, hormones, and neural impulses.

stressor A specific event that disrupts equilibrium and initiates complex biochemical responses.

general adaptation syndrome (GAS) The theory proposed by Hans Selye in which there are three distinct phases to the body's reaction to stress: alarm reaction, resistance, and exhaustion.

alarm reaction The first stage of the general adaptation syndrome; the body mobilizes its forces to meet a threatening situation.

resistance The second stage of the general adaptation syndrome; the body relaxes and returns to its normal state after the immediate threat has disappeared.

exhaustion The final stage of the general adaptation syndrome; it occurs when the body does not have a chance to restore itself to a state of equilibrium.

lactate A substance formed in the blood when muscles contract.

adrenaline A hormone that speeds up heartbeat and other responses to alarm; also called epinephrine.

noradrenaline A hormone that causes blood vessels to constrict and other responses to anger; also called norepinephrine.

How We React to Stress

The grandfather of stress research, University of Montreal biologist Hans Selye, developed a theoretical basis for the stress response in 1956. In what he called the **general adaptation syndrome (GAS),** Selye theorized that there are three distinct phases to the body's reaction to stress: **alarm reaction, resistance,** and **exhaustion.**

The first stage of the general adaptation syndrome is shock, or an alarm reaction to the stressful situation. The body mobilizes its forces to meet the threatening situation. It is like a call to arms. Muscles tighten, particularly those in the face and neck. **Lactate,** a substance formed when muscles contract, appears in the blood. **Adrenaline** and **noradrenaline**—also called epinephrine and norepinephrine respectively—the hormones that speed up heartbeat and constrict blood vessels, are also secreted into the bloodstream. Blood pressure rises, breathing accelerates, blood sugar increases, and so does general alertness. The full force of physical and mental resources of the individual is brought to bear on the stress-producing situation.

The next stage of adaptation is called resistance. At this point, calming chemicals are produced, and the body relaxes and returns to its normal state after the immediate threat has disappeared. Most people go through these first two stages time and time again, and they become a way of adapting to the conflicts of everyday life.

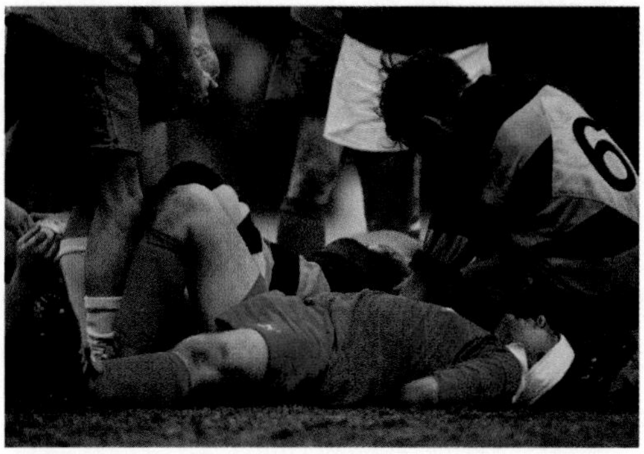

Physical stressors: strenuous physical activity, hunger, thirst, pain, cold, lack of sleep, illness, injury, temporary disability.

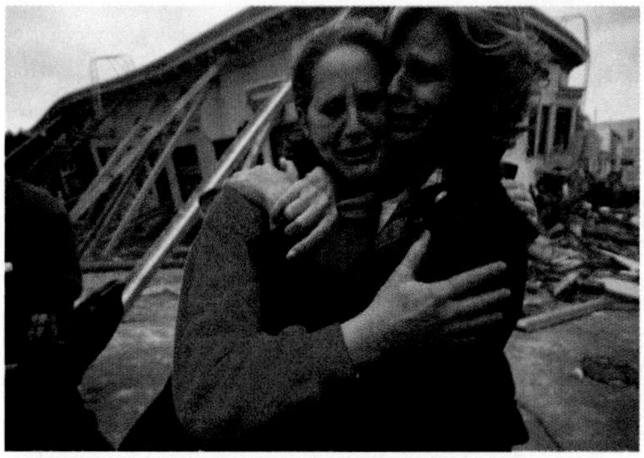

Environmental stressors: polluted air and water, extremes in temperature, noise, crowding and overpopulation, lack of privacy, natural disasters.

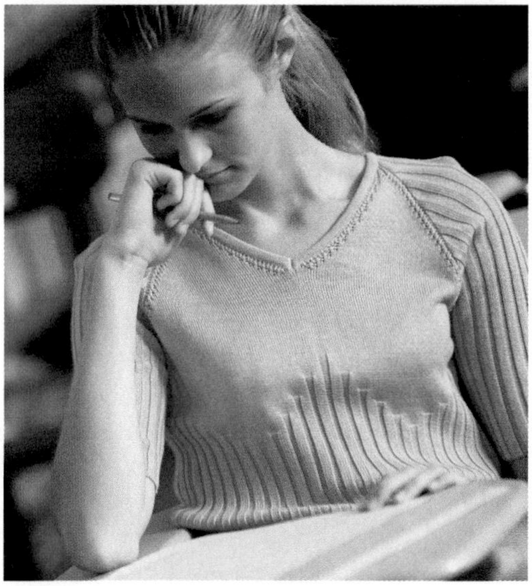

Psychological stressors: test taking, academic failure, boredom, graduation from college, frustration, anger, guilt, worry, anxiety, marriage, loss of a friend, vacation, threats to self-esteem, death of a relative, extreme joy, excitement in anticipation of an event.

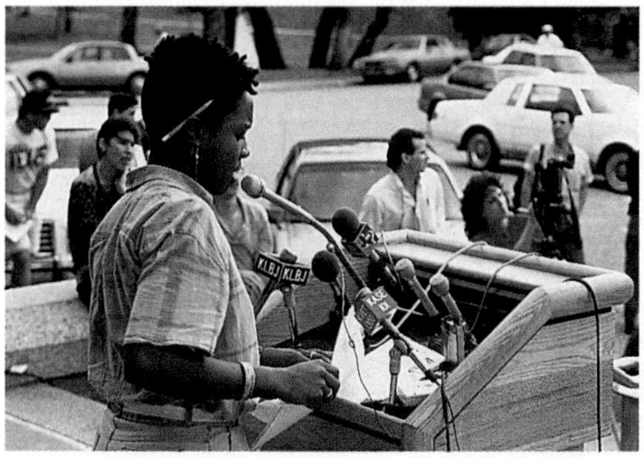

Social stressors: racial and religious prejudice, sexual harassment, underemployment and unemployment, public speaking, class reunion, isolation.

Figure 3.1 **Sources of Stress**

However, sometimes there are so many stressors that a person cannot react to them. When stress is persistent and chronic, the body may not have a chance to restore itself to a state of equilibrium, or its prestressed state. When this happens, a person enters the exhaustion stage. It is in this stage that you are more susceptible to illness and disease.

Stressors: Where Do They Originate?

Some stressors are obvious and are related to a specific event, such as writing a major research paper or being evaluated for your work performance. Others are hidden, such as worrying about your finances or the health of your parents. A **primary stressor** (the assignment of a research paper) initiates the stress response. A **secondary stressor** (worry) keeps the stress response activated.

There are four basic sources of stress in society today: physical stressors, environmental stressors, psychological stressors, and social stressors. The examples shown in Figure 3.1 illustrate the kinds of situations that can trigger stress.

primary stressor Something that initiates the stress response.

secondary stressor An additional stressor that continues the stress response.

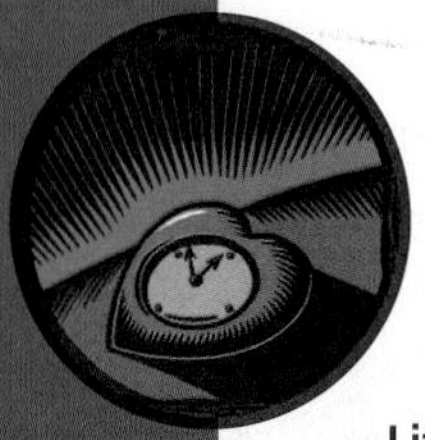

Rating the Stressors in Your Life

Stress can play a powerful role in your life. Often, when we think of personal stressors, we think of major events or even catastrophes. But even little daily things can bring about stress when added together. Use the following scale to test your stress level. Consider each of the following events and, in Column A, indicate the number of times you have experienced each one during the last twelve months.

Life-change event	Column A	Column B	Column C
1. Entered college	_____	50	_____
2. Married	_____	77	_____
3. Trouble with your boss	_____	38	_____
4. Hold a job while attending school	_____	43	_____
5. Experienced the death of a spouse	_____	87	_____
6. Major change in sleeping habits	_____	34	_____
7. Experienced the death of a close family member	_____	77	_____
8. Major change in eating habits	_____	30	_____
9. Change in or choice of major field of study	_____	41	_____
10. Revision of personal habits	_____	45	_____
11. Experienced the death of a close friend	_____	68	_____
12. Found guilty of minor violations of the law	_____	22	_____
13. Had an outstanding personal achievement	_____	40	_____
14. Experienced pregnancy, or fathered a pregnancy	_____	68	_____
15. Major change in health or behavior of a family member	_____	56	_____
16. Had sexual difficulties	_____	58	_____
17. Had trouble with in-laws	_____	42	_____
18. Major change in number of family get-togethers	_____	26	_____
19. Major change in financial state	_____	53	_____
20. Gained a new family member	_____	50	_____
21. Change in residence or living conditions	_____	42	_____
22. Major conflict or change in values	_____	50	_____
23. Major change in church activities	_____	36	_____
24. Marital reconciliation with your mate	_____	58	_____
25. Fired from work	_____	62	_____
26. Were divorced	_____	76	_____
27. Changed to a different line of work	_____	50	_____
28. Major change in number of arguments with spouse	_____	50	_____
29. Major change in responsibilities at work	_____	47	_____
30. Had your spouse begin or cease work outside the home	_____	41	_____
31. Major change in working hours or conditions	_____	42	_____
32. Marital separation from mate	_____	74	_____
33. Major change in type and/or amount of recreation	_____	37	_____
34. Major change in use of drugs	_____	52	_____
35. Took on a mortgage or loan of less than $10,000	_____	52	_____

Life-change event	Column A	Column B	Column C
36. Major personal injury or illness	____	65	____
37. Major change in use of alcohol	____	46	____
38. Major change in social activities	____	43	____
39. Major change in amount of participation in school activities	____	38	____
40. Major change in amount of independence and responsibility	____	49	____
41. Took a trip or a vacation	____	33	____
42. Engaged to be married	____	54	____
43. Changed to a new school	____	50	____
44. Changed dating habits	____	41	____
45. Trouble with school administration	____	44	____
46. Broke or had broken a marital engagement or steady relationship	____	60	____
47. Major change in self-concept or self-awareness	____	57	____
Total			____

To find your score on this scale, multiply the number in Column A by the number in Column B and place the product in Column C. Finally, add the rows in Column C. If your score totals 1,435 or higher, you are in the "high" category for developing an illness. If your total is 347 or less, you fall into the "low" category. The "medium" score is 890.

Source: Reprinted with permission of Elsevier Science Inc. from M. T. Mark, et al., "The Influence of Recent Life Experiences on the Health of College Freshmen," *Journal of Psychosomatic Research* 19: 87–98, 1975

Positive and Negative Stress

The effects of stress appear to be similar whether they are experienced in response to positive or negative events. This is why when medical researchers Thomas Holmes and Richard Rahe devised their list of major stressors, they put positive experiences as well as negative events near the top. For example, getting married and experiencing the death of a parent are high on the list. The student life-change rating scale in the Assess Your Health box is adapted from the original Holmes-Rahe Social Readjustment Rating Scale. Research suggests that people with high stress scores on evaluations such as this tend to be more vulnerable to illness.

Special terms differentiate between bad stress (**distress**) and good stress (**eustress**). Distress is the type of stress that brings about negative mental or physical responses. After experiencing distress, people are often wound up and have trouble relaxing or calming down. Examples of events that cause distress are a major exam or a fight with a roommate, as well as major life events such as family celebrations and moving to a new city.

In addition, the minor daily hassles of life can wear a person down by overstimulating the body. These hassles might include concern about weight, the health of a family member, money, too many things to do, and fear of crime.

In contrast to distress, eustress is the type of stress that is a healthy part of daily living. After experiencing eustress, people are able to relax and enjoy a feeling of peacefulness and calm. Examples of events that cause eustress are a vacation, a personal achievement, or an exciting classroom or workplace experience. Eustress can help you channel nervous energy into better performance.

Personality and Stress

There are at least two personality types that affect how different individuals respond to stress. In 1974, Drs. Meyer Friedman and Ray Rosenman identified these personalities as Type A and Type B. The **Type A personality** is described as being excessively hostile, competitive, aggressive, driven, and impatient. Someone with this personality would find it stressful to be stuck in a traffic jam or to wait in a supermarket or bank line. The **Type B personality,** in contrast, is described as being

distress The type of stress that brings about negative mental or physical responses; also known as bad stress.

eustress The type of stress that is a healthy part of daily living; it can result in the ability to relax and enjoy a feeling of peacefulness and calm.

Type A personality Competitive, aggressive, driven, and impatient.

Type B personality Less competitive and more relaxed and patient than Type A personality.

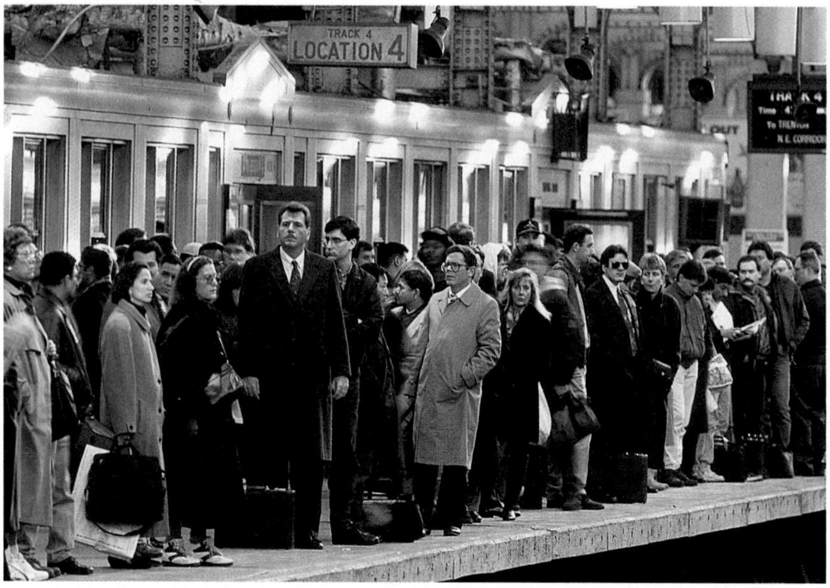

People with Type A personalities are described as being competitive, driven, and impatient. For these people, waiting for a train can be very stressful.

relatively more relaxed and patient. There is some indication that Type A's tend to be more prone to heart disease. However, this finding is controversial because of the influence on Type A's of other risk factors associated with coronary disease, including age, sex, family history, and occupation. Overall, smoking and high cholesterol predict coronary disease among Type A's more strongly than does personality.

The Impact of Stress on Health

The primary reason that it is important to understand the underlying source of stress and to come to grips with it is that there is a well-established scientific connection between too much stress and the incidence of disease. Research has demonstrated a relationship between stress and several biochemical changes, such as changes in adrenaline and cholesterol levels. Physiological effects of stress have been documented as well, including increased heart rate, blood pressure, and muscle tension. Finally, psychological responses to stress have been documented, including anxiety and depression.

Surveys show that stress-related disorders account for a significantly high number of visits to primary care physicians. Typical of these symptoms are irritability, insomnia, heart palpitations, headaches, stomachaches, and skin rashes. Although these are not life-threatening conditions, they should not be discounted, because if they continue they can cause more serious problems.

Stress Symptoms Seen in the Physician's Office

Some of the stress-related symptoms that bring people to a physician's office are listed here in three categories:

1. **Health effects:** Asthma, amenorrhea, back pains, chest pains, diarrhea, dizziness, heart palpitations, heartburn, headaches, hives, insomnia, loss of sexual interest, nightmares, psychosomatic disorders, skin rashes, ulcers, and weakness.
2. **Subjective effects:** Anxiety, apathy, boredom, depression, fatigue, frustration, guilt, irritability, inability to make decisions, moodiness, nervousness, and tension.
3. **Behavioral effects:** Being accident prone, drug use, emotional outbursts, excessive eating and drinking, impulsive behavior, lack of concentration, loss of appetite, nervous laughter, restlessness, and trembling.

Clearly, you don't go to the physician to complain about the fact that you are having difficulty making decisions or that you are bored and restless. But if these problems are coupled with other symptoms—perhaps weight loss or gain or a skin rash—your physician may diagnose a stress-related disorder.

Research Findings on Stress and the Immune System

Several recent studies have found that stress can result in a weakening of the immune system. One study demonstrated that the level of important immune system cells in the body measurably decreased among a group of medical students in response to the stress of taking final exams. These cells are important in fighting diseases ranging from the common cold to cancer.

- When healthy volunteers were exposed to cold viruses in an experiment at the University of Pittsburgh School of Medicine and the University of Virginia Health Sciences Center, researchers found that those who had been having ongoing work problems or interpersonal difficulties with family and friends for a month or more were most likely to catch a cold—that is, stress made them less resistant to the cold virus.

- Researchers at the University of California, San Francisco, found a correlation between positive psychological characteristics—low levels of tension, depression, fatigue, and anger—and increased numbers of disease-fighting immune system cells in patients with AIDS. Of the patients studied, those who coped better with the distress associated with their illness had higher numbers of such cells. It is possible, the researchers concluded, that adaptive coping styles might modify the course of immunological-related diseases such as AIDS.
- Some researchers believe that having good, positive thoughts—even laughter—can boost the immune system because it promotes the release of protective chemicals in the brain. This is called mind-body healing. An area of research involving mind-body healing is **psychoneuroimmunology,** the study of how the brain affects the immune system.

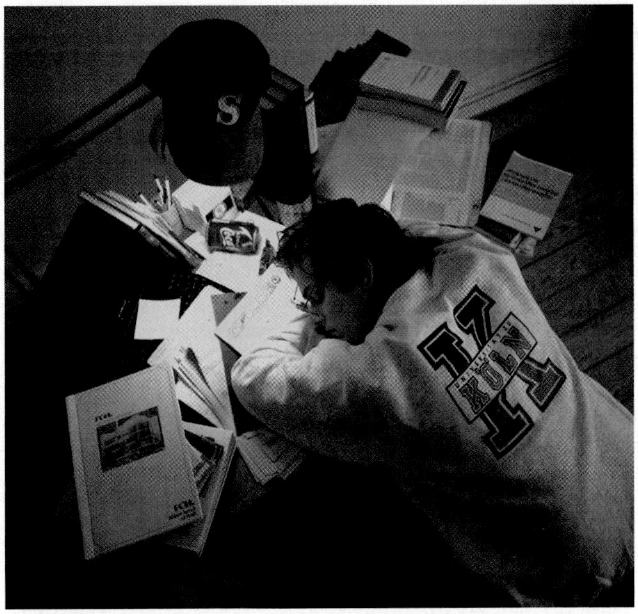

The stress of taking final exams can result in exhaustion and can reduce the number of immune cells, which are necessary for fighting diseases such as the common cold.

Stressors of Everyday Living

Stress is a part of every phase of life. Prenatal heart rates have been found to increase and decrease in response to the mother's listening to various forms of music. This suggests that a fetus senses the stress levels of the mother. Predictable stressors occur at different stages throughout life. For children, the first day of school is a classic stressful experience. For young adults, the passage from the world of college to the world of work is a predictable period of stress. And for older adults, retiring from work can be extremely stressful.

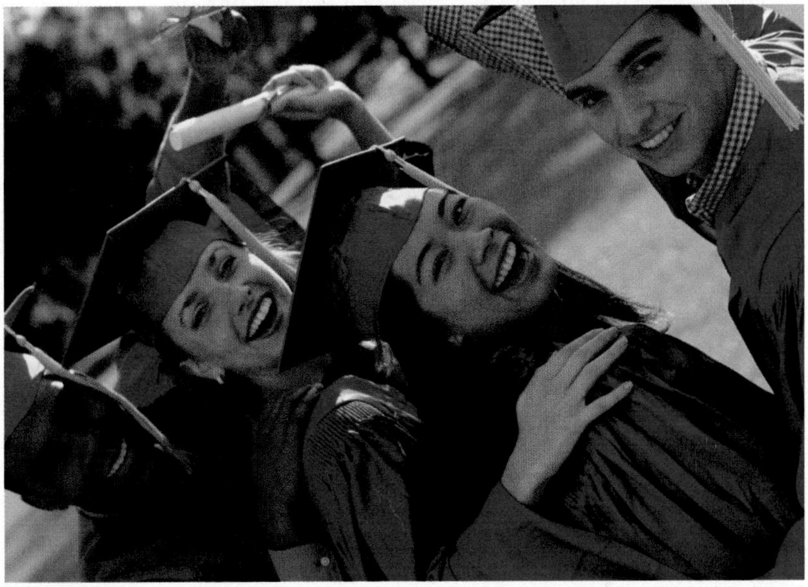

College includes many stressors—including graduating, leaving close friends, and even the excitement of heading out into the "real" world. Coping involves dealing constructively with stress.

At College

The transition from high school to college presents numerous potentially stressful demands. Prominent among stressors are:

- leaving your parents, siblings, and friends—perhaps for the first time
- making a new network of friends
- assuming responsibility for yourself, including buying clothes and balancing a budget
- making decisions about drugs, alcohol and sexual behavior
- facing new intellectual challenges
- juggling the pressures and time constraints of working while going to school.

One of the reasons that college life is so stressful is that many of the decisions that students make can have

psychoneuroimmunology The study of how the brain affects the immune system.

long-term consequences. Choosing a major, for example, can be especially stressful because this decision affects a student's course selection for the remainder of college life. It may also affect eventual career choice.

Not all college students go to school directly from high school. An increasing number of college students have worked for a while. Some go to school and work in the evenings, or work in the day and go to school at night. Older students face some of the same stressors as younger students. But older students also face the stress of fear of failure: How can I keep up with younger people? Can I successfully juggle school with the other parts of my life—my children, my job, my spouse, my sick parents?

At Work

Stress in the workplace is pervasive. More than 40 percent of American workers say they are either very or extremely concerned about stress from work demands. The number one source of stress among those surveyed is worry about the ability to balance work and family.

In contrast to the stereotype of a high-pressured executive having a heart attack, in reality a receptionist or junior assistant is more prone to get sick. What these nonexecutives have in common—and what makes their jobs particularly stressful—is a lack of control over their work. Workers in jobs with little chance for decision making have a 50 percent higher rate of heart disease, compared with workers who have a high level of control on their job.

What is the key to getting sick—or staying healthy—on a stressful job? A University of Chicago researcher studied 200 executives over a three and one-half year period when the company was undergoing major corporate changes. Half of the executives took ill, whereas the other half stayed well. Why? It is hypothesized that the group that stayed well had **personality hardiness**—that is, they had a clear sense of who they were. They looked at the tensions on the job and saw them as challenges, not threats. In a word, they felt they were in control.

As for the relationship between hardiness and health, the group of 100 executives who were well at the time of the study stayed well during the next two years. They developed only half as many symptoms of illness as a control group of less hardy people.

personality hardiness A state of resilience due to clear self-concept.

coping Adaptation to stress.

fight-or-flight reaction The body's reaction to stress in which it becomes physically ready to resist or fight a stressor or to run from it.

defense mechanisms Coping strategies by which people defend themselves against negative emotions.

stressor identification Recognizing stress in order to begin effective management.

coping skills Strategies used to deal constructively with stressors.

Adapting to Stress

Although there will always be some stress in your life, that does not mean you cannot do anything about it. In fact, the best medicine for stress appears to be learning how to adapt to or cope with it.

Coping is adaptation to stress. In primitive times, coping with stress meant little more than exercising the basic **fight-or-flight reaction** to threatening situations. For example, if a tiger threatened a primitive man, he would either stand and fight (and do so with added strength and cunning brought about by the stress reactions described by the general adaptation syndrome) or run from the threat (also with the added strength and cunning brought about by the stress reaction).

Today, we are not threatened by tigers. Threats come instead from difficult school, work, or social situations, unexpected bills, and disappointing news. Although survival is still at issue, it is not as much the survival of an individual as maintaining self-esteem in stressful situations. The fight-or-flight response still works well in some cases, as do **defense mechanisms,** such as avoidance and denial. These responses, however, are usually effective only for the short term. Fleeing or denying a stressful situation might be very useful in diminishing the acute pain of an unhappy event, but it does not help you deal with the source of the stress over the long run.

Coping with Stress

There are several ways you can effectively minimize the negative effects of everyday stress, whether it is in school, on the job, or at home. One preventive action is to make sure that you take good care of your physical health. You do this by eating nutritiously, exercising, not smoking or using drugs, and getting an adequate amount of sleep. You will find tips on how to develop good health habits in the related chapters in this textbook. Being in good physical health can help your body fight the negative health effects that can accompany stress.

Another preventive way to deal with stress is to recognize it so that you can begin to manage it effectively. Stress researchers call this process **stressor identification.** Once you identify a stressor, it is possible to develop coping strategies.

There are many things you can do to deal constructively with stressors. Collectively, these are called **coping skills,** and they fall into one of three categories: changing perception, managing time, and managing emotion.

1. **Changing perception:** This involves changing the way you perceive and define a stressful event. One way to do this is by improving communications so that you can better understand the nature of the stressor and how it occurred. Another is to remove yourself from the stressor by depersonalizing it. An accident that causes a traffic tie-up doesn't occur just to harass you. Similarly, if someone gets angry with you, it might be because he or she is distressed over something that has nothing to do with you.

Developing Health Skills

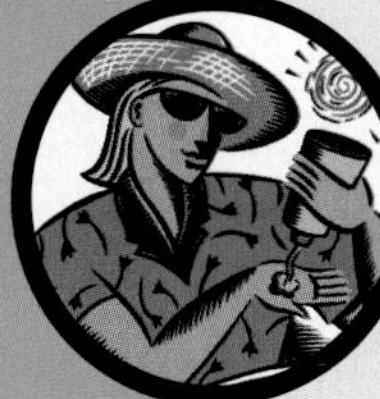

Managing Time

Using time well is one of the best ways to manage stress. Some good tips for managing time are:

- Set long-term goals.
- Make a daily "to do" list.
- Rank items on that list.
  - A—Absolutely must do today
  - B—Do as soon as possible
  - C—Needs to be done sometime
  - D—Really doesn't matter if it ever gets done (scratch it)
- Start with A items, number in order.
- Then B items, number in order.
- Recognize that not every task demands the same quality performance.
- If possible, complete one job before going on to another. Do it right the first time.

Cultural View

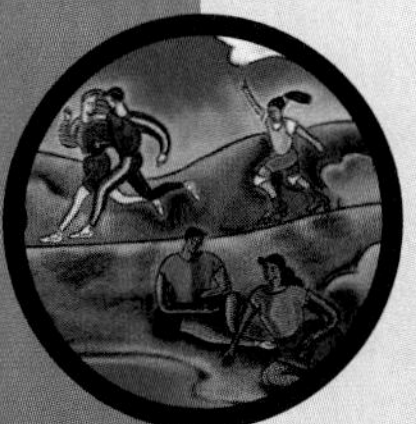

Managing Stress through T'ai Chi

Chi (pronounced CHEE) is a Chinese term representing the life force; t'ai chi is a form of exercise that regulates this energy to improve balance, strength, and flexibility. The Chinese have been practicing t'ai chi for thousands of years as a way to live in harmony and balance with the world. Today, groups of thousands of people gather in various parts of Beijing, Shanghai, and other Chinese cities to practice t'ai chi in the early morning hours before work. Even visits to American cities with large Chinese populations provide an opportunity to witness this ancient martial art. An early-morning stroll through parks in or near San Francisco's Chinatown district or Boston's Public Garden provide passersby with a basic demonstration of t'ai chi. Non-Chinese people are also practicing t'ai chi, now that the word of its benefits has spread.

Studies show that people who practice t'ai chi have a marked decrease in their resting heart rate and stress hormones for the rest of the day, and feel less physical tension, fatigue, anxiety, and anger than those who do not practice t'ai chi. This holds true for beginners of the technique as well as long-time practitioners.

Even though it is a branch of martial arts, t'ai chi is well known for its calming effects. In fact, it is often called a "moving meditation." With the proper training, t'ai chi teaches you how to live in harmony with aggression, fear, and other stressors, rather than fight them. As one instructor said, "T'ai chi teaches you how to be relaxed in all aspects of your life and how to stay relaxed in the face of stress."

Using more than 100 positions or movements, t'ai chi embraces four basic philosophical concepts:

- Finding comfort in solitude.
- Returning to the joys of childhood, such as embracing laughter and play.
- Moving with the flow of nature, as exemplified by a Ping-Pong ball in water—when you push it under, it always pops back up with little or no energy.
- Acknowledging failure as the first step to success.

T'ai chi classes are offered at many colleges, community centers, and health clubs. Before signing up, make sure the instructor's philosophy is similar to yours. Some instructors focus on t'ai chi as a form of martial arts; others teach it as a form of meditation; others emphasize health and fitness. The key is finding the right class for your needs.

Developing Health Skills

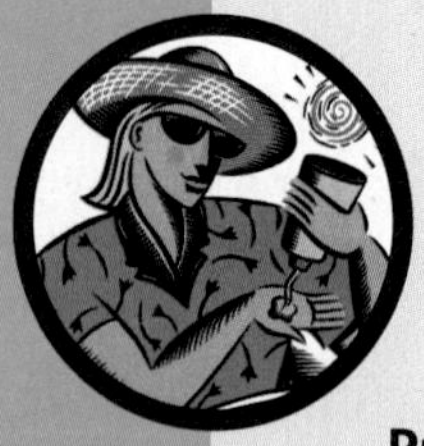

Learning to Relax

Relaxation is another way to reduce stress. The following are examples of two different kinds of relaxation exercises that have been used to reduce stress. You might want to try one.

Progressive Muscle Relaxation

Relaxation and muscle tension are incompatible. Therefore, reducing muscle tension leads to a reduction in anxiety and stress levels. The relaxation technique described here involves focusing attention on muscle activity, learning to identify even small amounts of tension in a muscle group, and practicing releasing tension from the muscle.

- Make a tight fist with one of your hands for several seconds. Focus on the tension; become aware of it. Gradually ease the tension. Feel the relaxation rising up your arm and slowly spreading over your entire body. Close your eyes and rest. Repeat the tensing and relaxing process with the muscles in your midsection, holding each muscle tight for five to ten seconds.
- Tense your arm, raise your shoulders, and tighten your stomach muscles, calves, and feet. Ease the tension, and relax.
- Lastly, furrow your brow, close your eyes tightly and clench your jaw. Ease the tension, and relax.

Note: Always remember to relax each muscle for at least fifteen seconds before tensing the next muscle.

Meditation

Meditation takes many forms. In its simplest form, it amounts to little more than calm thinking. You can try this form of meditation, also referred to as breathing relaxation. Relax quietly with your eyes closed and focus on your breathing. Each time you inhale, fill your lower abdomen with air first and allow your stomach to expand upward until your chest is full of air. Exhale at half the rate that you inhaled, slowly and completely, each time thinking about the word *calm.* Stretch out the word so that it becomes *caaaaallllmmmmm.* If thoughts arise or your attention wanders, simply focus on your breathing.

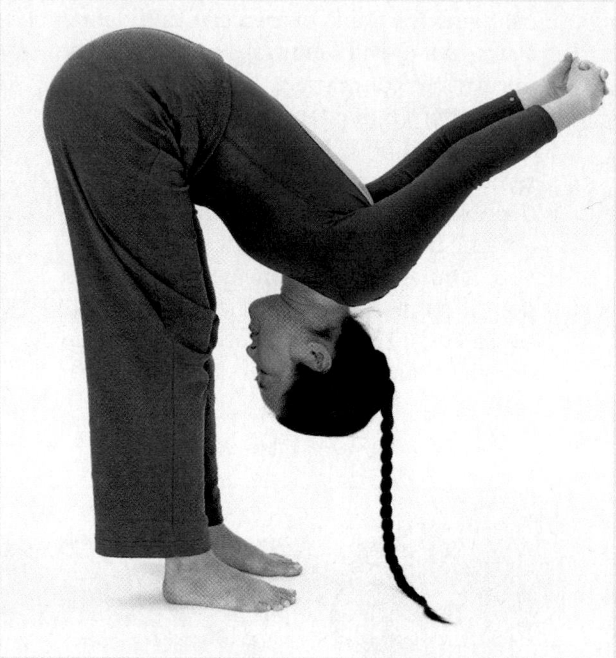

2. **Managing time:** By setting personal priorities, you can control the stressors in your life rather than allow them to control you. In addition to preventing stressors from building up, time management can lead to changes in behavior that better meet your personal needs and enhance your sense of self-esteem and general well-being (see the Developing Health Skills box).
3. **Managing emotion:** The emotional aspects of stress—whether they be happy or sad—need to be managed. If you are angry about something, it is usually better to recognize that anger and express it rather than to suppress it. Once an emotion is honestly labeled, actions can be undertaken to release it. In the case of anger, this might mean laughing it off, talking it out, seeking support or solace from another person, or in some cases crying.

Most coping skills also involve **interpersonal skills,** because many stress-producing situations involve relations with other people. Interpersonal skills include getting help from others, sharing feelings, effective communication, conflict resolution, active listening, assertiveness, and team building. These skills help to build a network of personal support that can be used to manage the stress in your life and help you cope competently. Conflict resolution—a way to deal with feelings that could escalate into violent encounters—is discussed in further detail in Chapter 9.

A strong social support system of family and friends not only can help you in times of stress but also can lower your risk for serious illness. One reason for this, according to researchers, is that social relationships can facilitate health-promoting behaviors such as proper sleep, diet, exercise, or seeking appropriate medical care when needed.

interpersonal skills The techniques involved in relating to other people.

Exercise: A Stress Reducer

There is evidence that exercise functions as a stress reducer. Most people report that they "feel good" or "feel better" following vigorous exercise. It may well be that exercise reduces stress through an individual's increased sense of well-being or by simply providing a "time out" (see the Cultural View box).

Depending on your lifestyle, there are many ways to exercise to reduce stress. For people who like to jog, a run before or after school can be an excellent way to get the day's stressors under control. This can be attributed to a release of tension or the so-called runner's high (which is thought to result from the release of brain hormones called endorphins). Meditation can also have a soothing effect on emotions (see the Developing Health Skills box). It can provide an excellent opportunity to clearly contemplate and solve problems. Conversely, a run or meditation can distract you from your problems and give your mind a rest so that you can better tackle the problems at hand (see Chapter 6). Researchers are also finding that exercising the spirit—for example, by volunteering—can make people feel good physically and emotionally and can reduce their levels of stress.

A final word: Positive and negative stressors are everyday experiences. It is not the existence of stressors but how you respond to them that is important for your overall health. A healthy response to stressors begins with an overall healthy approach to living. "Take good care of yourself!" is good advice because people who lead healthier lives also do a better job of managing the normal stress of day-to-day living.

CASE STUDY 3: Coping with Stress

George knew it would be a bad day. It started out wrong as soon as he woke up and saw that it was raining hard. Traffic would be backed up, and he hated getting stuck like that. In fact, George was right. There was a tie-up, and he arrived late for class—and fuming. George was still angry at lunch time, when he gulped down a sandwich and a cup of black coffee before rushing off to the library. Later, he took two aspirin for his "stress" headache, which he said he knew was coming. This is George's way of coping with things out of his control—getting angry and letting the daily hassles of life bother him for hours.

When Juan woke up and saw that it was raining hard, he got dressed quickly, ate breakfast, and began driving to school early. He knew from experience that he was likely to get caught in a traffic jam, and he had a lot to get done in the library and didn't want to lose any time. He also knew how stressful it could be sitting in a car that was going nowhere. But Juan had his way of dealing with this, too—books on tape, which allowed him to use the "dead" time productively, and more important, enjoyably. He arrived at school feeling good and on time to get his work done.

Juan usually handles stress well. Instead of getting angry at things, such as the traffic, he tries to find ways to deal positively with frustrating situations that are out of his control.

In Your Opinion

George and Juan faced the same stressor—the promise of a long line of slow-moving traffic. From the start, George mismanaged his stress, while Juan managed his situation well.

- What steps did George take that started him on his downward spiral?
- At what point could he have reversed the situation?
- After experiencing eustress people are able to relax and enjoy a feeling of peacefulness. Which of these two young men, Juan or George, experienced eustress? Why?
- What message do you get from Juan's way of handling stress?
- What would you have done in this situation?

KEY CONCEPTS

1. Stress is a perception of an external situation that brings about an internal response.
2. A stressor is an event or circumstance that brings about stress.
3. According to the classic theory of stress, the general adaptation syndrome, there are three distinct phases

to the body's reaction to stress: alarm reaction, resistance, and exhaustion.
4. Stressors can be psychological, physical, environmental, social, or a combination of two or more of these.
5. Not all stress is bad. Harmful stress is referred to as distress and may result in serious health problems. The good kind of stress is called eustress and is considered an important aspect of healthy living.
6. Stress-related disorders account for a high percentage of all visits to primary care physicians.
7. Being in good physical condition can help your body fight the negative health effects that can accompany stress.
8. Coping involves dealing constructively with stress.
9. Coping skills fall under one of three categories: changing perception, managing time, and managing emotion.
10. Physical exercise and relaxation techniques can reduce levels of stress. Relaxation techniques include breathing relaxation, muscle relaxation, and visualization relaxation.

REVIEW QUESTIONS

1. Describe the three stages of Hans Selye's general adaptation syndrome theory.
2. List four types of stressors and give examples of each.
3. Differentiate between eustress and distress.
4. Describe the impact of stress on physical health.
5. Cite examples of stressors that occur in the college environment, at home, and at work.
6. Describe the fight-or-flight reaction. How does it help and/or hinder daily living?
7. Name three coping skills that are useful in dealing with the normal stress of daily living.
8. Describe the role of exercise in stress management.
9. Explain how volunteering can serve as a stress management strategy.
10. Explain the processes of progressive muscle relaxation and meditation as each relates to stress reduction.

CRITICAL THINKING QUESTIONS

1. We all experience eustress, the "good stress," when we attend joyful events, share happy occasions, or feel accomplishment. Is it possible, however, to have too much eustress? If you believe it is not possible, explain your beliefs. If you believe it possible, then what eustress management steps should you take? How might you monitor your eustress level to assure health benefits and reduce health risks?
2. To what extent should public health policy be used to control stressful environments? For example, should a government agency monitor stress levels at work sites? Should employers be held responsible for stress-related illnesses that are caused by stress on the job? After all, it is not the environment but rather the reaction to the environment that produces stress.
3. *Healthy People 2010* contains an objective of reducing the proportion of homeless adults who have serious mental illness. How is homelessness related to stress? Does a homeless person experience unusual stress? Or could a homeless person be homeless due to an inability to manage the day-to-day stressors of living? Do you believe there is a connection between stress and serious mental illness?
4. Despite reports of effectiveness, meditation is not widely practiced. To what extent could this be the result of its association with religion? To what extent could this be the result of simple lack of appropriate health skills?

JOURNAL ACTIVITIES

1. List stressors that you routinely experience in college life. For each of these, give three ways of coping.
2. Look at your schedule for this semester. How stressful do you think it will be? Draw a timeline from the beginning of the semester to the end. With a red pen, identify those periods you think will be highly stressful; with a green pen, identify those periods that you think will have less stress. How can this exercise help you plan your semester?
3. Go to a popular place on campus and identify someone who on the surface seems highly stressed. What makes you believe that person is under stress? Now identify someone who appears relaxed. Differentiate between these two people by listing the visual characteristics of each. How many of these characteristics are related to health?
4. Sometimes just taking a walk in a quiet place can have a calming effect. Contact your local parks and recreation department to find out what facilities and activities are available for members of the community.

SELECTED BIBLIOGRAPHY

Davis, M., and M. McKay. *The Relaxation and Stress Workbook* (5th Ed.). Oakland, CA: New Harbinger Publications, Inc., 2000.

Goldberger, L., and S. Brent. *Handbook of Stress: Theoretical and Clinical Aspects.* New York: The Free Press, 1986.

Holmes, T. H., and R. H. Rahe. "The Social Readjustment Scale." *Journal of Psychosomatic Research* 11 (1967): 213–218.

Lazarus, R. S. *Psychological Stress and the Coping Process.* New York: McGraw-Hill, 1966.

Murphy, L. R. "Stress Management in Work Settings: A Critical Review of the Health Effects." *American Journal of Health Promotion 11,* 2 (1996):112–135.

Rosenman, R. H., and M. Friedman. "Neurogenic Factors in Pathogenesis of Coronary Heart Disease." *Medical Clinics of North America* 58 (1967): 269–276.

Selye, H. "The General Adaptation Syndrome and Diseases of Adaptation." *Journal of Clinical Endocrinology* 6 (1946): 217–230.

Selye, H. Stress Without Distress. New York: Signet, 1974.

HEALTHLINKS

Websites for a Better Understanding of Stress

You can access better health as it relates to this chapter by checking out some of the following sites on the Internet. These sites can be accessed directly from the *Decisions for Healthy Living* Website located at www.aw.com/pruitt.

American Psychological Association Help Center

Identifies and discusses six myths about stress.

Center for Anxiety and Stress Treatment

Provides resources and services regarding a broad range of stress-related topics.

Medical Basis of Stress

Excerpts from a publication by two practitioners in stress reduction work.

HEALTH HOTLINES

Coping with Stress

American Institute of Stress
(914) 963-1200
124 Park Avenue
Yonkers, NY 10703

Association for Applied Psychophysiology and Biofeedback
(800) 477-8892
10200 West 44th Avenue, Suite 304
Wheat Ridge, CO 80033

TEST YOUR KNOWLEDGE ANSWERS

1. False. There is no such thing as a stress-free life. In fact, some stress is important as a stimulus for a high quality life.
2. False. Eustress is actually considered "good stress." This type of stress is a healthy part of daily living produced by personal achievement, workplace experiences, or events such as vacations. It is not related to physical symptoms.
3. True. Distress has been associated with a weakened immune system.
4. True. The list of the physical manifestations of stress goes far beyond those listed to include among other symptoms: heartburn, loss of sexual interest, nightmares, skin rashes, and ulcers.
5. False. Stress in the workplace is found to be higher among workers who feel no control over their jobs. Therefore, receptionists or junior assistants are among those workers with less control and therefore are in higher stress jobs.

CHAPTER

4

Eating Smart

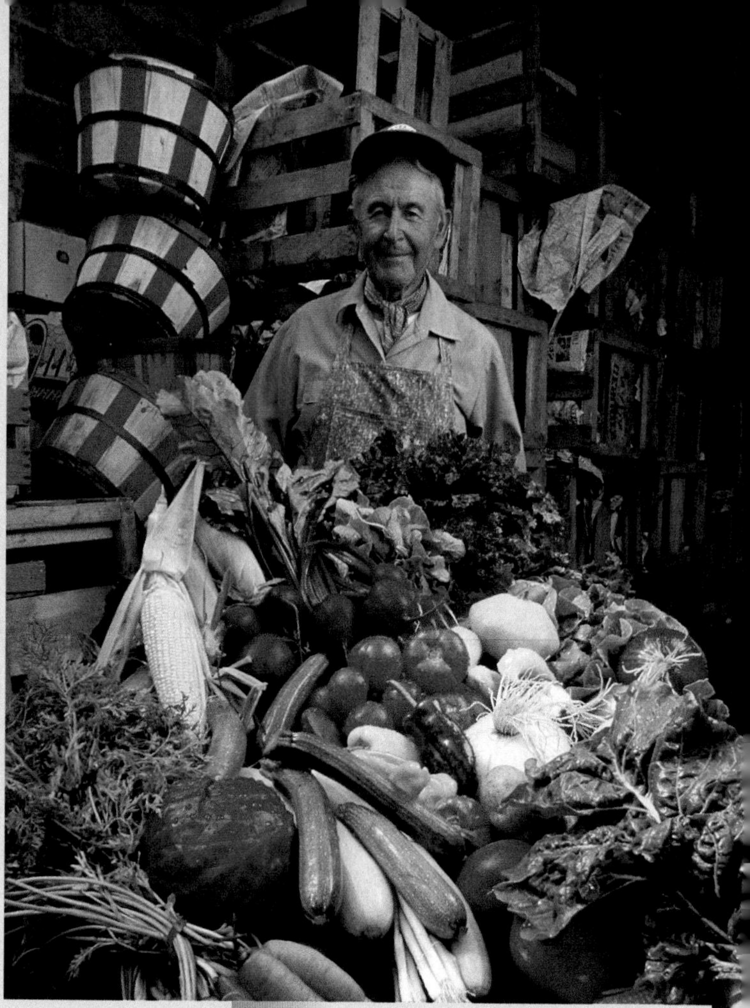

OBJECTIVES

When you finish reading this chapter, you will be able to:

1. List the essential nutrients that make up food.
2. Describe the primary sources for each nutrient and give examples of how each contributes to overall health.
3. Know the difference between a complete protein and an incomplete protein.
4. Explain how blood cholesterol is affected by diet.
5. Identify the minerals essential to a healthy diet and differentiate among "major" minerals and "trace" minerals.
6. Describe the Dietary Guidelines currently available from the U.S. Department of Agriculture, and demonstrate how those guidelines can lead to a healthy diet.
7. Describe several eating styles and cite examples of how each contributes to or detracts from overall health.
8. Identify common eating habits that present a threat to the health of college students.
9. Read a food label and understand how it describes the nutritional value of a food.
10. Explain how food preparation both enhances and detracts from the quality of food.

TEST YOUR KNOWLEDGE

1. Older people (around 65 years old and over) generally have more healthful diets than younger people (around 25 years old and under). True or False?
2. All amino acids are synthesized (made) from foods containing proteins. True or False?
3. Vitamin supplements provide a healthy addition to most diets and present little risk because excess vitamins are simply passed from the body in the urine. True or False?
4. Choosing a diet using the four food groups—meat, milk, fruits and vegetables, and bread—assures a healthy variety of foods. True or False?
5. A vegetarian diet can meet all nutritional needs. True or False?

Answers found at end of chapter.

Most Americans are not smart eaters. We eat too much fat and too little fiber, consume excesses of salt, sugar, and meat, and do not get enough of all the essential vitamins and minerals from our diets.

Because of these nutritional habits and other dietary and lifestyle factors, there has been an increase in the incidence of diet-related diseases in the United States, such as heart disease, obesity, and certain cancers. The good news is that you can do something about it. Nutritionists are finding that, in some cases, the effects of these diseases can be reversed or slowed down considerably just by a change in diet. By developing the skills of healthy food selection and preparation, you can break many unhealthy habits.

The choices are vast—an elegant four-course meal in a fine restaurant, dinner at the student cafeteria, grabbing a bite on the run. No matter what your pace of life or taste in food, your diet can be healthy—or unhealthy. It depends on what you choose to eat and how you choose to prepare it. Because there is no such thing as a food instinct in humans—eating is a learned behavior—it requires skill to have a good diet. With a better understanding of nutritional needs and healthy ways to meet those needs, your choices can become smarter choices that benefit your health now and in the future.

What You Need to Eat: The Essential Nutrients

A recent survey by the U.S. Department of Agriculture's Center for Nutrition Policy and Promotion showed that only 23 percent of Americans were interested in improving their diet, compared to 37 percent who were not interested. This, despite the fact that poor diet is known to be a contributing factor in at least four of the ten leading causes of death for this country. Scientists know that women generally have a more healthful diet than men; older people generally have more healthful diets than younger people; and those with more schooling generally have more healthful diets than those with less schooling. One fact seems to explain these differences. People with more healthful diets generally have a greater store of nutrition information and are more aware of the links between poor diet and certain diseases. The intention to eat a healthy diet begins with an understanding of the basic structure of foods and the essential nutrients that they provide.

All foods are composed of chemical compounds. The body's digestive system breaks down the complex compounds into substances that the body can use for building tissue and creating energy. The basic chemical compounds that make up food are generally referred to as **nutrients.** Nutrients that are essential to health include carbohydrates, fiber, proteins, fats, vitamins, minerals, and water. (Although water contains no nutritious value, it is essential for life; therefore it is considered an essential nutrient.)

Foods provide not only nutrients for building tissue, but also energy for daily activities. Energy is measured in the form of calories. A **calorie** is a unit measuring the energy produced by food when oxidized in the body. A constant concern, particularly with weight-conscious individuals, is healthy caloric intake—that is, consuming enough calories for daily activity but not consuming so many calories that it results in weight gain. (For more on weight control, see Chapter 5.)

Carbohydrates

Carbohydrates are made up of sugars and starches. Sugars such as table sugar (sucrose), honey, and corn syrup are **simple carbohydrates** and contain molecules made of only one or two sugar units. Starches found in whole grains, fruits, and vegetables are **complex carbohydrates;** chemically, they are composed of chains of many sugar units.

Carbohydrates represent the body's primary source of energy. However, there is a big difference between

nutrients The basic chemical compounds that make up food.

calorie A unit measuring the energy produced by food when oxidized in the body.

carbohydrates Nutrients made of sugars and starches; the body's primary source of energy.

simple carbohydrate A basic nutritional compound made of short chains of simple sugars that are broken down quickly in the body.

complex carbohydrate A basic nutritional component made of long chains of simple sugars that are slowly broken down in the body.

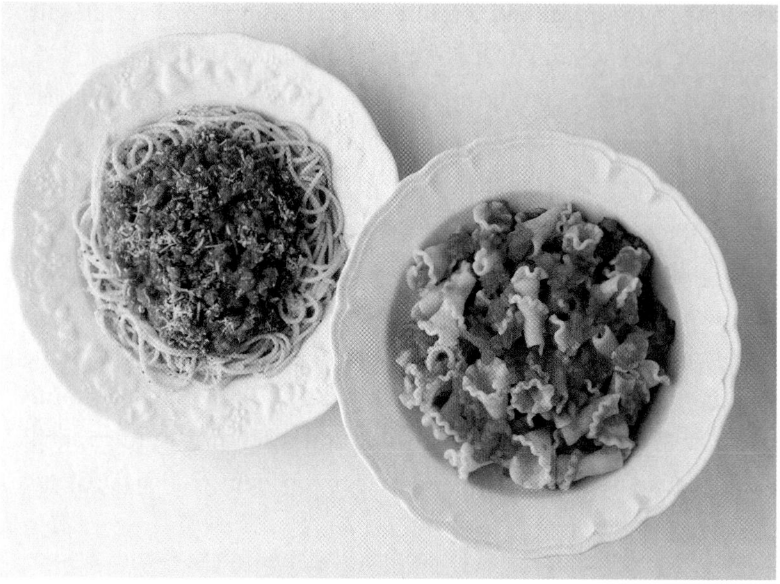

Pasta is a good source of carbohydrates. About 60 percent of your daily calories should come from carbohydrates.

getting energy from sugar (simple carbohydrates) and from starches (complex carbohydrates). Energy derived from simple carbohydrates, such as those found in a candy bar, lasts only a short period of time. Energy from complex carbohydrates, such as those found in an apple, lasts for a longer period of time. Unfortunately, most people's diets are high in sugar and low in starches.

Sugar is often found in desserts and soft drinks, but it is also in processed foods including breakfast cereals, canned soups, and main dishes. Although sugar supplies energy, or calories, foods high in sugar provide few nutrients. This is why high-sugar foods are called **empty calories.** Eating too much sugar can fill you up and keep you from eating nutritious food; it can also contribute to tooth decay and excess weight.

Starches are a better way to get carbohydrates because in addition to providing energy, they are a source of many vitamins and minerals. Examples of starches are grain products such as bread, pasta, rice, and cereal, and vegetables such as potatoes, peas, and beans. Many people think that starchy foods are fattening. Actually, eating starchy foods can be a low-calorie way to fill up with good nutrients. What are fattening are the additions, such as butter and sour cream heaped into a baked potato or cream cheese smeared on a bagel.

Fiber

Fiber is a complex carbohydrate. Starchy vegetables and whole-grain breads and cereals are rich in fiber. Fiber plays a particularly important role in the digestive system. It cannot be broken down by human digestive enzymes, so it passes down the intestinal tract and contributes bulk to the stool. It binds to water in the digestive process and aids in moving your bowels, producing softer, bulkier stools and more rapid movement of wastes through the intestines. Easy bowel movements are normal for people who consistently choose a high-fiber diet.

A diet that is high in fiber and low in fat may reduce the risk of cancer. Studies show that cancer of the large bowel (**colon cancer**) is very common in economically developed countries such as the United States, Canada, and Western Europe. In contrast, colon cancer is relatively rare in less developed areas of Africa, where the diet consists of high-fiber, unprocessed plant foods. (Other factors in the African diet have to be considered, including the fact that it is also usually low in fat and animal protein.) The possible benefits of fiber for heart disease, diabetes, and obesity are also being studied.

Given this scientific uncertainty, how much fiber should your diet include? The National Cancer Institute recommends eating between twenty and thirty grams a day—considerably more than the average of eleven grams that Americans consume. The old adage, "an apple a day keeps the doctor away," might prove to have a scientific basis, at least as far as the apple's fiber content (3.3 grams) is concerned. Fiber is found in fruits, vegetables, beans, and grains.

Proteins

Proteins are the building blocks of the body. They provide the structural framework for the skin, hair, nails, cartilage, tendons, and muscles. They provide an important structural part of the bones and are essential for the body's growth as well as maintenance, the regulation of body processes, and the replacement of body cells. In fact, proteins are a vital part of every cell.

Proteins are made up of over twenty **amino acids.** Most of these amino acids can be made, or synthesized,

empty calories Foods high in calories but with few nutrients; largely made up of sugar.

starches White, tasteless substances found in potatoes, rice, corn, wheat, and other vegetable products.

fiber A complex carbohydrate that is indigestible by humans.

colon cancer Cancer of the large bowel.

protein A group of complex compounds containing amino acids that are essential for growth and repair of tissue.

amino acids A class of organic compounds that are the building blocks of proteins.

by the body. Nine amino acids cannot be synthesized by the body yet are considered essential for health, so they must be consumed every day to ensure an adequate protein supply. A second reason that proteins must be consumed every day is that, unlike other nutrients such as fat, proteins are not stored. They are used up by the body to make structures such as muscles in a matter of hours.

A **complete protein** in food is one that contains all nine of the essential amino acids in amounts that correspond to human needs or amounts needed to make body protein. Complete proteins are found in animal products such as eggs, meat, milk, poultry, fish, and cheese. Unfortunately, many of these sources of protein are also high in fat and cholesterol. Soy protein, a low-fat alternative, is found in tofu and tempeh.

An **incomplete protein** is one in which one or more of the essential amino acids are missing or in short supply relative to the need for protein synthesis. Plants contain incomplete proteins and are divided into three groups: grains, legumes (starchy peas, beans, and lentils), and vegetables. Foods from the grain group must be combined with foods from the legume or vegetable group to form a complete protein. Examples are beans and rice, a bean burrito, or a bean tostada. Any legume plus any grain, or a legume plus nuts and seeds, will give you a complete protein. The concept of **complementary protein relationships** is especially important to **vegetarians,** who must continually combine nonanimal sources of protein to ensure adequate complete protein intake.

Fats

Fats are the most concentrated source of energy in your diet. They also add flavor to foods and are essential for the body's absorption of fat-soluble vitamins (A, D, E, and K). Fatty substances in the body, which are called lipids, also provide insulation from temperature extremes.

There are different kinds of dietary fat. **Saturated fats** are found in animal products such as meat, eggs, milk, and dairy products, as well as in palm oil and coconut oil, which come from plants. This is the type of fat that is deposited along the walls of your arteries. The accumulation of this fat is a contributing factor to diseases of the cardiovascular system such as high blood pressure and heart attacks.

Unsaturated fats are either polyunsaturated or monounsaturated. Both types of unsaturated fats can lower body cholesterol. Examples of **polyunsaturated fats** are corn oil, soybean oil, and cottonseed oil. Some fish are also sources of polyunsaturated fat. **Monounsaturated fats** are found in peanut oil, olive oil, and canola oil. Although beef fat, lard, and chicken fat have quite a bit of monounsaturated fat, they are also very high in saturated fat. Margarine contains both saturated and unsaturated fat. During the process of making margarine, **trans fatty acids** are formed, which researchers now believe are the worst type of fat because they increase **low density lipoproteins (LDLs),** the "bad" cholesterol and decrease **high density lipoproteins (HDLs),** the "good" cholesterol.

Cholesterol is a fatlike substance that is manufactured by the liver and is necessary for certain bodily processes, including the formation of sex hormones, vitamin D, and bile. Cholesterol is also taken into the body when you eat animal products such as meat, milk, eggs, and dairy foods. Plant foods do not contain cholesterol.

Cholesterol in the body circulates in the blood stream. Eating a diet high in saturated fats causes blood cholesterol levels to rise because once saturated fats enter the body they are not easily used up. Conversely, substituting unsaturated fats for saturated fats (olive oil instead of butter) can cause blood cholesterol levels to drop. Total cholesterol should be below 200 milligrams per 100 milliliters

complete protein A protein containing all nine essential amino acids.

incomplete protein A protein in which one or more of the essential amino acids is missing.

complementary protein relationship The idea that two foods, neither of which when taken alone would provide a complete protein, can be combined at a meal to provide complete protein.

vegetarian A person who follows a diet consisting of no meat, chicken, or fish; all nutrition is obtained from vegetables, fruits, and grains. Some vegetarians eat dairy products.

saturated fat The type of fat that has all hydrogen sites occupied and is usually solid at room temperature; usually comes from animal sources and is thought to encourage plaque build-up.

polyunsaturated fat The type of fat that has several hydrogens available to bind and is soft at room temperature; usually comes from plant or fish sources.

monounsaturated fat The type of fat that has one hydrogen available to bond and is liquid at room temperature; usually comes from plant or fish sources.

trans fatty acids Fatty acids formed as a part of the hydrogenation process when making margarine that increase LDLs (bad cholesterol) and decrease HDLs (good cholesterol).

low density lipoproteins (LDLs) A fatty substance that is the type of cholesterol that is considered bad and that promotes atherosclerosis.

high density lipoproteins (HDLs) A fatty substance that is the type of cholesterol that is considered good and that prevents atherosclerosis.

cholesterol A white, crystalline substance found especially in animal fats, blood, nerve tissue, and bile; in excessive amounts, a factor in atherosclerosis.

of blood serum, according to the National Cholesterol Education Program of the National Heart, Lung and Blood Institute. Cholesterol levels above that limit may put you at higher risk for heart disease. You can have too much cholesterol in your blood because your liver overproduces it—a genetically determined factor—and/or because you eat too many foods that contain saturated fat or cholesterol.

HDLs and LDLs transport cholesterol through the body to cells. HDLs are called the "good guys" because they carry cholesterol in the bloodstream to the liver, where it is used to produce bile. LDLs are called the "bad guys" because they pick up the excess cholesterol and deposit it in the walls of the arteries. If there is a rough spot in an artery, the lipoprotein carrying the fat may get stuck there. When the protein dissolves, the cholesterol is left in the artery. This buildup of cholesterol is called **plaque.** If this process continues for years, it causes **atherosclerosis,** a hardening of the arteries.

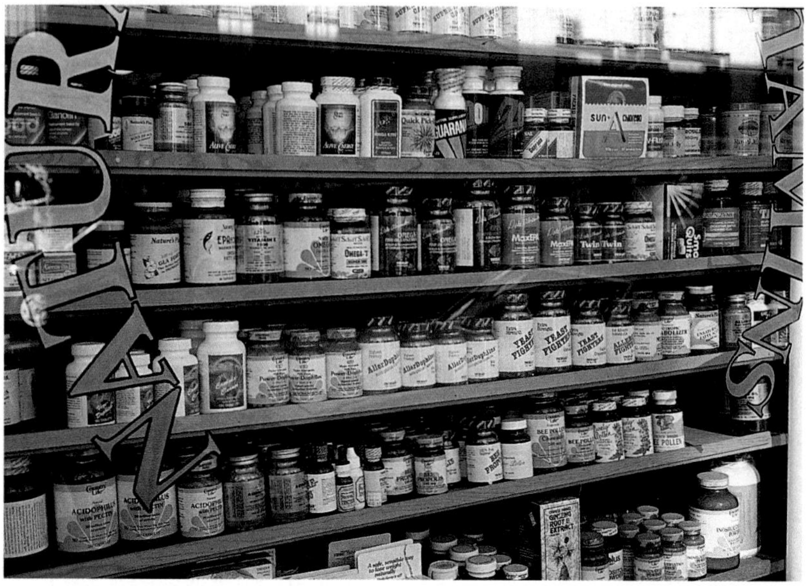

Vitamins, minerals, and other dietary supplements line the shelves of drug and health food stores. The best source of nutrients for you, however, is in the food that you eat—not supplements from bottles.

Plaque causes narrowing of the vessels, which results in reduced blood flow and can cause heart disease. If this occurs in the arteries feeding the heart muscle, a heart attack may occur.

Researchers believe that a healthy blood cholesterol ratio should be one HDL to three LDLs. The best way to lower your cholesterol overall and at the same time raise the number of HDLs is through diet, aerobic exercise, and not smoking. In some cases, drug therapy is needed to bring the total cholesterol level down. This is particularly true for people with a genetic predisposition to high cholesterol. Given the complexities of cholesterol, only your physician can tell which is the best way to keep your cholesterol levels in check.

Vitamins

Vitamins are the tools used by the body to process food. They do not supply energy, but they help release it from carbohydrates, proteins, and fats. They occur in foods as either fat-soluble or water-soluble substances. In general, the **fat-soluble** vitamins (A, D, E, and K) are stored by the body's fat cells. The **water-soluble vitamins** (the B vitamins and vitamin C) are not stored by the body, and amounts not used by the body are excreted in urine. This is why water-soluble vitamins must be consumed daily. The B vitamins include thiamine, riboflavin, niacin, pyridoxine (B_6), cyanocobalamin (B_{12}), folic acid, pantothenic acid, and biotin. Table 4.1 describes the effects and sources of eleven major vitamins. Are the foods you eat listed?

A large percentage of the public purchases vitamin and mineral supplements. Such expenditures are often a waste of money. Taking large doses of vitamin C has never been proven effective for curing conditions ranging from cancer to the common cold. Because vitamin C is a water-soluble vitamin, what is not used by the body is excreted in the urine, so there are few harmful effects to taking it. This is not the case with all vitamins. Taking large amounts of fat-soluble vitamins A and D, which are stored in the body, can lead to toxicity, serious illness, and even death.

In special circumstances, some people need to take supplemental vitamins. Included in this group are pregnant women and nursing mothers; strict vegetarians; elderly people who do not eat balanced meals; and people recovering from major wounds such as burns or from specific vitamin deficiency diseases, malabsorption, or prolonged illness. Most healthy people, however, do not need supplements. The best sources of vitamins are found in foods.

Some vitamins are best known as **antioxidants**—substances that interfere with LDL cholesterol lipoprotein ox-

plaque A buildup of cholesterol in the arteries, which over time can restrict blood flow.

atherosclerosis Hardening of the arteries due to a buildup of fatty plaque.

fat-soluble vitamins Vitamins that are transported and stored by the body's fat cells; examples are vitamins A, D, E, and K.

water-soluble vitamins Vitamins that are not stored in the body, (and excesses are excreted in the urine); examples are B-complex vitamins and vitamin C.

antioxidant A substance that inhibits oxidation; in nutrition, a substance that interferes with LDL cholesterol lipoprotein oxidation.

Table 4.1 How Vitamins Help You

Vitamin	Effects	Sources
A	Maintains skin and eyes; is needed for normal growth of bones and teeth, and for good night vision	Milk, liver, fish, eggs, butter, green and yellow vegetables, cheese
B_1	Helps in normal metabolism of carbohydrates; helps in the release of energy from food	Meat, whole-grain cereals, nuts, soybeans, peas, potatoes, and most vegetables and fruits
B_2	Helps the body cells use oxygen; assists in repair of tissue and healthy skin, maintains nervous tissue	Milk, cheese, liver, fish, poultry, yeast, fruits, lean meats
Niacin	Is needed for cell metabolism of carbohydrates; helps maintain healthy skin	Liver, yeast, lean meat, enriched breads and cereals
B_{12}	Is essential for red blood cell development; helps proper function of nervous system	Eggs, meat, milk, milk products
K	Is essential for normal blood clotting	Leafy vegetables; made by intestinal bacteria
Biotin	Maintains the circulatory system and healthy skin	Eggs, liver, kidney, most fresh vegetables; available in a great variety of foods
Folic acid	Essential in the production of red blood cells	Green leafy vegetables, yeast, meat, liver
C	Essential for growth and maintenance of bones and teeth; needed for tissue metabolism and wound healing	Citrus fruits, tomatoes, raw cabbage, potatoes, strawberries, green peppers, cantaloupe, other vegetables
D	Essential for calcium and phosphorus metabolism	Fish liver oils, fortified milk, eggs, tuna, salmon, sunlight on the skin
E	Helps maintain heart and skeletal muscles and may help maintain the reproductive system	Whole-grain cereals, lettuce, vegetable oils

idation. This process has been associated with atherosclerosis. Because atherosclerosis is a leading cause of heart attacks and strokes, many Americans have begun supplementing their diet with antioxidants in hopes of preventing heart disease. In fact, according to the American Heart Association (AHA), about 30 percent of Americans are taking some form of antioxidant supplement, usually as vitamin tablets. The most common antioxidants are vitamins E, C and beta carotene (a form of vitamin A).

Despite the encouraging research on antioxidants and their preventive effects on atherosclerosis, clinical trials designed to provide conclusive evidence of the value (or lack of value) of antioxidant supplements in reducing cardiovascular disease are not yet complete. Therefore, rather than take antioxidant supplements, the AHA recommends that the best way to prevent heart disease through diet is to choose healthy foods. A diet low in saturated fat and cholesterol and that includes lots of fruits and vegetables will provide a rich natural source of antioxidants—the same antioxidant vitamins but without the additional cost of supplements. Most healthy people do not need supplements.

Minerals

Minerals form healthy bones and teeth, regulate body functioning, and help nerves and muscles react normally. Minerals are divided into two categories: major and trace. Major minerals are needed in the diet in amounts of 100 milligrams or more per day. **Trace minerals** are essential to healthy living but are needed in smaller amounts.

Major minerals	Trace minerals
Calcium	Chromium
Chloride	Cobalt
Magnesium	Copper
Phosphorus	Fluoride
Potassium	Iodine
Sodium	Iron
Sulfur	Manganese
	Molybdenum
	Selenium
	Zinc

As with vitamins, daily needs can generally be met by eating a balanced diet. Milk products and vegetables

trace minerals Minerals that are essential for proper growth and functioning but are needed in very small amounts.

Food product	Serving Size	Calcium (mg)
Yogurt, plain, low-fat	1 cup	400
Sardines, with bones	3 ounces	370
Milk, all types	1 cup	300
Orange juice, enriched	1 cup	290
Swiss cheese	1 ounce	270
Pizza	1 slice (4 ounces)	250
Salmon, with bones	3 ounces	225
Turnip greens	1 cup cooked	200
Ice cream or ice milk	1 cup	175
Cottage cheese	1 cup	150
Cereal, fortified	3/4 cup	150–250
Baked beans, canned	1 cup	140
Tofu	2 ounces	115
Broccoli	1 cup cooked	70

Figure 4.1 Foods Rich in Calcium
Here's how to get the calcium your body needs. Dairy products are rich in calcium—but often high in fat—so try to get your calcium through a low-fat or no-fat variety of milk, yogurt, or cheese or through nondairy alternatives.

are particularly important sources of minerals. Some groups of people have difficulty meeting their needs for certain minerals in their diet. For example, children under four years old and women up to age fifty often lack sufficient iron in their diets. Supplements are often recommended in these instances, particularly for pregnant women and those who are breast-feeding.

Many diets are also not sufficient in **calcium,** a mineral important for building strong bones and teeth in growing children and for helping maintain the bones of adults. A condition that may be related to insufficient calcium intake throughout life is **osteoporosis,** a disorder in which bone density decreases and bones become more likely to break. The risk for osteoporosis is greater for women than for men, especially after women experience menopause. Many health researchers believe that consuming adequate calcium in the diet or in supplements may help prevent or slow osteoporosis.

Dairy products are usually the first calcium-rich foods that come to mind, but these can be high in fat content. Calcium can also come from nondairy foods. See Figure 4.1 for a list of nondairy and low-fat dairy sources of calcium.

Since most people reach their peak bone mass by the time they are thirty years old, it is important to begin to take action earlier in life to retard the progress of or prevent the disease. You can read more about preventing osteoporosis through exercise in Chapter 6 and the effects of it later in life in Chapter 14.

Sodium is a puzzling mineral. It is essential to health and at the same time it can cause health problems—at least in the amounts consumed by many Americans. It is the only mineral that is too abundant in most American diets. Sodium draws water into the body's blood vessels and therefore helps maintain normal blood volume and blood pressure. It is also needed for the normal function of nerves and muscles. The body needs only a small amount of sodium to carry out these functions—perhaps as little as 500 milligrams per day. High sodium intake is of concern because it may be linked with **hypertension** (high blood pressure), a condition that affects about one quarter of the population and leads to higher risk for stroke, heart attack, and kidney failure.

calcium A mineral important for building strong bones and teeth in growing children and for helping maintain the bones of adults.

osteoporosis A disorder in which bone density decreases, making the bones more likely to break.

hypertension A chronic disease better known as high blood pressure.

Water

Often called the "forgotten nutrient," water is essential to life. Without it, you could live only about one week. About 65 to 70 percent of your body weight is made up of water in the form of blood, saliva, sweat, urine, cellular fluids, and digestive enzymes. In all these various forms, water helps transport nutrients, remove wastes, and regulate body temperature.

Water carries nutrients along the digestive path and to the cells. First, it does this by liquefying food and moving it through the stomach, small intestine, and large intestine. When the food is absorbed into the blood, water plays an important role by regulating the concentration of nutrients on both sides of the cell walls.

Water needs vary, depending on the climate and a person's activity level. In a cold climate, the body's demand for water is less than in a warm climate. An active person's demand for water is much greater than a sedentary person's demand. Also, more water is needed at higher altitudes than at lower altitudes. Bodily water is lost through perspiration and respiration.

There are many ways to get liquid from your diet. The most obvious source is a glass of water. Most authorities agree that six to eight glasses of water per day provide an adequate supply to the average adult. Other healthy beverages are skim or low-fat milk and fruit juices. In addition, many fruits and vegetables are excellent sources of water.

Beverages containing alcohol, although water-based, are not a good source of water in the diet. This is because the health risks of alcohol consumption far outweigh the risks of low water intake. Furthermore, alcohol may inhibit the body's effective use of vitamins and minerals, compounding the health risks associated with this substance (see chapter 7).

Conditions such as high fever, nausea, or diarrhea may result in an abnormal loss of water called **dehydration.** Extended periods of dehydration resulting in as much as a 10 percent reduction in intracellular water concentration can lead to death.

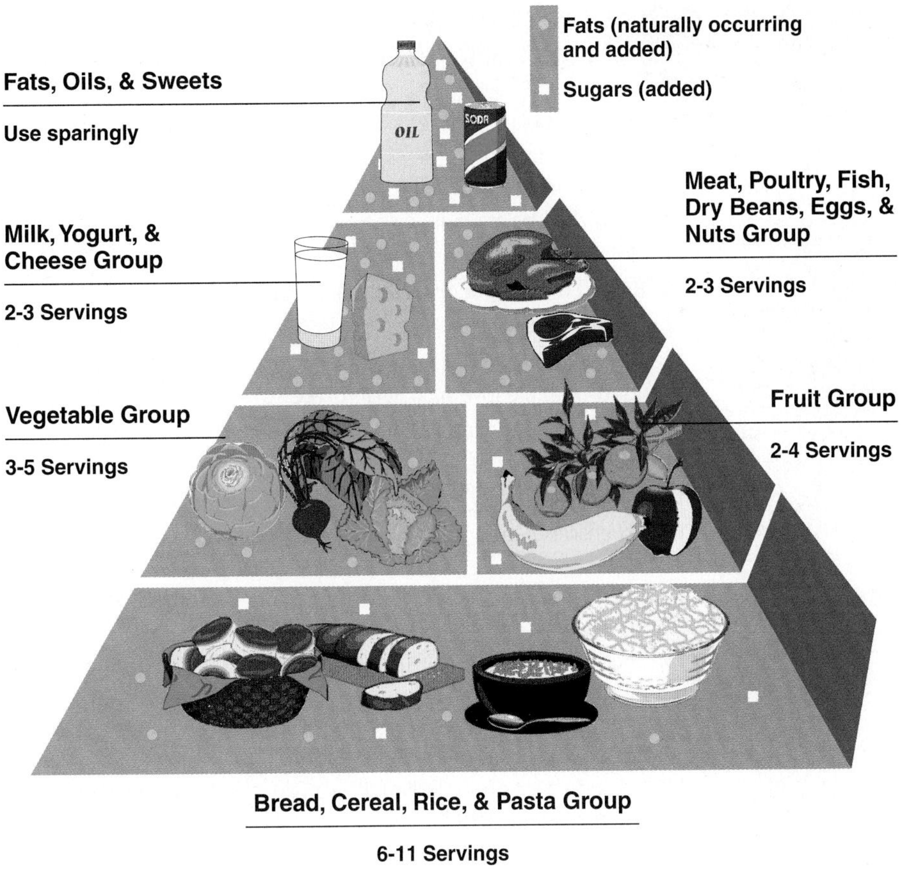

Figure 4.2 The Food Guide Pyramid
The Food Guide Pyramid is a general guide of what to eat each day. It recommends you eat a variety of foods to get the nutrients you need and the right amount of calories necessary to maintain a healthy weight. Note that the smallest segment of the pyramid—the tip— represents the foods we should eat the least of: fats and sweets.

Dietary Guidelines: How Much Do You Need?

You may have heard of the four food groups. For years, nutritionists used these groups to measure what has been called a balanced diet. Balanced referred to the amount of nutrient intake based on the following groupings: the meat group (meat, poultry, fish); the milk group (milk, yogurt, cheese); the fruits and vegetables group; and the bread group (bread, cereal, rice). This convenient grouping of foods was a very successful marketing device for the meat and milk products industries. But the four food groups did not accurately measure nutritional balance in a diet. In fact, with what we know about nutrition today, the emphasis on meat and milk could be considered unhealthy.

In the early 1990s, a more accurate device—the Food Guide Pyramid—was developed by the Department of Agriculture as a part of its *Dietary Guidelines for Americans.* The pyramid provides a general guide of what to eat daily. It recommends that you eat a variety of six different kinds of foods to get the nutrients you need and the right amount of calories to maintain proper weight. The Food Guide Pyramid is a little more complicated than the four food groups model, but it is based on scientifically derived guidelines, not on business interests.

Look at the illustration of the Food Guide Pyramid in Figure 4.2. Notice how the meat and milk groups receive a much smaller emphasis than do breads and cereals. Also notice what is meant by a serving size. The fast food industry might suggest "supersize" fries and a 64-ounce soft drink. But according to the *Dietary Guidelines,* serving sizes are smaller than what you might usually eat. For example, many people eat a cup or more of pasta in a meal, which, according to the Food Guide Pyramid, is equal to two or more servings. Look at Table 4.2 to see how many servings of each component of the Food Guide Pyramid you need.

One way to understand how big a serving size is with reasonable accuracy is to compare it visually to something common. Consider the following serving sizes:

dehydration An abnormal loss of water.

Assess Your Health

Testing Your Nutritional Knowledge

	True	False	Don't Know
1. One way for people to increase the amount of fiber in their diets is to eat more fruit.	_____	_____	_____
2. Cooking chicken without the skin reduces its fat content.	_____	_____	_____
3. Flavorings such as soy sauce, mustard, and garlic salt are good low-sodium substitutes for table salt.	_____	_____	_____
4. Most cheeses are high in salt.	_____	_____	_____
5. Hot dogs are a good source of protein.	_____	_____	_____
6. Broiled foods have more fat than fried foods.	_____	_____	_____
7. A breaded pork chop has more fat than a broiled pork chop.	_____	_____	_____
8. Chicken nuggets are much lower in fat than a hamburger.	_____	_____	_____
9. Foods that are low in cholesterol are naturally low in fat.	_____	_____	_____
10. Butter and margarine have about the same amount of cholesterol.	_____	_____	_____
11. Pizza is high in fat.	_____	_____	_____
12. Dry cooked beans are a good source of fiber.	_____	_____	_____
13. Expensive brands of ice cream usually have less fat than the cheaper brands.	_____	_____	_____
14. Most people should eat fewer starchy foods, such as bread and potatoes.	_____	_____	_____
15. Eating a lot of salt may increase a person's chance of developing high blood pressure.	_____	_____	_____
16. Eating starchy foods, such as crackers, between meals increases a person's chance of developing tooth decay.	_____	_____	_____
17. Drinking a lot of alcohol interferes with the body's ability to use vitamins and minerals.	_____	_____	_____
18. Being overweight does not affect a person's chance of developing coronary heart disease.	_____	_____	_____
19. Diets that are very low in calories can cause serious health problems.	_____	_____	_____
20. Most people should take a multivitamin every day.	_____	_____	_____

Answer Key

1 T; 2 T; 3 F; 4 T; 5 F; 6 F; 7 T; 8 F; 9 F; 10 F; 11 T; 12 T; 13 F; 14 F; 15 T; 16 T; 17 T; 18 F; 19 T; 20 F

Source: U.S. Public Health Service

Table 4.2 How Many Servings Do You Need Each Day?

Food Group	Suggested number of daily servings for teen girls, active women, and most men (about 2,200 calories)	Suggested number of daily servings for teen boys, and active men (about 2,800 calories)
Grains (especially whole grains), cereal, rice, and pasta group	9	11
Vegetable group	4	5
Milk (preferably fat-free or low-fat), yogurt and cheese group	3	4
Fruit group	3	4
Meat (preferably lean or low-fat), poultry, fish, dry beans, eggs, and nuts group	2 (total of 6 ounces)	3 (total of 7 ounces)

Source: U.S. Department of Agriculture, *Dietary Guidelines for Americans*

- 1 ounce of meat = matchbook
- 3 ounces of meat = bar of soap
- 8 ounces of meat = tennis ball
- 1 cup of vegetables or fruit = your fist
- 1 cup of dry cereal = large handful
- 1 teaspoon of butter or margarine = tip of your thumb
- 1/2 cup of cooked pasta = scoop of ice cream

To check your nutritional knowledge, see the Assess Your Health box.

Eating Styles

The fast pace of today's lifestyle has led to eating patterns that often present health problems. For the college student, breakfast is often skipped or consists of coffee and sweet rolls, and lunch may be only a large soft drink. Snacks often take the place of missed meals. Most college students are eating on their own for the first time and have no parents around to remind—or nag—them to eat a balanced diet.

Throughout the life cycle, people must meet special nutritional needs. For example, teenagers require calcium and iron because they are growing rapidly, undergoing hormonal changes, and often have high levels of physical activity. As people get older, adjustments generally need to be made in eating habits. Part of this is due to a natural slowing of the metabolic processes. Another reason is that most people tend to exercise less as they age. More sedentary people need to eat less food. Specific adjustments, such as low-salt or low-fat diets, may be prescribed by a physician due to a particular risk factor.

Runners, bikers, swimmers, volleyball and basketball players, and weekend athletes of any age need extra calories to accommodate their high-intensity exercise needs. However, athletes do not need extra protein and, despite what some advertising suggests, should avoid protein drinks as a source of energy.

Eating at Home

Most people learn their eating behaviors around the family table. African Americans and Hispanics, for example, are more likely to have a lifelong habit of eating fruits and vegetables than are whites. However, whites eat vegetables cooked in fat to a lesser degree than do the other two ethnic groups. The type of food prepared, the atmosphere in which it was consumed, and the amount of food eaten often can be traced to past experiences.

Historically, many of the foods consumed at home had an ethnic tie. Today, eating styles are far more alike than different. You do not have to be Jewish to eat bagels and cream cheese. Fresh tortillas are sold in supermarkets across the country. And a huge percentage of Americans eat pizza—both at home and in restaurants.

Another aspect of life that is changing is dinner as a relaxed family affair including time for communication. Increasingly, family dinners are eaten at fast food restaurants, and when they are eaten at home, they are often consumed while the family watches television. Around the world, American-type fast food establishments are changing traditional eating habits.

Fast Food Living

People are eating out in restaurants more than they have ever done before. More than two of every five dollars spent on eating out goes to fast food restaurants. For the most part, consumers are willing to pay for the convenience of fast food even though they most often do not get good nutritional value for their money. Fast food hamburgers, fried chicken, and milk shakes are usually high in fats, salt, and sugar.

Not all fast food is synonymous with junk food. Most fast food restaurants now include some healthier options on their menus. A grilled chicken sandwich or a salad with light vinaigrette dressing, for example, is healthier than a hamburger or french fries. (See the

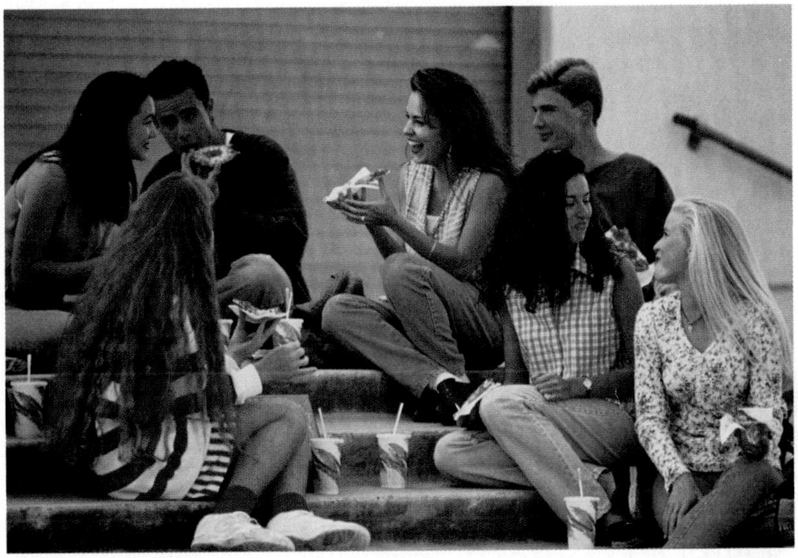

Pizza is a favorite fast food for college students, but it can be high in saturated fat if you go heavy on the cheese, sausage, and pepperoni. Ask for mushrooms, green peppers, or other vegetable toppings, instead.

Developing Health Skills

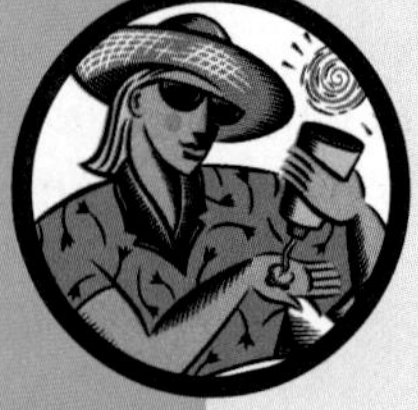

Consumer Health: Fast Food Choices

Depending on what you choose from the menu, fast food restaurants can provide more nutritious food than in the past. Among the offerings are lower-calorie and lower-fat vegetarian burgers, salad dressing, and even chili. The following table shows what you can get—for better or worse—at five popular fast food chain restaurants.

	BETTER (Calories/Fat grams)	WORSE (Calories/Fat grams)
McDonald's	McSalad Shaker/grilled chicken with fat-free herb vinaigrette dressing (140/3)	Big Mac (590/34)
	Fruit & Yogurt Parfait with granola (380/5)	Large Shake (1,010/29)
Burger King	Veggie Burger (330/10)	Double Whopper with cheese (1,020/65)
	BK Broiler Chicken Sandwich/ no mayo (390/8)	Fries, kingsize (600/30)
Subway	6-inch Veggie Delite/no cheese (200/3)	6-inch tuna sub (660/44)
	6-inch turkey breast sub (220/4)	6-inch classic meatball sub (500/25)
Wendy's	Small Chili (210/7)	Classic Triple with everything (1,030/65)
Taco Bell	Bean, Chicken Fiesta, or Steak Fiesta Burrito (370/12)	Mucho Grande Nachos (1,320/82)

Source: Michael Jacobson and Jayne Hurley. *Restaurant Confidential.* Washington, DC: Center for Science in the Public Interest, 2002. Reprinted with permission.

Developing Health Skills box.) To help health-conscious customers, more and more restaurants are providing nutritional information on their menus.

Vegetarianism

The vegetarian diet has gained popularity in recent years, particularly among college students. There have always been vegetarians who, for religious or ethical reasons, choose not to eat meat. But now people are choosing a vegetarian diet on health grounds alone. A recent analysis of five large studies found that, compared with those who regularly eat meat, vegetarians had 34 percent lower risk of heart disease. Those who just occasionally ate meat had a 20 percent lower risk.

True vegetarians, also called **vegans,** have no meat, chicken, fish, eggs, or any milk products in their diet. They get all of their protein from vegetables, fruits, and grains. **Lactovegetarians** eat dairy products but no other animal products. Another variation of vegetarians is **ovolactovegetarians,** who eat eggs as well as dairy products.

Selecting a healthy vegetarian diet is far more complicated than just deciding not to eat meat or animal products. Because vegetarians do not eat animal products, which are a source of complete protein, they must combine the incomplete proteins in plant foods to get the proper amount of all essential amino acids. This is important at all times, but especially during periods of rapid growth, such as childhood and adolescence, and during pregnancy. Vegetarians also must make sure they get enough minerals, such as calcium and iron, and must guard against long-term vitamin B_{12} deficiency, which can cause mild, (and if untreated, irreversible) nerve damage. Holding to a strict vegetarian diet can be a healthy way to live, but it requires a specific health skill based on a good understanding of the principles of nutrition and on giving considerable attention to your daily diet.

A vegetarian diet can meet all nutritional needs, according to the American Dietetic Association. The key—as with any other diet—is to eat a wide variety of foods and to limit your intake of sweets and fatty foods.

vegans Vegetarians who do not eat any food of animal origin.

lactovegetarians Vegetarians whose diet includes dairy products but no other animal products.

ovolactovegetarians Vegetarians whose diet includes eggs as well as dairy products.

Vegetarian diets are usually lower in fat than a traditional diet, but even so, vegetarians can further decrease fat consumption by substituting fruit juices or water for oil in recipes and by using soy lecithin sprays instead of oil when sautéing. Since cholesterol is only found in animal products, vegetarians do not have to be as concerned as meat eaters about their cholesterol levels. However, they should limit consumption of coconut and palm oils and other foods that are high in saturated fat, because these foods may increase cholesterol levels.

For a balanced diet, vegetarians should eat:

Foods	**Suggested Daily Serving**
Breads, cereals, rice, and pasta	6 or more
Vegetables	4 or more
Legumes and other meat substitutes	2 to 3
Fruits	3 or more
Dairy products	Optional—up to 3
Eggs	Optional—3 to 4 a week

How Eating Habits Become Unhealthy . . . and How to Correct Them

For the most part, eating is a healthy activity. But some eating habits, if repeated for long enough, become very unhealthy. Three such habits are skipping meals, eating too many snacks, and taking too many vitamins.

Skipping meals. Unfortunately, many college students skip meals. How many times have you heard your classmates say, "I don't want to gain weight," or, "I'm simply too busy to eat." Breakfast seems to be the most frequently missed meal of the day. Some studies have suggested that missing breakfast can affect your concentration as well as your overall health. In addition, most people who skip breakfast tend to substitute a less nutritious, midmorning snack because they feel hungry. Another common habit is to skip dinner. Whether in order to write a paper or to reduce your intake of calories, skipping dinner is not a good idea. Eat nutritious meals on a regular schedule. You will find that you are better equipped to meet the demands of school or work and that you will be less hungry for snacks.

Eating too many snacks. Most commercial snack foods are high in fat, sugar, or salt and have few healthy nutrients. Apart from not making much of a contribution to your dietary needs, as outlined by the Food Guide Pyramid, they can lead to excess weight, dental caries (cavities), and other health problems. Occasional snacking is fine, especially when you need extra energy, but don't overdo it. Snacks of low-fat yogurt, vegetables, fruits, unsalted nuts, whole-grain rolls or crackers are tasty, healthy, and nutritious alternatives.

Taking too many vitamins. "I know I don't have a good diet, so I'll make up for it by taking vitamins." Many college students make this mistake in logic. As you read earlier, vitamins serve to help other nutrients (proteins, carbohydrates, fats, and minerals) function effectively and efficiently. Vitamins do not replace the need for other nutrients. It is a mistake to attempt to rectify a poor diet by taking vitamin supplements. In fact, a real health hazard can result. Taking too many vitamins can cause toxicity, illness, and, in extreme cases, even death. If you eat a healthy diet, vitamin supplements are usually not necessary. If in doubt, ask a physician for an opinion.

Selecting and Preparing Healthy Foods

Selecting foods based on their nutritional content can be a daunting task. After all, there are so many nutrients in so many different foods. Yet shoppers always want good value for their money; this increasingly means that they want good nutritional value, not just a bargain. By knowing the meaning of a few key terms, you can make your food selection easier—and, by making the right selections, you can make your diet more healthy. Here are several terms you should know when shopping for food:

Processed food. Food that has been cooked, frozen, or otherwise treated to preserve it for a period of time or to improve its taste is referred to as processed food. Processing often destroys many of the nutrients, such as vitamins, normally found in foods, and usually adds large quantities of salt.

Vitamin-enriched food. Vitamin-enriched food tries to make up for the vitamins destroyed by processing. Sometimes it contains supplemental vitamins—that is, vitamins that are not naturally found in the food.

Organically grown food. Food grown without the use of pesticides or fertilizers is referred to as organically grown. There is probably little difference in the nutritional quality of such food, but products labeled "100 percent organic" carry an assurance that additives and certain contaminants are not present. Other categories in the new standards set by the Department of Agriculture are "organic" (is at least 90 percent organic), "made with organic ingredients" (is at least 70 percent organic), and "contains organic ingredients" (is less than 70 percent organic).

Fat-free food. To comply with FDA regulations, any food labeled "fat-free" must contain less than half a gram of fat per serving.

Low-fat food. To comply with FDA regulations, any food labeled "low-fat" must contain three grams of fat or less per serving.

Light food. To comply with FDA regulations, any food labeled "light" must have less than half the fat or at least one-third fewer calories than the regular version of the food.

Lower-, reduced-, or less-fat food. To comply with FDA regulations, any food labeled "lower fat," "reduced fat," or "less fat" must contain 25 percent less fat than a regular version of the product or some other logical reference food.

Healthful Shopping

When you enter a supermarket, the first things you see are rows and rows of canned, frozen, and packaged goods. These products are usually located in the center of the store. Look along the walls for foods that have not been highly processed: meats, poultry, and fish; vegetables and fruits; and milk and dairy products. Salad bars, like the other low-process foods, are located near the walls. The foods near the walls require careful handling and refrigeration and have rapid turnover. The foods in the center of the store can generally stay on the shelf for months or even years.

What does a healthy shopper do? Shop along the walls for foods that have undergone little processing and have high nutritional value. Shop carefully throughout the store to select the more highly processed foods that may be needed to complement a healthy diet.

Reading a Food Label

Food labels have become popular reading. A nationwide survey found that about four out of five adults "pay attention" to ingredient lists and that two out of three say that they use the list to avoid or limit consumption of certain items.

Food labels list ingredients in order of their prominence by weight, from the greatest to the least. Therefore, you can recognize that a product is high in sugar when the label lists sugar or other sweeteners—or lists several sugars—near the top of the list of ingredients. Similarly, a product is likely to be salty if sodium-based products—salt, onion salt, MSG, baking soda—are high on the list.

There is also nutrition information on the labels of all packaged goods. This information, required by the federal government, includes the amount per serving and the percent daily value of sodium, total fat (including saturated fat), cholesterol, proteins, total carbohydrates (including dietary fiber and sugars), vitamins, and minerals. In addition, the label lists the number of servings per container and number of calories per serving. Fresh meat, poultry, fish, and produce are not required to have nutritional labels. Look at the label in Figure 4.3. How can it help you the next time you shop at the supermarket?

Nutrition Facts

Serving Size 1 cup (228g)
Servings Per Container 2

Amount Per Serving

Calories 260 Calories from Fat 120

	% Daily Value*
Total fat 12g	20%
Saturated Fat 5g	25%
Cholesterol 30mg	10%
Sodium 660mg	28%
Total Carbohydrate 31g	10%
Dietary Fiber 0g	0g
Sugars 5g	
Protein 5g	

Vitamin A 4% • Vitamin C 2%
Calcium 15% • Iron 4%

*Percent Daily Values are based on a 2,000 calorie diet. Your daily values may be higher or lower depending on your calorie needs:

	Calories:	2,000	2,500
Total Fat	Less Than	65g	80g
Sat Fat	Less Than	20g	25g
Cholesterol	Less Than	300mg	300mg
Sodium	Less Than	2,400mg	2,400mg
Total Carbohydrate		300g	375g
Dietary Fiber		25g	30g

Calories per gram:
Fat 9 • Carbohydrate 4 • Protein 4

Figure 4.3 Nutrition Label
This label provides you with information about the levels of fat, cholesterol, sodium, fiber, and other nutrients in the product. It can be used as a guide to help you eat a healthy diet.

Preparing Healthy Meals

You don't have to be a gourmet chef to know how to prepare healthy foods. Even the healthiest of foods, such as a baked potato, can be made unhealthy by adding things such as butter or sour cream to it. Here are some common sense skills for preparing healthy meals:

- Serve as much unprocessed food as possible.
- Bake, steam, or broil food. Don't fry it.
- Baste roasted food with tomato juice or broth in place of oil or butter.
- Have a variety of colors on the plate. Choose from green (spinach), red (beets), yellow (corn), orange (salmon), purple (cabbage), black (beans), brown (bread), beige (chicken), white (rice)—and so on. The variety helps assure that there is a full range of nutrients in the meal.

In fact, pay attention to how food is presented. Healthier foods can look and smell delicious. Spend a little extra time and make the meal look attractive—for example, add fresh orange slices to a chicken or pork dish. You will enjoy eating healthy food if it looks good.

CASE STUDY 4: Eating Smart

Fred was rushing out to his first class of the day. He was running late, as usual, but stopped by the cafeteria for his breakfast—a cup of coffee. His lunch usually isn't nutritious either—a candy bar or two and a can of soda.

By dinnertime, Fred is starved and eats whatever the main course is in the cafeteria—beef tacos, chicken casserole, meat loaf with sauce. Two or three times a week, he goes to a fast food place for dinner with friends: burgers and fries, pizza, submarine sandwiches, or deep-fried chicken. Fred's daily diet is high in cholesterol and fats, low in essential vitamins and minerals, and he eats no fruits or vegetables.

Now consider what Antonio eats. He, too, has an early-morning class, but gets up in time to have breakfast in the cafeteria. He drinks a glass of juice while going through the line, then selects a low-sugar cold cereal with skim milk. Sometimes he has a bran muffin or whole-wheat toast with jam.

For lunch, Antonio usually gets something from the salad bar. He goes heavy on the vegetables—tomatoes, green peppers, cucumbers, radishes, lettuce, beans—and lighter on cholesterol-rich foods such as sliced eggs and cheese. He bypasses the artificial, high-sodium bacon bits and the creamy salad dressings. If there is fresh fruit, he might take a piece or two for a mid-afternoon snack.

For dinner, he chooses fish or chicken when it is offered in the cafeteria—and asks for a serving without the rich sauce it always seems to be swimming in. Just like Fred, Antonio and his friends go out to fast food places a few nights a week but he orders broiled fish, not fried chicken sandwiches. And if he orders pizza, his "extras" are vegetables—onions, mushrooms, peppers, and tomatoes—not sausage, meatballs, and cheese.

In Your Opinion

Fred and Antonio have two different nutritional health styles.

- What do you think of Fred's food choices?
- What can he do to eat more nutritiously while on the run?
- Fred is not worried about his diet now, but he plans to change his habits when he gets older. After reading this chapter, do you believe Fred will follow-through with dietary changes as he ages?
- Why is Antonio's diet healthier?
- How do you rate your nutritional health style?

KEY CONCEPTS

1. A diet that is high in fiber and low in fat may reduce the risk of cancer.
2. Proteins are the building blocks of the body and are essential for growth, maintenance, and replacement of body cells.
3. Fats are the most concentrated source of energy in your diet. Fats are found in saturated and unsaturated forms.
4. Vitamins are the tools used by the body to process food. They do not supply energy, but they help release it from carbohydrates, proteins, and fats. Minerals form healthy bones and teeth and help nerves and muscles react normally.
5. Between 60 and 70 percent of the body is made up of water. Without drinking it, you could live only about one week.
6. Throughout the life cycle, nutritional needs change. This means that a teenager's diet should be different from a nursing mother or an older adult.
7. Vegetarians need to combine vegetables, grains, and fruits in careful amounts to ensure adequate consumption of complete protein.
8. Three common eating habits that are unhealthy are skipping meals, eating too many snacks, and taking too many vitamins.
9. The ingredients on a food label are listed in order of their prominence by weight, from the greatest to the least.
10. When shopping for food at a grocery store, look along the walls for the unprocessed foods. The center of the store is where you will find the more processed foods.

REVIEW QUESTIONS

1. List six nutrients found in food and describe the primary function of each.
2. How does the Food Guide Pyramid serve to improve food selection? Explain how it represents an improvement over the old four-food-groups model.
3. Describe how consumption of fat can actually lower blood cholesterol.
4. Describe the health hazards of taking high doses of vitamin supplements.
5. What is the difference between major minerals and trace minerals?
6. Identify both the health benefits and health risks of sodium in the diet.
7. Identify three common eating habits that can lead to unhealthy results.
8. Explain the difference between a vegan and an ovolactovegetarian.
9. Explain why one ingredient on the food label is listed before another.
10. Describe how food preparation can enhance—or lessen—the nutritional quality of food.

CRITICAL THINKING QUESTIONS

1. An objective in *Healthy People 2010* is to "increase the proportion of persons aged 2 years and older who consume at least two daily servings of fruit." What strategies do you think public health officials should undertake to bring about the successful accomplishment of this objective? To what extent is the barrier to this objective a lack of health knowledge, health skills, and health values?
2. The four food groups were, at one time, our best guide to proper nutrition. This guide was successfully used by the meat and milk products industries to increase sales. The six-part Food Guide Pyramid now replaces the four food groups. How might different food industries take advantage of this new guide to nutrition? What industries stand to gain the most from the new guide? What industries will be harmed?
3. An objective of *Healthy People 2010* is to: "increase the proportion of children and adolescents aged 6 to 19 years whose intake of meals and snacks at school contributes to good overall dietary quality." Should schools help meet this goal by banning snack-food vending machines? Should schools allow students to drink soft drinks? Are there reasons why these convenience snacks should be provided at school? Eating habits begin early. How can public health educators, parents, and others teach children to choose food wisely?
4. Good nutrition might be made much simpler if tighter controls were placed on the food industries. Why, for example, do we continue to produce masses of junk food despite the clear understanding that such food products are not nutritious? How do you think we can best balance the freedom to choose with what is in the best interest of the public's health?

JOURNAL ACTIVITIES

1. Keep a record of everything you eat for a week. Determine the relative healthiness of your diet. In your estimation, did you meet the requirements as set out in the *Dietary Guidelines for Americans*? To know for sure, what additional information do you need (e.g., calories, fat and cholesterol content, amount of salt, etc.)?
2. Numerous computer-assisted dietary analyses are available. Your library or computer lab might have such a program, or you can find one on the Internet. Locate at least one program and analyze the diet you recorded in the first activity above.
3. Interview the director of food services, the manager of the snack bar, or some other person responsible for food on your campus. Ask what is being done to promote good nutrition. What does this person think are the main nutritional problems facing the students on your campus?
4 Find evidence of how poor eating habits affect health in your community. You may find an article in the newspaper on malnutrition or see evidence of obesity.

SELECTED BIBLIOGRAPHY

Diet and Health: Implications for Reducing Chronic Disease Risk. Washington, DC: National Academy Press, 1991.

Dietary Guidelines for Americans. Washington, DC: U.S. Department of Agriculture and Department of Health and Human Services, 2001.

Duffy, R. S. *American Dietetic Association Complete Food and Nutrition Guide.* Hoboken, NJ: John Wiley & Sons, Inc., 2002.

FDA Consumer. Food and Drug Administration (published monthly).

Food Guide Pyramid. Hyattsville, MD: U.S. Department of Agriculture, Human Nutrition Information Service, 2002.

Griffith, H. Winter. *Vitamins, Herbs, Minerals, and Supplements: A Complete Guide.* Tucson, AZ: Fisher Books, 1998.

Tufts University Diet and Nutrition Letter (published monthly).

HEALTHLINKS

Websites for a Better Understanding of Nutrition

You can access better health as it relates to this chapter by checking out some of the following sites on the Internet. These sites can be accessed directly from the *Decisions for Healthy Living* Website located at www.aw.com/pruitt.

American Dietetic Association (ADA)

Provides information on a full range of dietary topics, including sports nutrition, healthful cooking, and nutritional eating. Also links to scientific publications and provides information on scholarships and public meetings.

International Food Information Council

The International Food Information Council (IFIC) Foundation provides sound, scientific information on food safety and nutrition to journalists, health professionals, educators, government officials, and consumers.

Dietary Guidelines for Americans

The Department of Agriculture's guidelines are based on scientifically derived information and are the best guide to food choice available.

Physicians Committee for Responsible Medicine

Provides information about vegetarian diets ranging from clinical findings to recipes.

U.S. Food and Drug Administration (FDA)

Provides information and web links for consumers and professionals on nutrition, food information, food safety, and supplements.

HEALTH HOTLINES

Eating Smart

Food Allergy and Anaphylaxis Network
(800) 929-4040
10400 Eaton Place, Suite 107
Fairfax, VA 22030-2208

National Center for Nutrition and Dietetics
American Dietetic Association
(800) 366-1655
216 West Jackson Boulevard
Chicago, IL 60606-6995

TEST YOUR KNOWLEDGE ANSWERS

1. True. Older people do have more healthful diets than younger people. In addition, women generally have a more healthful diet than men, and those with more schooling generally have more healthful diets than those with less schooling.
2. False. Proteins are made up of amino acids and most amino acids can be synthesized by the body. Nine amino acids, however, cannot be synthesized and thus must be consumed (through food intake) in some form on a regular basis.
3. False. Many vitamins pass out of the body in urine, but fat-soluble vitamins (A, D, E, and K) are stored by the body's fat cells. Excess intake of these vitamins can present health problems.
4. False. The four food groups were an excellent marketing campaign by the meat and dairy industries, but provide a poor tool for judging the quality of a diet. A much better guide is the Food Guide Pyramid developed by the U.S. Department of Agriculture.
5. True. Eating a healthy vegetarian diet is complicated, but certainly possible.

CHAPTER

5

Maintaining Proper Weight

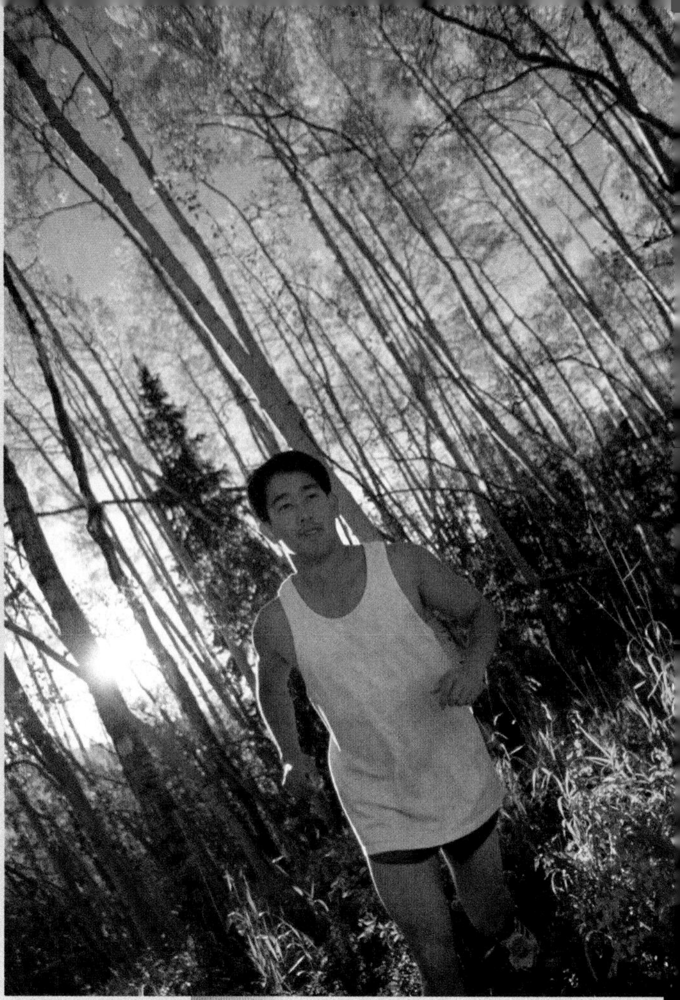

OBJECTIVES

When you finish reading this chapter, you will be able to:

1. Explain the benefits of maintaining your proper weight and the health risks associated with being overweight.
2. Describe the health risks of being underweight.
3. Accurately assess your body weight as well as approximate your body mass.
4. Explain why some people become overweight more easily than others.
5. Describe how eating behaviors influence body composition and how eating behaviors are learned.
6. Explain why fat in the diet is essential for health and why excess fat leads to health risks.
7. Explain the relationship between exercise and weight control.
8. Understand the nature of anorexia and bulimia, two eating disorders that can be fatal.
9. Describe ways to control your weight and maintain health.
10. Identify fad diets and describe how they can be harmful to your health.

TEST YOUR KNOWLEDGE

1. The number of overweight adults who use exercise and dieting to lose weight has decreased in recent years. True or False?
2. Infants of obese mothers show evidence of obesity themselves by age one. True or False?
3. Eating low-fat food is the best way to lose weight. True or False?
4. A thin person has approximately the same number of fat cells as an obese person. An obese person's fat cells, however, are much larger than those of a thin person. True or False?
5. Bulimia is found in about 2 percent of the population and is a primary cause of extreme obesity. True or False?

Answers found at end of chapter.

One of the first announcements made when a baby is born is "...and she weighs eight pounds, three ounces." Children learn early to make jokes about body weight and to label at least one classmate "fatso" and another "skin and bones." And for adults, scores of greeting cards poke fun at the person who has a weight problem.

Having a weight problem—and this can mean being underweight as well as being overweight—is not a laughing matter. It can contribute to heart disease, diabetes, cancer, and many other unhealthy conditions.

Weight—or more precisely, the inability to maintain proper weight—is a serious public health problem in the United States. According to the Surgeon General, more than 60 percent of American adults are overweight. In addition to those who are seriously overweight, millions more want to lose a few pounds. At any given time, nearly 30 percent of men and more than 40 percent of women are trying to lose weight. In spite of this obsession with weight, the prevalence of overweight has actually increased in recent years and the proportion of overweight adults who use exercise and dieting to lose weight has decreased.

How Weight Can Be Harmful to Your Health

Concerns about being overweight are based on more than vanity. Too much weight is harmful to your health and may significantly increase your risk for hypertension, cancer, stroke, heart disease, and adult-onset diabetes, which together account for about 70 percent of U.S. deaths.

Obesity is not a synonym for overweight. Obesity refers to **adiposity,** a surplus of body fat—more than 30 percent for women and 25 percent for men. **Overweight,** on the other hand, refers to a simple excess of body weight relative to a specified standard for height. Neither term involves accurate measurements. A person may be overweight—for example, a bodybuilder who has a lot of muscle—but not obese.

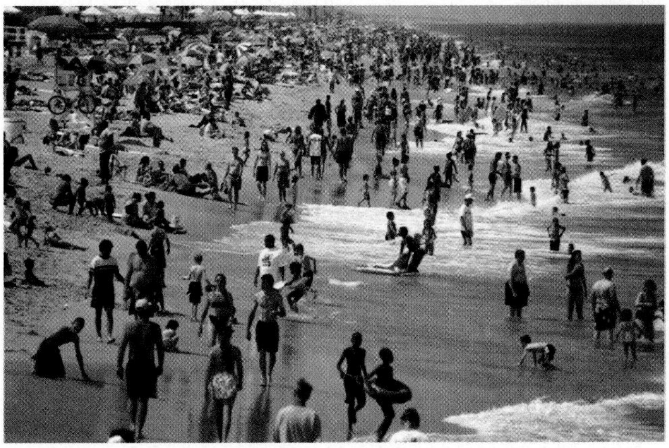

At any given point, nearly 30 percent of men and more than 40 percent of women in the United States are on a diet, although not all need to be. People who are overweight are more likely to have health problems, such as hypertension and heart disease.

Problems of Being Overweight

Obese people are at increased risk for a wide range of health conditions including hypertension, high cholesterol, heart disease, stroke, gallbladder diseases, diabetes, asthma, osteoarthritis, depression, and complications in pregnancy. The Framingham (Massachusetts) Heart Disease Epidemiology Study has been looking at the health of men and women between the ages of thirty and sixty for more than sixty years. This highly respected study reported that the risk for suffering from **angina** (chest pain resulting from a lack of blood supply to the heart) rises significantly as weight increases.

Some overweight people may be at greater risk than others, depending on where the fat is. Research shows that people who tend to have their fat concentrated in the waist and abdomen rather than in the thighs and buttocks are more prone to high blood pressure, diabetes, early heart disease, and certain types of cancer.

obesity An excessive amount of body fat relative to body weight.

adiposity A surplus of body fat.

overweight An excess of body weight relative to a specified standard for height and age.

angina Chest pain resulting from a lack of blood supply to the heart.

Assess Your Health

Are You at Risk for an Eating Disorder?

Losing your appetite on occasion is normal—for example, you may have butterflies in your stomach before a big exam and not want to eat much. But having a serious eating disorder that results in a life-threatening weight loss is totally different: It is not safe, and you should seek out a health care professional who is experienced in working with people who have eating disorders. The student health office should be able to direct you to appropriate care for this problem.

Review the following common symptoms of eating disorders, and ask yourself if you—or someone you know—needs professional help in dealing with eating problems.

Symptom	Anorexia	Bulimia	Binge eating
Excessive weight loss in a relatively short period of time	✓		
Continuation of dieting although bone thin	✓		
Dissatisfaction with appearance; belief that body is fat even though severely underweight	✓		
Loss of monthly menstrual periods	✓	✓	
Unusual interest in food and development of strange eating rituals	✓	✓	
Obsession with exercise	✓	✓	
Eating in secret	✓	✓	✓
Serious depression	✓	✓	✓
Binging—consumption of large amounts of food		✓	✓
Vomiting or use of drugs to stimulate vomiting, bowel movements, and urination		✓	
Binging but no noticeable weight gain		✓	
Disappearance into bathroom for long periods of time to induce vomiting		✓	
Abuse of alcohol or drugs		✓	✓

Source: National Institute of Mental Health

Underweight: A Problem Too

Anyone who is more than 10 percent lighter than average for his or her height and build may be at an increased health risk. In general, thin men and women have higher mortality rates than do well men and women of average weight. Thin smokers are at a higher risk for developing a serious disease and dying from it than are smokers of average weight.

Taken to an extreme, **underweight** due to compulsive eating behaviors may become a life-threatening condition. **Anorexia nervosa,** a condition characterized by starvation behavior, primarily affects women (fewer than 1 percent of all women)—most particularly adolescent girls, but it also occurs in men. A person suffering from anorexia usually diets and exercises excessively in an effort to approach a distorted body weight goal that seems progressively out of reach. Factors that appear to be related to the disease include susceptibility to social pressures to be thin, problems in family interaction, and a strong need for control.

A person with anorexia can lose up to 30 percent of total body fat. Left untreated, such weight loss can result in starvation and death. Treatment usually involves a combination of medical intervention and psychotherapy.

Bulimia is another eating disorder that affects between 1 and 3 percent of young women. It is character-

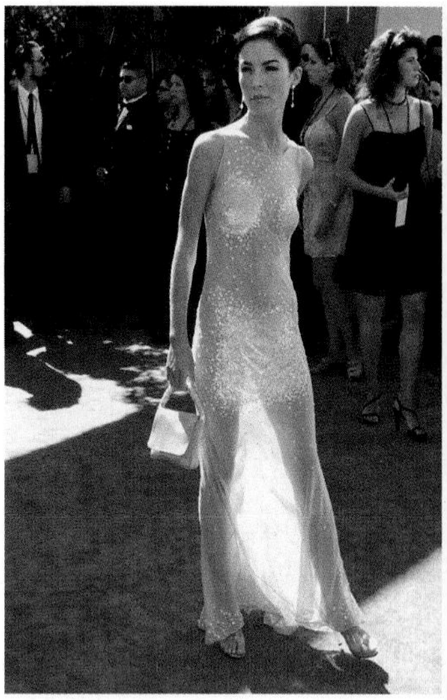

The ideal body image portrayed in the media is often unrealistic. Social pressure to be thin is one of several factors related to eating disorders.

underweight Less body weight relative to a specified standard for height and age.

anorexia nervosa An eating disorder characterized by starvation behavior brought on by a preoccupation with thinness.

bulimia An eating disorder characterized by the extreme behavior of binge eating and vomiting.

ized by the extreme behavior of **binge eating** and **purging.** Binge eating refers to eating excessively, consuming greater than the normal amount of food usually taken in one sitting, such as a gallon of ice cream and two large pizzas. A bulimic person can eat 10,000 calories or more at one time—usually when she (or occasionally, he) is alone. To avoid the weight gain that normally results from such eating behavior, the bulimic engages in excessive exercise and follows a binge with self-induced vomiting and/or the use of laxatives, enemas, syrup of ipecac, and/or **diuretics** to purge the stomach and bowels. Bulimics tend to be perfectionists and have feelings of inadequacy and low self-esteem. Although bulimia is typically a disease of young women, young men are at risk as well—particularly wrestlers, runners, dancers, and models.

Left untreated, the bulimic is at risk for a variety of complications, including nutritional deficiencies, reproductive problems, and, in extreme cases, death. The treatment for bulimia is similar to that for anorexia—a combination of medical intervention and psychotherapy.

Binge eating disorder, which is found in about 2 percent of the population, resembles bulimia because it involves periods of uncontrolled eating. People with this disorder consume enormous quantities of food and stop eating only when they are uncomfortably full. Unlike bulimics, people who have binge eating disorder do not purge themselves afterwards to get rid of the excess food. And in contrast to both anorexics and bulimics, one fourth to one third of all people who have binge eating disorder are men. One reason for this kind of binge eating is related to dieting. Recent research shows that it occurs in about 30 percent of people in medically supervised weight-control programs.

Most people who have eating disorders share certain personality traits:

- Low self-esteem
- Feelings of helplessness
- A fear of becoming fat

Are you, or someone you know, at risk for an eating disorder? See the Assess Your Health box for a list of symptoms.

Assessing Weight

Proper weight varies from person to person, and even in one person throughout his or her life. Accurately assessing your body weight is a health skill that you will use your entire life. It is not as simple as stepping on a bathroom scale and reading from the dial, but must be considered in relation to other factors such as age, height, body type, and level of exercise. For example, it is not necessarily unhealthy to weigh 170 pounds. It depends on who weighs that 170 pounds. For a 5-foot-tall woman, 170 pounds would be considered obese and thus unhealthy. For a 6-foot-tall man, 170 pounds might be considered ideal.

Measuring Body Mass

The **body mass index** (BMI) is a measure of weight in relation to height. It is a good indicator of weight-related health risks because it is an easy way to compare the fatness of people of different heights. BMI is calculated as your weight in pounds divided by the square of your height in inches, multiplied by 703. Use the following formula to calculate your BMI:

$$\text{BMI} = \frac{\text{weight (in pounds)}}{\text{height (in inches)}^2} \times 703$$

In general, if your BMI is in the 19–24 range, consider yourself healthy; if it is in the 25–29 range (20 to 30 pounds above the norm for your height), you may be considered overweight; and if it is 30 and above (roughly 30 or more pounds overweight), you are considered obese. BMI may not accurately measure all body types. For example, it can overestimate body fat in persons who are very muscular.

What is your BMI? Look at Table 5.1 to see if you are in the normal zone or if you are moving toward the high-risk area.

Measuring Body Fat

The most accurate way to measure the health risks of body weight is to determine how much fat tissue you have. There are three ways to do this.

binge eating Eating excessively; consuming much much more than the normal amount of food taken in at one sitting.

purging Self-induced vomiting and/or otherwise ridding the body of excessive food; often done after binges by a bulimic person.

diuretic A medication that promotes the excretion of excess body fluids and salt in the urine.

binge eating disorder An eating disorder characterized by periods of uncontrolled eating.

body mass index (BMI) A numerical representation of the relationship of height and weight; it correlates positively with measures of body composition such as underwater weighing and the pinch test.

Table 5.1 Body Mass Index

	Normal						Overweight					Obese										Extreme Obesity														
BMI	**19**	**20**	**21**	**22**	**23**	**24**	**25**	**26**	**27**	**28**	**29**	**30**	**31**	**32**	**33**	**34**	**35**	**36**	**37**	**38**	**39**	**40**	**41**	**42**	**43**	**44**	**45**	**46**	**47**	**48**	**49**	**50**	**51**	**52**	**53**	**54**
Height (inches)												**Body Weight (pounds)**																								
58	91	96	100	105	110	115	119	124	129	134	138	143	148	153	158	162	167	172	177	181	186	191	196	201	205	210	215	220	224	229	234	239	244	248	253	258
59	94	99	104	109	114	119	124	128	133	138	143	148	153	158	163	168	173	178	183	188	193	198	203	208	212	217	222	227	232	237	242	247	252	257	262	267
60	97	102	107	112	118	123	128	133	138	143	148	153	158	163	168	174	179	184	189	194	199	204	209	215	220	225	230	235	240	245	250	255	261	266	271	276
61	100	106	111	116	122	127	132	137	143	148	153	158	164	169	174	180	185	190	195	201	206	211	217	222	227	232	238	243	248	254	259	264	269	275	280	285
62	104	109	115	120	126	131	136	142	147	153	158	164	169	175	180	186	191	196	202	207	213	218	224	229	235	240	246	251	256	262	267	273	278	284	289	295
63	107	113	118	124	130	135	141	146	152	158	163	169	175	180	186	191	197	203	208	214	220	225	231	237	242	248	254	259	265	270	278	282	287	293	299	304
64	110	116	122	128	134	140	145	151	157	163	169	174	180	186	192	197	204	209	215	221	227	232	238	244	250	256	262	267	273	279	285	291	296	302	308	314
65	114	120	126	132	138	144	150	156	162	168	174	180	186	192	198	204	210	216	222	228	234	240	246	252	258	264	270	276	282	288	294	300	306	312	318	324
66	118	124	130	136	142	148	155	161	167	173	179	186	192	198	204	210	216	223	229	235	241	247	253	260	266	272	278	284	291	297	303	309	315	322	328	334
67	121	127	134	140	146	153	159	166	172	178	185	191	198	204	211	217	223	230	236	242	249	255	261	268	274	280	287	293	299	306	312	319	325	331	338	344
68	125	131	138	144	151	158	164	171	177	184	190	197	203	210	216	223	230	236	243	249	256	262	269	276	282	289	295	302	308	315	322	328	335	341	348	354
69	128	135	142	149	155	162	169	176	182	189	196	203	209	216	223	230	236	243	250	257	263	270	277	284	291	297	304	311	318	324	331	338	345	351	358	365
70	132	139	146	153	160	167	174	181	188	195	202	209	216	222	229	236	243	250	257	264	271	278	285	292	299	306	313	320	327	334	341	348	355	362	369	376
71	136	143	150	157	165	172	179	186	193	200	208	215	222	229	236	243	250	257	265	272	279	286	293	301	308	315	322	329	338	343	351	358	365	372	379	386
72	140	147	154	162	169	177	184	191	199	206	213	221	228	235	242	250	258	265	272	279	287	294	302	309	316	324	331	338	346	353	361	368	375	383	390	397
73	144	151	159	166	174	182	189	197	204	212	219	227	235	242	250	257	265	272	280	288	295	302	310	318	325	333	340	348	355	363	371	378	386	393	401	408
74	148	155	163	171	179	186	194	202	210	218	225	233	241	249	256	264	272	280	287	295	303	311	319	326	334	342	350	358	365	373	381	389	396	404	412	420
75	152	160	168	176	184	192	200	208	216	224	232	240	248	256	264	272	279	287	295	303	311	319	327	335	343	351	359	367	375	383	391	399	407	415	423	431
76	156	164	172	180	189	197	205	213	221	230	238	246	254	263	271	279	287	295	304	312	320	328	336	344	353	361	369	377	385	394	402	410	418	426	435	443

Source: Adapted from *Clinical Guidelines on the Identification, Evaluation, and Treatment of Overweight and Obesity in Adults: The Evidence Report.* National Institute of Health: National Heart, Lung, and Blood Institute

- A **pinch test**, conducted by a technician using special skin-fold calipers, pinches layers of fat at specific body sites. This provides a fairly accurate measure of your percentage of body fat. This method does not account for inherited variations in fat distribution.
- **Underwater weighing** involves total submersion in a swimming pool or special tank. After the person being weighed exhales as much air as possible, body density is measured and the percentage of body fat is calculated. This calculation process does not correct for age and body type and can result in as much as 5 percent error, depending on how much air is exhaled.
- Using small electrodes attached to a person's wrists and ankles, **bioelectrical impedance** measures the body's water content. Only fat-free tissues contain water, and the water content information is used to calculate the percentage of body fat. Results can vary, depending on how much food and water a person has recently ingested.

The most common way of determining weight, however, is not scientific but may be as effective for most people. It involves simply looking in the mirror. If you appear and feel overweight, you may indeed be overweight. A major drawback of this method of weight assessment is that it is difficult for some people, such as anorexics, to visually assess their own weight accurately. Before beginning weight-control strategies, you should confirm your weight through other measurements. Regardless of the measurement technique applied, the assessment of weight is an important first step in the weight-control process.

Why Do Some People Become Obese?

"I just look at food and I gain weight." How many times have you heard someone say that? Of course, that doesn't actually happen. It just seems so. But the fact remains that some people can eat enormous amounts of food and maintain a constant body composition and weight whereas others who have similar characteristics—for example, the same sex, age, height, and basic body build—gain weight even when they eat small amounts of food.

Why is this so? There are a number of endocrine-related diseases such as **hypothyroidism** (not enough thyroid activity) and some forms of diabetes that may be responsible for obesity. But for the most part, the tendency to be overweight appears to be related to heredity, eating behavior, and exercise patterns.

Genetic Linkage

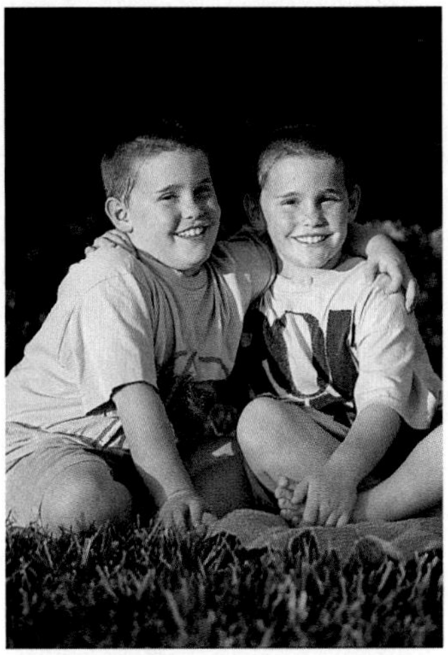
There is a genetic susceptibility to obesity, but not all family members —even identical twins—show the same degree of it.

Obesity is known to run in families, but the cause—genetics or environment—has long been debated. For example, one study divided a group of 540 adopted men and women into four groups: thin, median weight, overweight, and obese. When researchers compared the adoptees to their biological parents, a clear relation was noted between their BMIs. However, there was no such relationship between the adoptive parents and the adoptees. This suggests that genes play a leading role in determining weight, and that childhood family environment alone has little effect.

Researchers have found a gene that is thought to be responsible for at least some types of obesity in mice—and possibly in humans. The gene, which acts only in fat cells, normally controls appetite by sending a message to the brain that there is enough fat in the body. When the gene malfunctions, however, it fools the brain into thinking that there is not enough fat and that more food is needed. This discovery supports the theory that some people are destined to be overweight.

Other scientific theories about a genetic trigger for obesity point toward:

- A susceptibility to form fat cells.
- Too much or not enough of one or more hormones, which leads a person to overeat.

pinch test A test that uses special skin-fold calipers to pinch layers of fat at specific body sites; a measure of body fat.

underwater weighing A test of body fat that weighs a person underwater to determine body composition.

bioelectrical impedance A test that uses a weak electrical current to measure the body's fat content.

hypothyroidism Not enough thyroid activity.

- A low activity level of the **vagus nerve,** which runs between the posterior part of the brain stem and the stomach. (This means that it takes more food in your stomach to give your brain the message that you are full.)

If overweight or obesity runs in your family, these research findings do not mean that you should give up trying to control your weight. People who have a genetic susceptibility to fatness can lose weight and stay slim, but they have to work hard at it by maintaining a high level of physical activity and watching what they eat.

Some researchers believe that each person has a particular weight at which his or her body functions normally. This is called a **set point.** According to the set point theory, people who lose weight will return to their set points once they begin eating in response to hunger. Fortunately, a person's set point can change, so overweight people are not locked into their current body weights. Again, exercise plays a role. When an inactive person starts to exercise regularly, his or her set point will decrease.

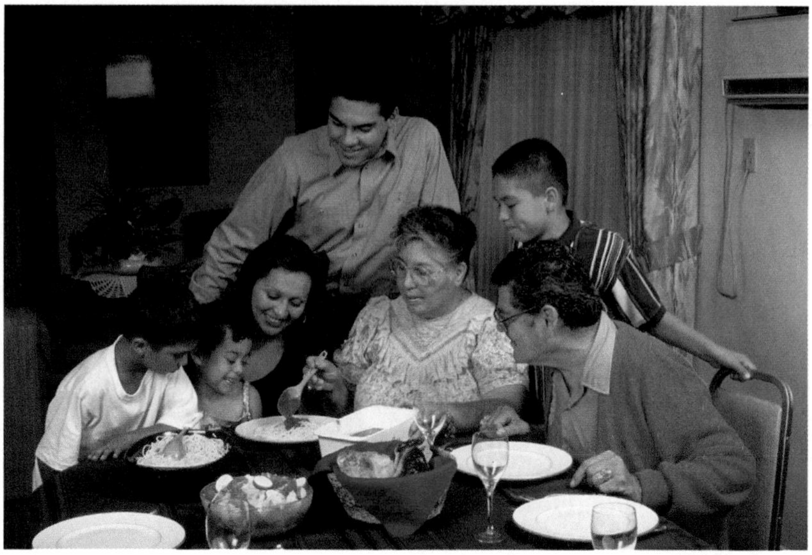

Family traditions can play an important role in maintaining proper weight. Sitting down together for a healthy and well-balanced dinner promotes healthy habits in children.

Eating Behaviors Learned at Home

Eating behaviors established in childhood and reinforced throughout life can lead to an overweight condition. For example, childhood obesity is influenced by a number of factors, including parents' weight, age, marital status, socioeconomic class, and race.

A study of eighteen infants, half from obese mothers and half from thin mothers, found that by the time the infants from obese mothers were one year old, most were showing signs of an overweight condition. The researchers determined that at three months of age, the infants from very fat mothers were burning nearly 21 percent fewer calories than the infants from very thin mothers, even though no signs of overweight were observable. The infants of obese mothers were also less active than infants of thin mothers. Researchers can only speculate about whether such inactivity was the result of modeling behavior or triggered by some genetic code.

Family traditions also play an important role. Many families have eating rituals, such as a big breakfast on the weekends, eating together in front of the television, or having a snack just before going to bed. Cultural and geographic influences also affect a family's eating habits, including the selection and preparation of food. For instance, deep-fried cooking is a popular feature of many classic southern recipes.

Television advertisers spend considerable money promoting high-calorie foods such as beer and hamburgers but give less attention to healthier, low-calorie alternatives. Television provides yet another link to being overweight. It is speculated that the number of hours spent watching television contributes to obesity because watching is sedentary and requires no expenditure of calories. Therefore, the more a person—particularly a child—watches television, the greater the risk of obesity.

There are also unconscious and emotional reasons for eating. For example, some people try to eat their way out of loneliness, boredom, or stress. This does not help the underlying problem and can result in unwanted weight gain. An important health skill is learning how to be in tune with your hunger. This involves respecting your natural hunger instincts and accepting the way you look (see the Assess Your Health box).

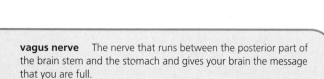

vagus nerve The nerve that runs between the posterior part of the brain stem and the stomach and gives your brain the message that you are full.

set point A particular weight at which a person's body functions normally.

How the Body Stores and Uses Energy

Food is the body's source of energy. As you learned in Chapter 4, some sources of energy are more nutritious

Assess Your Health

Are You Hung Up about Your Weight?

Eat when you're hungry, stop when you're full, and choose foods that are good for you. Oh, and while you're at it, learn to love your body, whatever its shape or size. If only it were so simple. But experts say that until we learn to respect our natural hunger signals and to accept the way we look, we'll never be able to kick the dieting habit. To find out how close you are to that healthy goal, pick up a pencil and circle true or false for each of the following statements.

My life would be better if only I could lose some weight.	True or False
I often eat when I am upset, depressed, anxious, or angry as a way of feeling better.	True or False
I tend to overeat in social situations.	True or False
I avoid mirrors.	True or False
I keep eating even when I'm full.	True or False
If I ate whenever I wanted to, I would get very fat.	True or False
I choose clothes that hide the size of my body.	True or False
I often feel guilty after I eat.	True or False
I'm afraid to have even a taste of dessert because I might lose control and eat too much.	True or False
I have tried many diets.	True or False
I prefer to make love in the dark because I'm embarrassed about my body.	True or False
I eat even when I don't feel hungry.	True or False
I compare my body unfavorably with those of others.	True or False
I eat normally when I'm with friends; when I'm by myself I tend to pig out.	True or False
I think about food nearly all the time.	True or False
I'm embarrassed about the fact that I like to eat.	True or False

Total number of true responses _______

Five or fewer true
Congratulations. You're in tune with your hunger, and you've resisted the pressures—cultural or otherwise—that make so many people dissatisfied with their bodies.

Six or more true
You probably realize that your relationship with food and your view of your body are somewhat troubled. Try to ease up on yourself and take steps to relearn a more natural way of eating.

Source: "Are You Hung Up about Your Weight?" *Health,* April 1997, p. 61. Reprinted by permission of Time Inc. Health

than others. Table sugar, for example, is an energy source that is virtually devoid of nutrition. The body uses energy for basic functions such as breathing, blood circulation, and growth. When the amount of food consumed is not burned in the performance of these normal bodily processes, it is stored for future use in the form of fat. When the body needs more energy than the amount provided by food, it uses the energy stored in fat tissue.

The Relationship Between Calories and Pounds

Fattening foods do not make you fat. What makes you fat is eating more calories than your body needs. A **calorie** is a unit measuring the energy produced by food when oxidized in the body. A simple way to measure how many calories your body needs is to multiply your desirable weight by eighteen if you are a man and by sixteen if you are a woman. This means that a woman weighing 125 pounds uses up about 2,000 calories a day (125 x 16). Be cautious, however, because the number of calories each person needs depends on several factors in addition to gender, including age, body frame, and, of course, exercise or activity level.

Compare a high-carbohydrate meal of spaghetti and tomato sauce with a high-calorie steak dinner. Carbohydrates and proteins contain approximately four calories per gram; fat contains approximately nine calories per gram. Moreover, you can fill up with calories from carbohydrates quicker than you can with calories

calorie A unit measuring the energy produced by food when oxidized in the body.

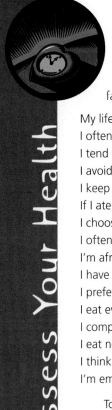

Developing Health Skills

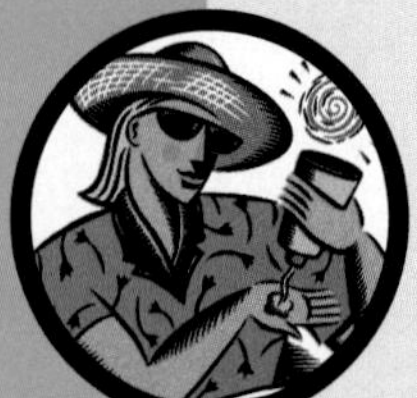

How Not to Gain Weight . . . When You Eat Low-Fat Foods

Almost every day another low-fat food appears on supermarket shelves. So why aren't Americans getting thinner? It may be human nature: Many people seem to feel that it's okay to eat more since they're making low-fat choices. In other words, a person who would normally eat six Oreos might eat a whole box of fat-free cookies—which adds up to less fat, sure, but more calories. To test how a low-fat or non-fat label affects food intake, Barbara Rolls, professor of nutrition at Penn State University, gave 48 women (healthy and not currently dieting) three indistinguishable raspberry-flavored yogurts:

Yogurt (per cup)	*Fat (grams)*	*Calories*
1 High-fat, high-calorie	18	240
2 Low-fat, high-calorie	2	240
3 Low-fat, low-calorie	2	105

The women ate about a cup and a half of one of the yogurts 30 minutes before lunch; on the next two days, they ate one of the two other types of yogurt before lunch. For half the women, the yogurt was labeled simply "high-fat" or "low-fat"; the others ate unlabeled yogurt. The result: When the women ate the yogurts labeled "low-fat," they consumed significantly more calories during the subsequent lunch and dinner than they did after eating the yogurt labeled "high-fat." When the yogurts weren't labeled for fat content, these differences did not occur.

That's a classic dieting scenario. People eat low-fat foods, pat themselves on the back, and feel they can indulge. Some even think they can eat unlimited amounts of a food if it's low in fat. Low-fat foods can help promote weight loss—but only if they are also low in calories, are eaten in "normal" portions, and don't serve as a license to overeat later. It seems obvious, but many people just don't get it: If they don't cut down on calories (and/or exercise more) over the course of the day, they won't lose weight.

Source: "How Not to Gain Weight When You Eat Low-Fat Foods," reprinted with permission from the *University of California at Berkeley Wellness Letter,* April 1997. © Health Letter Associates, 1997

from fat. A two-ounce piece of a chocolate bar has the same number of calories (21 percent of them from fat) as three medium-sized bananas that together weigh more than a pound (no calories from fat).

Two recent studies dramatically illustrate the relationship between carbohydrates and fat and weight gain. In one study conducted in a Vermont prison, a group of male prisoners had difficulty gaining weight on a high-carbohydrate, low-fat diet despite an enormous caloric intake. A second group gained weight easily on a low-carbohydrate, high-fat diet. In another study, a group of men were fed 2,000 calories of carbohydrates at one meal. When tested ten hours later, each subject had stored only 81 calories of fat. Further testing showed that the men actually lost body fat over the next ten hours because their normal metabolism burned more than the 81 calories of fat that they had gained.

Far from being fattening, carbohydrates from starches, fruits, and vegetables are excellent sources of food for weight reducers. They fill you up, give you something to chew on, can satisfy a sweet craving (at least in the case of fruits), and supply you with nutrients, too. Studies have shown that eating bread with meals—long considered a no-no for dieters—makes eaters feel full before they consume their usual quota of calories.

Switching to a low-fat diet, however, won't help if you still consume a lot of food (see the Developing Health Skills box).

Fat as Essential, Fat as Excess

Fat is a general term that can refer to a group of foods or a type of body tissue. In either case, the main components of fat are carbon, hydrogen, and oxygen.

As food, fat is essential to health: without fats in the diet, deficiencies of the fat-soluble vitamins A, D, E, and K would result. Of particular importance to good health are three fatty acids: linoleic, linolenic, and arachidonic acids. Linoleic acid cannot be manufactured by the body but is present in many kinds of foods and is abundant in some oils, including walnut and linseed oil, and some nuts and soybeans.

As tissue, fat is found in all parts of the body. It serves to insulate, cushion, and lubricate the anatomy, but most importantly, it stores energy. The body of the average, healthy man is 15 percent fat; for the healthy woman, 23 percent body fat is average.

One factor related to obesity is the number of fat cells in the body. The number and size of fat cells in the body seem to proliferate naturally in the first year of life. At one year, the fat cells in children begin to decrease in size (but not number). Fat cells increase in both size and number again in early adolescence. Studies show that obese children do not experience the normal drop in fat cell size at age one. Instead, the cells continue to grow and multiply. By the time they are nineteen years old, they have twice as many fat cells as does an average person of the same age. Moreover, these fat cells are between 30 and 40 percent larger. Given these findings, a critical factor in controlling obesity is limiting the number of fat cells, particularly in childhood and adolescence. This can be achieved through healthy eating.

Your Body's Energy Needs

Energy needs differ depending on body composition, size, and age. It is obvious that a large person needs more calories to keep the body going than does a small person. Generally, men have higher calorie needs than women, not only because they are larger but also because they have a greater proportion of muscle tissue. The more muscle tissue a person has, the more energy that person uses. Calorie needs also differ at various stages in life. Calorie requirements are greatest during infancy, adolescence, pregnancy, and lactation (breast feeding). As adults get older, they need fewer calories to keep their bodies functioning. One reason for weight gain in middle age is that most people do not alter their intake of food.

There are three major reasons why the body needs less energy with age. To begin with, the demand for food energy is reduced by a drop in the **basal metabolic rate**—the speed with which the body expends calories on basic functions such as breathing. Calorie requirements decrease between 2 and 8 percent for each decade of life past age twenty. At the same time, the adult body converts more food into fat than it did in earlier years, and fat tissue uses less energy than the same weight of muscle tissue would use. On top of this, most people have a tendency to become less active as they grow older.

The Importance of Exercise

Without exercise, it is difficult to lose weight—and keep it off. The reason why so many diets are not successful is that they do not include a program for exercising, and the reason a diet without exercise does not work well has to do with the body's metabolism. When you decrease the amount of food you normally eat—that is, when you go on a diet—the body's natural tendency is to conserve energy. This results in a 15 to 30 percent decrease in basal metabolic rate. Exercise is a counteracting force: It speeds up metabolism.

Exercise is another way of burning up calories. If you want to cut your calories by 500 a day, you can do this by consuming 200 fewer calories and burning off 300 calories by walking, jogging, biking, playing tennis, or engaging in many other forms of exercise.

The number of calories burned depends on four factors:

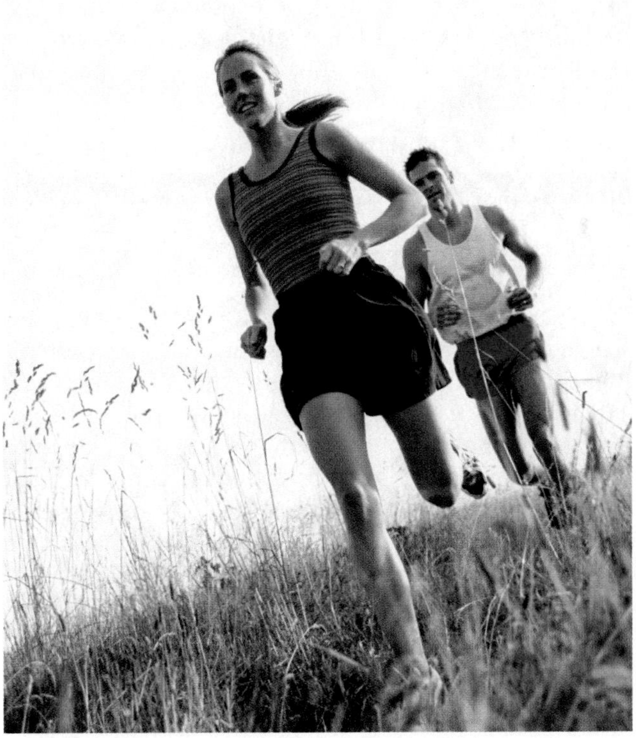

Without doing some form of exercise, it is difficult to lose weight and keep it off. Exercise burns calories and increases metabolism.

- The degree of the activity (twenty minutes of running burns more calories than twenty minutes of walking).
- The length of the activity (the longer the activity continues, the more calories burned).
- Air temperature (exercising in colder weather burns up more calories).
- Your weight (a heavier person uses more energy than a lighter person for the same activity).

Exercise does not have to be strenuous in order to have an impact. There are many ways to burn calories during the day. Stand rather than sit; use the stairs instead of the elevator; walk or bike instead of taking the car. A leisurely walk burns around 300 calories, which is more than twice the number of calories burned when merely standing. In one study, obese women who added a half-hour walk to their daily routines lost twenty pounds in a year's time—even without dieting.

Physical activity also improves a person's sense of well-being and reduces stress. The relationship of this

basal metabolic rate The speed with which the body expends calories on basic functions at a resting state.

to weight control is that many people eat more when they are under stress. Finally, when people are involved in an exercise program, they are otherwise occupied and cannot be tempted to snack.

The Reality of Weight Control

There is simply no magic bullet that can take away unwanted fat. Instead, think of weight control as a combination of three factors: (1) a healthy diet, (2) appropriate exercise, and (3) healthy eating behaviors. Before beginning a weight-control program, consult a physician to make sure you do not have a medical condition that would preclude doing exercise or going on a special diet. Consulting with a health professional can also help you plan a safe weight-control program.

Controlling Your Weight

A complete weight-control program begins with a **balanced diet.** This means an emphasis on whole grains, fresh fruits, and vegetables and a de-emphasis on high-fat foods, processed foods, red meats, and rich desserts. The best advice from nutritionists calls for consuming about 1,200 calories a day for women and about 1,500 for men trying to lose weight.

Note the word *balanced.* Eating a variety of foods is important. But remember that certain foods can help you lose weight whereas others may hinder weight loss. For example, high-fiber foods are more filling and have fewer calories than do fatty foods. Chapter 4 is a good source of information about how different foods affect your weight.

You have already read about the importance of exercise in a weight-loss program. For maximum benefits, exercise four or five days a week, starting slowly—perhaps with a five-minute workout—and build up to thirty minutes. Do not forget to do your warm-up and cool-down exercises. Chapter 6 provides more information about exercising to maintain proper weight.

Finally, to help you succeed with a new health style of eating right and exercising, you may need to make some changes in how you eat. Most eating habits were learned a long time ago, and it will take time to unlearn them and to learn new ones. Basically, this involves substituting "thin" strategies for "fat" ones. Consider some of the following ideas:

- Serve yourself on a smaller plate. Smaller portions will fill it up, and you are less likely to feel deprived by a skimpy serving.
- Do not put serving bowls on the table.
- Let your family and friends know that you are changing your eating habits. Ask them not to offer you seconds.
- Get someone else to clear the table and put away the leftovers. Alternatively, clear plates directly into the garbage. Either way, you will be less tempted to nibble after eating.
- Keep a supply of low-fat snacks on hand—raw vegetables, for example.
- Drink a glass of water before meals, and sip water while eating. This will help you fill up without overloading on calories.

Dangers of Fad Diets

No diet works quickly, and most of them do not work over the long run. Fewer than 5 percent of the people who have lost weight while on a diet have maintained that loss for more than one year. Moreover, people who do **yo-yo dieting**—going on and off diets year after year—may actually be inhibiting future weight loss. In a study of patients enrolled for the second time in a university weight-loss clinic, the dieters lost markedly fewer pounds on the second diet (2.1 pounds per week) than on the first (3.1 pounds per week). There is some

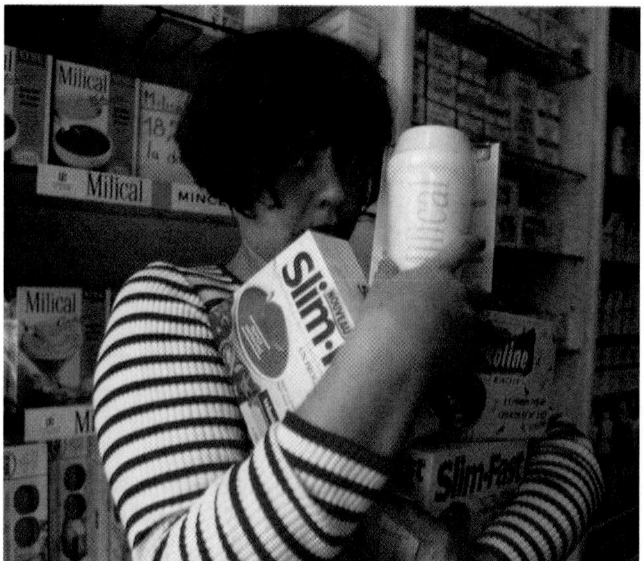

There is no magic pill for losing weight. Most fad diets are nutritionally unbalanced, and some can be very dangerous.

balanced diet An eating pattern that includes a variety of foods in amounts that result in health enhancement.

yo-yo dieting Going on and off diets.

Developing Health Skills

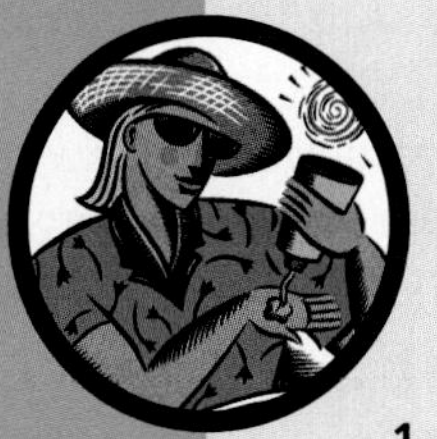

Consumer Health: Ready to Go on a Diet?

Questions to Ask Before Going on a Diet

1. Does the diet provide a reasonable number of calories? This means no fewer than 1,200 calories for the average-sized woman and 1,600 for the average-sized man.
2. Does it provide enough, but not too much, protein? It should have at least the recommended dietary allowance (RDA) but not more than twice that amount.
3. Does it provide enough, but not too much, fat? No more than 30 percent of the calories in the diet should come from fat.
4. Does it provide enough carbohydrates, particularly complex carbohydrates? No more than 20 percent of the calories should come from concentrated sugar.
5. Does it offer a balanced assortment of vitamins and minerals from whole-food sources in all food groups? If a food group is omitted (for example, meat), is a suitable substitute provided?
6. Does it offer variety? Can different foods be selected each day?
7. Does it consist of ordinary foods that are available locally at the prices people normally pay, or does the dieter have to buy special, expensive foods to adhere to the diet?

Note: You may want to refer to Chapter 4 for a review of nutritional information and what constitutes a healthy diet.

Source: From *Understanding Nutrition,* 5th edition by Whitney/Hamilton/Rolfes. © Reprinted with permission of Wadsworth, a division of Thomson Learning: www.thomsonrights.com. Fax 800-730-2215

indication that repetitive dieters tend to gain weight back in fat tissue, which is harder to lose.

From a nutritionist's point of view, it is a good thing that **fad diets** fail and that most people do not stick with them for very long. Virtually every fad diet is nutritionally unbalanced in one way or another because they emphasize eating only a limited number of foods. No combination of only a few foods can provide the essential nutrients (see the Developing Health Skills box).

High-protein, low-carbohydrate diets. These are based on the theory that when, in the absence of carbohydrates, the body burns fat as its major energy source, acidic products called ketones develop, and these are supposed to induce weight loss. However, the accumulation of ketones in the blood **(ketosis)** can cause nausea, vomiting, apathy, fatigue, and low blood pressure.

Low-protein, high-carbohydrate diets. These consist of a lot of cereal, pasta, fruit, and vegetables. But they are so limited in protein and essential minerals such as calcium and iron that the body is forced to break down its own muscle tissue in order to meet its protein needs. At least one low-protein diet calls for eating so much fruit that it can cause severe diarrhea and result in high fever, muscle weakness, rapid pulse, a severe drop in blood pressure, and shock.

Protein-sparing diets. These are near-starvation diets. They involve a caloric intake of 300 to 500 calories in a liquid protein formula. Some of these formulas are fortified with minerals and vitamins, but others are not. Weight loss is rapid, averaging between three and five pounds a week. These diets were originally designed for use by extremely obese individuals and were intended to be carried out under strict medical supervision. Their widespread use among people with little or no medical supervision has resulted in deaths.

In addition to weight-loss plans, a variety of drugs are used as diet aids, but these carry the problems associated with any drug use: adverse drug reactions. A combination of fenfluramine and phentermine, commonly known as fen/phen, was used by some two million dieters before the Food and Drug Administration pulled it off the market in the late 1990s because of evidence that as many as one third of those using the prescription medications may develop a rare form of heart valve damage that could lead to weakening of the heart—and even death.

Water pills or diuretics dehydrate the body, and depending on how much water was in the body, a person may lose three to ten pounds this way. Weight lost due to use of laxatives is also essentially water weight (most laxatives work by increasing the amount of water in the stool). Amphetamines can reduce hunger pangs, but the weight lost is regained as soon as one stops taking the drug. Some people take thyroid pills to lose weight,

fad diets Diets that are popular for brief periods of time then lose popularity; the loss of popularity usually results when the effectiveness of a fad diet is questioned.

ketosis An accumulation of chemical compounds called ketones in the blood.

based on the belief that obese people suffer from a malfunctioning thyroid gland. The fact is that less than one percent of overweight people have abnormal thyroid function. The dangers of taking thyroid hormones include heart palpitations and increased heart rate.

Several other gimmicks are advertised as avenues to weight loss. Body wraps, for example, are sold as a method of removing inches from your waistline by means of temporary fluid loss or perspiration. Health spas advertise machines that shake away cellulite—lumpy fat deposited near the external tissue on hips and thighs. However, shaking fat doesn't make it go away.

Weight-loss organizations such as Weight Watchers and TOPS (Take Off Pounds Sensibly) promote the use of well-balanced meals, and Overeaters Anonymous offers encouragement for dieters. This can be useful for people who can benefit from group support. However, the quality of leadership varies from group to group.

A Final Word on Weight Loss

It would be nice if weight loss were simple—if you could take a pill or purchase a product and have the pounds come off. But the fact remains that there is no quick and easy way to lose weight. Anyone who attempts to do so takes risks. It takes time to develop an overweight problem, and it takes time to get yourself back to your desired weight. If you want to lose weight, take the advice of a health professional—a nurse, health educator, nutritionist, physician, or dietician—not a zealot. Remember: A good weight-control program is one that you want to live with for the rest of your life.

CASE STUDY 5: Dieting

Sarah has had a weight problem most of her life. When she was in grade school, she bought clothes for "chubby girls." As a college student, she wears clothes for "larger-sized women." Yet Sarah dreams of being thin, and over the years has gone on diet after diet. She thought she had won the battle after spending a few weeks on a liquid diet and dropping twenty pounds. But as soon as she went back to eating solid foods, nearly all the weight came back.

Sarah does not know how to say no to food or yes to exercise. She claims she doesn't have time for exercise, but because she has led a sedentary, "fat girl's" life, she is afraid that she will be clumsy in an aerobics class.

Kishia has also had a longtime battle with weight. Although she wasn't taunted as a "fatty" as a child, she was always saying, "I just want to lose a few pounds." Instead, she gained the standard "freshman fifteen" pounds in college. She, like Sarah, went on numerous quick-weight-loss diets, but she always put the weight back on.

Her last diet, however, really was her last diet because it became a lifelong diet. She lost twenty pounds—and has kept them off for nearly two years. To do this, Kishia changed her eating habits: what she eats, when she eats, and how much she eats. She also exercises regularly. What motivated Kishia to lose weight? Her physician. He warned her of the health implications of her high cholesterol levels, which resulted from a rich diet and lack of exercise. Her other motivation was her overweight uncle, who had had a minor heart attack.

In Your Opinion

Sarah and Kishia are both fighting the same problem, but one is winning the battle, the other is losing it.

- Why was Sarah so unsuccessful in losing weight permanently? What was wrong with her attitude?
- What behavior was she trying to change?
- What are the reasons behind Kishia's success story?
- What conscious decisions did Kishia make concerning weight loss?
- What steps would you take if you wanted to lose weight?

KEY CONCEPTS

1. The inability to maintain proper weight is a serious public health problem in the United States. According to the Surgeon General, more than 60 percent of American adults are overweight.
2. Obesity refers to a surplus of body fat. Overweight, on the other hand, refers to an excess of body weight.

3. Anyone who is more than 10 percent lighter than average for his or her height and build is considered underweight and at increased risk of mortality. This is especially true in the case of smokers.
4. The tendency to overweight appears to be related to heredity, eating styles, and exercise patterns.
5. Overweight parents tend to have overweight children, and thin parents tend to have thin children.
6. A calorie is a unit measuring the energy produced by food when oxidized in the body.
7. As food, fat is essential to health. Without fats in the diet, deficiencies of the fat-soluble vitamins A, D, E, and K would result.
8. Weight control results from a lifelong commitment to healthy eating as well as from an appropriate level of exercise, not from going on a diet.
9. Virtually every fad diet is nutritionally unbalanced in one way or another because fad diets emphasize eating only a limited number of foods.
10. Fewer than 5 percent of the people who lose weight while on a diet have maintained that loss for more than one year.

REVIEW QUESTIONS

1. Explain the difference between overweight and obesity.
2. List five chronic diseases that have been associated with overweight.
3. Al is six feet two inches tall and weighs 192 pounds. What is his approximate body mass index? Is Al overweight?
4. Explain the difference between fat as an essential food and fat as excess body tissue.
5. Overweight parents often have overweight children. Explain why this may occur.
6. Describe how exercise is an important element of a weight-control program.
7. List characteristics of anorexia and bulimia. What is the prognosis if such diseases are left untreated?
8. Explain the difference between body weight and body mass.
9. Define yo-yo dieting and explain the health risks associated with this eating behavior.
10. List several specific actions you can take to help maintain a weight-control program of healthy eating and exercise.

CRITICAL THINKING QUESTIONS

1. The bathroom scale is a common means of monitoring body weight, yet many weight management experts consider it your worst enemy. Why might this be? How healthy is this tool for weight assessment?
2. In *Healthy People 2010,* the following objective is listed: "Reduce the proportion of adults who are obese." If we were to reach this objective by 2010, what are the implications for society? Would there be economic impact? Would there be a public health impact? What would these impacts be?
3. *Healthy People 2010* seeks to "increase the proportion of adults who are at a healthy weight." What is the relationship of *knowing* about healthy weight and *being* at a healthy weight? Why is nutrition education an important strategy for achieving this weight-control objective?
4. The goal of fad diets is weight loss—not health enhancement—and they are part of a multimillion-dollar industry. How might they be a symptom of modern lifestyles? Why do they continue to be followed even when proven to be unhealthy?

JOURNAL ACTIVITIES

1. Using the formula on page 67, calculate your body mass index (BMI). Are you in the normal zone? What do the results suggest about your diet and exercise habits? Should they change, and if so, how?
2. What is your favorite food? How much do you consume of it at one sitting? Estimate the number of calories you consume each time you eat your favorite food. You will find a calorie chart in nutrition books in the library or on the Internet.
3. Being overweight or underweight is related to one's health, but it does not deter from the worth of the individual. Write a paragraph explaining why you agree or disagree with this statement.
4. Spend one-half hour "people watching" in a heavily trafficked place on campus. Using your best judgment, count the number of people who are overweight, normal weight and underweight. Compare your findings with those presented in the text.

SELECTED BIBLIOGRAPHY

American Anorexia Bulimia Association, Inc. *Facts on Eating Disorders.* New York, NY, 1998.

Dietary Guidelines for Americans. Washington DC: U.S. Department of Agriculture and U.S. Department of Health and Human Services, 2001.

Flegal, K. M., et al. "Overweight and Obesity in the United States: Prevalence and trends, 1960–1994." *International Journal of Obesity* 22 (1998): 39–47.

Graves L. *Why Diets Don't Work.* Wellesley, MA: National Eating Disorders Screening Program, 1998.

Obesity: Preventing and Managing the Global Epidemic. Geneva, Switzerland: World Health Organization, 1998.

The Surgeon General's Call to Action to Prevent and Decrease Overweight and Obesity. Rockville, MD: 2001. U.S. Department of Health and Human Services, Public Health Service, Office of the Surgeon General.

"Update: Prevalence of Overweight among Children, Adolescents, and Adults—United States, 1988–1994." *Morbidity and Mortality Weekly Report* 46 (March 7, 1997).

HEALTHLINKS

Websites for Maintaining a Healthy Weight

You can access better health as it relates to this chapter by checking out some of the following sites on the Internet. These sites can be accessed directly from the *Decisions for Healthy Living* Website located at www.aw.com/pruitt.

Duke University Diet and Fitness Center

Visit one of the best programs in the country that focuses on helping people live healthier, fuller lives through weight loss and lifestyle change. This site provides detailed information about weight management and links to related programs.

Healthtouch Online

Collection of articles and resources from multiple organizations on eating disorders.

HEALTH HOTLINES

Maintaining Proper Weight

National Association of Anorexia Nervosa and Associated Disorders
(847) 831-3438
P.O. Box 7
Highland Park, IL 60035

TEST YOUR KNOWLEDGE ANSWERS

1. True. Nearly 30 percent of men and more than 40 percent of women report attempting to lose weight, yet the percentage of overweight individuals using diet and exercise as a means of weight loss has decreased.
2. True. Research comparing infants of thin mothers to those of obese mothers, found that the infants of obese mothers were less active, burned fewer calories, and showed signs of overweight by age one.
3. False. Although eating foods low in fat content is recommended as a part of a weight-loss program, it is possible to eat such foods in large enough quantities or at the expense of a balanced diet, thus producing health risks. A good weight-loss program includes a balanced diet with some fat intake, and an appropriate exercise program.
4. False. An obese person actually has more, and larger, fat cells than a thin person. The number and size of fat cells in the body proliferate naturally in the first year of life and again during adolescence. Through healthy eating, the number of fat cells in a person's body can be reduced.
5. False. Bulimia is a cause of being extremely underweight, not overweight. It is a disorder characterized by the consumption of enormous quantities of food followed by purging. Left untreated, a bulimic person faces a variety of health threats.

CHAPTER

6

Keeping Fit

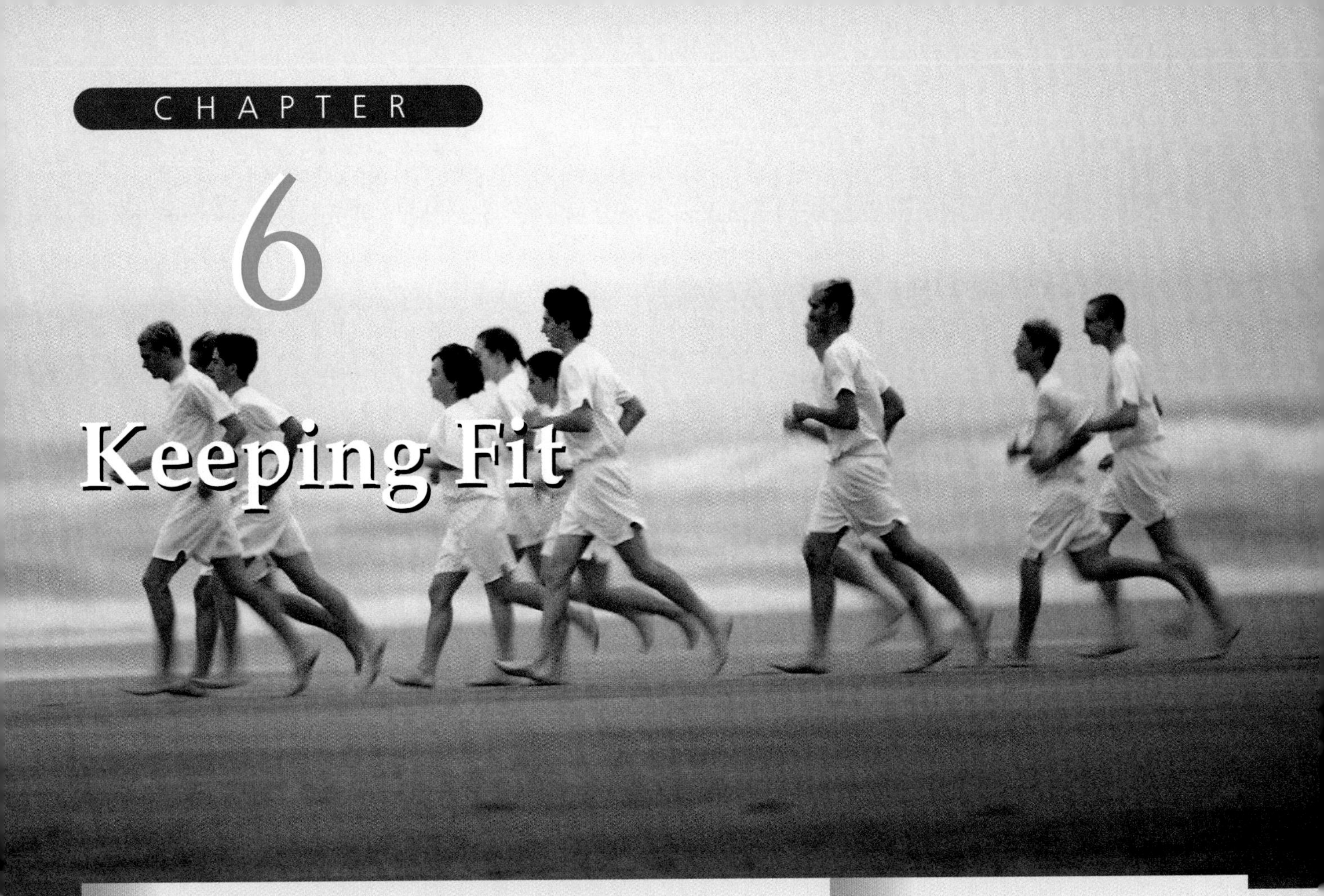

OBJECTIVES

When you finish reading this chapter, you will be able to:

1. Examine the extent to which people exercise and give reasons for the apparent low level of exercise.
2. Describe the physical health benefits of exercise.
3. Describe the effect of exercise on psychological well-being.
4. Explain the three major components of fitness: strength, flexibility, and endurance.
5. Differentiate between isokinetic, isotonic, and isometric exercises.
6. Differentiate between aerobic and anaerobic activities.
7. Explain the importance of intensity, duration, and frequency of exercise sessions.
8. Determine your target heart rate for exercise as well as your maximal heart rate.
9. Plan a personal fitness program including warm-up, conditioning, and cool-down periods.
10. List several tactics for maintaining a fitness program.

TEST YOUR KNOWLEDGE

1. Studies consistently show that people who exercise have a greater bone mineral content than those who do not. True or False?
2. Very strenuous anaerobic exercise contributes to muscle strength, but does little to enhance cardiovascular health. True or False?
3. The training effect is accomplished by raising the heart rate during exercise to 150 to 160 beats per minute. True or False?
4. Research suggests that warming up prior to exercise is not necessary and that stretching provides an adequate preparation. True or False?
5. The Surgeon General's *Report on Physical Activity and Health* suggests that physical activity need not be strenuous in order to achieve health benefits. True or False?

Answers found at end of chapter.

Interest in sports in the United States is at perhaps its highest point in history—but the interest is in spectator sports rather than participation sports. The reason: Most people who do not engage in physical activity say they do not have enough time. In addition, advances in technology have contributed to the increasingly sedentary lifestyle of Americans. More and more, work sites are mechanized and automated, making physical fitness no longer a requisite for earning a living. Telecommunications and easy transportation have reduced the need for walking.

At home, television viewing requires little or no physical exertion, especially when a remote control device is used for changing channels. Even people who work out in front of their television sets often do so not to achieve fitness, but rather in pursuit of the promise of "looking good." Good looks, however, do not always translate into good health and well-being.

Exercise as Part of Your Lifestyle

Evidence suggests that, as a nation, we are not very fit. According to the most recent National Center for Health Statistics report on physical activity and health, more than 70 percent of American adults are not regularly physically active. And as many as one in four are not active at all. Of those who do **exercise,** few do so at what is considered an appropriate level of activity.

The appropriate level involves physical activity that is both regularly vigorous and regularly sustained (see the Physical Activity Pyramid in Figure 6.1). Note the importance of the word regularly. On most—if not all—days of the week, you should spend thirty minutes

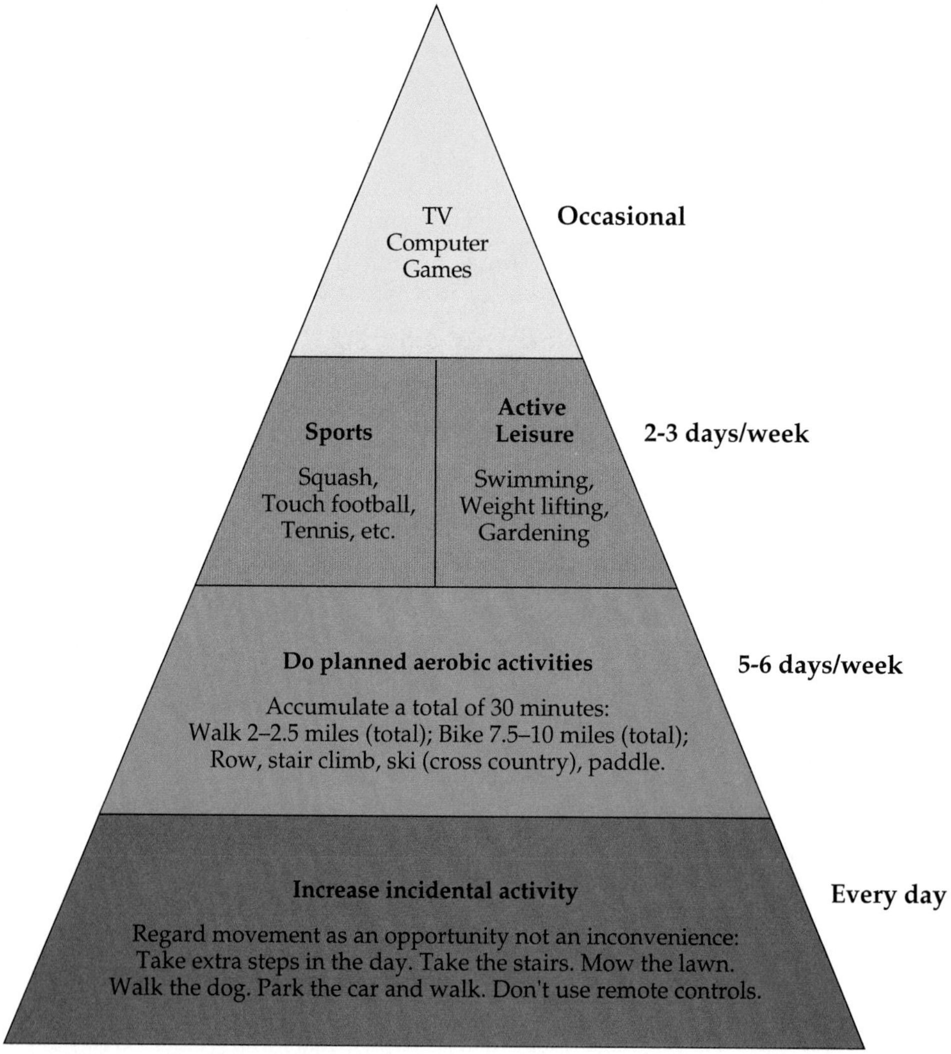

Figure 6.1 **Physical Activity Pyramid**
The Physical Activity Pyramid is a general guide to activities to do every day as well as a couple of times a week. Note that playing computer games, which is popular with college students, is listed as an "occasional" activity on the pyramid.
Source: Rauramaa, R., and Leon, A.S. (1996). Physical activity and risk of cardiovascular disease in middle aged individuals. *Sports Medicine* 22(2):65–69

exercise Bodily movement undertaken to improve or maintain one or more of the components of physical fitness.

Less vigorous, more time

Washing and waxing a car for 45–60 minutes
Washing windows or floors for 45–60 minutes
Playing volleyball for 45 minutes
Playing touch football for 30–45 minutes
Gardening for 30–45 minutes
Wheeling self in wheelchair for 30–40 minutes
Walking $1\frac{3}{4}$ miles in 35 minutes (20 min/mile)
Basketball (shooting baskets) for 30 minutes
Bicycling 5 miles in 30 minutes
Dancing fast (social) for 30 minutes
Pushing a stroller $1\frac{1}{2}$ miles in 30 minutes
Raking leaves for 30 minutes
Walking 2 miles in 30 minutes (15 min/mile)
Water aerobics for 30 minutes
Swimming laps for 20 minutes
Wheelchair basketball for 20 minutes
Basketball (playing a game) for 15–20 minutes
Bicycling 4 miles in 15 minutes
Jumping rope for 15 minutes
Running $1\frac{1}{2}$ miles in 15 minutes (10 min/mile)
Shoveling snow for 15 minutes
Stairwalking for 15 minutes

More vigorous, less time

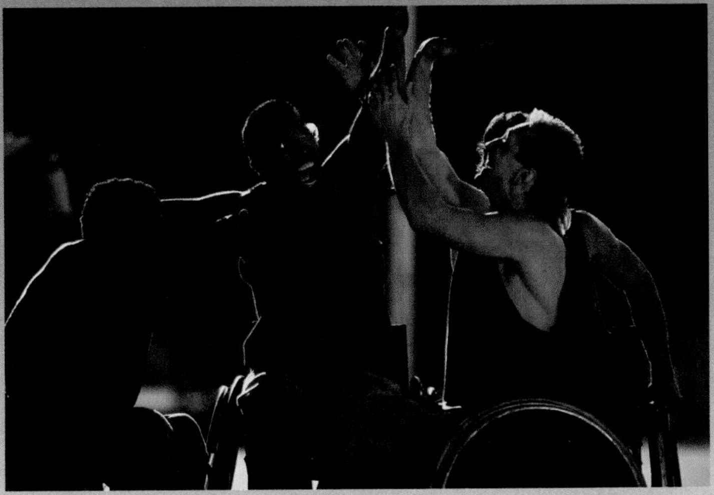

Significant health benefits can be obtained with a moderate amount of physical activity, preferably daily. The same moderate amount of activity can be obtained in longer sessions of moderately intense activities (such as 30–40 minutes of wheeling oneself in a wheelchair) or in shorter sessions of more strenuous activities (such as 20 minutes of wheelchair basketball).

Figure 6.2 Examples of Moderate Amounts of Activity
From washing your car to walking up and down the stairs, there is a wide range of physical activity that you can do on a regular basis. (*Source: Physical Activity and Health: A Report of the Surgeon General,* 1996)

or more on moderate-intensity physical activity, such as brisk walking (see Figure 6.2 for more examples of moderate amounts of activity). Does this sound possible, given your busy student life? The answer is yes, once you make being physically fit a part of your lifestyle.

What will it take to get people who are leading sedentary lives to change their habits? For one thing, people need to know that being out of shape can increase health risks, whereas being in shape can reduce those risks. People who exercise regularly already know this. When asked why they exercise, many say they feel and look better when they are physically fit. They have more self-confidence and a better self-image. Others say they are physically active for social reasons—that is, they like to participate in exercise programs such as aerobic dancing or spinning because their friends are doing it. Some report that they have simply gotten into the exercise habit and enjoy it. Most physically active individuals, however, say they exercise for the "health" of it.

The Health Benefits of Exercise

It is unfortunate that so few people exercise because exercise is a critical component of a healthy lifestyle. In fact, exercise may well be the single most important thing you can do if you want to live a long and healthy life. Researchers have persistently found that higher levels of physical activity and physical fitness lead to longer life—and a higher quality of life. Regular exercise also helps to control weight. To lose one pound every two weeks from exercise alone, the average person must burn 200 to 250 calories a day in physical activity. Consult Table 6.1 for the number of calories burned while performing various physical activities.

The U.S. Surgeon General recognizes that physical activity

- Reduces the risk of dying prematurely.
- Reduces the risk of dying from heart disease.

Table 6.1 Burning Calories: The Average Caloric Expenditure by Activity (per hour)

	Body Weight		
	110 lbs.	**154 lbs.**	**198 lbs.**
Baseball/softball			
Infield/outfield	220	280	340
Pitching	305	390	475
Basketball			
Moderate	435	555	675
Vigorous	585	750	910
Bicycling			
On level 5.5 mph	190	245	295
13 mph	515	655	790
Bowling (nonstop)	210	270	325
Bricklaying	160	205	250
Calisthenics	235	300	365
Canoeing (4 mph)	490	625	765
Chopping wood	355	450	550
Gardening	155	215	280
Gardening and weeding	250	315	380
Golf			
Twosome	295	380	460
Foursome	210	270	325
Handball/racquetball	610	775	945
Hill climbing	470	600	730
Hoeing, raking, and planting	205	285	370
Housework	175	245	320
House painting	165	210	255
Motorcycling	165	205	250
Mountain climbing	470	600	730
Mowing grass			
Power, self-propelled	195	250	305
Not self-propelled	210	270	325
Rowing (20 strokes/min)	515	655	795
Running			
5.5 mph	515	655	795
7 mph	550	700	850
9 mph	720	920	1120
Sailing (calm water)	120	155	190
Sawing wood	180	230	280
Shoveling snow	475	610	745
Skating (ice)			
Moderate	275	350	425
Vigorous	485	620	755
Skiing			
Downhill	465	595	720
Cross-country (5 mph)	550	700	950
Soccer	470	600	730
Swimming			
Backstroke 20 yds/min	165	235	305
Breaststroke 10 yds/min	210	295	380
Butterfly (per hr)	490	630	760
Crawl 20 yds/min	235	300	365
Sidestroke (per hr)	230	320	420
Tennis			
Moderate	335	425	520
Vigorous	470	600	730
Volleyball (moderate)	275	350	425
Walking			
2 mph	145	185	225
4.5 mph	325	450	550
Downstairs	355	450	550
Upstairs	720	920	1120
Waterskiing	335	475	610
Yard work	155	215	275

- Reduces the risk of developing diabetes.
- Reduces the risk of developing high blood pressure.
- Helps reduce blood pressure in people who already have high blood pressure.
- Reduces the risk of developing colon cancer.
- Reduces feelings of depression and anxiety.
- Helps control weight.
- Helps build and maintain healthy bones, muscles, and joints.
- Helps older adults become stronger and better able to move about without falling.
- Promotes psychological well-being.

tissue plasminogen activator A natural enzyme that prevents blood from clotting.

Helping the Heart

Perhaps the most important effects of physical activity relate to the heart. Exercise affects your heart in a number of ways. It increases the plasma, thus thinning the blood and allowing it to move smoothly through the vessels. It also stimulates the release of a natural enzyme that prevents

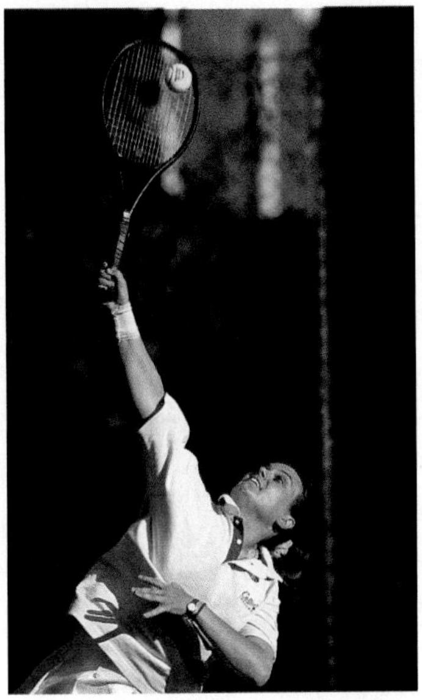

Women who participate in intensive regular exercise—swimming or playing tennis twice a week or running 2 miles five days a week—are less likely than nonathletes to develop breast cancer, other cancers of the reproductive system, or diabetes.

blood from clotting—**tissue plasminogen activator.** These effects are immediate and provide protection for up to one and a half hours after exercising. Over the long term, exercise can increase the size of the major coronary arteries.

Exercise contributes to lowering blood pressure and reducing the risk for **hypertension** by increasing the number as well as the capacity of capillaries, which carry blood to arteries. In addition, exercise improves the levels of blood cholesterol by raising the "good" cholesterol, the **high density lipoproteins (HDLs),** and lowering the "bad," plaque-forming cholesterol, the **low density lipoproteins (LDLs)** (see Chapter 4). It can also help lower blood sugar levels and increase the body's sensitivity to insulin. This is particularly important to diabetics, 70 percent of whom die from heart disease.

Preventing Osteoporosis

Another health benefit of physical activity is that it helps strengthen bones. Without sufficient weight-bearing exercise, bones become demineralized—that is, they lose their calcium and become brittle. Walking, running, aerobics, and racquet sports are all examples of weight-bearing exercise.

Osteoporosis is a condition that is characterized by a thinning of the bones. In women, bones reach their maximum density and strength at around age thirty. After that, bone mass begins to diminish at a rate of about 10 percent per decade. By age seventy, about 35 percent of the total amount of bone mass has been lost. In men, bone mass loss begins approximately twenty years later and proceeds at about half the rate as in women.

One of the best defenses against osteoporosis is a lifelong history of weight-bearing exercise. Studies consistently show that people who exercise have a greater bone mineral content than those who do not exercise. Moreover, the greater the load borne during exercise, the greater the bone density. Weight lifters have a greater bone mass than throwers, throwers greater than runners, runners greater than soccer players, and soccer players greater than swimmers. Recent studies report that physiologists have found that exercise can help increase bone mass even among a very elderly and sedentary population. One 3-year study of elderly women aged sixty-nine to ninety-six showed that bone mass content increased 4.2 percent among a group doing mild exercise and decreased 2.5 percent among a control group of nonexercisers.

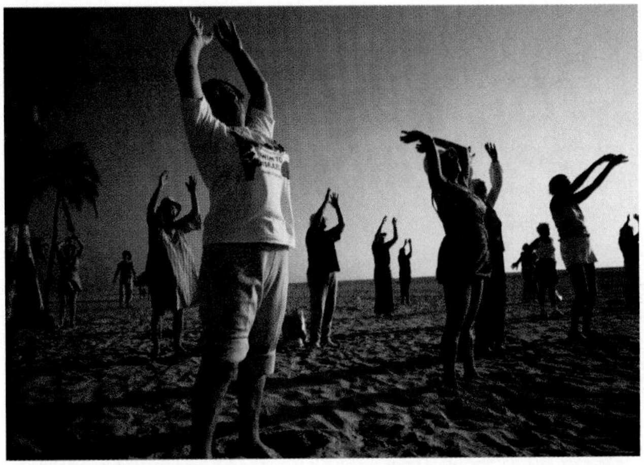

Exercise helps to strengthen bones, thereby reducing the risk of developing osteoporosis, a thinning of bones. It's never too late to benefit: Studies show that bone mass content increases in elderly people who do mild exercise.

As discussed in Chapter 4, diet also plays a role in preventing osteoporosis. Especially important is the intake of the bone-building mineral calcium.

Psychological Well-Being

Vigorous exercise has psychological benefits as well. People who exercise regularly tend to feel better and to have more energy and less trouble sleeping than do people who do not exercise regularly. Symptoms of anxiety and mild to moderate depression can be reduced through regular exercise. Exercise can reduce stress, and some people claim it gives them a "high." The so-called **runner's high** is due to an increase in the production of

hypertension High blood pressure.

high density lipoproteins (HDLs) A fatty substance that is the type of cholesterol that is considered good and that prevents atherosclerosis.

low density lipoproteins (LDLs) A fatty substance that is the type of cholesterol that is considered bad and that promotes atherosclerosis.

osteoporosis A disorder in which bone density decreases, making the bones more likely to break.

runner's high The feeling of euphoria due to an increase in the production of the hormone endorphin during or following exercise.

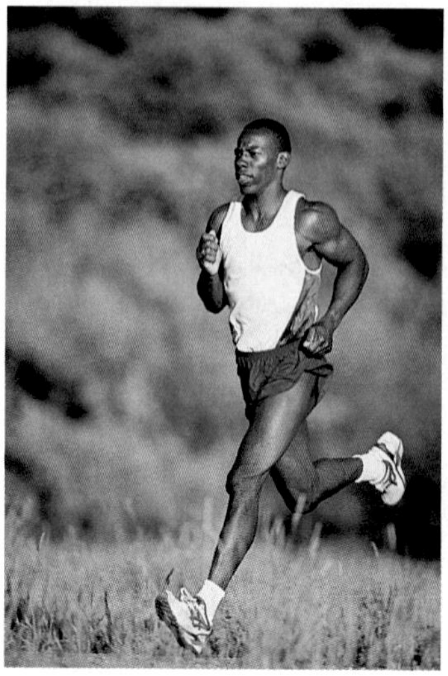

The so-called "runner's high"—a feeling of euphoria—can come after a half hour or so of running.

the hormone **endorphin,** which is thought to cause a feeling of euphoria. This can take place after about thirty minutes of running. Other types of physical activity can induce an endorphin release as well.

The mental health benefits of exercise are clearly shown in the psychological well-being scores of a group of participants in a twelve-week exercise class that met three times a week. According to researchers from the Department of Sports and Leisure Studies at the University of Connecticut, the participants, who were thirty-six years old on average, reported having less anxiety, greater job satisfaction, and/or better self-esteem after the twelve weeks. In contrast, a control group of people who did not participate in the exercise class reported having more anxiety, less job satisfaction, and/or reduced feelings of self-esteem over the same twelve-week period.

The Fitness Triangle

The goal of an exercise program is physical fitness. When you think of being physically fit, what do you have in mind? Having muscles? Being able to swim 100 laps or lift 100 pounds? Actually, **physical fitness** is a measure of how efficiently your body works. **Strength, flexibility,** and **endurance** are three major components of fitness that contribute both to the level of exercise performance and to health (see Figure 6.3). These components dynamically interact to ensure that an individual is able to:

- Meet the day-to-day demands for movement of the body.
- Have a reserve available for unexpected events requiring movement.
- Reduce the risk of certain chronic and degenerative diseases.

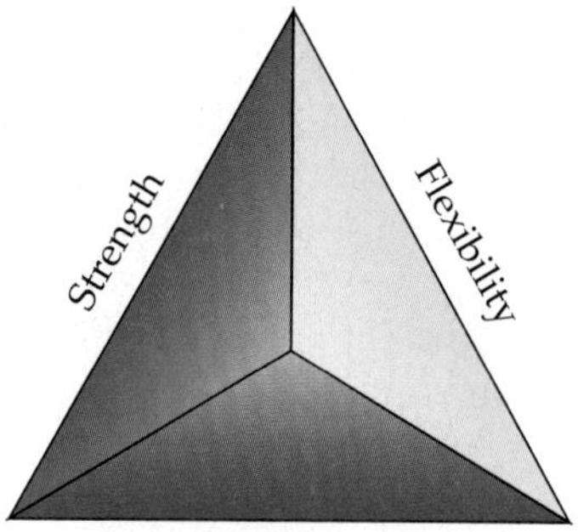

Figure 6.3 The Fitness Triangle
Strength, flexibility, and endurance are three major components of fitness.

endorphin A hormone produced in the brain that helps give a sense of pleasure and satisfaction.

physical fitness How efficiently the body works as measured by strength, flexibility, and endurance.

strength The extent to which an individual is capable of exerting force in one effort, as needed.

flexibility The range of movement an individual can achieve around a joint or group of joints.

endurance The ability to exercise vigorously at a sustained level for a period of time.

absolute strength The total force that an individual can exert when flexing muscles; usually measured in pounds.

relative strength A measure of strength determined by dividing absolute strength by body weight.

isokinetic exercise An exercise in which there are slow-moving contractions throughout a full range of movement against a constant resistance.

Strength

Strength is the extent to which you are capable of exerting force as needed. For example, if you are riding a bicycle, you must be able to exert enough force against the pedals to sustain movement. Most of us have enough strength to ride a bicycle but not enough to bench-press a heavy weight. You do not have to be a weight lifter to be considered physically fit. You need only enough strength to respond to the day-to-day demands on your body.

Strength is measured in many ways. **Absolute strength** refers to the total force exerted in one effort—for example, lifting a 100-pound weight. This can be an important factor in sports such as football, baseball, and bowling. **Relative strength** takes the effect of body size into account. Larger people generally have larger muscles and therefore tend to have more absolute strength than do smaller people. Relative strength is determined by dividing absolute strength by body weight. Gymnastics is an example of a sport in which relative strength is more important than absolute strength. Generally, women do not have as much strength as men do. In part, this is due to the fact that about 45 percent of men's body weight is muscle whereas women's bodies are about 36 percent muscle.

Three types of exercise contribute to strength development. **Isokinetic exercise** involves slow-moving contractions throughout a full range of movement against a constant resistance. This form of exercise requires spe-

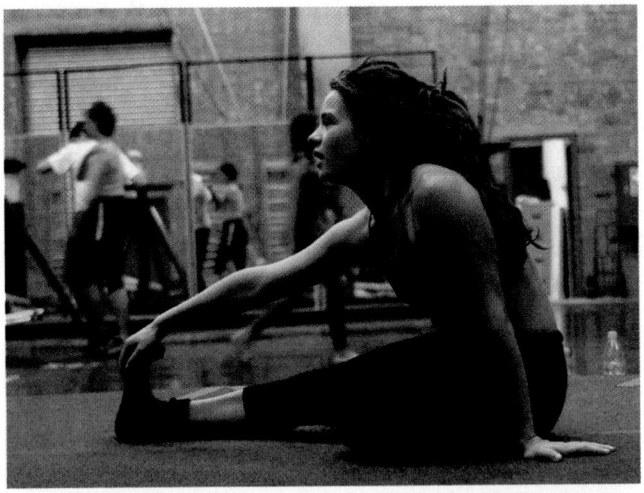

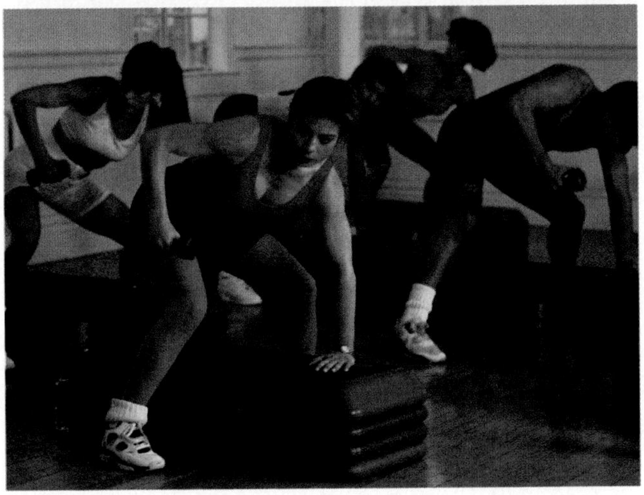

Stretching helps develop flexibility, while weight training helps tone muscles and increase muscular strength.

cial heavy equipment in a gym. **Isotonic exercise** involves contracting muscles against a movable resistance, as in lifting weights. **Isometric exercise** involves muscle contractions performed against an immovable object, such as a wall. No special equipment is needed for isometric exercise.

In recent years, a great deal of publicity has focused on the use of anabolic steroids to build strength and enhance athletic performance. While these drugs can contribute to the development of body mass and strength, the adverse health effects far outweigh the benefits of taking them. People who use steroids are at higher risk for heart attacks and liver cancer as well as some physically unattractive effects, such as acne and breast development in men. The best advice is to avoid the nonmedical use of steroids. (For more on steroids and other drugs, see Chapter 8.)

Flexibility

Flexibility is the range of movement an individual can achieve around a joint or group of joints. It is usually determined by muscle elasticity. A physically fit person is flexible enough to meet the day-to-day demands for movement of the joints, from reaching for a book on a high shelf to serving a tennis ball.

Good muscular elasticity can increase your agility and your speed, but more importantly, it can reduce your chance of injury to muscles, tendons, and ligaments. Flexibility appears to decrease with age in sedentary people, but there is some consensus among exercise physiologists that flexibility does not decrease significantly in people who do stretching exercises regularly.

Endurance and Aerobic Capacity

Endurance is a term for the ability to exercise vigorously at a sustained level for a period of time. A fit person can maintain vigorous activity for at least 20 minutes without taking a break. **Aerobic capacity** is the best way to measure whether you can meet the physiological demands of strenuous exercise. It is usually expressed as maximal oxygen uptake, or VO_2 max. By evaluating how much oxygen you use in a minute, an exercise physiologist can measure your body's respiratory and circulatory ability to support exercise.

Aerobic (meaning "with oxygen") is short for aerobic metabolism, a process of energy production through which carbohydrates, fats, and proteins are used to produce energy, and carbon dioxide and water are given off as by-products. Because the cells of the body continuously produce energy, aerobic metabolism is under way even when you are sleeping. Aerobic activities include those that can be maintained continuously through rhythmical and repetitive motions. Activities such as running, swimming, biking, walking, dancing, and jumping rope are aerobic exercises. In a fit person, the body's respiratory and circulatory systems can keep up with the muscles' demand

isotonic exercise An exercise involving the contraction of muscles against a movable resistance.

isometric exercise An exercise involving the contraction of muscles performed against an immovable object.

aerobic capacity The largest volume of oxygen that your body can consume in one minute; also called maximal oxygen uptake, or VO_2 max.

aerobic To be "with oxygen"; the process of energy production through which carbohydrates, fats, and proteins are used to produce energy and carbon dioxide and water are given off as by-products.

for oxygen during aerobic exercise, thus allowing nutrients to metabolize to meet energy needs.

Aerobic capacity is not a fixed point: It can change for better or worse depending on how much and how often you exercise. If you exercise regularly, you can maintain your aerobic capacity and perhaps even increase it. If you stop exercising regularly, your aerobic capacity decreases. (You can regain it, once you exercise regularly again.) Smoking adversely affects aerobic capacity. It decreases the amount of air that can be taken into the lungs as well as the amount of oxygen the blood can carry.

Anaerobic (meaning "without oxygen") refers to the process of energy production in which surges of energy are needed for a brief amount of time. Sprinting and weight lifting are examples of anaerobic exercise. The respiratory and circulatory systems cannot keep up with the demand for oxygen during anaerobic exercise.

Very strenuous anaerobic exercise contributes to muscle strength but does little to enhance cardiovascular health. This is primarily due to the short duration of anaerobic activity. The body simply does not endure anaerobic exercise for periods lasting longer than one or two minutes. Exhaustion is reached, causing an immediate and involuntary reduction in exercise intensity. Both aerobic and anaerobic exercises contribute to the fitness of an individual, but aerobic exercise is much more valuable from an overall health perspective.

Fitness Through Exercise

Exercise is bodily movement undertaken to improve or maintain one or more of the components of physical fitness. A planned exercise program has three components: intensity, duration, and frequency. According to the National Health Interview Survey, most Americans do not know how vigorously, how long, and how often they should exercise in order to achieve an appropriate level of activity.

anaerobic To be "without oxygen"; the process of energy production in which surges of energy are needed for a brief amount of time.

exercise intensity The degree of energy that is exerted during exercise.

heart rate The number of heartbeats per minute.

exercise duration The length of time a person exercises.

exercise frequency How often an exercise is done.

resting heart rate The number of heart beats per minute in a resting state.

Exercise intensity refers to how hard you exercise. Exercise should be intense enough to be effective but not so intense as to be unsafe for you. For an exercise session to be effective, you need to stimulate your heart, lungs, and muscles to work beyond their normal resting state. You can achieve this state without straining your muscles or forcing your heart to the point of maximum output. The best overall indicator of exercise intensity is **heart rate.** As exercise intensity increases, so does the heart rate, or the number of heartbeats per minute. You can monitor your intensity of exercise by monitoring your heart rate.

Exercise duration refers to how long a person exercises. It is directly related to the intensity of exercise as well. **Exercise frequency** means how often an exercise is done. Because the purpose of exercise is to improve or maintain cardiorespiratory fitness, exercise should be done frequently enough to accomplish this purpose. According to the Surgeon General, the best advice concerning duration and frequency is to work out at your target heart rate at least three times per week for thirty minutes. Not all exercise physiologists believe that such a rigorous exercise plan is necessary to gain health benefits. There is agreement, however, that such a plan is well within the ability of most people and represents a reasonable target for exercise frequency and duration. (See how to calculate your target heart rate on page 87.)

If you're just beginning an exercise program, you might want to consider walking. Read the Developing Health Skills box to learn about the exercise intensity, duration, and frequency involved in a walking program for becoming fit.

Monitoring Your Exercise Intensity

A practical health skill, and one that you may use nearly every day, is measuring your heart rate. The heart is the muscular pump that circulates blood throughout the body. Each contraction, or beat, produces pressure inside the arteries that causes blood flow and thus the delivery of energy-producing nutrients to the cells.

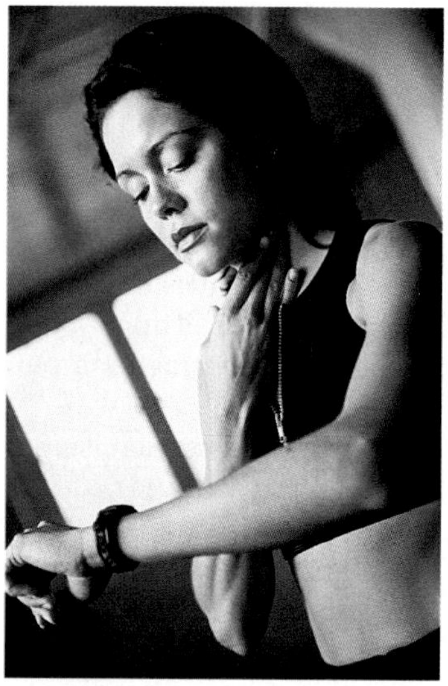

Learning how to take your pulse is a practical skill to learn. You can use it to measure your heart rate before and after exercise to determine your exercise intensity and to monitor one of your vital statistics.

At rest, a normal person's heart beats anywhere from 60 to 100 times per minute. This number is called the **resting heart rate.**

Developing Health Skills

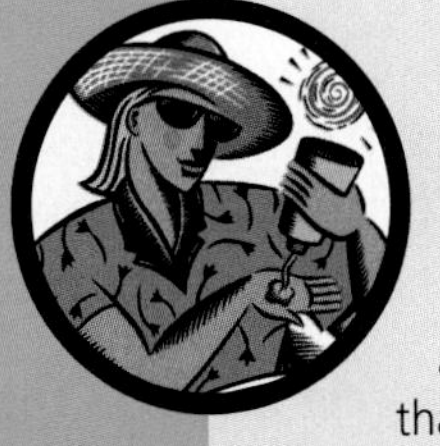

Starting Out: A Walking Program

What is the simplest, safest, least expensive exercise? Walking. Research has shown that walking at speeds of between 3.5 and 5 miles an hour—that's brisk walking, not strolling—produces cardiovascular benefits. A woman of average size can walk comfortably at brisk speeds of between 3.5 and 4 miles an hour and the average man can walk between 4.5 and 5 miles an hour. Slower walking (2 miles an hour) can be advantageous for older people, cardiac patients, or people recuperating from an illness. Walking at a speed of 5 miles an hour can burn as many calories as moderate jogging, but even slow walking can burn 60 to 80 calories per mile. If weight control is one of your primary goals, a minimum of 30 minutes three times a week is required for significant results.

Here are tips for a walking program:

1. Find a partner. Walking is an excellent social activity that can be done almost anywhere. Social support will help you adhere to your program and make it more enjoyable.
2. Wear a pair of shoes that provide a comfortable fit, adequate support, and cushioning.
3. Your walking style should be relaxed and efficient. To increase your pace, swing your arms more and maintain a heel-to-toe foot plant.
4. In order to experience an aerobic benefit, your exercise heart rate should be elevated to between 110 and 120 beats per minute for a minimum of twenty to thirty minutes.
5. The use of small hand weights (between 1 and 5 pounds) can increase your workload and provide muscular conditioning to the arms and shoulders. To avoid possible shoulder injury, it is important not to exaggerate your movements by swinging your arms across your body or by using weights that are too heavy.

A physically fit individual has a resting heart rate in the lower range, whereas an unfit individual has a higher resting heart rate. People who do aerobic exercises for at least thirty minutes three times per week experience what is called a **training effect.** The exercises actually train the heart to be more efficient—to pump more blood per stroke. The training effect of regular exercise can result in a decline in resting heart rate by as much as twenty beats per minute.

Your heart rate is most easily measured by taking (counting) your pulse. To take your pulse, place your index and middle fingers lightly over an artery at the wrist or neck. The throbs you feel correspond exactly to the beats of the heart. To measure your resting heart rate, the number of beats per minute at a resting state, use a digital watch or a watch with a second hand to count the throbs for ten seconds and multiply by six. The resulting number is the number of beats your heart makes every minute. To be more accurate, take two or three measures of your resting heart rate and calculate an average.

Maximal heart rate denotes the highest number of beats per minute that may safely be achieved during an exercise period. The maximal heart rate for a healthy person is about 220 minus his or her age. This is true for about 70 percent of the U.S. population. Exercise physiologists know that a training effect is accomplished by raising the heart rate during exercise to between 60 percent and 80 percent of the maximal heart rate. This means that for a healthy twenty-year-old—a typical college student—the average maximal heart rate is 200 beats per minute, and a training effect is achieved at between 120 and 160 beats per minute.

Achieving a training effect is the goal of an exercise period, thus the term **target heart rate range** is used to denote heart activity high enough to bring about a training effect and low enough to be safe. The target heart rate range of the typical college student is between 120 beats per minute and two-hundred beats per minute. What is your target heart rate?

To determine your approximate target heart rate range, complete the following formula:

Step 1: 220 – ________ = ________________
(your age) (maximal heart rate)

Step 2: ________ × 0.60 = ________________
(maximal heart rate) (lowest heart rate for exercising)

Step 3: ________ × 0.80 = ________________
(maximal heart rate) (highest heart rate for exercising)

training effect Health benefits, most notably increased heart efficiency, produced by exercising for a sufficient duration and intensity.

maximal heart rate The maximum number of heartbeats per minute that should be reached during exercise; usually equal to 220 minus the person's age.

target heart rate range Heart activity high enough to bring about a training effect and low enough to be safe.

The range between the lowest and highest heart rate for exercising will provide a training effect. If a training program is designed for weight reduction, it may surprise you to know, it should aim to achieve a training effect toward the *lower* end of the heart rate range.

Planning and Maintaining a Personal Fitness Program

One place to start in personalizing your fitness program is with a complete physical examination conducted by a physician. This is essential for anyone over age thirty-five, but can be important regardless of age. Once you get the go-ahead from your physician, you are ready to measure your fitness level.

There are two important reasons for measuring fitness before beginning a new fitness program:

- Unknown physical problems can be detected in order to design a modified program that will reduce risk.
- Baseline data can be established so that progress can be measured.

The skill of measuring your fitness level will be valuable not only now but also for the rest of your life because your fitness level will no doubt change. A skill as simple as measuring your heart rate, for example, can provide a means of monitoring such change. As you become more fit, the readings on your heart rate assessment will likely go down. After a period of not exercising, you may discover that your heart rate rises. You may also seek professional help and have clinical assessments to monitor change.

Three Phases of Exercise: Warm-Up, Conditioning, and Cool-Down

An exercise session, often referred to as a workout, always involves three segments: the warm-up, the conditioning period, and the cool-down.

During the **warm-up period,** no effort is made to achieve target heart rate. Rather, its purpose is to prepare the body for the exertion that will soon follow. More importantly, the warm-up period is a means of avoiding unnecessary injury and may be related to a reduction in muscle soreness.

When the body warms up, muscle fibers and tendons become more fluid and stretch more easily. The warm-up should consist of jogging in place, riding a stationary bicycle, or stretching exercises (see the Developing Health Skills box). When stretching, take care not to bounce. Bouncing during a stretch can tear muscle fibers. Instead, slowly stretch the muscle and maintain that position for ten to thirty seconds. Start off slowly. Experts say that stretching when muscles are cold could result in injury.

How long should a warm-up last? A good sign that the body is ready for more intense exercise is when body temperature increases by one and a half to two degrees, which is usually the point at which you begin to sweat. About five to ten minutes of warm-up may be sufficient, but it may take as much as fifteen to twenty minutes.

The **conditioning period** varies greatly from individual to individual. For a beginner, the conditioning period may consist of alternating brisk walking and leisurely walking. Someone slightly more fit may alternate periods of jogging and walking. For the fit individual, vigorous exercise sustained for thirty minutes is appropriate. Always remember that a conditioning period is tailored to personal ability and needs. Fitness results from regular exercise, not extreme exertion. Therefore, it is more important to exercise regularly than to exercise vigorously. With regular exercise, the ability for vigorous exercise will increase.

An often overlooked segment of an exercise period is the **cool-down period.** This involves reducing the intensity of exercise to allow the body to recover partially from the conditioning period. During vigorous exercise such as jogging, a lot of blood is pumped to the legs, and there may not be enough to supply the heart and brain. Failure to cool down properly may result in dizziness, fainting, and in rare instances, a heart attack. Walking and stretching are common cool-down activities. In fact, the same procedures used in the warm-up are appropriate for the cool-down. By reducing the level of physical exertion gradually, blood flow is redirected back to the heart and brain.

How long should you cool down? Again, as with the warm-up, about five to ten minutes may be sufficient, but a longer cool-down may be necessary, particularly in warm weather.

warm-up period The period of exercise in which the body becomes prepared for exertion.

conditioning period The period of exercise in which a training effect is reached and maintained.

cool-down period The period of exercise in which the intensity of exercise is reduced to allow the body to recover partially from the conditioning period.

Raising Your Safety Consciousness

Despite the benefits of exercise, you need to recognize some risks before embarking on a program. A host of injuries can be attributed to overzealous exercise.

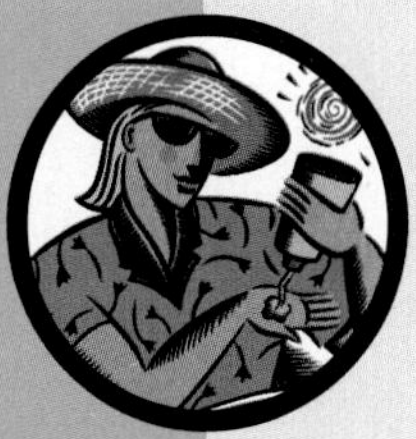

The Basic Stretching Session

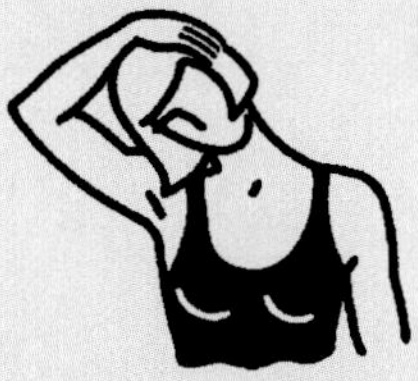

1. **Neck Stretch.** Tilt head to right, keeping shoulders down. Place right hand on left side of head. Gently pull head toward right shoulder and hold for 10 to 30 seconds. Switch sides and repeat.

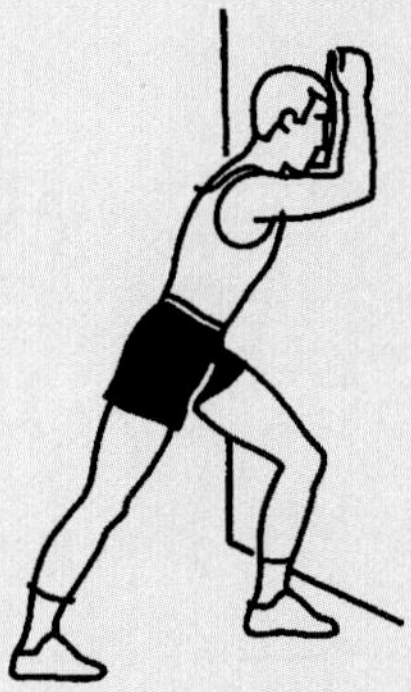

2. **Calf Stretch** (for gastrocnemius and soleus muscles). Stand 2 to 3 feet from a wall, with feet perpendicular to wall in the position shown, and lean against wall for 10 to 30 seconds. Keep feet parallel to each other; make sure rear heel stays on floor. Switch legs and repeat. Variation: keep rear knee slightly bent during stretch.

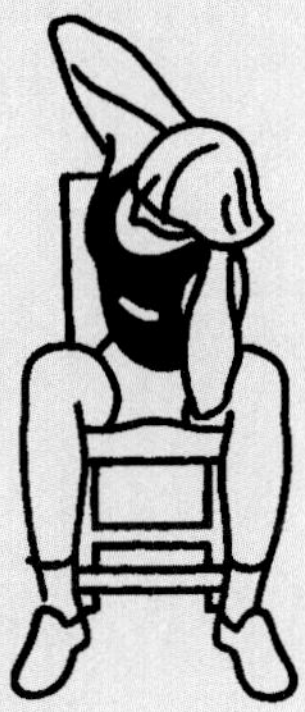

3. **Spinal Stretch**. Sit in a chair with your back straight, feet firmly on floor, toes pointing up slightly. Lock hands behind head, with elbows out and chin down. Contract abdominal muscles. To loosen up, twist upper body to one side as far as you can, then repeat 4 times in the same direction. The last time, rotate, hold, and then flex your torso forward, leaning toward floor with elbow. Hold for 2 seconds. Return to upright position. Repeat 8 to 10 times. Do same routine on other side.

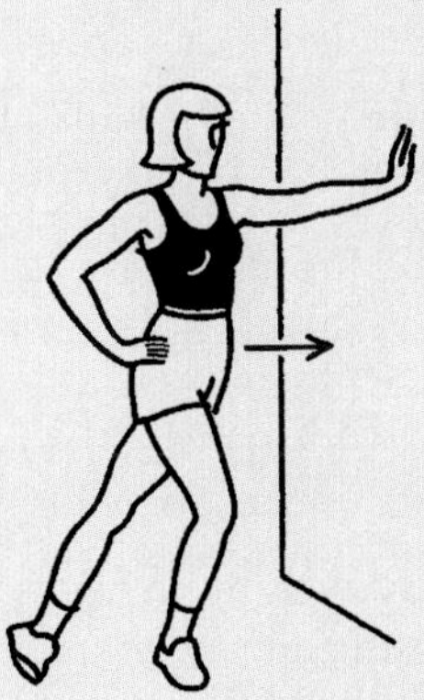

4. **Outer Thigh Stretch** (for iliotibial band). Placing left hand against wall for balance, place left foot behind and beyond right foot. Bend left ankle and lean into wall. Hold for 10 to 30 seconds, then switch and repeat.

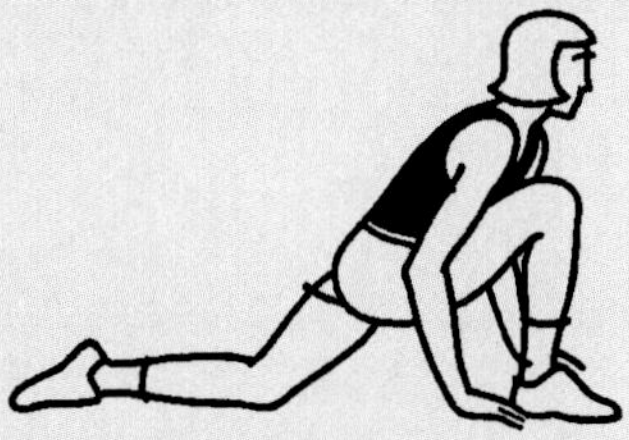

5. **Hip Stretch** (for hip flexor). From a kneeling position, bring right foot forward until knee is directly over ankle; keep right foot straight. Rest left knee on floor behind you. Leaning into front knee, lower pelvis and front of left hip toward floor to create an easy stretch. Hold for 10 to 30 seconds, then switch legs and repeat.

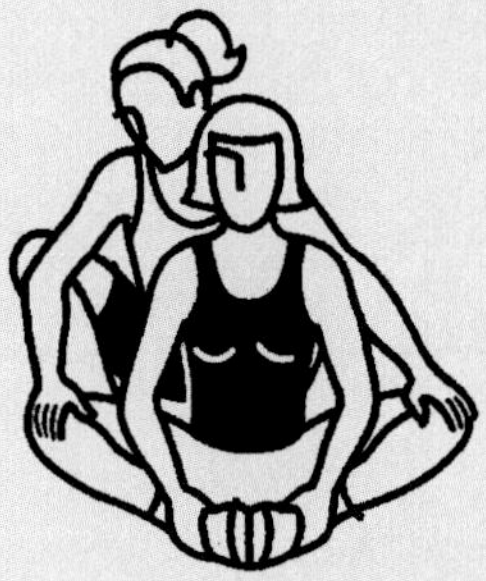

6. **Butterfly Stretch** (for adductor muscles in groin). Sit on floor, bringing heels together near groin and holding feet together by the ankles. Have a partner gently push your knees down; hold for 5 seconds. Try to bring your knees upward as partner provides resistance. Relax, then have partner gently push down again for a greater stretch. Repeat. You can do the first part without a partner, simply by lowering your knees as far as possible.

7. **Thigh Stretch** (for quadriceps, in front of thigh). Lie on stomach. Have a partner grasp your lower leg and bend it until you feel the stretch on front of thigh. While partner provides resistance, try to push leg back for 3 to 5 seconds. Relax while partner bends your leg again until you feel a stretch again. Switch legs.

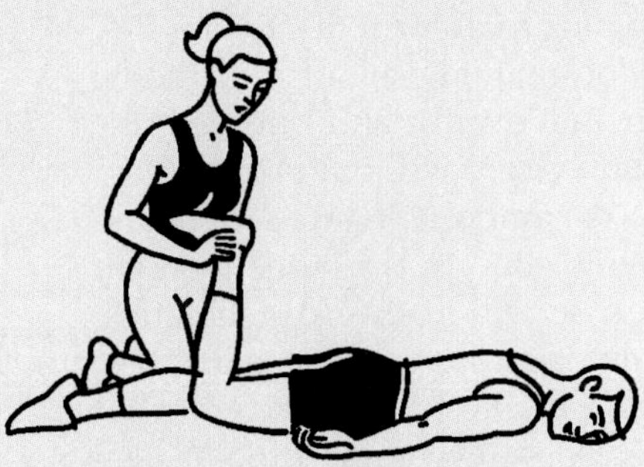

(continued on following page)

8. **Crossover Stretch** (for lower back). Lying on back, bend left knee at 90° and extend arms out to sides. Place right hand on left thigh and pull that bent knee over right leg. Keeping head on floor, turn to look toward outstretched left arm. Pull bent left knee toward floor; keep shoulders flat on floor. Hold for 10 to 30 seconds, then switch sides and repeat.

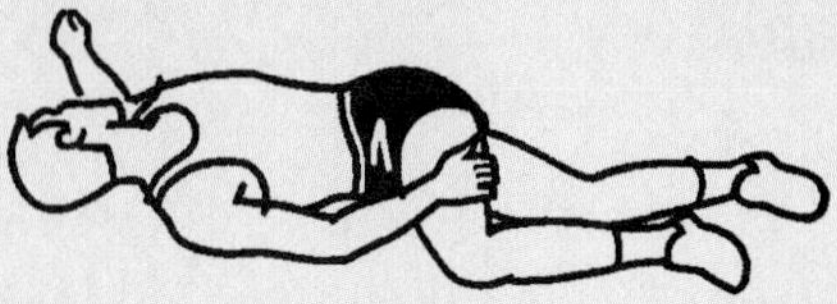

9. **Thigh Stretch** (for hamstrings, in back of thigh). Lie on back. Place a rope loosely around sole of one foot, grasping both ends with both hands. Contracting front of thigh, lift that leg as high as possible, aiming your foot toward the ceiling. "Climb" hand over hand up the looped rope to lift your leg gently, keeping upper body on floor. Keeping tension on the rope and using it for gentle assistance, hold stretch for 2 seconds. Don't pull your leg into position—that can

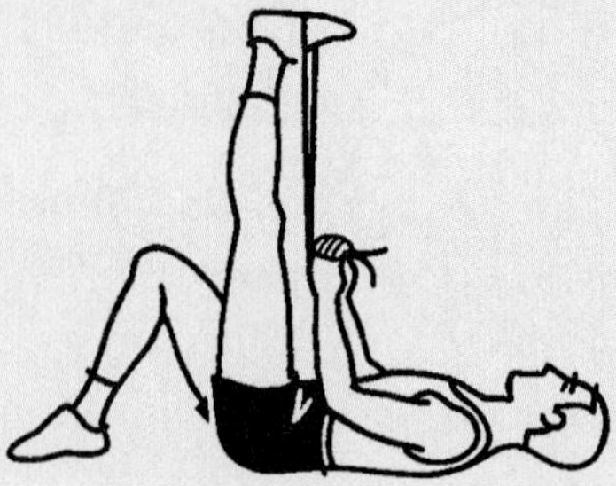

cause knee problems. Repeat 8 to 10 times, then switch legs.

10. **Lumbar Stretch** (for lower back). Lying on back, clasp one hand under each knee. Gently pull both knees toward chest, keeping lower back on floor. Hold for 10 to 30 seconds, relax, then repeat.

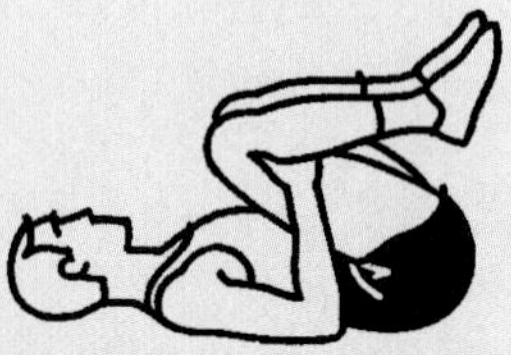

Source: www.wellnessletter.com UC Berkeley Wellness Letter, © December 1998. Susan Blubaugh, illustrator

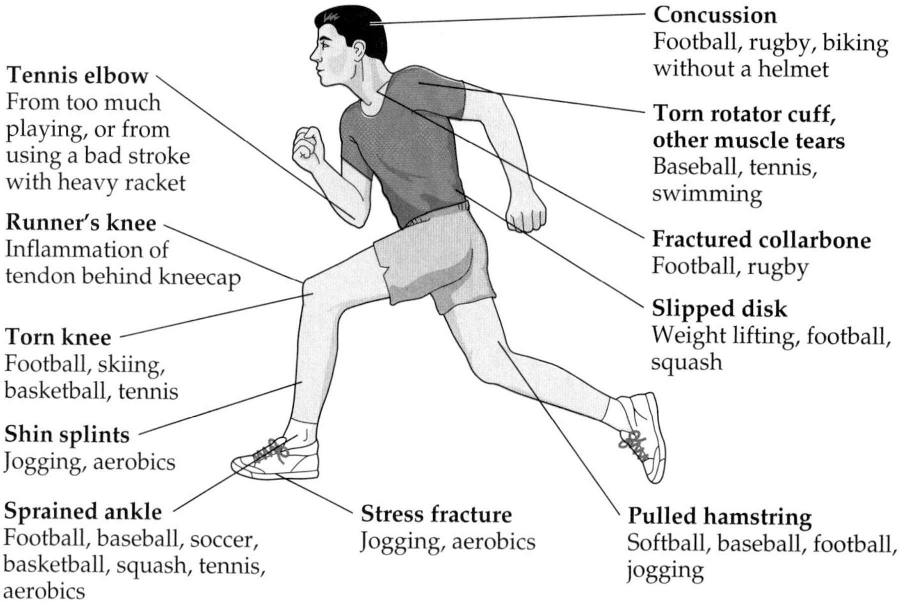

Figure 6.4 Train, Don't Strain
Injuries, such as muscle strains and stress fractures, can bring your exercise program to a standstill.

When designing your personal exercise program, remember the saying, "Train, don't strain." Initiating a strenuous exercise program too fast can produce injuries such as muscle strains and stress fractures that can bring your exercise program to a standstill. Figure 6.4 points out common athletic and exercise injuries along with the sports with which each is associated. For some injuries, simple first-aid treatment can help. Resist the urge to return to your usual form of exercise until the injured part of your body can move fully and support the usual weight without pain.

An important but still unanswered concern is whether regular exercise will lead to degenerative joint disease, or osteoarthritis. Many biomechanical factors may predispose exercisers to joint disease. When a runner leaves the ground momentarily, the leg he or she lands on has to absorb a load two to three times the body weight. When a tennis or basketball player leaps in the air, he or she lands with a force of up to seven times the body weight.

Poor consumer decisions can result in injury. Jogging or walking in improper shoes, for example, can produce injuries to the feet, ankles, and knees. Exercising in cold weather in inappropriate attire can

hypothermia A loss of body temperature that can result in mental confusion, unconsciousness, and death.

result in frostbite and **hypothermia,** a loss of body temperature that can lead to mental confusion, unconsciousness, and in extreme cases, death.

Another safety issue relates to hydration. It is important to drink enough water before, during, and after strenuous exercise. In hot weather, experts advise to not go for more than twenty minutes without drinking water, and to drink even if you do not feel thirsty. Fluids are needed in the winter, as well, since colder air is drier air, and water is lost with each breath. More than a quart of water may be lost in a day of skiing or snowshoeing.

Perhaps one of the most important safety precautions for joggers and bikers is to wear reflective gear when running or biking at night. Bicycling accidents cause approximately 1,300 deaths and 60,000 injuries a year. Head trauma is the most frequent cause of death in these cases. Wearing a helmet, using hand signals, and abiding by traffic laws can result in safer exercise programs on bicycles. (See Chapter 9 for more about unintentional injuries.) As with most health-promoting behavior, the watchwords for a safe exercise program are moderation and common sense.

Patience and Adherence

Few quick results can be expected from a program of physical activity. Over time, however, you will notice clear evidence of improved fitness. Therefore, be patient. How long do you have to wait to see results? This varies from individual to individual, but younger exercisers will see evidence of improved fitness levels more quickly than will older exercisers. Establishing baseline data on your strength, flexibility, and aerobic capacity before exercising can help you monitor subtle and otherwise not visible improvements in your fitness level. This will help reinforce your adherence to a fitness program.

For a variety of reasons—including a mismatch between the person and the activity—more than 50 percent of exercisers do not adhere to an exercise program for more than twelve months. The key to success is finding the right match with an exercise activity that you will enjoy and continue to do. Sometimes, this involves a period of experimentation. Care also needs to be taken to design an exercise program that fits the time you have available—or are willing to make available—and that will meet your expectations for short-term and long-term effects.

Tactics for Maintaining a Fitness Program

Here are some tips on how to create a fitness program that works for you.

- Choose an activity that you like and that you feel competent and safe doing.
- Set a regular time and place for your exercise. Make sure it is easily accessible to you on a regular basis.
- Establish realistic goals that you can achieve.
- Choose an exercise program that fits your schedule and your budget.
- Alternate the physical activities you do—brisk walking one day, swimming another.
- Be aware of physical activities you can do as part of your day-to-day living, such as cleaning your room or walking up and down the stairs.
- Don't overdo it. Avoid injury by gradually working up to fitness.
- Feel good about what you are doing. Reward yourself when you reach significant goals.
- Guard against giving yourself excuses for not exercising, such as, "I'm too busy."

The Surgeon General's *Report on Physical Activity and Health* suggests that people who are usually inactive can improve their health and well-being by becoming even moderately active on a regular basis. It also points out that physical activity need not be strenuous to achieve benefits. Moreover, it states that great health benefits can be achieved by increasing the duration, frequency, or intensity of physical activity. In other words, physical activity is well within the reach of everyone.

CASE STUDY 6: Fitness

Every weekend, Gilda is seen doing one sport activity or another—tennis, swimming, running, rollerblading. It may look like she is serious about her exercise program, but Gilda is a weekend warrior, doing all her exercise in one or two days a week. Because she does not exercise on a regular basis, she is not in shape for the 10K run or half-mile swim that she takes on the weekend. She often ends up with sore joints or blisters and wonders why. She sees herself as a jock. But in reality, Gilda has no true exercise plan for herself, and although she is active, she has no real commitment to fitness.

Toshio has an exercise plan, which he follows carefully. He meets the same group of friends to do brisk walking three mornings a week. No matter how busy he is, Toshio finds time for his walk because he knows that physical fitness results from frequency as much as from intensity. Throughout the day, Toshio builds in additional exercise. He takes the stairs rather than the elevator; he walks to an off-campus building rather than take the free shuttle bus. Toshio has clearly made a choice about his level of fitness. He has established a lifelong commitment to exercise.

In Your Opinion

Gilda and Toshio both look fit, as well they should. Each spends several hours a week in some form of exercise.

- What is wrong with Gilda's fitness program?
- Does it make her physically fit?
- Do you think she will still be fit ten years from now?
- What do you see Toshio doing in ten years?
- How is his current health style related to decisions concerning exercise that he made earlier in his life?

KEY CONCEPTS

1. Most Americans do not exercise on a regular basis, and of those who do, few exercise at the appropriate level of activity.
2. The benefits of regular exercise include reduced risk for coronary artery disease, hypertension, and osteoporosis and increased psychological well-being.
3. Exercisers report feeling better and having more energy and less trouble sleeping. Some evidence suggests that physically fit people learn better and stay mentally alert longer than those who are less fit.
4. Fitness involves the efficient use of muscles and bones to bring about movement, maintain posture, and sustain a healthy appearance.
5. Strength, flexibility, and endurance are three major components of fitness.
6. A planned exercise program has three components: desired intensity of exercise (how much), desired duration of exercise (how long), and frequency of exercise (how often).
7. A good measure of fitness is the resting heart rate. Physically fit individuals tend to have a lower resting heart rate than those who are less fit.
8. The best fitness programs are personalized and begin with a complete physical examination conducted by a physician.
9. An exercise session consists of the warm-up, the conditioning period, and the cool-down, three relatively distinct and important stages.
10. Few dramatic changes result from an exercise program. The health benefits of fitness develop over time.

REVIEW QUESTIONS

1. Describe the exercise pattern of most American adults.
2. Identify three chronic diseases associated with a sedentary lifestyle and explain the impact of exercise on each disease.
3. Support this statement: People who exercise regularly tend to feel better.
4. What are the three major components of fitness? Describe the types of exercise that develop each component.
5. Differentiate between isokinetic, isotonic, and isometric exercises.
6. Give examples of both aerobic and anaerobic activities.
7. How do exercise intensity, exercise duration, and exercise frequency affect the quality of an exercise session?
8. What is the difference between a resting heart rate, a maximal heart rate, and a target heart rate?
9. Why is a warm-up period important to an exercise plan? What about a cool-down period?
10. List several tactics for maintaining a fitness program.

CRITICAL THINKING QUESTIONS

1. *Healthy People 2010* established the following objective: "Reduce the proportion of adults who engage in no leisure-time physical activity." Baseline data show that 40 percent of adults aged 18 and older engage in no leisure-time physical activity. What can be done to change this? How can health educators, health promoters, and government officials encourage people to exercise during their leisure time?

2. How can psychological well-being be measured? If you were designing a study of how a person feels after exercise, how might you measure these feelings? How do you know that you can trust your information?
3. *Healthy People 2010* established the following objective: "Increase the proportion of adults who engage in vigorous physical activity that promotes the development and maintenance of cardiorespiratory fitness 3 or more days per week for twenty or more minutes per occasion." Three days per week, 20 minutes per day doesn't seem like much time. Why do you think so many Americans have difficulty being physically active for a total of only one hour per week? Are they too busy to be active? Do they dislike the effects of activity (e.g., sweat, heat, etc.)? Or are they simply uninformed about the value of physical activity?
4. New research indicates that individuals who know the risks of personal lifestyle factors are more inclined to change their behavior. Do you believe that knowing the risks of a sedentary life (i.e., increased heart disease, decreased psychological well-being) causes people to take part in physical activity? Or do people exercise because it is a popular thing to do?

JOURNAL ACTIVITIES

1. For a period of two weeks, chart your resting heart rate in a notebook. Do this by counting the number of times your heart beats in the two-minute period when you first awake in the morning (before you stand up from bed). At the end of the semester chart your resting heart rate again for two weeks. Did your overall fitness level improve or decline during the semester?
2. In the vicinity of your dorm or home, measure a walking or running course and identify mile markers. A marker of the first miles of your course might be an unusual tree that you pass; the marker for the second mile might be a building. As you undertake your walking or running programs this semester, make a mental note of how you feel each time you pass these markers. Do you feel better on days when you got plenty of sleep? Do you feel better as the semester and your exercise program progress? Can you feel your fitness level improving?
3. Interview several people to determine the role of exercise in their lives. From this information, make two lists: (1) the actual health values people derived from exercise and (2) the myths they believe about how exercise will help them. What percent of the people you interviewed exercise because they truly understand the health values they gain from it?
4. Make a list of health clubs in your community. Develop a comparative table of services offered at each location (e.g., aerobic dance, lap swimming). Then investigate similar services available at no charge, perhaps on your campus, at the local high school, or at another community facility.

SELECTED BIBLIOGRAPHY

American College of Sports Medicine Fitness Book. Champaign, IL: Human Kinetics Press, 1998.

American Heart Association. *Fitting in Fitness.* New York: Random House, 1997.

Anderson, R. E., et al. "Relationship of Physical Activity and Television Watching with Body Weight and Level of Fatness among Children: Results from the Third National Health and Nutrition Examination Survey." *Journal of the American Medical Association* 279 (1998): 938–942.

Journal of Physical Education, Recreation and Dance. Reston, VA: American Alliance for Health, Physical Education, Recreation and Dance (published monthly).

Pate, R. R., et al. "Physical Activity and Public Health: A Recommendation from the Centers for Disease Control and Prevention and the American College of Sports Medicine." *Journal of the American Medical Association 273,* 5 (1995): 402–407.

Physical Activity and Cardiovascular Health (Consensus Development Conference Statement). Bethesda, MD: National Institutes of Health, 1995.

Physical Activity and Health: A Report of the Surgeon General. Atlanta, GA: Centers for Disease Control and Prevention, 1996.

Powers, S., and S. Dodd. *Total Fitness.* Boston: Allyn & Bacon, 1999.

Research Quarterly for Exercise and Sport. Reston, VA: American Alliance for Health, Physical Education, Recreation and Dance (published quarterly).

HEALTHLINKS

Websites for Keeping Fit

You can access better health as it relates to this chapter by checking out some of the following sites on the Internet. These sites can be accessed directly from the *Decisions for Healthy Living* Website located at www.aw.com/pruitt.

American College of Sports Medicine Online

A link with the American College of Sports Medicine and all their resources.

American Alliance for Health, Physical Education, Recreation, and Dance

Home page for the national organization dedicated to the advancement of health, physical education, recreation, and dance education standards.

HEALTH HOTLINES

Keeping Fit

American Running Association
(800) 776-2732
4405 East-West Highway, Suite 405
Bethesda, MD 20814

Women's Sports Foundation
Information and Referral Service
(800) 227-3988
Eisenhower Park
East Meadow, NY 11554

TEST YOUR KNOWLEDGE ANSWERS

1. True. In fact, the greater the load borne during exercise, the greater the bone density. For example, weight lifters have greater bone density than swimmers.
2. True. The body simply cannot endure anaerobic exercise for periods lasting long enough to contribute to cardiovascular health.
3. False. The training effect of exercise is different for each individual. Some individuals achieve a training effect when the heart rate is raised to 150 to 160 beats per minute, while others require a much higher heart rate for the same training effect.
4. False. Exercise physiologists consistently recommend a warm-up period prior to vigorous movement to avoid injuries due to the strain of exercise. Stretching is an important element of the warm up, but stretching alone is not considered sufficient.
5. True. In fact, people who are usually inactive can improve their health and well-being by becoming even moderately active on a regular basis. The health benefits of physical activity are within everyone's reach.

CHAPTER 7

The Health Effects of Smoking and Drinking

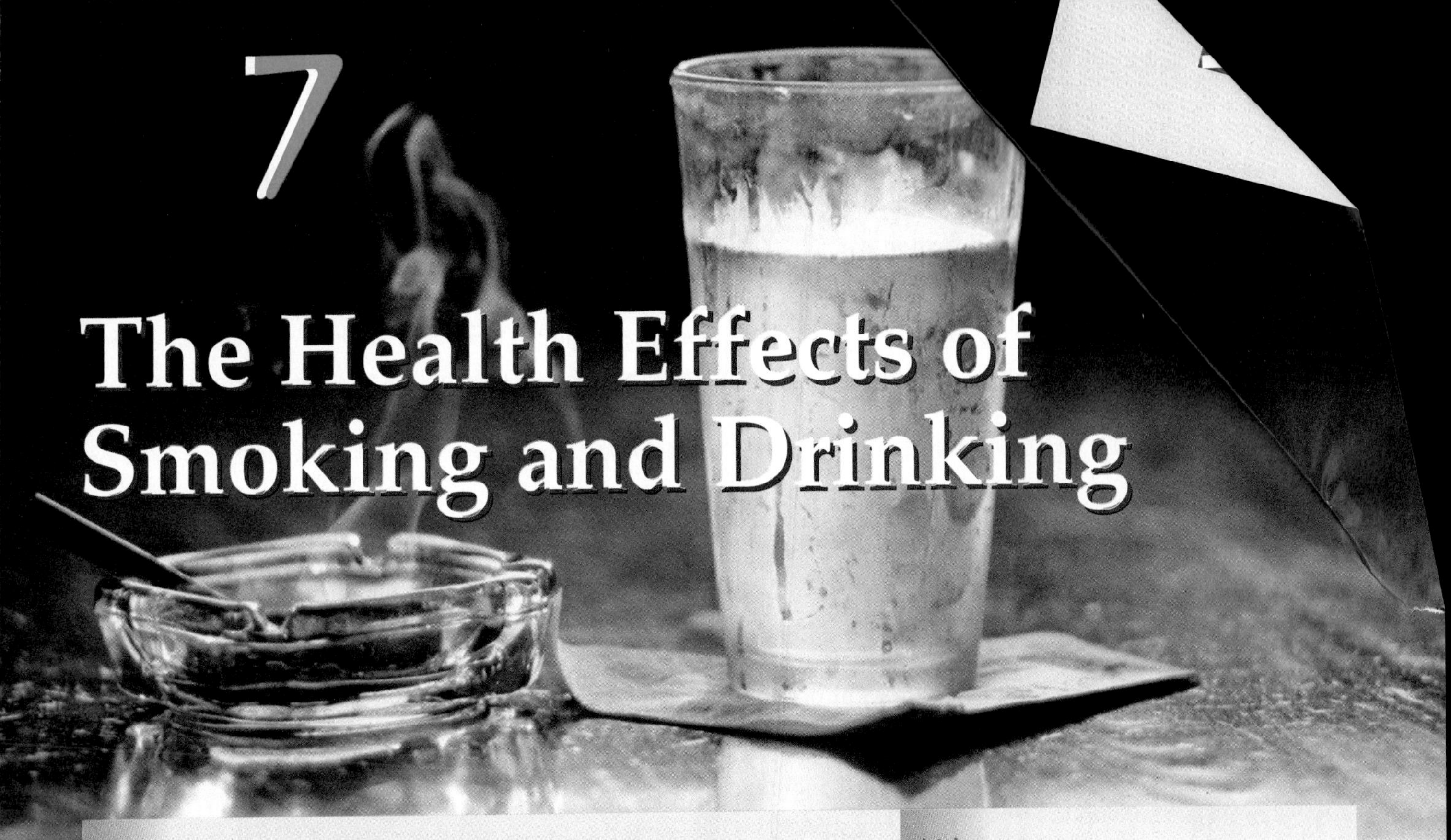

OBJECTIVES

When you finish reading this chapter, you will be able to:

1. Identify the similarities between addiction to tobacco and addiction to alcohol.
2. List three major components of cigarette smoke and identify the health risks of each.
3. Describe how tobacco use contributes to cancer, heart disease, and lung disease.
4. Differentiate and compare the effects of smoking and the use of smokeless tobacco.
5. List three means of smoking cessation and compare the advantages of each.
6. Describe the dangers of binge drinking.
7. Define alcoholism as a disease.
8. Differentiate between the occasional drinker, the social drinker, and the problem drinker.
9. Identify treatment options for alcoholism.
10. Explain how to avoid problem drinking. Include in your explanation the importance of social assertiveness skills.

TEST YOUR KNOWLEDGE

1. Nicotine reaches the brain in a matter of seconds after a smoker inhales. True or False?
2. College students smoke at a rate significantly lower than the general population with less than 10 percent having smoked in the last month. True or False?
3. Small amounts of alcohol may actually reduce the risk of heart attacks in both men and women. True or False?
4. The number of college students who abstain from drinking alcohol has declined steadily to less than 15 percent in 2002. True or False?
5. A single dose of alcohol, if large enough, can be lethal. True or False?

Answers found at end of chapter.

W…e think of **substance abuse,** they think of marijuana, cocaine, heroin, LSD, and a host of …iscussed in Chapter 8. But substance abuse also includes tobacco and alcohol, which cause …s, illnesses, and disabilities than any other preventable health condition. Smoking and **side-stream sm**… comes from the burning end of cigarettes, cause cancer and lung and heart disease. And while alcohol i… with an increased incidence of certain forms of cancer and liver disease, its greatest toll comes from th… and disabilities associated with alcohol-related motor vehicle accidents (see Chapter 9).

Wh… of such grim findings, does 24 percent of the adult population smoke? Why is binge drinking a major publ… problem on many college campuses? The reasons are myriad—from social to environmental to genetic. But …derlying reason is that the **nicotine** in tobacco and the **ethyl alcohol** (ethanol) in alcohol are addictive drugs.

Why People Smoke

Each day, more than three thousand American teenagers start smoking. More than 60 percent of seniors in high school have smoked at least once, according to national surveys. And by the time they are in college, at least one third report smoking in the last month. Young smokers also tend to be heavy smokers. Teenage smoking trends are important to future public health, because 90 percent of smokers pick up the habit—the **addiction**—in adolescence (in contrast to adulthood). Teenagers also are more likely to become heavy smokers than are those who begin smoking as adults.

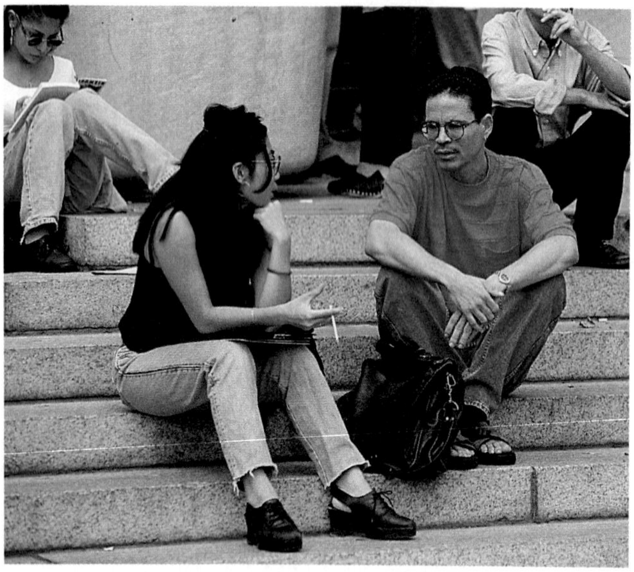

Despite the negative health effects, smoking among young people continues to pose a serious problem. By the time they are ready for college, more than 60 percent of high school seniors have smoked at least once.

Addiction to Nicotine

Once they start smoking cigarettes, people continue because they are addicted to the nicotine in them. Within seconds after a smoker inhales a cigarette, nicotine reaches the brain. Over time, a chemical change takes place that causes the smoker to feel the need for additional nicotine. As with addiction to other drugs, such as cocaine and heroin, people who have a **nicotine addiction** smoke in spite of the clear harm. They talk about the desire to quit, but the addiction makes it difficult for them to do so. Those who do quit go through withdrawal—that is, they develop **withdrawal symptoms** such as irritability.

Many smokers say, "It's just tobacco—not a drug." But the nicotine in tobacco is a drug, and addiction to nicotine has the same characteristics as alcohol and heroin addiction.

Primary Characteristics of Tobacco, Alcohol, and Drug Addiction

- The individual displays a highly controlled or compulsive pattern of use.
- The individual experiences **psychoactive** or mood-altering effects from use.
- The individual finds that use leads to further use.

Additional Characteristics of Tobacco, Alcohol, and Drug Addiction

- The user experiences **tolerance** (increased doses are either tolerated without discomfort or are needed to achieve desired effects).
- The individual experiences physical **dependence** (he or she cannot live comfortably without it).
- The individual uses the substance(s) despite harmful effects.

- The individual experiences a relapse following abstinence.
- The individual experiences recurrent cravings.

Influence from Family, Peers, and Advertising

Typically, children first become exposed to smoking at home or through friends. Children of smoking parents are more likely to smoke than are children of nonsmoking parents. Studies consistently support the notion that peers also play an important role in the questions of whether to smoke and whether to use smokeless or chewing tobacco. Smoking teenagers are more likely to have friends who smoke than are nonsmoking teenagers.

An even greater influence on teenagers is cigarette advertising. A study published in the *Journal of the National Cancer Institute* found that teens are twice as likely to be influenced to smoke by cigarette ads as by peer pressure.

The Components of Cigarette Smoke

Each time a smoker inhales a cigarette, he or she gets a dose of nicotine, tar, carbon monoxide, hydrogen cyanide, and other dangerous particles and gases. Overall, tobacco smoke contains more than four thousand separate substances, many of which have some biological activity. At least forty-three are known to be **carcinogens**—that is, agents capable of causing cancer. The following are the three primary harmful ingredients in tobacco smoke.

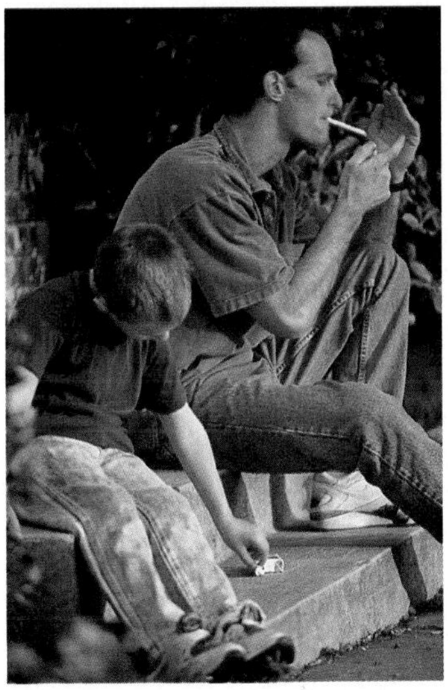

Many children first become exposed to smoking at home. Teenagers are more likely to smoke if their parents do.

Nicotine

The major reason nicotine is harmful is that it is the ingredient in tobacco smoke that causes addiction. For smokers who inhale, 90 percent of the nicotine is absorbed in the bloodstream. Even if you don't smoke, nicotine can get into your bloodstream if you are exposed to sidestream smoke. Nicotine causes the heart to beat faster and coronary blood flow and blood pressure to increase. These effects create additional oxygen requirements by the heart muscle and are associated with increased risk of a heart attack.

Tar

Tar is the gummy mixture left over from burning tobacco. It consists of more than two hundred chemicals and is the most carcinogenic substance in cigarettes. Smoking damages the cilia, which are hairlike structures in the respiratory system that sweep debris, such as tar, out of the lungs. With the cilia damaged, tar and other debris can easily enter the lungs and remain there. Tar also affects the respiratory system by blocking the normal action of mucus. As a result, foreign materials are not screened from the lungs and irritants attack lung tissue.

Carbon Monoxide

Most of the compounds in cigarette smoke are gaseous, and many of them are toxic. By far the most hazardous of these gases is **carbon monoxide,** the same gas that is

substance abuse Patterns of increasing levels of use of tobacco, alcohol, and other drugs that result in health consequences or impairment in social, psychological, and/or occupational functioning.

sidestream smoke The smoke originating from the burning end of the cigarette between puffs, which adversely affects the health of individuals nearby.

nicotine The ingredient in tobacco smoke that causes addiction.

ethyl alcohol The ingredient in alcohol that causes addiction; also called ethanol.

addiction A strong desire or need to continue using tobacco, alcohol, or another drug.

nicotine addiction The state of being physically and emotionally dependent on nicotine.

withdrawal symptoms The symptoms ranging from mild discomfort to very traumatic events when a person stops taking a drug.

psychoactive Affecting the mind or behavior.

tolerance The progressive change in the body's reaction to tobacco, alcohol, or another drug, causing an individual to need more and more of the drug to achieve the same effect.

dependence A condition in which a person is so physically and/or psychologically attached to a drug that he or she cannot live comfortably without it.

carcinogen An agent capable of causing cancer.

tar The most carcinogenic substance in cigarettes; the gummy mixture left over from burning.

carbon monoxide A dangerous, poisonous, odorless gas produced in the burning process.

Assess Your Health

The Physical Effects of Smoking

This test consists of twenty statements about the effects of smoking. Put a check to show whether you think each statement is true or false. If you don't know whether a statement is true or false, put a check under "Don't know."

	True	False	Don't know
1. Smoking low-tar and low-nicotine cigarettes reduces the risk of all smoking-related diseases.	_____	_____	_____
2. Carbon monoxide is inhaled when a person smokes.	_____	_____	_____
3. How deeply a smoker inhales is not related to his or her chance of developing lung cancer.	_____	_____	_____
4. Most experts agree that the harmful effects of smoking on health are not as great for women as for men.	_____	_____	_____
5. Cigarette smoking increases the risk of developing breathing problems.	_____	_____	_____
6. Cigarette smoke can increase air pollution in homes and offices.	_____	_____	_____
7. Cigarette smoking increases the health dangers associated with taking birth control pills.	_____	_____	_____
8. Frequent pipe and cigar smokers are more likely than nonsmokers to develop lung cancer.	_____	_____	_____
9. The average life expectancy of a smoker is the same as that of a nonsmoker.	_____	_____	_____
10. People who smoke filter cigarettes inhale less carbon monoxide than do people who smoke nonfilter cigarettes.	_____	_____	_____
11. Most people gain weight when they quit smoking.	_____	_____	_____
12. Smokers have an increased risk of developing a lung infection after an operation.	_____	_____	_____
13. Smoking during pregnancy does not increase a baby's risk of death.	_____	_____	_____
14. Pipe smokers have a greater risk of developing cancer of the mouth than do cigarette smokers.	_____	_____	_____
15. Smoking causes the heart to beat more slowly.	_____	_____	_____
16. The health risks due to smoking do not change even after a person stops smoking.	_____	_____	_____
17. The more a person smokes, the greater the chance of developing heart disease.	_____	_____	_____
18. Cigarette smoke in the air can cause eye soreness in nonsmokers.	_____	_____	_____
19. On average, babies born to mothers who smoke during pregnancy are smaller than babies born to nonsmokers.	_____	_____	_____
20. Nicotine does not cause dependence similar to other addictive drugs.	_____	_____	_____

Answers

1 F; 2 T; 3 F; 4 F; 5 T; 6 T; 7 T; 8 T; 9 F; 10 F; 11 T; 12 T; 13 F; 14 T; 15 F; 16 F; 17 T; 18 T; 19 T; 20 F

Source: U.S. Department of Health and Human Services, Office of Disease Prevention and Health Promotion

emitted from the exhaust pipe of a car. The amount of carbon monoxide that stays in a smoker's blood is related to activity levels. During the day, carbon monoxide remains in the blood for two to four hours; during sleep, however, it remains for up to eight hours. Carbon monoxide affects the hemoglobin's ability to carry oxygen. This causes smokers to get out of breath when doing exercise—running, playing tennis, or even walking. It also causes problems for people already suffering from or at risk for cardiovascular diseases.

Why Smoking Is Dangerous to Your Health

Every pack of cigarettes and cigars sold in the United States carries a health warning, but a label cannot document just how dangerous smoking is. Cigarette smoking is responsible for nearly one out of every five deaths in the United States. Each year, some 440,000 people die from cigarette-related diseases. These deaths often result from a variety of cancers, including lung cancer, and from heart and lung disease. About one half of all regular smokers will die due to this addictive behavior. To test your knowledge of the physical effects of smoking, see the Assess Your Health box.

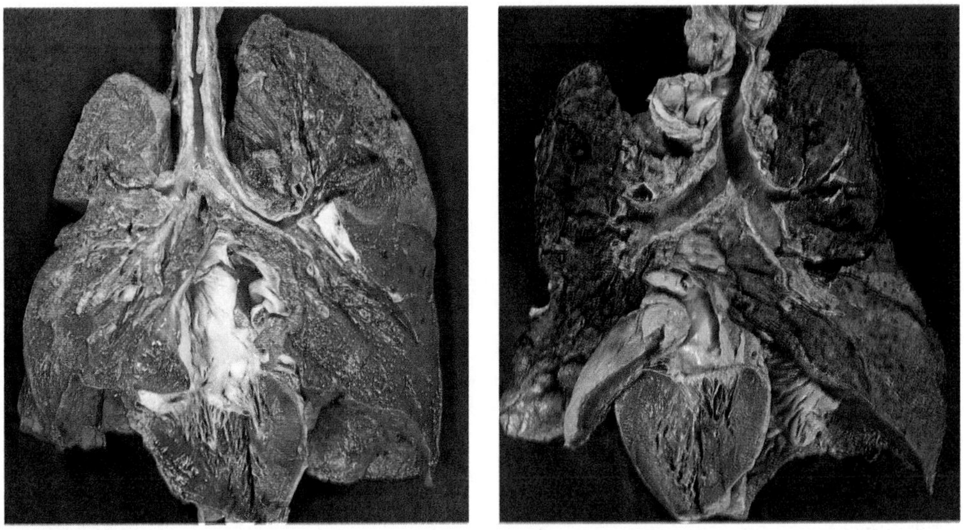

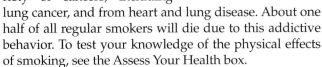

Figure 7.1 Most Lung Cancer Deaths Are Attributable to Smoking. Compare the healthy lungs of a nonsmoker on the left with the cancerous lungs of a smoker on the right.

Links to Cancer

Cigarette smoking is the leading cause of cancer deaths in the United States. Lung cancer has long been the most common form of cancer in men, and starting in 1986, lung cancer caught up with and has now surpassed breast cancer as the leading cause of cancer deaths in women. Most lung cancer deaths—87 percent—are attributable to cigarette smoking (see Figure 7.1).

As one would expect, the likelihood of dying from lung cancer increases with the number of cigarettes a person smokes, the deeper the smoke is inhaled, and the younger the initiation age. The good news is that quitting helps (see the Developing Health Skills box).

After twenty years of not smoking, a former smoker's risk of dying of lung cancer is nearly equal to that of someone who has never smoked.

Smokers also are at increased risk for cancer of the mouth, larynx, esophagus, kidney, bladder, pancreas, stomach, and cervix.

Heart Disease and Stroke

Heart disease is a term that refers to a broad range of conditions from **atherosclerosis** (hardening of the arteries) to **myocardial infarction** (major heart attack). It results from many factors, one of which is cigarette smoking. Cigarette smoking accounts for about 20 percent of all coronary heart disease deaths. Smoking also decreases cerebral blood flow, which can cause stroke.

Although smoking does not actually cause heart disease, it contributes to nearly every physiological factor associated with it. For example, smoking increases the risk for having **angina** (chest pains that occur when the heart muscle does not get enough blood supply), having a heart attack at an earlier age, and dying of a heart attack.

The two major components in smoke that contribute to heart disease are nicotine and carbon monoxide. Nicotine increases blood pressure, heart rate, the amount of blood pumped by the heart, and the blood flow in the arteries; carbon monoxide reduces the amount of oxygen available to the heart and other parts of the body.

Lung Damage

Smoking is a major cause of emphysema, chronic bronchitis, and other lung diseases. **Emphysema** is a disease of the lungs, particularly affecting the small air sacs. Over time, the lungs lose their ability to expand as a result of

atherosclerosis Damage to the circulatory system brought about by a buildup of plaque on the inner walls of arteries; sometimes called hardening of the arteries.

myocardial infarction Damage of heart tissue caused by an interruption of blood supply to the heart that can result in death.

angina Chest pain that occurs when the heart muscle does not get enough blood supply.

emphysema A disease of the lungs, particularly of the small air sacs, in which the lungs lose their ability to expand as a result of an accumulation of fluid in the tissue.

Developing Health Skills

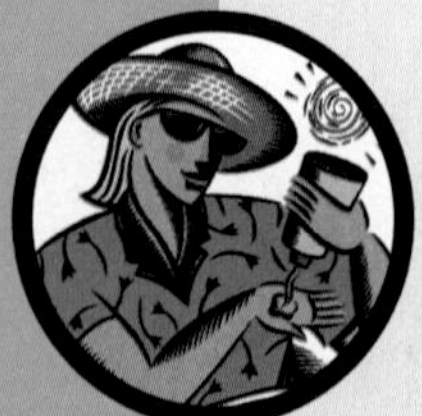

The Benefits of Quitting Smoking

Did you know that you could notice the health benefits in less than one hour after quitting smoking? If you were to quit smoking right now…

In 20 minutes

- Your blood pressure would decrease.
- Your pulse rate would drop.
- The body temperature of your hands and feet would increase.

In 8 hours

- The carbon monoxide level in your blood would drop to normal.
- The oxygen level in your blood would increase to normal.

In 24 hours

- Your chance of heart attack would decrease.

In 48 hours

- Your nerve endings would start regrowing.
- Your ability to smell and taste would enhance.

In 2 weeks to 3 months

- Your circulation would improve.
- Walking would become easier.
- Your lung function would increase.

In 1 to 9 months

- Coughing, sinus congestion, fatigue, and shortness of breath would decrease.

In 1 year

- Your excess risk of coronary heart disease would decrease to half that of a smoker.

In 5 years

- From 5 to 15 years after quitting, your risk for stroke would be reduced to that of people who have never smoked.

In 10 years

- Your risk of lung cancer would drop to as little as one-half that of continuing smokers.
- Your risk of cancer of the mouth, throat, esophagus, bladder, kidney, and pancreas would decrease.
- Your risk of ulcer would decrease.

In 15 years

- Your risk of coronary heart disease would be similar to that of people who have never smoked.
- Your risk of death would return to nearly the level of people who have never smoked.

Source: Reprinted with permission © American Lung Association. For more information on how you can support to fight lung disease, the third leading cause of death in the U.S., please contact The American Lung Association at 1-800-LUNG-USA (1-800-586-4872) or visit the website at www.lungusa.org.

the accumulation of fluid in the tissue. **Chronic bronchitis** is a condition in which the bronchial tubes become inflamed as a result of irritation. One cause of bronchial irritation is smoke. About as many people die each year from these lung diseases as from lung cancer.

Complications During Pregnancy

Two of the most basic things in life—getting pregnant and having a baby—are compromised for women who smoke cigarettes. To begin with, women who smoke take longer to conceive than do nonsmoking women. Once pregnant, a smoker seriously harms her growing fetus in many ways. The carbon monoxide in cigarette smoke crosses the placenta and is transported into the fetal blood. Carbon monoxide reduces the flow of oxygen and nutrients to the fetus, which slows down the fetal growth process. With the baby's growth compromised, the risk for having a spontaneous abortion (miscarriage), stillbirth, neonatal death, or premature birth are greater.

The good news is that if a mother gives up smoking early during pregnancy, her baby will probably develop normally.

chronic bronchitis A condition in which the bronchial tubes become inflamed as a result of irritation.

Other Health Effects of Smoking

Smokers are at risk for increased illness and death from a range of other health conditions, including digestive diseases (cigarette smoke stimulates more digestive acid secretions from the stomach) and circulatory diseases (the carbon monoxide in smoke constricts the already damaged blood vessels).

Smoking contributes to many problems that, although not life threatening, reduce the quality of life. For example:

- Smoking is associated with an increase in upper respiratory infections such as colds and influenza.
- Smoking contributes to allergy symptoms such as coughing and sneezing.
- Smoking reduces the effects of medications, especially antianxiety drugs and painkillers.
- Smoking damages cells and tissues, which can result in delayed wound healing, poor circulation in the lower legs, and psoriasis (an unsightly and discomforting skin condition).

Noncigarette Exposure to Tobacco

So far, this chapter has discussed the health effects of smoking cigarettes. However, there are other ways to be exposed to tobacco, including inhaling the cigarette smoke around you, smoking cigars and pipes, and chewing tobacco.

Passive Smoking

Passive smoking—inhaling environmental tobacco smoke—is an acknowledged health hazard. Sidestream smoke, the smoke that comes from the burning end of the cigarette between puffs, can cause lung cancer in healthy nonsmokers. This is because passive smokers inhale the same chemicals and carcinogens as smokers do.

Young children are especially affected by sidestream smoke. One reason for this is that they breathe faster and inhale more air for their body size than do adults. Another is that they have not yet fully developed their natural immunities to fight disease. Another vulnerable group are people who have heart conditions. For example, angina patients are more prone to attacks when they are in smoke-filled rooms.

Cigar and Pipe Smoking

Cigar and pipe smokers have higher lung cancer rates than do nonsmokers but lower rates than do those who smoke only cigarettes. Cigar and pipe smokers are more at risk than cigarette smokers for cancer of the mouth, lips, and tongue. This is due to the way people smoke pipes and cigars. Most do not inhale; rather, they hold the smoke in their mouths and release it. As with users of other tobacco products, National Cancer Institute studies show that cigar smokers are more likely than nonsmokers to develop chronic obstructive lung disease and heart attacks.

Smokeless Tobacco

Even though it is not inhaled, **smokeless tobacco**—chewing tobacco and snuff—is still harmful. It contains carcinogens that cause oral cancer. It also causes **leukoplakia** (white patches on the oral mucosa that can become malignant) and periodontal diseases, including gingivitis and receding gums. In addition, smokeless tobacco is highly addictive. Although it takes longer for the nicotine to reach the brain from smokeless tobacco than from cigarettes, users are exposed to blood levels of nicotine equal to those of cigarette smokers.

Smokeless tobacco is more popular with men than women. About twenty percent of male high school seniors have used it. If you ever used smokeless tobacco, be sure to see the Developing Health Skills box.

Kicking the Habit: How to Stop

Most smokers want to quit, and surveys show that 70 percent of current cigarette smokers have tried to stop at least once. These statistics clearly illustrate the addictive nature of nicotine.

Physical Problems of Quitting

The initial problems that smokers have to face when they stop smoking are symptoms related to withdrawal from nicotine. As with any drug withdrawal, these symptoms can cause great discomfort. Withdrawal symptoms—which are experienced in varying degrees from mild to severe—include craving for tobacco, irritability, anxiety, restlessness, dry mouth, difficulty sleeping, and impaired concentration, judgment, and motor coordination. These symptoms usually last one

passive smoking Inhaling tobacco smoke from the environment, as a result of someone else smoking.

smokeless tobacco Tobacco products that are chewed, placed in the mouth, and/or sniffed through the nose.

leukoplakia White patches on the oral mucosa that can become malignant.

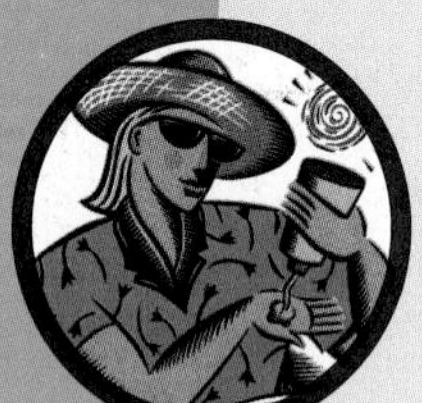

Developing Health Skills

Smokeless Tobacco Users: Check Monthly for Early Signs of Disease

The early signs of cancer of the mouth and tongue may be detected by self-examination. Dr. Elbert Glover, director of the Tobacco Research Center at West Virginia University, and the American Cancer Society recommend that the following self-check procedures be conducted every month:

- Check your face and neck for lumps on either side. Both sides of your face and neck should be the same shape.
- Look at your lips, cheeks, and gums. Look for sores, white or red patches, or changes in your gums by pulling down your lower lip. Check your inner cheeks, especially where you hold your tobacco. Gently squeeze your lip and cheeks to check for lumps or soreness.
- Put the tip of your tongue on the roof of your mouth. Place one finger on the floor of your mouth and press up under your chin with a finger from your other hand. Feel for bumps, soreness, or swelling. Check around the inside of your teeth from one side of your jaw to the other.
- Tilt your head back and open your mouth wide. Check for color changes or bumps or sores in the roof of your mouth.
- Stick out your tongue and look at the top. Gently grasp your tongue with a piece of cloth and pull it to each side. Look for color changes. Feel both sides of your tongue with your finger for bumps.

If you use smokeless tobacco and find anything that looks or feels unusual, see your dentist or physician as soon as possible.

to two weeks. In some cases, however, they can last several months.

In addition to the problem of nicotine addiction and physical dependence, many people also have a psychological dependence on smoking. Cigarettes are used automatically along with simple everyday activities such as walking to class or reading, watching television or studying. These events are called triggers because they trigger the urge to smoke.

Another reason some people have a problem quitting is that they think they will gain a lot of weight. The fact is that most people will gain some weight when they stop smoking—on average fewer than 10 pounds—but health researchers note that this weight gain is a negligible health threat compared with the risks of continued smoking.

smoking cessation The process of breaking a smoking habit; stopping the use of tobacco.

behavior modification Therapy designed to change the learned behavior of an individual.

nicotine replacement Therapy in which a person who smokes gets nicotine by means other than tobacco.

transdermal nicotine patch A form of nicotine replacement that, when applied to the skin, releases nicotine into the system at a constant rate.

Cessation Approaches

As difficult as it is to stop smoking, nearly half of all people who have ever smoked have quit. Most—90 percent—did it on their own, but help with **smoking cessation** is available for those who want it.

One approach is **behavior modification,** in which smokers learn to change their behavior pattern of smoking. Taking a short walk after dinner, for example, is one way to break the pattern of having a cigarette at the end of the meal. Other tactics include calling a friend when you are tempted to smoke and forcing yourself to break patterns by smoking only on the odd hour—for example, 7, 9, 11. About 40 percent of smokers completing behavior modification classes sponsored by the American Cancer Society, the American Lung Association, and private groups such as Smokenders are free from cigarettes a year later.

Hypnosis helps about 20 percent of the people who try it to stop smoking. When the smoker is in a trance state, the hypnotist coaches him or her how to stop. Motivation is the key to making hypnotism work, and researchers say that the more a smoker wants to quit, the better hypnosis works. There is no solid evidence that acupuncture lessens the physical symptoms of withdrawal, yet many people who try it are able to stay off cigarettes.

Nicotine replacement is also successful in getting smokers to quit. Through this technique, the smoker gets nicotine by means other than tobacco, and the urge to smoke is lessened. Nicotine is available in a gum that is chewed, a **transdermal nicotine patch** applied to the skin (usually the upper torso or upper arm), and a nasal spray. By itself, the gum helps 11 percent of smokers to quit for at least a year. Using the gum in conjunction with counseling, 29 percent remain smoke-free. Twenty-five percent of smokers who use the patch or nasal spray are smoke-free a year later.

The Changing Climate of Public Acceptance of Tobacco Use

The social and political climate concerning smoking has changed substantially over the years. Nonsmokers are less willing to accept smoke in their environment, and smoking has been banned in many places where people congregate. Almost every state requires smoke-free indoor air to some degree. There are even smoke-free jails.

The legal and regulatory environment has also changed. States sued tobacco companies for reimbursement for Medicaid costs of treating indigent smokers with tobacco-caused diseases, and received $206 billion in compensation. Some states are using this money for Medicaid costs, and others for smoking prevention messages aimed at teenagers and other public health needs; still others are using it as general operating income for the state.

It is against the law in every state to sell and distribute tobacco products to anyone under age eighteen, but most teenagers—an estimated two-thirds—report having no problem buying cigarettes. To help enforce these laws, the Food and Drug Administration requires retailers to get identification showing proof of age before selling tobacco products to young people.

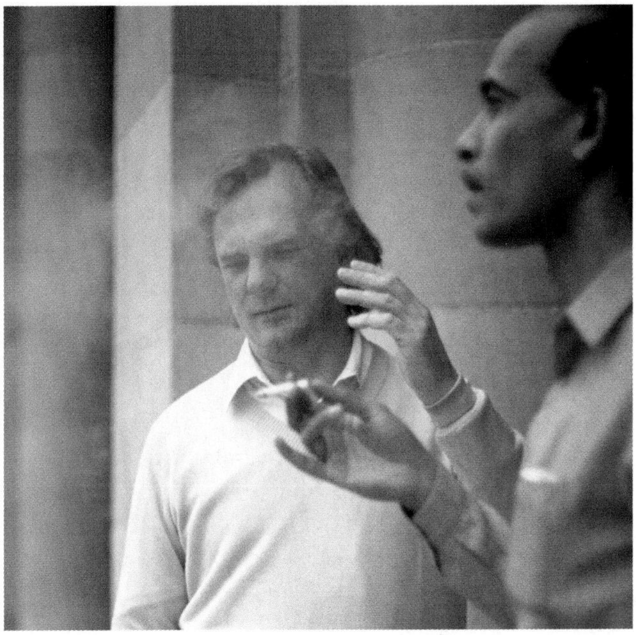

In an effort to protect employees from sidestream smoke, many businesses ban smoking inside their buildings, forcing smokers to smoke outside.

Drinking at College

According to the National Household Survey on Drug Abuse, almost half of all Americans drink. College students, however, are more likely to drink than the national average—just as they are more likely to smoke cigarettes. Studies show that more than 60 percent of undergraduates choose to drink alcohol. Alcohol is two to three times as popular among college students as the next leading drug, marijuana. (Although college age varies, most students are under age twenty-one, and every state requires that a person be twenty-one years old in order to purchase alcohol. As with cigarettes, most underage students are still able to purchase alcohol.)

College students also tend to drink more often—and more often to excess—than the general adult population. A study conducted at 140 campuses by researchers at the Alcohol Studies Program at the Harvard School of Public Health found that 44 percent of college students are **binge drinkers.** Binge drinking is defined as having five drinks in a row for men or four in a row for women on at least one occasion in the two weeks before the survey. (Because women generally have more fat in their bodies than do men, it takes women longer to metabolize alcohol; they are therefore affected by lesser amounts.)

Binge drinking can cause significant health and social problems. According to the study, binge drinkers were far more likely to have unprotected sex, drive after drinking, and fall behind in school than nonbinge drinkers. It is not fully understood why college students drink alcohol more than the general public does,

binge drinking Having five drinks in a row for men or four in a row for women on at least one occasion in the past two weeks.

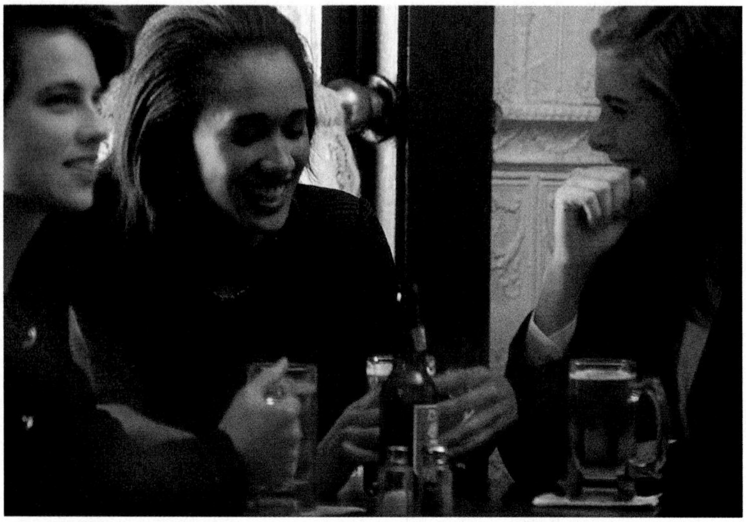

Drinking habits are changing among women. Many young women are consuming alcohol about as frequently as young men.

but factors such as newly found independence and social pressure likely contribute.

At the same time that binge drinking is taking place on college campuses more students are abstaining from drinking. Nearly 20 percent of students surveyed report that they do not drink, up from 15 percent in 1993. There are several possible reasons for this:

- There is a perceptible change in attitude.
- College students have grown up with tough drunk driving laws and are aware of the consequences of drinking and driving.
- For African American and other students following Muslim tenets, drinking is forbidden, and many do not want to be around people who are drinking.
- The average age of college students has risen. Priorities change, and for many older students, spending time and money drinking is not at the top of their list—or even on it.

Why People Drink

People choose to drink alcohol for a variety of reasons. Some people drink because of social circumstances ("All my friends do it") or as a way to release inhibitions ("I just want to let loose after a rough day"). Others drink to celebrate special occasions such as the end of the school year, a promotion, or a birthday. Some people, however, do not make a conscious decision to drink. Rather, they drink because of a compulsion to do so—they are addicted to alcohol.

alcohol addiction Extensive dependence on alcohol; this dependence is so acute that the acquisition and use of alcohol becomes the focus of everyday life.

Social Reasons

Many college students drink because they believe it will increase their interpersonal skills, allow them to be more socially assertive, produce feelings of power, and reduce tension. Such logic is erroneous. Drinking does not lead to social assertiveness—in fact, social assertiveness is one of the best means of controlling drinking, as you will read later in this chapter. College students may also believe that drinking alcohol will increase sexual feelings. Again, this is erroneous. Studies show that alcohol can result in less sexual arousal. It can cause testosterone levels in men to fall as much as five times below normal and can hinder women's ability to have satisfying sexual interactions.

Alcohol Dependence

Alcohol dependence occurs when a person is so physically attached to alcohol that he or she cannot live comfortably without it. Dependence usually develops over a long period of time and after a pattern of excessive alcohol consumption. In some individuals, however, it may develop in an extremely short time and after limited alcohol consumption. The need for alcohol may vary from a mild craving to a compulsion to use the drug.

The term **alcohol addiction** refers to a severe degree of alcohol dependence. The person addicted to alcohol is so dependent on the drug that the acquisition and use of alcohol become the focus of his or her life.

Health Hazards of Alcohol

Alcohol can affect nearly every part of the body. It can alter memory and reflexes, lower sex drive, lead to birth defects, cause heart muscle deterioration, and produce fatal liver damage. Cancers of the tongue, mouth, esophagus, larynx, and liver occur in higher numbers among alcohol users than among nonusers. At the same time, there is evidence that moderate drinking has health benefits. According to the 2000 *Dietary Guidelines for Americans,* moderate drinking—defined as no more than one drink a day for women and no more than two drinks a day for men—may lower the risk of heart attacks for men over age 45 and women over age 55. However, moderate consumption provides little—if any—health benefit for younger people.

Central Nervous System Effects

Alcohol has its most significant impact on the central nervous system. It depresses, or slows down, the activities of the central nervous system. Within minutes after consumption, the brain's normal functioning changes. Alcohol alters judgment, increases the time it takes to react to something, reduces muscle control, and affects reasoning.

Alcohol acts primarily on four parts of the brain: the **cerebrum**, the **cerebellum**, the **thalamus,** and the **medulla.** The cerebrum is the part of the brain that is responsible for reasoning and inhibitions. When alcohol sedates this area, thought processes can become disorganized and memory and concentration are dulled. The cerebellum, a portion of the brain that contributes to the control of movement, also becomes restricted, often resulting in the impairment of motor processes and quick changes in moods.

The thalamus plays a part in controlling the senses. Accordingly, alcohol levels in the blood can affect vision, hearing, smell, taste, and touch. Specifically, it becomes more difficult to hear and see. The medulla controls breathing. In extreme cases, drinking can cause impaired respiration and can result in death.

A **hangover** is characterized by nausea, upset stomach, anxiety, and a headache. The symptoms normally appear a few hours after heavy drinking and disappear over time. Hangovers have no permanent damaging effect.

Blackouts may occur with almost any level of alcohol in the body, although they usually are experienced by people who have consumed high levels of alcohol and/or are **intoxicated.** A blackout is a temporary form of **amnesia.** The individual appears to be conscious of what he or she is doing but the next day cannot remember much or any of what happened. Blackouts are a clear warning sign of problem drinking.

One of the most serious central nervous system impairments is the **Wernicke-Korsakoff syndrome,** a form of alcohol-related amnesia and personality disorder. It usually is not reversible. Other mental disorders associated with alcohol use are alcohol psychosis, delirium tremens (DTs), and acute alcoholic hallucinosis.

Liver Problems

Alcohol is processed by the liver. It eventually handles virtually all the alcohol in the bloodstream, but it does so at a constant pace—usually about 0.5 to 1 ounce per hour. This is why the amount of alcohol consumed is directly related to how long it takes a person to become intoxicated.

Cirrhosis of the liver is a condition that is seven times more common in heavy drinkers than in nondrinkers and results at least in part from the strain placed on the liver by excessive amounts of alcohol. What happens is that blood is diverted to those areas of the liver that are processing the alcohol. Cells in other parts of the liver are deprived of blood and eventually die. The process of filling in these regions with scar tissue leads to cirrhosis.

Fetal Alcohol Syndrome

Alcohol in the blood of a pregnant woman passes readily through the placental membranes and into the fetus's circulation system. Because alcohol is present in fetal blood in about the same concentration as in maternal blood, the amount of alcohol that a pregnant woman drinks is an important indicator of the risk for birth defects.

A pregnant woman who drinks moderately (four or five drinks per week) has a much higher chance of having a spontaneous abortion or a low-birth-weight infant

cerebrum The part of the brain responsible for reasoning and inhibitions.

cerebellum The part of the brain that contributes to the control of movement.

thalamus The part of the brain that plays a part in controlling the senses.

medulla The part of the brain that controls breathing.

hangover A condition caused by excess alcohol consumption and characterized by nausea, upset stomach, anxiety, and headache.

blackout A temporary form of amnesia in which the individual appears to be conscious of what he or she is doing but later cannot remember much, if any, of what happened.

intoxicated Having consumed enough alcohol to experience its effect, usually indicated by a high blood alcohol concentration, delayed muscle coordination, and impaired judgment.

amnesia Partial or total loss of memory.

Wernicke-Korsakoff syndrome A form of alcohol-related amnesia and personality disorder associated with central nervous system impairment; usually not reversible.

cirrhosis of the liver A disease in which scar tissue replaces normal liver tissue and interferes with the liver's ability to function.

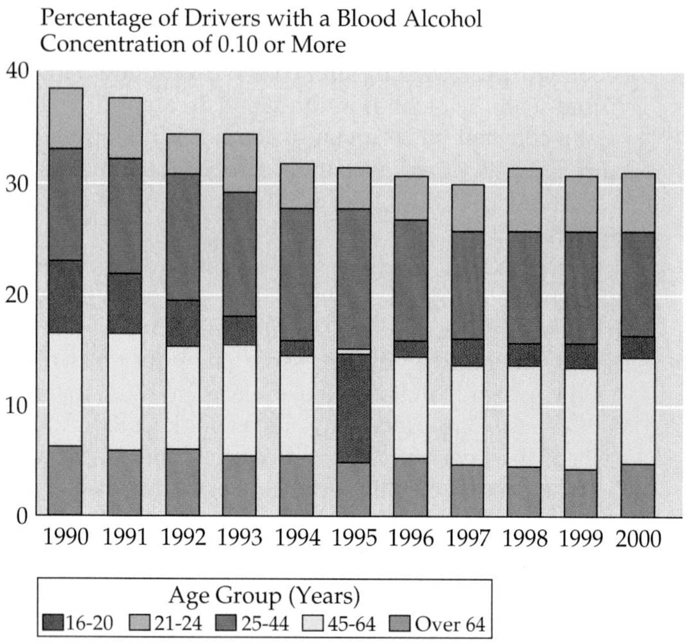

Figure 7.2 **Intoxicated Drivers in Fatal Crashes by Age Group, 1990–2000.**

College students and other young adults are at a higher risk of dying in car accidents due to drunk driving than people in any other age group.

Source: U.S. Department of Transportation

than a pregnant woman who does not drink. Large amounts of alcohol consumption by a pregnant woman significantly increase the risk for having a baby who has **fetal alcohol syndrome (FAS).** This syndrome includes irreversible mental retardation, poor motor coordination, hyperactivity in childhood, facial deformities, and other abnormalities. It is the third leading cause of birth defects accompanied by mental retardation, and it is the only one of the top three causes of birth defects that is preventable.

More than 16 percent of American women drink at some point when they are pregnant. Because a safe level of alcohol consumption during pregnancy is not known, the office of the Surgeon General, the National Council on Alcoholism and Drug Dependence, and other health-related groups recommend complete abstinence during this time.

fetal alcohol syndrome (FAS) A constellation of birth defects caused by alcohol consumption during pregnancy that is characterized by mental retardation, poor motor coordination, hyperactivity in childhood, facial deformities, and other abnormalities.

blood alcohol concentration (BAC) A measure of the amount of alcohol in the blood.

alcoholism A progressive disease related to the uncontrolled use of alcohol that interferes with the drinker's health and social functioning.

alcoholic Someone who suffers from alcoholism and who has lost control over his or her drinking.

casual drinker A person who drinks an alcoholic beverage every now and then but seldom consumes enough alcohol to become intoxicated.

Drinking and Death

In contrast to the chronic health conditions discussed above, which develop over time, sometimes drinking too much can result in immediate death. A single dose of alcohol, if large enough, can be lethal. Each year during freshman hazing season, several students usually die from alcohol poisoning. For example, one freshman died of alcohol poisoning after drinking a gallon of wine in forty-five minutes during a hazing session. As with most depressant drugs, death due to alcohol poisoning usually results from respiratory failure. Generally a **blood alcohol concentration (BAC)** of 0.40 percent is considered lethal, but some individuals may be at risk for alcohol poisoning at a lower level.

Perhaps the most life-threatening use of alcohol occurs when an individual chooses to drink and then to drive. Alcohol is closely linked with about 40 percent of all traffic fatalities, or more than 12,000 motor vehicle deaths each year; in addition, millions more are injured (see Figure 7.2). See Chapter 9 for other injuries associated with drinking.

Alcoholism as a Disease

Alcoholism is a primary, chronic progressive disease influenced by genetic, psychosocial, and environmental factors. It is characterized by impaired control over drinking, preoccupation with alcohol, use of it despite adverse consequences, and distortions in thinking, most notably denial. It also results in impaired social or occupational functioning. The disease is often progressive and fatal. Of adults who drink today, between 7 percent and 10 percent will become chronic **alcoholics.**

Alcoholism begins gradually, when the **casual drinker** (someone who drinks an alcoholic beverage

Assess Your Health

A Self-Assessment of Your Drinking

	Yes	No
1. Are you unable to stop drinking after a certain number of drinks?	____	____
2. Do you need a drink to get motivated?	____	____
3. Do you often forget what happened while you were "partying" (have blackouts)?	____	____
4. Do you drink or "party" alone?	____	____
5. Have others annoyed you by criticizing your alcohol use?	____	____
6. Have you been involved in fights with your friends or family while you were drunk?	____	____
7. Have you done or said anything while drinking that you later regretted?	____	____
8. Have you destroyed or damaged property while drinking?	____	____
9. Do you drive while drunk?	____	____
10. Have you been physically hurt while drinking?	____	____
11. Have you been in trouble with the school authorities or the campus police because of your drinking?	____	____
12. Have you dropped or chosen friends based on their drinking habits?	____	____
13. Do you think you are a normal drinker despite friends' comments that you drink too much?	____	____
14. Have you ever missed classes because you were too hungover to get up on time?	____	____
15. Have you ever done poorly on an exam or assignment because of drinking?	____	____
16. Do you think about drinking a lot?	____	____
17. Do you feel guilty or self-conscious about your drinking?	____	____

If you answered yes to three or more of these questions, or if your answer to any of the questions concerns you, you may be using alcohol in ways that are harmful. Do not waste your time blaming yourself for past binges or any other alcohol-related behavior. If you think you have or might be developing problems in which drinking plays a part, act now. You can get help.

For more information and counseling, contact your campus health or counseling center community mental health facility, or Alcoholics Anonymous (AA). Information about local AA meetings may be available from your local library or telephone directory as well as from the national AA office at P.O. Box 459, Grand Central Station, New York, NY 10163.

Source: Reprinted from the brochure *Alcohol: Decisions on Tap* with permission from the American College Health Association, P.O. Box 28937, Baltimore, MD 21240-8937

once in a while) or **social drinker** (someone who drinks regularly in social settings) becomes a **problem drinker.** Using alcohol in a manner that causes physical, psychological, or social harm to the drinker or others is considered problem drinking. The problem drinker often does not exercise control over how much he or she drinks. An alcoholic is someone who has lost at least some, and often total, control over his or her drinking behavior. You can assess your drinking behavior by responding to the questions posed in the Assess Your Health box.

Genetics and the Environment

Researchers looking for a genetic link to alcoholism have found a lot of evidence, but no one gene. It is likely that alcoholism involves a number of genes at two or more chromosome locations.

Particularly compelling data supporting a genetic linkage come from studies of sons of alcoholic mothers or fathers who had been adopted by other families at an early age. These sons have about a threefold greater chance of becoming alcohol abusers or alcoholics than do adopted sons of nonalcoholics. Because most of the alcoholic adoptees studied had been separated from their biological parents within the first few months of life, they presumably were removed from any of the

social drinker A person who drinks regularly in social settings but seldom consumes enough alcohol to become intoxicated.

problem drinker A person who uses alcohol in a manner that causes physical, psychological, or social harm to the drinker and/or others.

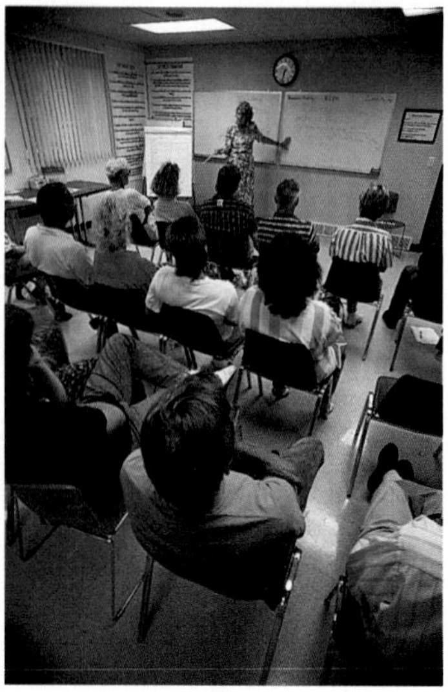

Members of Alcoholics Anonymous (AA) meet regularly with the goal of attaining sobriety one day at a time.

predisposing environmental influences of an alcoholic home. Other studies show abnormal brain patterns among both young sons of alcoholics and their fathers. These abnormalities are present in the sons long before they begin to drink.

Studies on twins also suggest a strong genetic link. In a review of current research, the National Institute of Alcohol Abuse and Alcoholism reports that identical twins—who are genetically alike—tend to develop more similar drinking patterns and problems than would fraternal twins—who are no more genetically alike than regular siblings.

Does this settle the case for a genetic component? Not entirely. Environment alone can also cause alcoholism. More than 35 percent of alcoholics have no family history of alcohol abuse. A significant relationship has been found between a person's self-esteem and alcoholism. Researchers have found that alcoholics often have dependent personalities and lack a good self-image. However, many people who have low self-esteem never become alcoholics. It is now widely accepted by researchers in the field that alcoholism can result from the interaction of heredity and environment.

Treatment Options

A variety of treatment programs and approaches are designed to help the alcoholic control his or her disease. More than half a million people are in treatment on any one day in the year. Hospitals and private facilities offer services for alcoholics and their families, including detoxification, drug treatment, and social support. These services are available on an inpatient and outpatient basis.

For many alcoholics, the first step in the treatment process is **detoxification.** This process of removing all alcohol from the person's body is usually an inpatient treatment conducted in a hospital or similar medical facility. The complete process can take days, or even weeks, depending on the amount of alcohol the individual has consumed. Once alcohol has been removed from the body, other treatments are possible.

Disulfiram (Antabuse) is a widely prescribed drug and has been required by courts for some cases involving alcohol abuse. It causes severe reactions to the ingestion of alcohol, including nausea, vomiting, accelerated heart rate, and severe dizziness. Disulfiram has demonstrated some effectiveness with alcoholics who voluntarily enter a drug therapy program. Similar results, however, have not been produced when the alcoholic involuntarily enters a program.

Perhaps the most widely known and successful treatment program is **Alcoholics Anonymous.** AA, as it is commonly called, is a self-help approach for the problem drinker. Members attending AA meetings are required to admit that they are alcoholics and that they desire to stay sober while helping other alcoholics do the same. The goal of AA is sobriety—not for a lifetime but for one day at a time. Evidence exists that attendance at AA meetings is positively correlated with maintaining **abstinence.** A review of the literature on outcomes in AA suggests that between 26 percent and 50 percent of its members are fully abstinent after one year of sobriety.

One of the most controversial topics in alcoholism treatment is whether alcoholics can go back to social drinking once they are cured. Moderation Management (MM) is a treatment program and support group for problem drinkers based on the belief that some—but not all—people who abuse alcohol can learn to moderate their drinking. MM begins with thirty days of abstinence followed by limits on how much alcohol can be consumed in any one week. The number of problem drinkers who can learn to drink in moderation is believed to be very small—between 4 percent and 14 percent of those who try it.

detoxification The process of removing all alcohol from an individual's body.

Alcoholics Anonymous A membership organization of recovering alcoholics who provide social support for avoiding the use of alcohol.

abstinence The choice of not consuming alcoholic beverages in any form.

Avoiding Problem Drinking

Avoiding the problems associated with the consumption of alcohol is not complicated. It does, however, re-

Table 7.1 Blood Alcohol Concentration (BAC): A Measure of Drunk Driving

Within minutes after having a drink, the brain's normal functioning is changed. One measure of how your brain, vision, and decision making might be impaired is how much alcohol is in your blood. This is called the blood alcohol concentration.

Your Weight	Number of drinks (over a two-hour period) 1.5 oz. 80 proof liquor or 12 oz. can of beer											
100	1	2	3	4	5	6	7	8	9	10	11	12
120	1	2	3	4	5	6	7	8	9	10	11	12
140	1	2	3	4	5	6	7	8	9	10	11	12
160	1	2	3	4	5	6	7	8	9	10	11	12
180	1	2	3	4	5	6	7	8	9	10	11	12
200	1	2	3	4	5	6	7	8	9	10	11	12
220	1	2	3	4	5	6	7	8	9	10	11	12
240	1	2	3	4	5	6	7	8	9	10	11	12

Social	Warning	Intoxicated
Drive with caution	Driving impaired	Do not drive
BAC to 0.05%	0.05–0.09%	0.10% and up

This table is only a guide. Information presented is based on averages and may vary according to particular circumstances or from individual to individual.

Source: U.S. Department of Transportation, National Highway Traffic Safety Administration

quire knowing the effects of alcohol on the body, how those effects can be minimized, and the skills needed to handle the social settings in which drinking takes place.

Pace Your Drinking

When alcohol is consumed at the pace of one drink per hour, the body is generally able to process the alcohol. One drink is measured as one and a half ounces of eighty-proof liquor, five ounces of 12 percent wine, or twelve ounces of five percent beer (this usually means one shot of liquor, one glass of wine, or one bottle of beer). **Proof** equals two times the percentage of pure alcohol in a beverage. Therefore, a one and a half ounce drink of eighty-proof liquor would contain 40 percent alcohol.

If a 150-pound man has one drink, his blood alcohol concentration will be 0.01 percent (see Table 7.1). In one hour, nearly all the alcohol from one drink is eliminated from the blood through sweating, respiration, urination, and metabolism in the liver. If this same, 150-pound man consumed four drinks within a one-hour period, his BAC could rise to 0.07. Six drinks could bring his BAC up to 0.11, higher than the 0.10 legal limit in most states. It takes a person more than six hours to eliminate six ounces of alcohol from the blood.

Alcohol begins to influence the brain, vision, and decision making at BAC levels of 0.02, and from this point on, driving is impaired. Between 0.10 and 0.20, an individual may have difficulty walking a straight line or touching his or her fingers together, two common tests used during highway sobriety checks. Blood concentration levels of 0.40 can be lethal.

The Full Stomach Factor

If you choose to drink, make sure you have had something to eat. Drinking on a full stomach has a different effect than drinking on an empty stomach. Alcohol consumed on an empty stomach may be absorbed directly

proof Two times the percentage of pure alcohol in a beverage.

through the stomach wall into the bloodstream. The fuller the stomach, the longer it takes alcohol to be absorbed. When alcohol mixes with food, it passes more slowly into the small intestine and from it into the blood. On the other hand, alcohol taken together with carbonated beverages—gin and tonic, rum and cola, scotch and soda—is usually absorbed more rapidly.

Be Socially Assertive

The primary skill necessary for reducing the health risk of alcohol is social assertiveness, which in this case means following your own agenda on drinking. The most effective way to be socially assertive is to know exactly how much alcohol you will consume before entering into a social situation where drinking takes place. By doing so, you are assured that your limits are based on clear thinking, not social pressure. You need to decide how you will answer the following questions:

- How much are you going to drink?
- How fast will you have those drinks?
- What type of alcohol will you drink?
- With whom are you going to drink?
- With whom are you not willing to drink?
- How will you get home after attending a function where you have been drinking?

Once you have made your decisions and set limits on your drinking, stick to them. If you don't set limits for yourself, make sure someone else in your group sets limits for him- or herself. Identify a designated driver—someone who agrees not to consume alcohol during the evening and who will drive you and the others who do drink home.

A Word about Prevention

Preventing health and social problems associated with alcohol use is a major personal and public health task. Prevention programs for college students are designed to raise awareness of the dangers of alcohol abuse and encourage the social skills needed to avoid alcohol abuse. At a growing number of schools, student–administration coalitions are working together to develop—and enforce—policies such as banning kegs at football games and at fraternity house parties, and enforcing drinking-age laws.

It is hoped that prevention strategies such as these will create a climate for college students in which alcohol consumption does not lead to the costly and deadly public health problems seen in today's society.

CASE STUDY 7: Tobacco Use

Manuel had tried to quit smoking several times, but each time, he went back to smoking. This time, he had not had a cigarette in three weeks, and here he was—stuck in his car in a traffic jam while driving to school. He was frustrated and he was alone. He reached into the pocket where he used to keep his cigarettes, but none were there. He reviewed some of the techniques he had learned in a smoking-cessation clinic: Think of something enjoyable—sailing, listening to music, a world without traffic jams; remind yourself that smoking won't change the situation.

Manuel tried these techniques, but he got too frustrated and pulled into a gas station to buy a pack of cigarettes. Once he had them in his hand, his resolution to stop smoking left him immediately. He smoked. "Maybe next time," he said, "I'll really quit."

Donetta was also taking a smoking-cessation class, and she, too, had tried to quit before without much success. But this time, she was really determined to do it after nine smoke-free days. Her will was tested one night after studying when she and three friends were at a popular coffee bar. They were having a good time when suddenly, Donetta started feeling jumpy and on edge; she wanted to smoke. What worried her was that she knew she could bum a cigarette from one of her friends.

Just as Manuel did, Donetta reviewed some of the tricks she had learned in smoking-cessation class. She reminded her friends that she was no longer a smoker and asked them not to offer her a cigarette. She got up twice from the table when she felt the urge to smoke and went to the ladies room, where she washed her face and combed her hair. She played with her spoon to keep her hands busy and even chewed gum at the table. But she didn't smoke.

That evening was a turning point for Donetta. After that, she knew she would not go back to smoking. And she was right.

In Your Opinion

Manuel and Donetta both wanted to quit smoking, but only one of them succeeded—at least for the time being.

- What do you think was the most important factor in Donetta's ability to quit? Why?
- Should Manuel take a different approach the next time he tries to quit? If so, what approach should he take?
- If you had just quit smoking, what would you do in the situations in which Manuel and Donetta found themselves? If you had had beer or wine instead of coffee, do you think you would still be as strong as Donetta?
- Is there a way you can help a friend who is trying to quit?

KEY CONCEPTS

1. Tobacco and alcohol cause more deaths, illnesses, and disabilities than any other preventable health condition.
2. Currently, about 24 percent of Americans smoke.
3. The main reason people smoke is the addictive nature of nicotine.
4. Cigarette smoking is the leading cause of cancer deaths and is related to nearly every risk factor associated with heart disease.
5. Nearly half of all people who have ever smoked have quit.
6. Smoking-cessation approaches include behavior modification, hypnosis, and nicotine replacement.
7. Nearly 50 percent of the adult population drinks. Studies of college populations show that more than 60 percent of college students drink and 44 percent are binge drinkers.
8. Alcohol has its most significant impact on the central nervous system. It depresses, or slows down, the activities of the central nervous system.
9. A problem drinker is a person who uses alcohol in a manner that causes physical, psychological, or social harm to the drinker or to others.
10. The primary skill necessary for reducing the health risks of alcohol is social assertiveness. Prior to beginning to drink, a socially assertive person decides how much and under what conditions he or she is going to drink and with whom he or she is not willing to drink.

REVIEW QUESTIONS

1. Compare dependence that results from tobacco use with that resulting from alcohol use.
2. Give three reasons why people smoke.
3. Explain the health risks of nicotine, tar, and carbon monoxide.
4. Describe how tobacco use contributes to cancer, heart disease, and lung disease.
5. Identify three approaches to smoking cessation.
6. Describe how alcohol acts on the central nervous system.
7. Differentiate between a hangover and a blackout.
8. Identify and discuss three different treatment options for alcoholism.
9. Explain the importance of the pace of consumption and the full stomach factor in avoiding the problems associated with alcohol use.
10. Explain how being socially assertive can help prevent the problems associated with alcohol use.

CRITICAL THINKING QUESTIONS

1. In *Healthy People 2010,* the following objective is listed: "Reduce the proportion of nonsmokers exposed to environmental tobacco smoke." How can this best be accomplished? Should laws be passed to restrict where smoking can take place (i.e., citywide bans on smoking in public places), or should nonsmokers be taught how to avoid environmental tobacco smoke?
2. Tobacco companies have begun paying large sums of money to states as a result of legal action intended to recover the costs of providing health care for smokers. Some states have spent the tobacco settlement monies to repair roads, build bridges, and on other day-to-day operations of the state. Is this an appropriate use of tobacco settlement funds, or should those funds be dedicated to tobacco-related health care and the prevention of tobacco use?
3. *Healthy People 2010* contains the following two objectives: "Increase abstinence from alcohol, cigarettes,

and illicit drugs among pregnant women," and "Reduce the occurrence of fetal alcohol syndrome (FAS)." How can these objectives best be accomplished? Through educational efforts of the state or federal government? Through policies and/or laws restricting the consumption of alcohol and other drugs by pregnant women? Through prenatal classes for pregnant women? How would you propose to accomplish these objectives?

4. The Eighteenth Amendment to the Constitution, passed in 1919 and in effect until 1933, prohibited the manufacture, sale, and transport of intoxicating liquors in the United States. Prohibition, as it was called, was considered a failure. Why do you believe that this law failed? Are there drugs for which another Prohibition should be considered?

JOURNAL ACTIVITIES

1. If you smoke, make a list of all the reasons why you smoke and all the reasons why you should stop smoking. Read this list every day for a week. Make additions if you think of other reasons why you smoke or why you should stop. At the end of a week, do the reasons for stopping seem more compelling than they did at the beginning of the week? Why? Why not?
2. Look through a stack of popular magazines from the library, such as sports or women's magazines. What percent of ads are for cigarettes? Explain how these ads are designed to capture your attention. Find examples of misleading ads.
3. Answer the following questions concerning blood alcohol concentration using Table 7.1 on page 109.
   - John weighs 140 pounds and Mike weighs 200 pounds. Each man drinks one 12-ounce beer. Who has the greater percentage of alcohol in the blood and by how much?
   - Mario, Jeff, and Karl have four glasses of wine each. If Mario weighs 120 pounds, Jeff 160 pounds, and Karl 140 pounds, could any of them be considered legally intoxicated? How much would Karl's blood alcohol concentration increase if he had one more glass of wine?
   - Leslie has two beers. She weighs 120 pounds. How much will her blood alcohol concentration increase if she drinks two more beers? Would she be considered legally intoxicated?
4. Contact the local chapters of the national office of four sororities and fraternities. Find out if their charter says anything about drinking, and what they are doing to promote responsible drinking on campus. If you have attended a party given by any of these Greek clubs, were they following the rules set down in the charter?

SELECTED BIBLIOGRAPHY

Alcohol and Health, 10th Special Report to the U.S. Congress from the Secretary of Health and Human Services. Rockville, MD: National Institute on Alcohol Abuse and Alcoholism, 2001.

Houston, T., and N. J. Kaufman. "Tobacco Control in the 21st Century: Searching for Answers in a Sea of Change." *Journal of the American Medical Association 284,* 6 (2000).

Monitoring the Future Study. Rockville, MD: National Institute on Drug Abuse, 2001 (published annually).

Morse, R. M., et al. "The Definition of Alcoholism." *Journal of the American Medical Association* 268, (1992): 1012–1014.

Substance Abuse: The Nation's Number One Health Problem. Princeton, NJ: The Robert Wood Johnson Foundation, 2001.

Wechsler, H., et al. "Underage College Students' Drinking Behavior, Access to Alcohol, and the Influence of Deterrence Policies." *Journal of American College Health 50,* 5 (2002): 223–236.

Women and Smoking: A Report of the Surgeon General. Washington, DC: U.S. Department of Health and Human Services. 2001. See also other reports of the Surgeon General.

HEALTHLINKS

Websites for The Health Effects of Smoking and Drinking

You can access better health as it relates to this chapter by checking out some of the following sites on the Internet. These sites can be accessed directly from the *Decisions for Healthy Living* Website located at www.aw.com/pruitt.

American Cancer Society

The home page for the largest private organization dedicated to fighting cancer. The site includes anti-smoking games, news, and other information.

American Lung Association

The home page for the largest private organization dedicated to the prevention of lung disease and respiratory disorders, as well as tobacco control and environmental health.

National Institute on Alcohol Abuse and Alcoholism

This national government agency provides information on the latest findings in alcohol research, including direct links to statistical information, abstracts, and surveillance reports.

Office on Smoking and Health: Tobacco Information & Prevention Sourcepage (TIPS)

The federal agency dedicated to eliminating tobacco use, primarily among young people. This site provides numerous links to educational materials and resources, as well as providing tips for cessation.

Alcohol and Drug Information

A special site from the National Clearinghouse for Alcohol and Drug Abuse. PREVLINE offers electronic access to searchable databases and substance abuse prevention materials that pertain to alcohol, tobacco, and drugs.

QuitNet

A smoking cessation service affiliated with Boston University. The site provides quit guides, self-assessments, online support community and more.

HEALTH HOTLINES

The Health Effects of Smoking and Drinking

National Clearinghouse for Alcohol and Drug Information
(800) SAY-NOTO (729-6686)
11426 Rockville Pike, Suite 200
Rockville, MD 20852

National Drug and Alcohol Treatment Routing Service
(800) 662-HELP (662-4357)
107 Lincoln Street
Worcester, MA 01605

TEST YOUR KNOWLEDGE ANSWERS

1. True. Over time, chemical changes take place in the brain that cause a smoker to feel a need for more nicotine.
2. False. Thirty-three percent of college students report smoking in the last month.
3. True. While one drink a day for women over age fifty-five and no more than two drinks a day for men over age forty-five may lower risk of heart attacks, moderate consumption provides little—if any—health benefit for younger people.
4. False. Nearly 20 percent of students surveyed report that they do not drink, up from 15 percent in 1993.
5. True. Respiratory failure is generally the cause of death due to alcohol poisoning.

CHAPTER

8

Understanding the Dangers of Drug Use

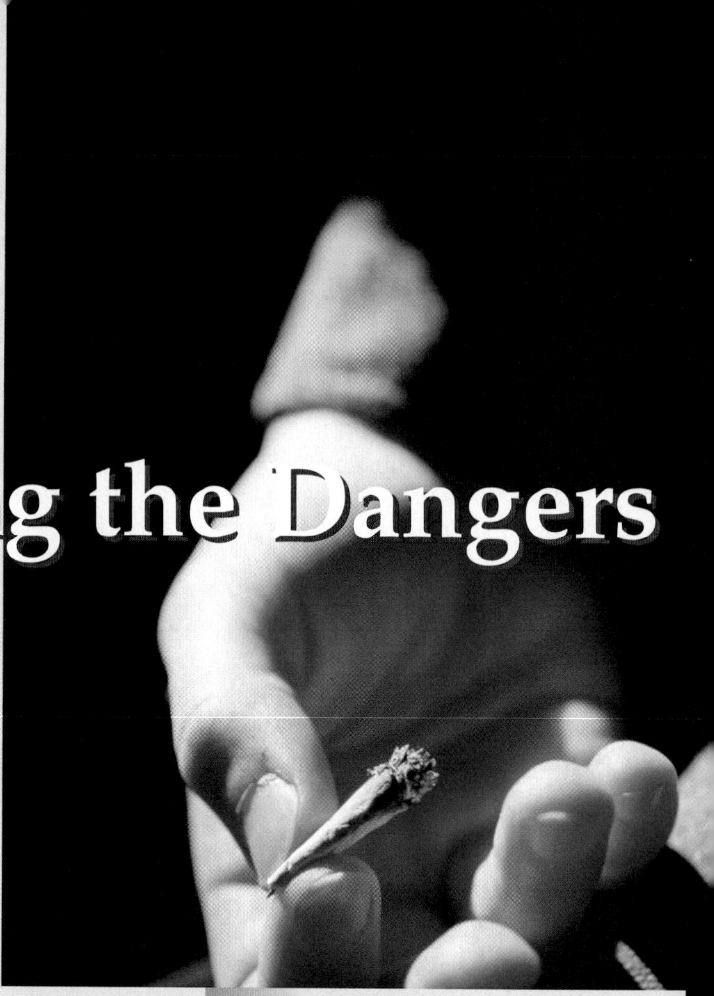

OBJECTIVES

When you finish reading this chapter, you will be able to:

1. Cite the most often used drugs among college students.
2. Differentiate between over-the-counter drugs, prescription drugs, and dangerous or illegal substances.
3. Explain the concept of staging as it relates to drug use.
4. Differentiate between main effects and side effects of drugs.
5. Explain the dangers of mixing drugs and describe additive, inhibitory, and synergistic effects.
6. Group drugs by their psychoactive effects.
7. Describe the health risks associated with drug abuse.
8. Describe the cost to society of drug abuse.
9. Describe three treatment alternatives for individuals experiencing a drug problem.
10. Suggest specific actions you can take to avoid drug abuse.

TEST YOUR KNOWLEDGE

1. Rohypnol is referred to as the date-rape drug because it is often used to incapacitate an unsuspecting person. True or False?
2. Marijuana use by college students does not tend to lower students' academic performance (as measured by grades). True or False?
3. The brain makes its own natural opiates that produce pleasure and mask pain. True or False?
4. The most commonly used drug classified as a hallucinogen is cannabis, usually referred to as marijuana. True or False?
5. Treatment success rates for drug abusers are similar to those suffering from asthma, diabetes, and hypertension. True or False?

Answers found at end of chapter.

From morning through night, some form of **drug** seems to be used—or abused. A drug is any chemical substance that causes a change in the body's functioning, including physiological and psychological activity. Coffee helps people wake up in the morning, and sleeping pills help them sleep at night. Aspirin is used to get rid of headaches during the day, and beer, wine and other alcoholic drinks are used to wind down in the evening. In addition, crack, heroin, uppers and downers, poppers and snappers, and hundreds more **illicit**—that is, illegal—drugs are available. Because drugs can be addictive, their use has enormous consequences for your personal health and safety and for that of the American public.

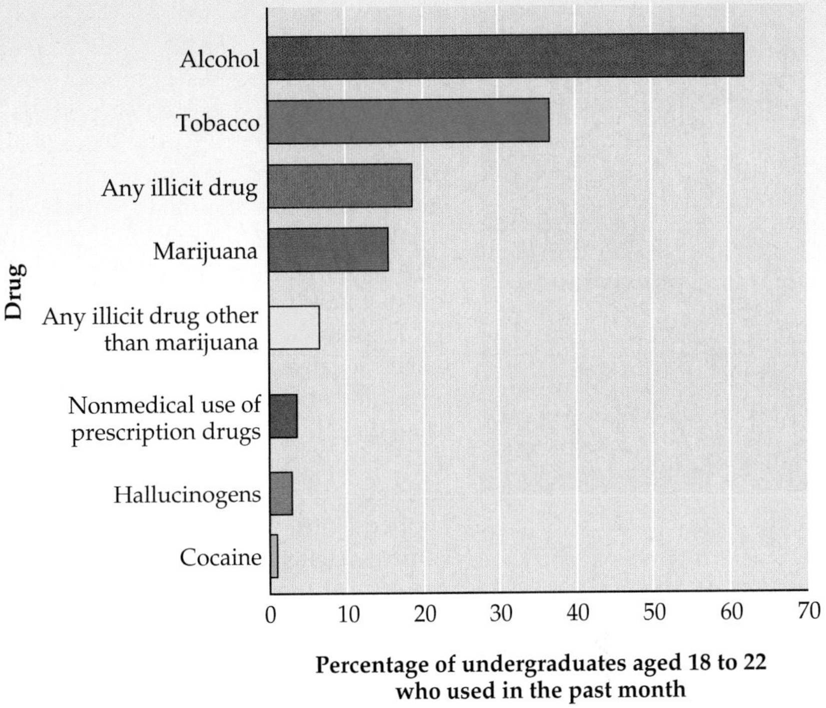

Figure 8.1 Drugs of Choice for College Students

Source: Substance Abuse and Mental Health Services Administration, 2000, *National Household Survey on Drug Abuse*

People from virtually all economic, racial, and ethnic backgrounds use drugs. Figure 8.1 shows the primary drugs used by college students. Some have experimented with drugs in high school—particularly marijuana—and the increased availability of drugs on the college campus plus the absence of parental guidance make further experimentation tempting.

From Drug Use to Drug Abuse

Some drugs are safe to use—for example, drugs prescribed by your physician for a specific condition—but any drug can be misused and abused. **Drug use** is the use of a chemical substance for the purpose intended. **Drug misuse** is taking prescribed medication without consulting a physician—for example, using someone else's prescription for menstrual cramps. **Drug abuse** is the intentional misuse of a chemical. The person who misuses tranquilizers by taking them to feel at ease socially becomes a drug abuser when he or she can't get through the day without several doses of tranquilizers. Although people who abuse tranquilizers usually obtain them illegally, drug abuse is more often associated with illicit drugs such as cocaine and heroin.

Tolerance and dependence/addiction to drugs were discussed in Chapter 7, on tobacco and alcohol. They are reviewed here with specific reference to the use of illegal drugs. **Tolerance** is a physical adaptation

drug A chemical substance that causes a change in the body's functioning, including physiological and psychological activity.

illicit Illegal.

drug use The use of a chemical substance for the purpose intended, to bring about a change in the way the body functions.

drug misuse The use of a prescribed medication without consulting a physician.

drug abuse The intentional and chronic misuse of a chemical substance.

tolerance The progressive change in the body's reaction to a drug causing an individual to need more and more of the same drug to achieve the same effect.

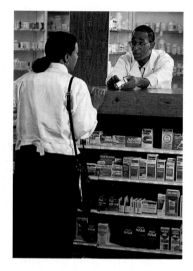

Your pharmacist can explain the safe use of a prescription drug. Prescription drugs can be considered dangerous if they are used for purposes other than the one intended by your physician.

to a substance that causes it to become less effective with repeated use. As a result, a person has to take more of the drug to get the intended effect. For example, a heroin user may go from a 3-mg dose to a 1,000-mg dose in a few months.

Dependence occurs when a person is so physically attached to the drug that he or she cannot live comfortably without it. When this happens, the body becomes accustomed to the presence of the drug and requires the drug to function normally. Another term for physical dependence is **addiction.** A person who has a physical dependence on a drug goes through **withdrawal** symptoms when he or she stops taking the drug. Withdrawal symptoms are usually unpleasant and sometimes dangerous. For example, withdrawal from heroin can include nausea, vomiting, joint and muscle pains, heightened blood pressure, racing pulse, tremors, and fever. Psychological dependence occurs when the person believes that he or she needs a drug to function normally. A person who is psychologically dependent may not experience physical withdrawal symptoms when the drug is not taken, but the process of stopping the drug use is still very difficult.

What the Term *Drug* Means

The word *drug* refers to a chemical substance that causes a change in the body's functioning, including physiological and psychological activity. This definition encompasses over-the-counter and prescription drugs; legal substances such as beer, wine, and coffee; and illegal substances such as marijuana, cocaine, and heroin (see the Developing Health Skills box). A drug is considered dangerous when it is believed to be a threat to the health of the user.

Over-the-counter drugs (OTCs) are chemical compounds that can be bought in pharmacies and supermarkets without restriction. They include analgesics (pain relievers) such as ibuprofen and aspirin and any number of aspirin compounds. Other examples of OTCs include cold capsules used to reduce the symptoms of colds and the flu; cough syrups used to reduce coughing and the symptoms of sore throat; laxatives used to treat irregular bowel activity; vitamin and mineral supplements used to enhance nutrition; and ointments used for the treatment of burns, minor abrasions, and fungal infections. There are thousands of over-the-counter drugs, and they all have one thing in common—they are available without restriction. This lack of restriction presents the possibility of health risks if the drugs are overused or used in certain combinations with other drugs.

Prescription drugs are chemical compounds that can be acquired legally only under a physician's direction. When a prescription is written, the physician gives the pharmacist specific information about which drug and how much of it to provide and gives the patient directions on how and when the drug is to be taken. When taken in a manner other than that prescribed or when taken by someone other than the person receiving the prescription, they may be considered dangerous drugs. It is illegal to sell prescription drugs for other than the primary intended purpose. (For more on medicinal drugs, see Chapter 16.)

Some substances are not thought of as drugs, yet they are abused substances and are often included when identifying drugs of abuse. For example, freon, glue, gasoline, and correctional fluids are abused substances when they are inhaled. Because such substances are easily available and legal to buy, they are often thought of as harmless. However, when abused they can result in respiratory failure and death.

Availability and Legality of Drugs

A person who wants illicit drugs can get them in almost any community in the United States. To a great extent, the small-time pusher assures the availability of illicit drugs to college students. At its simplest level, this is the person who buys beer for friends under the drinking age at the local convenience store. Other pushers buy marijuana, LSD, crack, and other drugs from dealers and then sell them in the dorms and other student hangouts. Availability and accessibility of drugs are more a matter of demand than of law.

The drug Rohypnol (Roofies), for example, is not approved for medical use in the United States, yet is available on the streets, where it is referred to as the

dependence A condition in which a person is so physically and/or psychologically attached to a drug that he or she cannot live comfortably without it.

addiction Physical or psychological dependence on a drug, often involving tolerance and withdrawal.

withdrawal The symptoms ranging from mild discomfort to very traumatic events when a person stops taking a drug.

Developing Health Skills

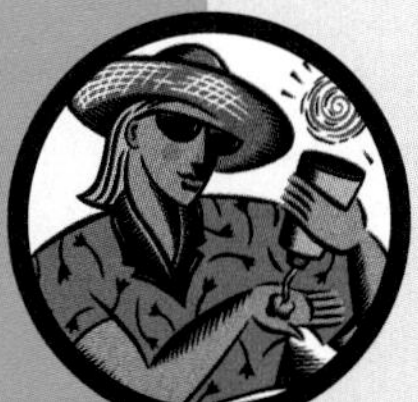

Consumer Health: The Caffeine High

Caffeine is the most popular and widely consumed drug in the world. It is in coffee, tea, soft drinks, chocolate, and medications, including cold pills. Like all drugs, caffeine causes an array of physiological changes.

As a stimulant, caffeine has a direct effect on the brain and the central nervous system. It can ward off drowsiness, improve alertness, and speed reaction times in people who are tired, and it can increase the muscles' capacity for work. It can also lead to nervousness, anxiety, jitteriness, and loss of sleep.

Like other stimulants, caffeine is addictive. People develop a tolerance for it and need more to get through the day. According to researchers at the Center for Science in the Public Interest, coffee drinkers tend to become dependent on caffeine at daily doses of about three and a half cups of coffee. As with other drug-related dependencies, caffeine produces withdrawal symptoms when regular users stop drinking coffee. These symptoms include lethargy, irritability, nervousness, and severe headaches.

Some people can consume large amounts of caffeine without noticing any effect. Others become jittery after one cup of coffee or a can of cola. Similarly, people differ in the duration of caffeine's effect. Caffeine has a half-life of three to seven hours for the typical nonsmoking adult. This means that half its effects wear off in that time. For reasons not fully understood, the half-life is shorter for smokers and longer for pregnant women.

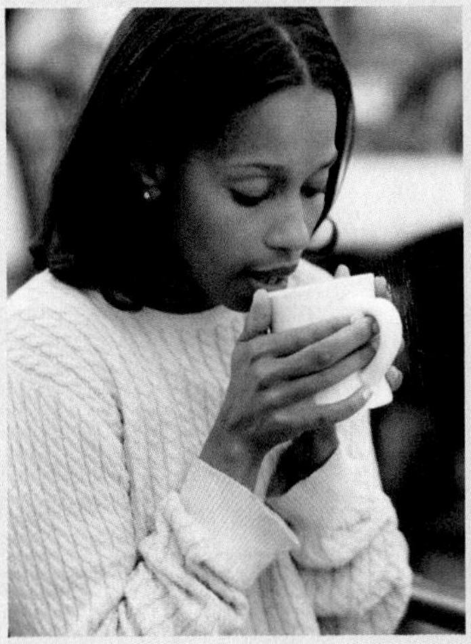

Coffee is a legal, socially accepted substance, but you can still become addicted to it.

Most experts agree that two cups of coffee a day pose little or no health hazard to adults. But the scientific evidence about high use is unclear. Some animal studies have implicated caffeine in birth defects, heart disease, and cancer. Even without conclusive evidence, the Food and Drug Administration recommends that women avoid or significantly reduce their intake of caffeine during pregnancy.

Alternatives to caffeine include decaffeinated coffee (which is not without health hazards itself because it contains additives that may cause liver cancer in mice), herbal tea, and grain-based drinks. For those who need their daily fix of junk food, there are caffeine-free sodas and chocolates.

date-rape drug because it impairs mental judgment, results in amnesia, and is used to incapacitate innocent people who are then exposed to violent assaults such as rape. As long as a demand exists for a certain drug, there will be a way to get it. Perhaps the best indicator of the availability of drugs is the price, because the drug business—like any other business—is subject to the economics of supply and demand. As the availability of drugs increases, the price drops. Currently, the price of drugs has reached a level at which only a few dollars buys a "hit."

Even though drugs are widely available, it is illegal in all states to possess, deliver, or manufacture controlled substances or dangerous drugs. A **controlled substance** is a drug or chemical that has been identified through legal review as a threat to an individual or to society. There are five categories (called "schedules") of drugs based on their potential for abuse, medical use, and standards for safe use.

- Schedule I drugs have a high potential for abuse and addiction and no accepted medical use.
  Examples: Heroin, LSD, marijuana, and PCP.
- Schedule II drugs have a high potential for abuse and addiction and some restricted medical use.
  Examples: Cocaine, methadone, morphine, and opium.
- Schedule III drugs have some potential for abuse and addiction and have accepted medical use.
  Examples: Codeine and barbiturates (can also be Schedule II or IV, depending on use) and anabolic steroids.
- Schedule IV drugs have a low potential for abuse and addiction and have accepted medical use.
  Examples: Minor tranquilizers, phenobarbital, and Thorazine.
- Schedule V drugs have the lowest potential for abuse and have accepted medical use.
  Examples: OTC drugs such as cough medicine.

controlled substance A chemical that has been identified through legal review as a threat to an individual and/or to society.

California has made it legal to prescribe marijuana for medical use (for example, to relieve the pain of critically ill patients and to increase the appetites of patients wasting from cancer or AIDS), but this is being challenged by the federal government. Some European countries have decriminalized marijuana and certain other drugs.

Drug Use

In the typical progression of drug use, a person starts with cigarettes, beer, or wine (also referred to as the **gateway drugs**). He or she then moves on to marijuana and hard liquor and subsequently to other illicit drugs such as barbiturates, heroin, and cocaine. This concept is called **staging**. According to the National Institute of Drug Abuse, for someone who has ever smoked or drunk, the risk for moving on to marijuana is five times higher than for a person who has never smoked or drunk; the risk for moving on to cocaine is more than 100 times higher for someone who has smoked marijuana at least once in his or her lifetime than for a person who has never done so. This progression, however, is not inevitable. That is, it cannot be said that smoking and drinking are the cause of later drug use.

Drugs and College Students

Even though more people aged eighteen to twenty-four use illicit drugs than people in any other age group, the fact is that most college students do not take drugs. Why do some students experiment with drugs while others do not? Perhaps this is because the drug problem is essentially a people problem, and not all people are at risk for taking drugs.

Researchers have identified several risk factors for drug abuse among older teenagers and young adults, including college students. Peer pressure is the strongest and most consistent of all factors. In fact, two questions reveal much about the risk of drug use among teenagers and young adults: "Do your friends use drugs?" and "Do your close friends disapprove of your using drugs?" A positive answer to the first question coupled with a negative answer to the second question suggests a very high probability of drug use. Opposite answers suggest a low probability of drug use.

Families can influence drug use behavior. Children are more at risk for using drugs if their parents use drugs and alcohol. Being involved in their parents' habits—as in getting mom or dad a beer from the refrigerator or lighting a cigarette for them—also increases their likelihood of using alcohol, cigarettes, and marijuana. Parental influence also may be positive. Living at home with parents, in contrast to living in the dorm or other student housing arrangements, results in statistically lower rates of marijuana use by college students.

There is also a relationship between low grades and marijuana use. Researchers at the University of Maryland, College Park, found that students who had the lowest grade point averages (below 2.5) were four times more likely to have used marijuana in the past month than those students who had the highest grade point averages (3.6 and above). It could be that low grades are a risk factor for smoking marijuana, that marijuana use can result in low grades, or both.

Additional risk factors include rebelliousness and little commitment to school, psychological variables such as low self-esteem, and emotional variables such as stress, depression, and the need for excitement. As the number of risk factors increases, the chances of drug use also increase.

There is no simple answer to the question of why college students—or anyone else for that matter—take drugs. Among the reasons may be to escape, to reduce pain, to be less inhibited, to feel pleasure, to reduce stress, or to gain energy. The fact remains that some college students do choose to use drugs, often with harmful consequences. However, researchers at the University of Michigan recently reported that maturity—specifically the responsibilities of marriage and family—diminishes drug use. In what they called the marriage effect, the researchers found that marijuana use dropped on average by more than one third when young adults got married.

gateway drugs Drugs such as tobacco, alcohol, and marijuana that most users of illicit drugs have tried before their first use of cocaine, heroin, or other illicit drugs.

staging The use of drugs in a predictable progression beginning with gateway drugs, such as tobacco and alcohol, and progressing to hard drugs, such as crack, cocaine and heroin.

main effect The desired (intended) physical or mental response of the body to a drug; sometimes called the primary effect.

How Drugs Work

Drug actions are usually spoken of in terms of effect—the impact of the chemical substance on the body. The **main effect** of a drug is the intended effect, for which the drug is taken. In the case of diet pills, the main effect might be reduced hunger. Diet pills, however, are introduced through the stomach into the bloodstream, and thus throughout the system. They therefore cause other effects, some of which are not intended. A **side effect** is an effect that a drug has on the body that is not the intended effect. A side effect of diet pills might be anxiety, nervousness, or sometimes hallucinations.

Drugs don't act just anywhere in the body. They act on specific organs or tissues. A **receptor site** receives natural chemicals made and used by the body to carry out its day-to-day functions. A drug can attach itself to a receptor site if its molecules have the right size, shape, and chemical and electrical characteristics. The brain, for example, makes its own natural opiates—endorphins—that produce pleasure and mask pain. Heroin and other drugs in the opiate family are taken up by those same cells, or receptors (see Figure 8.2).

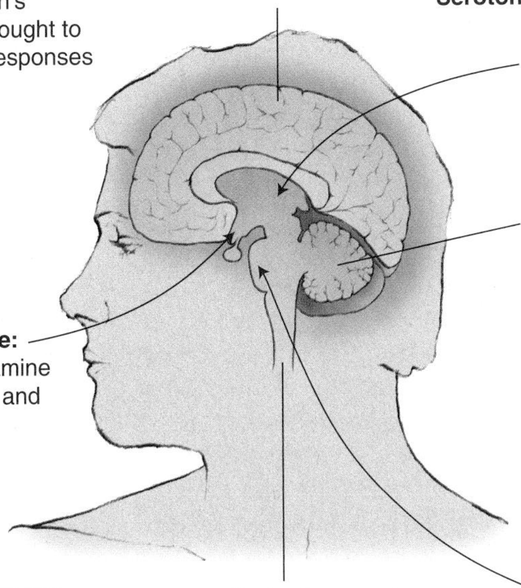

Figure 8.2 The Effect of Drugs on the Brain
Alcohol, cocaine, and heroin affect different parts of the brain. There are many theories about what happens in the brain and why.

Receptor sites may also hold some clues as to why users develop a tolerance to a drug and need increasing doses of it to get a high. According to one theory, chronic heroin use causes the brain to stop producing its own natural opiates, so highs have to come from outside the body. Another theory is that heroin users are more likely to have naturally underactive opiate systems.

Factors other than the drug itself or the receptor site can have a significant effect on the results of drug use. For example, the physical characteristics of the person taking a drug are critical to the actions of that drug. The same dosage of a drug taken by a 210-pound person may be far more potent if taken by a 120-pound person.

Without thinking much about the consequences, many people take more than one kind of drug a day—from a cold pill to marijuana. Taking more than one drug at a time is a very tricky business. The presence of two or more drugs in the body may result in an adverse **drug interaction.** Drugs may interact in three ways:

- *Additive effects.* The total effect of two drugs taken at the same time is equal to the simple sum of the two drugs' effects.
- *Inhibitory effects.* Two drugs are present at the same time, and the effect of one reduces or blocks the effect of the other.
- *Synergistic effects.* Two drugs present at the same time result in a total effect much greater than the simple sum of the two drugs' effects.

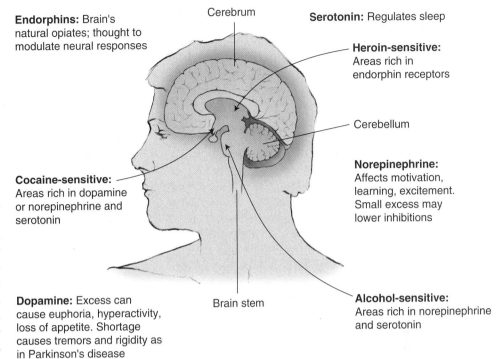

The additive effect of drugs can be seen when a cold remedy, which can be as much as 25 percent alcohol, is taken at the same time as an alcoholic beverage. This can lead to a blood alcohol content much higher than expected.

An example of the inhibitory effects of two drugs takes place when antibiotics are taken with birth control pills—the effectiveness of both is reduced. (The correct way to take prescription and over-the-counter drugs is discussed in Chapter 16.)

The synergistic effects are particularly potent when two **psychoactive** drugs, which have the potential to alter mood or behavior, are used. As an example of how

side effect An unwanted or even dangerous physical or mental effect caused by a drug or medicine.

receptor site The location in the body at which a drug triggers a response.

drug interaction The simultaneous presence of two or more drugs in the body, often having a detrimental effect.

psychoactive Affecting the mind or mental processes.

dangerous synergistic drug interactions can be, barbiturates (a depressant) and alcohol taken together have up to four times the depressant effect than either a barbiturate or alcohol would have alone. Mixing barbiturates and alcohol can result in death. Basically, the two drugs together can depress the central nervous system to the point that vital functions such as breathing cease.

A term often used to describe the undesired effects of taking a large amount of a single drug is **overdose**. An overdose can occur under two conditions: (1) when enough drug is consumed to produce exaggerated effects, or (2) when the person taking the drug is hypersensitive to the substance and thus physiologically or psychologically responds to even a small amount of the drug in an exaggerated manner. Most deaths attributed to cocaine use result from overdose. The fact that the drug is prepared without regulation means that concentrations of the drug vary from dose to dose because the purity of the product varies from purchase to purchase.

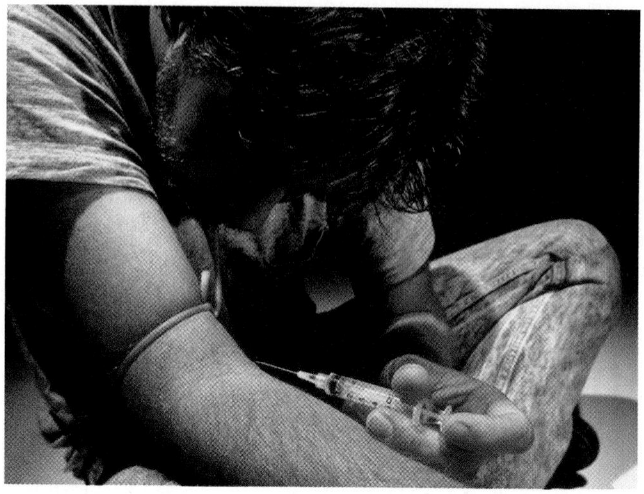

Illicit drugs are inhaled, smoked, swallowed, injected, or absorbed through the skin. Injecting illegal drugs carries the additional danger of contracting and spreading HIV.

Different Ways of Taking Drugs

Drugs may be inhaled, smoked, swallowed, injected, or absorbed through the skin. Drugs travel around the body differently, depending on how they are taken.

Some drugs are *inhaled* through the nostrils. In the case of legal drugs such as medication for asthma, the drug may be packaged in an inhaler to facilitate easy transmission. In the case of inhaled products such as airplane glue, which are taken to produce a high, the substance is put in a plastic or paper bag or on a rag and inhaled or sniffed. The results of inhaling a drug are almost immediate because the entry into the blood and in turn access to the brain is quick and easy through the lungs.

Inhalants are drugs that cause a quick rush to the brain. Popular abused inhalants are airplane glue, paint thinner, and dry cleaning solution. These substances are easily obtained at hardware stores. Restaurant and ice cream supply stores are the source of another abused inhalant—nitrous oxide capsules, which are used for making whipped cream. Some other inhalants have no commercial value other than to get the user high. An example of this type of inhalant is butyl nitrite. Because of their easy means of transmission, and in some cases easy access, children often abuse inhalants.

Marijuana and crack are two drugs that are usually *smoked.* The drug passes into the bloodstream and is carried to the brain in seconds.

When a drug is *swallowed,* as with most pills or in a marijuana brownie, the chemical reaches the brain more slowly because digestive processes are needed to release the psychoactive ingredients of the substance.

A more effective means of administering a drug is through *injection.* This occurs when a syringe is used to inject the drug directly into a vein. This is called an *intravenous injection.* Injections may also be *intramuscular* (into the muscle) or *subcutaneous* (under the skin). When a drug, such as heroin, is injected, it affects the brain within seconds. Injection, however, carries many health risks that are unrelated to the actual drug itself. HIV transmission, for example, can occur when unclean needles are used for administering illicit drugs.

Another means of transmission is *dermal* or *subdermal absorption*—often called topical application. Absorption, whether through use of a suppository, a transdermal patch, or a stamp, is a very effective means of transmitting drugs. LSD (lysergic acid diethylamide), for example, is often sold on stamp-like sections of paper to be placed on the tongue. The LSD on the stamp is absorbed through the tissue of the tongue. A transdermal patch with nicotine is used to transmit the drug to people who are trying to quit smoking yet still crave nicotine.

Effects of Drugs on the Mind and Body

Drugs are often classified by their psychoactive effects, or how they affect the mind. This provides a good way to compare and contrast drugs. There are five groups of substances: **stimulants, depressants,**

overdose A serious reaction to an excessive amount of a drug; it can result in coma or death.

inhalant A chemical that is inhaled through the nostrils to cause a quick rush to the brain; abused inhalants include airplane glue, paint thinner, and butyl nitrite.

stimulant A drug that speeds up the body's functions and movements.

depressant A drug that slows down the body's functions and movements.

Table 8.1 Drugs and Their Effects on Health

Stimulants	***Health effects of stimulants:*** Addiction, insomnia, excitability, hallucinations, severe mental disorders, malnutrition, and death.	
	What do they look like?	***How are they used?***
Amphetamines	Capsules, tablets, pills	Swallowed, inhaled, injected
Methamphetamines	White powder, pills, waxlike rock	Swallowed, injected
Cocaine	White powder	Inhaled, smoked, injected
Crack	Light brown or beige pellets, crystalline rocks	Smoked
Depressants	***Health Effects of Depressants:*** Addiction, decreased alertness, confusion, poor coordination and judgment, loss of appetite, drowsiness, irritability, nausea, and death.	
	What do they look like?	***How are they used?***
Barbiturates	Red, yellow, blue, or red-and-blue capsules	Swallowed
Methaqualone	Tablets	Swallowed
Narcotics	***Health Effects of Narcotics:*** Addiction, decreased alertness, confusion, hallucinations, stupor, slurred speech, nausea, vomiting, convulsions, unconsciousness, and death.	
	What do they look like?	***How are they used?***
Heroin	White to dark brown powder, tarlike substance	Injected, smoked, inhaled
Morphine	White crystals, injecting solutions	Injected, swallowed, smoked
Opium	Dark brown chunks, powder	Smoked, eaten
Hallucinogens	***Health Effects of Hallucinogens:*** Agitation, confusion, anxiety, changes in perception, impaired memory, anxiety, loss of coordination, hallucinations, delusions, vomiting, panic, severe mental disorders, and death.	
	What do they look like?	***How are they used?***
Phencyclidine	Liquid, capsules, pills, white powder	Swallowed, injected, smoked
Lysergic Acid Diethylamide	Colored tablets, blotter paper, thin squares of gelatin, clear liquid	Swallowed, licked off paper; gelatin and liquid can be put in eyes
Mescaline and Peyote	Tablets, capsules, hard brown discs	Chewed, swallowed, smoked
Psilocybin	Fried or dried mushrooms	Chewed, swallowed
Cannabis	***Health Effects of Cannabis:*** Psychological dependence, reduction of inhibitions, impaired memory, loss of interest and motivation, loss of coordination, changes in perception, panic, and paranoia.	
	What do they look like?	***How are they used?***
Marijuana	Dried parsley with stems and seeds	Smoked, eaten
Tetrahydrocannabinol	Soft gelatin capsules	Swallowed, smoked

narcotics, hallucinogens, and **cannabis.** Table 8.1 describes the major dangerous and illegal drugs, classified by psychoactive effects.

Stimulants. Stimulants speed up the body's functions and movements through actions on the central nervous system. They increase heart rate and raise blood pressure. In small doses they can improve alertness but with repeated use can cause restlessness and anxiety. A group of powerful stimulants is the amphetamines. These stimulants are available by prescription only and are considered safe when taken under a physician's

narcotic A drug that reduces pain and induces sleep.

hallucinogen A drug that causes a great change in perception.

cannabis Marijuana, hashish, ganga; the dried flowering tops of the hemp plant, *Cannabis sativa.*

supervision. But they may also be abused. Examples of amphetamines that are often abused are Benzedrine and Dexedrine. Closely related to the amphetamines are the *methamphetamines*—also called speed, meth, and ice. The effects of methamphetamine on the central nervous system are even greater than amphetamine, and users may become addicted quickly.

Methylphenidate, better known as Ritalin and used to calm hyperactive children, is another legally prescribed stimulant that is widely abused for its stimulant effects: appetite suppression, wakefulness, increased focus and attentiveness, and euphoria. Abusers take the tablets by mouth, crush and snort them, or dissolve them in water and inject the mixture.

Cocaine is a powerful but short-acting stimulant. Cocaine abusers sniff the drug into their noses, inject it into their bloodstreams, or smoke it. When smoked, crack—cocaine in its rock form, which vaporizes when heated—goes straight to the lungs and is released into the bloodstream, where it is pumped to every organ in the body within eight to ten seconds. In addition, crack is transported from the lungs to the brain directly. It bypasses the liver, which would normally detoxify the cocaine. Cocaine is highly addictive, and tolerance develops rapidly.

The effects of stimulants wear off quickly, so the abuser of these drugs may be left feeling depressed. Once depressed, the abuser may take more stimulants to counter the depression. Stimulants are habit forming and may be life threatening.

Depressants. Depressants slow down the body's functions and movements through actions on the central nervous system. Depressants relax a person and cause sleep. *Tranquilizers* such as Librium, Valium and Xanax are a form of depressant that slow nerve activity and relax muscle tension. They are safe when used as directed by a physician. They are used to treat anxiety, but can be habit forming. *Barbiturates* such as Nembutal and Seconal are also depressants considered safe when taken under a physician's supervision. Both tranquilizers and barbiturates are often abused. A tolerance for barbiturates or tranquilizers is developed quickly, causing the abuser to need more and more of the drug in order to feel the desired effects.

Narcotics. A narcotic is any drug made from or chemically similar to opium. Narcotics reduce pain and induce sleep. Opium is a drug obtained from the seed pod of a poppy plant. Morphine and codeine are natural narcotic compounds that are contained in opium. Heroin, a popularly used narcotic that is refined from morphine, is usually injected. Heroin addiction produces harsh withdrawal symptoms, including sweating, shaking, chills, nausea, and cramps. The user of heroin is always at risk for overdose because dealers often "cut," or dilute, the drug by adding other substances. This means that one purchase of heroin may be diluted while another may be pure. Codeine, an ingredient in some cough medicines, and pain killers such as OxyContin, Demoral, Percocet and Darvon, are other prescribed narcotics that are often abused.

Hallucinogens. Hallucinogens cause a change in perception, including causing people to see, hear, and feel things that are not really there. Hallucinogens are unpredictable—they may stimulate or depress the central nervous system. The strongest known hallucinogen is *LSD*. Users (all might be considered abusers) experience hallucinations in which they may see colorful visions and mistakenly feel that they have superhuman powers. Side effects are sometimes harsh, including unpleasant visions. The user of LSD may experience flashbacks, an unexpected return to the hallucinogenic state long after recovery from drug use. Other hallucinogens are mescaline, the psychoactive component of peyote cactus; psilocybin, which is obtained from a mushroom; and phencyclidine (PCP), an anesthetic used in veterinary medicine.

Cannabis. Cannabis, better known as marijuana, does not fit into any of the above categories because it can act like all of them. Under different circumstances, cannabis can be a stimulant, depressant, narcotic, or hallucinogen. This is because marijuana is not a single drug. It contains nearly 400 chemicals, at least 60 of which are unique to the *Cannabis sativa* plant. When marijuana is smoked, tetrahydrocannabinol (THC) enters the lungs, passes into the bloodstream, and is carried to the brain in seconds. Marijuana may act as a depressant because one or more chemicals having a depressing effect are present at a higher concentration at any given time in the body following marijuana use. It may act as a stimulant for similar reasons. Or it may cause a variety of reactions depending on the user's rate of metabolism of the various chemicals.

Designer drugs, like cannabis, do not fit in one specific class because they can mimic all of them. They look like drugs already on the market (both legal and illegal) but have something altered in their molecular structure so that they are "new" drugs. For example, one designer drug is a heroin substitute but is much more powerful and longer lasting. It has been linked to overdoses. Another designer drug, popularly called ecstasy, is similar to the stimulant methamphetamine and the hallucinogen mescaline. Its pleasurable effects include

designer drug A drug that looks like a drug already on the market but has something altered in its molecular structure so that it is a "new" drug. An example is ecstasy.

an enhanced sense of self-confidence, increased energy, and feelings of peacefulness. But it also produces hallucinations and can cause seizures, heart or kidney failure, and death.

Club drug is a term that refers to a wide variety of drugs, including ecstasy, Rohypnol ("roofies"), methamphetamine, and LSD. It refers to drugs used at all-night dance parties known as raves, at dance clubs, and at bars. While all of these drugs are dangerous by themselves, they can be even more dangerous—and lethal—when used in combination with alcohol. In addition, because some club drugs (such as roofies) are colorless, tasteless, and odorless, people who want to assault or sedate others can add them unobtrusively to beverages at a crowded party.

Anabolic steroids are another group of abused drugs. They promote tissue growth and lead to increased muscle mass and improved strength and power. While they are naturally in the body at safe levels, taking extra amounts of synthetic anabolic steroids can be dangerous.

Along with getting bigger, males who take steroids can experience numerous adverse side effects, including the development of breasts; hair loss; impotence and shrunken testicles; painful, prolonged erections; increased acne on the back, chest, and face; abnormally aggressive behavior, moodiness, and bodybuilders' psychosis; liver, kidney, and heart damage; stunted bone growth; cancer; and coma and death.

Steroid use isn't restricted to males, however. Recent indications suggest that more and more females are using steroids as well, and can have adverse reactions that include deepening of the voice, scalp hair loss, body hair growth, and clitoral enlargement.

Steroids are taken either by mouth in pill form or by injection. Sharing needles has resulted in a new health hazard associated with steroid use: HIV infection and AIDS.

The Impact of Drug Abuse

The cost of drug abuse is staggering: $160 billion a year. About 60 percent is associated with crime and the rest with illness, related medical care, and death. More than 25,000 people a year die from drug abuse; specific causes include hepatitis, homicide, suicide, and injury. Drug abuse ruins individuals, families, and neighborhoods. Drug abusers drop out of school and work, and the loss of their potential and self-esteem is immeasurable. The office of National Drug Control Policy estimates that typical heroin users spend $210 a week—about $11,000 a year on their habits. The only way for most people to get this kind of money is to do something illegal—stealing, pimping, prostituting, or selling drugs. It is estimated that an addict has to steal three to five times the actual cost of the drugs he or she abuses to maintain his or her habit. This means stealing about $33,000 to $55,000 worth of goods a year. There are no accurate figures on drug-related prostitution, but about one of every three or four prostitutes in major cities is thought to be a heroin addict.

The Health Toll from Drugs

Of all the drug-related health problems, AIDS exacts the greatest toll because of its impact on the individual involved as well as on society at large. AIDS is the fastest growing cause of all illegal-drug–related deaths. According to epidemiologists, injecting drug users who also smoke crack are seven times more likely to become infected than are injecting drug users not on crack. This is attributed to addicts swapping sex with their suppliers for crack or selling sex for money to buy the drug. This makes crack a significant contributing risk factor for AIDS.

People who inject drugs get the virus by sharing their needles, syringes, and other drug paraphernalia with users who already have HIV in their blood. AIDS is caused by a virus that destroys the body's immune system. It is passed from one person to another in bodily fluids, including blood, semen, and vaginal secretions. It can also be transmitted from an infected mother to her newborn baby.

In an effort to stop the increase in AIDS among injecting drug users, cities from New York City to Portland, Oregon, have experimented with programs in which free, clean needles are distributed to addicts. Researchers studying needle exchange programs are reporting positive results—that is, fewer cases of HIV infection and no increase in drug use. In addition, many communities have instituted programs that disseminate street information to drug users, and that provide them with condoms. These programs are controversial because they aid the continuation of an illegal activity—possession of heroin, cocaine, and other drugs that are injected.

club drug A term that refers to a wide variety of dangerous drugs used often in combination with alcohol at all-night dance parties known as *raves,* at dance clubs, and at bars. An example is ecstasy.

anabolic steroid A drug that promotes tissue growth and leads to increased muscle mass and improved strength and power.

Even noninjected drugs have a connection to AIDS. Drugs and sexual promiscuity often go together. Because drugs alter judgment, drug users are prone to engage in indiscriminate and unsafe sex, thus putting themselves and their partners at higher risk for getting HIV. Recent research indicates that HIV may require the presence of an already damaged immune system before it can cause disease. Some drugs, including amphetamines, marijuana, and inhalants, may first damage the immune system, leaving the user open to the further risk of AIDS. In addition, inhalants may be a cofactor in the development of Kaposi's sarcoma, a cancer associated with AIDS.

Special Concern for the Fetus

More than 10 percent of American babies are at risk for medical complications because their mothers abused drugs during pregnancy. The effect of a drug on a fetus depends on many factors, including the drug, the amount taken by the mother, and the stage of pregnancy at which it is taken. The fetus is in greatest danger during the first three months of pregnancy, when its major organs are developing.

Studies show that cocaine use at any time during pregnancy—even once—can cause lasting fetal damage. When cocaine crosses the placenta, a large proportion of it is converted into norcocaine, a water-soluble substance that does not leave the womb. It is thought that norcocaine is more potent than cocaine itself. At the very least, the fetus is continually exposed to it. Norcocaine is excreted into the amniotic fluid and the fetus swallows it and thus is re-exposed to the drug. Not only are many of these children born addicted to cocaine, but also they tend to suffer strokes and to have retarded growth, including smaller-than-normal-size heads and brains, and delayed motor development.

In general, pregnant women who are injecting drug users or sexual partners of injecting drug users greatly increase the risk of infecting themselves and their fetuses with HIV. About 30 percent of all babies born in the United States to mothers with HIV become infected.

Who should protect an unborn child from drugs? Lawsuits have been brought against women who have given birth to drug-addicted babies or have otherwise compromised their babies' lives by taking drugs during pregnancy. This has created much discussion within the legal community. Some of the issues involved in this controversy are an individual's right to privacy, the problem of proving intent to harm, and the conflict between fetal rights and women's rights.

maintenance program A treatment program that involves providing a less dangerous drug to prevent withdrawal symptoms.

detoxification program A treatment program that involves a gradual but complete withdrawal from an abused drug.

therapeutic community A residential treatment center where people who abuse drugs can live and learn to adjust to drug-free lives.

Harm Reduction: Preventing Drug Trafficking

One way to reduce the harm caused by illicit drugs is to reduce their entry into the United States. The number one point of entry of drugs is the United States–Mexico border, where cocaine, heroin, methamphetamine, and marijuana come in hidden among the millions of cars, people, and drugs that cross thirty-eight ports of entry spanning nearly 2,000 miles. The second largest drug trafficking route into the country is through the Caribbean, specifically via Puerto Rico and the U.S. Virgin Islands. Drugs, especially heroin, also come in from southeast Asia.

Each year, thousands of pounds of drugs worth millions of dollars are seized by U.S. government officials. Despite national and international efforts to disrupt trafficking—including reducing coca cultivation abroad and increasing arrests at home—drugs still come into the United States illegally. To consider different points of view on the drug issue, see the Developing Health Skills box.

Treatment Alternatives: The Long Road Back

A wide range of treatment alternatives are available for drug users, including **maintenance** and **detoxification programs, therapeutic communities,** hotlines, rap centers, and self-help groups. Drug abuse is a chronic, relapsing condition, which means that treatment is usually needed on more than one occasion. However, studies show that 30 percent to 50 percent of patients remained drug-free for one year after completing treatment—success rates that are comparable for people with other chronic, relapsing health conditions, such as asthma, diabetes, and hypertension.

Maintenance Programs

Maintenance programs involve substituting a more socially acceptable and less dangerous drug for the drug

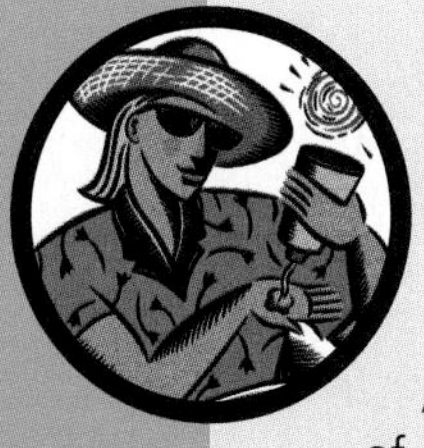

Developing Health Skills

Perspectives on Solving the Drug Problem: What Will Work?

Public opinion polls consistently show that Americans are greatly concerned about the extent of drug use in their country. There is no consistent response, however, on how to solve the drug problem. Attitudes toward drug use are diverse and conflicting and proposed solutions range from jailing all first-time offenders to legalizing drugs to making treatment and rehabilitation available to drug users.

Consider the following personal perspectives on the drug problem:

An Advocate of Stronger Law Enforcement

"What we need in this country are stronger laws, more laws, and more law enforcement officers. Test everybody for the presence of controlled substances within their system, and whoever fails should go to jail or pay a stiff fine. If we can simply get the pusher off the street and stop the flow of drugs across our borders, then our problems will be solved. The way to do this is to build more prisons and require that drug users and pushers serve time. In fact, we should take a hint from some of our foreign friends and cut off the hands of drug pushers. They would have a difficult time pushing so hard if they had no hands."

- Would the money spent on building jails and hiring law enforcement officers be better spent on drug rehabilitation and prevention?
- If everyone is tested for drug use, won't civil rights be abused?

An Advocate of Legalizing Drugs

"Make drugs legal, and the corruption and violence associated with them will disappear. Our cities will be safe again. The Prohibition Era proved that making a substance illegal simply doesn't work. That's why the eighteenth amendment was repealed. It was done with alcohol, and now it's time to legalize drugs."

- Won't this lead to more people taking drugs?
- Isn't there a big difference between legalizing marijuana and legalizing cocaine?

An Advocate of Education and Prevention

"The only answer lies in prevention. We must get to the children before they take their first drug. Let's tell them how to say no in social situations. Let's give them the facts about the dangers of drugs. If we are ever going to have a drug-free society, we must begin with a drug-free population—our children."

- Children recognize split messages such as, "Do as I say and not as I do." How can we ask them to say no to drugs when so many adults say yes?

A Former Addict

"Nobody knows what I know. When you take drugs you lose control. You forget about society, you forget about honesty, you forget your values and your moral upbringing. You'd kill your mother for a $5 hit. Nobody knows who has never been there. The answer is to provide treatment for the drug users—bring them back from the dead through intensive intervention and support. If we do that for everyone, then we'll be on the road to solving the drug problem."

- What does treatment cost, and who will pay for it—employers? The federal government?
- Can former addicts really be effective proponents of "say no" when they have said yes for so long?

of choice. The substitute is provided free or at low cost. Maintenance programs are mainly used for heroin addiction. Methadone, a synthetic drug, is used to alleviate an addict's craving for the natural drug heroin and to prevent withdrawal symptoms. There are many benefits of methadone:

- It is easy to administer (a pill).
- Its effects last twenty-four to thirty-six hours, compared with heroin's action of four to eight hours.
- It does not produce a feeling of euphoria.
- It is safe at maintenance levels.
- It frees users from a physical dependence on heroin so they can spend their energy putting their life back together—being part of a family, working, going to school.
- It is legal.

Methadone's primary purpose is to prevent withdrawal symptoms. It can help heroin addicts seeking another "hit" to avoid criminal behavior. The main disadvantage of methadone is that it substitutes one addiction for another. It does not change the underlying addictive behavior.

Detoxification Programs

The goal of a detoxification program is to reduce drug intake to zero and to give the addict medical and

Assess Your Health

How Would You React in These Situations?

Below are ten situations involving drugs. Read each situation, then circle the letter next to the action that you would most likely take.

1. During lunch, a friend claims that "everyone" should smoke marijuana, just to find out what it is like. This friend offers to get you high. What would you do in this situation?

- **A.** Tell your friend that you don't care what getting high is like.
- **B.** Avoid the subject by asking if anyone would like to go to a movie later.
- **C.** Point out to your friend that you know enough about marijuana to know that it's no good.
- **D.** Accept your friend's offer to try marijuana.

2. You are at a large party. You meet some people who are snorting cocaine. They invite you to sit down and "do some coke." What would you do in this situation?

- **A.** Sit down and snort the cocaine.
- **B.** Turn and leave without speaking.
- **C.** Sit down, but say, "Not right now," to the offer of cocaine.
- **D.** Explain that you don't use cocaine.

3. The actions of a close relative have made you extremely upset. When you discuss this with a friend, he offers you some tranquilizers to calm you down. What would you do in this situation?

- **A.** Accept the pills from your friend, but throw them away once your friend leaves.
- **B.** Accept the tranquilizers and take them.
- **C.** Refuse the pills and ask your friend to leave.
- **D.** Thank your friend for the offer, but refuse the pills.

4. You go out for the evening with a new friend whom you like very much. On your way to dinner, your friend asks if you would like to smoke some very good hashish. You can tell that your friend is trying to do something special for you. What would you do in this situation?

- **A.** End the evening right then and go home.
- **B.** Tell your friend that you're not ready to try smoking hashish yet.
- **C.** Smoke the hashish and make your friend happy.
- **D.** Decline the hashish and hope that you don't hurt your friend's feelings.

5. You must work many hours without rest to finish a project. A person working with you offers you some "speed" (amphetamines) to help you stay awake. What would you do in this situation?

- **A.** Say that you are concerned that taking speed would make you less able to do your work.
- **B.** Accept the pills, but throw them away when you go to get a glass of water.
- **C.** Say that you would rather keep drinking coffee to try to stay awake.
- **D.** Accept the speed, and take it.

6. A long-time friend asks you to try LSD. Your friend has never taken LSD and wants to find out what it is like. Your friend wants the two of you to take it together. What would you do in this situation?

- **A.** Tell your friend to take the LSD alone or with someone else.
- **B.** Take LSD with your friend, as long as you can find a safe time and place to do it.
- **C.** Suggest that the two of you find something safer to do than take LSD.
- **D.** Tell your friend that you might take LSD, but then hope that your offer is forgotten.

7. You are having dinner with several friends who are cigarette smokers. When the coffee is served, most of them light up. One offers you a cigarette. What would you do in this situation?

- **A.** Say that you don't smoke.
- **B.** Decline the offer, saying that you want to wait awhile.
- **C.** Have a cigarette.
- **D.** Tell the person that you can't smoke because you have a chest cold.

8. Your new neighbors invite you over for dinner. After dinner, one of them says that they sometimes smoke marijuana in the evening. They invite you to smoke with them. What would you do in this situation?

- **A.** Decline the offer and go home.
- **B.** Decline the marijuana, but stay and talk.
- **C.** Smoke the marijuana.
- **D.** Tell them that you would rather smoke it some other time.

9. You are under great pressure at work. You feel nervous all the time and have begun to lose sleep. A good friend suggests that you take some Valium (tranquilizers) until the pressure eases off. Your friend has a prescription for the drug and can easily give you the pills. What would you do in this situation?

- **A.** Try the pills to see if they help.
- **B.** Accept the pills, but throw them away.
- **C.** Refuse your friend's offer.
- **D.** Tell your friend that you would like to think about it.

10. You attend a party of people from work. To your surprise, several of your coworkers are snorting cocaine ("coke") together. It is apparent that they have done this before, and they encourage you to join them. These are people you work with every day, and you like them. What would you do in this situation?

A. Tell the group that your ride is leaving, so you don't have time to use the cocaine.

B. Snort the cocaine.

C. Tell the group that you don't use drugs.

D. Refuse the offer by saying that you're not in the mood to snort cocaine.

Below is a key to the answer choices that entail using drugs. For each of these selected, assign no points. For any other response selected, assign one point. Sum your scores.

Item no.	Drug use response
1	D
2	A
3	B
4	C
5	D
6	B
7	C
8	C
9	A
10	B

A maximum score of ten indicates that you believe strongly that you will not take drugs if offered. A minimum score of zero indicates that you believe strongly that you will take drugs if offered.

Source: U.S. Department of Health and Human Services, Office of Disease Prevention and Health Promotion

psychological assistance during withdrawal. This approach can work well, especially for alcoholics. The majority of heroin addicts who enter a detoxification program drop out after a few days because, even though the discomfort of withdrawal is minimized, the craving for heroin still remains. Some detoxification centers are housed in hospitals or clinics; others are in outpatient settings with the addicts attending programs and therapeutic sessions all day.

Therapeutic Communities

The goal of therapeutic communities is to deal with the psychological cause of drug dependence and to bring about a complete lifestyle change. This includes moving toward abstinence from drugs, developing employable skills or returning to school, self-reliance, and honesty. Part of the treatment includes encountering group therapy and group pressure. All members of the community are assigned jobs in the community and eventually on the "outside." Staff members are mostly former drug addicts who have been rehabilitated in the same or a similar therapeutic community.

One of the drawbacks of this approach is that it takes about fifteen months before a resident is ready to leave the community, and there is a high dropout rate. Some people get bored or frustrated with the program or aren't ready for such a complete change in their lifestyles. Among those who remain, there is a relatively high success rate.

Other Treatment Modalities

Although these results are not clinically documented, some people report successful treatment for drug addiction with acupuncture, biofeedback, and hypnosis. In addition, there are groups including Narcotics Anonymous, free clinics, and hot lines, which are used for self-help and crisis intervention and to direct people to appropriate resources in the community. The growth of drug abuse treatment facilities in recent years reflects an increase in the demand for such services.

Caution should be exercised when deciding to seek professional help for a substance abuse problem. A reliable way to check a treatment center's credentials is through your physician, college health clinic, a local medical school, or a psychiatric society.

Preventing Drug Abuse

Here are some strategies that health education specialists recommend for college students to prevent drug abuse. Think about how you can incorporate them as a part of your lifestyle (see the Assess Your Health box).

Build self-esteem and self-confidence. Drug abuse is a symptom of low self-esteem. For the person who values social acceptance above his or her own health, drug abuse is an option. For the person who values him- or herself above the all-too-brief social acceptance of a night out, drug abuse is not an option.

Make decisions about drugs rationally, not emotionally. Be proactive, not reactive. The decision to use or not to use a drug should not be a spur-of-the-moment choice. It should be done well ahead of the real-life confrontation with drugs. Good decision-making skills include (1) honestly assessing a situation and identifying the problems that might result, (2) examining solutions to the problems and the possible consequences of each solution, (3) taking action that is in the best interest of yourself and those around you, and (4) evaluating the choices.

Assertively resist peer pressure. Peer pressure exists at all levels of society and at all ages. Being assertive is important in dealing with many health-related behaviors. Whether the pressure is to drink or to become involved with harder drugs like crack cocaine, resistance is a matter of assertively standing up to people—and for yourself.

Reduce stress. Stress is one of the primary reasons people turn to drugs. By developing coping skills and learning breathing exercises and other techniques, you can reduce stress and, in turn, reduce the potential for succumbing to drug abuse.

Get involved in hobbies and recreational activities. Hobbies and recreational activities can provide excitement and challenge. The healthy nature of such activities leaves little room for the unhealthy activity of drug abuse.

Remain informed. Get accurate and up-to-date information about drugs, including the short- and long-term risks. By knowing the facts, you will be in a good position not to want to engage in health-compromising behaviors.

CASE STUDY 8: Drug Use

Suzy studies hard and usually gets good grades. After studying for a big exam she felt tense and "relaxed" by smoking marijuana with some friends. She started smoking cigarettes when she was in high school, so smoking marijuana was an easy move for her.

The next day, Suzy remembered very little of what she had reviewed. She didn't know that marijuana can affect short-term memory; instead, she rationalized that she hadn't studied enough—after all, she did take some time off to be with friends. She didn't associate the lower grade with her marijuana smoking.

James has to work hard to get B's and C's, so he takes all of his exams seriously. He studies his class notes ahead of time—not just the night before an exam. And he goes over review questions with classmates to help him feel more confident when answering the real test questions.

Like Suzy, he took some time the night before the exam to be with friends. But unlike Suzy he didn't do anything that would cloud his judgment and understanding about facts and concepts during the exam. He went to a popular coffee bar, listened to music, and just hung out and relaxed.

In Your Opinion

Suzy never questioned whether marijuana was responsible for her lower grade, and James never took the risk of smoking it before an exam.

- Suzy has progressed from smoking cigarettes to smoking marijuana, but vows that she would never try any other drug. Does the use of marijuana increase the chances to using other drugs? Why or why not?
- Suzy is not convinced that the joints she smoked affected her test score. What evidence would you suggest to convince her otherwise?
- On another night, Suzy smokes her usual joint, but instead of feeling relaxed, she becomes high-strung, excessively tense, and then very upset. Why would this reaction occur?
- How do you explain James's ability to avoid drug use?

KEY CONCEPTS

1. The term *drug* refers to a chemical substance that causes a change in the body's functioning, including physiological and psychological activity.
2. Drug abuse normally occurs in stages, with a typical progression starting with cigarettes, beer, or wine; moving on to marijuana and hard liquor; and subsequently moving on to illicit drugs such as heroin and cocaine.
3. Marijuana is the most frequently used illicit drug by college students.
4. When used properly, many drugs, such as antibiotics, offer great benefit. These drugs, however, can be misused in a way that leads to a threat to health and well-being.
5. Dependence occurs when a person is so physically and/or psychologically attached to a drug that he or she cannot live comfortably without it.
6. A drug may affect only a limited portion of the body,

or it may affect the entire body. Drugs also can be transmitted across the placenta and compromise the normal development of a fetus.

7. Drugs are grouped as stimulants, depressants, hallucinogens, and narcotics. Marijuana (cannabis) can act like all of them, and is in a class by itself.
8. Designer drugs can mimic all of the groups of drugs, and are a variation on illegal drugs. An example of a designer drug is ecstasy.
9. The National Institute on Drug Abuse estimates that typical drug users spend $210 a week—about $11,000 a year—on their habits.
10. Treatments for drug addiction include maintenance and detoxification programs, therapeutic communities, hot lines, and self-help groups such as Narcotics Anonymous.

REVIEW QUESTIONS

1. List the drugs most often used by college students.
2. Define the term *drug,* and explain how over-the-counter drugs, prescription drugs, and dangerous or illegal substances all fit the definition.
3. What is a gateway drug and how is it related to the concept of staging?
4. Differentiate between main effects and side effects of drugs.
5. Using mathematics, illustrate additive, inhibitory, and synergistic effects that result when two or more drugs are taken at the same time.
6. Explain the differences between stimulants, depressants, hallucinogens, narcotics, and cannabis.
7. List ways that injecting illegal drugs harms health.
8. Of all the health risks associated with drug abuse, why is the fetus in a most vulnerable position?
9. Describe three treatment alternatives for individuals experiencing a drug problem.
10. List specific actions you can take in order to avoid drug abuse.

CRITICAL THINKING QUESTIONS

1. The *Healthy People 2010* objectives include the following: "Increase the proportion of patients who receive verbal counseling from prescribers and pharmacists on the appropriate use and potential risks of medications." Perhaps "verbal counseling" can help prevent the accidental misuse of prescription drugs, but can it prevent the intentional abuse of such substances? What can be done to make sure prescription drugs are used *only* for their intended purposes?
2. The concept of staging in drug abuse has been understood for generations, yet much of the effort to address the drug problem focuses on the user of hard drugs, not the user of gateway drugs. Would our efforts to curb drug abuse be better spent addressing gateway drugs?
3. Needle exchange programs are designed to reduce the health threats that occur through the use of illegal drugs such as heroin or crack cocaine. Opponents to needle exchange programs insist that such action condones, and may even encourage, the continuation of an illegal activity. Supporters of such programs point to the scientific evidence of the reduction in disease transmission and the lack of evidence of increased drug usage that result. How do you feel about needle exchange programs? Should they be supported because they are scientifically sound? Should they be canceled because they condone illegal behavior?
4. The *Healthy People 2010* objectives include the following: "Increase the number of communities using partnerships or coalition models to conduct comprehensive substance abuse prevention efforts." What do "partnership" and "coalition" have to do with reducing the problems of substance abuse? Is substance abuse an individual problem? Or is substance abuse a problem that affects the community as a whole?

JOURNAL ACTIVITY

1. Think of a time you took a risk that you later realized could have been dangerous for you or someone else, or in fact was dangerous. Did that risk involve the use of drugs? Develop a check list for evaluating risk, and use it as a tool to help you "draw the line" on risk, particularly as it relates to drugs.
2. Make a list of places where you can go for information about drug treatments on your campus and in the community. Call three or four of them for information about their treatment program. For example, find out what the program includes, how long it usually lasts, and how much it costs. If you had a drug problem, which one would you go to first, and why?
3. Write the pros and cons of a child abuse conviction for a woman who took drugs during her pregnancy and gave birth to a child with drug-related birth defects. What sentence would you give her, and why?
4. Contact a local law enforcement agency to find out what laws relate to possession and use of illegal substances. Make a table or graph to show the incidence of drug-related arrests in your community over the past two weeks, and match the law with the arrests. Are you surprised at the findings, or are they what you would have expected given what you heard on news programs?

SELECTED BIBLIOGRAPHY

Cahalan, D. *An Ounce of Prevention: Strategies for Solving Tobacco, Alcohol, and Drug Problems.* San Francisco: Jossey-Bass, 1991.

The Economic Costs of Drug Abuse in the United States, 1992–1998. Rockville, MD: Office of National Drug Control Policy, 2001.

Hoyert, D. L., K. D. Kochanek, and S. L. Murphy. "Deaths: Final data for 1997." *National Vital Statistics Reports,* vol 47, no 19. Hyattsville, MD: National Center for Health Statistics, 1999.

Monitoring the Future Study. Rockville, MD: National Institute on Drug Abuse (published annually).

National Household Survey on Drug Abuse. Rockville, MD: Substance Abuse and Mental Health Services Administration (published annually).

Principles of Drug Addiction Treatment: A Research-Based Guide. Rockville, MD: National Institute on Drug Abuse, 1999.

Substance Abuse: The Nation's Number One Health Problem. Princeton, NJ: The Robert Wood Johnson Foundation, 2001.

HEALTHLINKS

Websites for Understanding the Dangers of Drug Use

You can access better health as it relates to this chapter by checking out some of the following sites on the Internet. These sites can be accessed directly from the *Decisions for Healthy Living* Website located at www.aw.com/pruitt.

Center for Substance Abuse Research (CESAR)

Based at the University of Maryland, the Center for Substance Abuse Research collects, analyzes, and disseminates information on the nature and extent of substance abuse and related problems.

National Institute on Drug Abuse

Home page of this national government agency with information on the latest statistics and findings in drug research, including community drug alerts on specific drugs.

Partnership for a Drug-Free America

This site includes information on the slang names of drugs, identification of different drugs, and tips on how to talk to youth about drugs.

HEALTH HOTLINES

Understanding the Dangers of Drug Use

National Clearinghouse for Alcohol and Drug Information
11426 Rockville Pike, Suite 200
Rockville, MD 20852
(800) SAY-NOTO (729-6686)

National Drug and Alcohol Treatment Routing Service
107 Lincoln Street
Worcester, MA 01605
(800) 662-HELP (662-4357)

TEST YOUR KNOWLEDGE ANSWERS

1. True. Rohypnol impairs mental judgment, results in amnesia, and is used to incapacitate innocent people who are then subjected to assaults such as rape.
2. False. Students who have lower grade-point averages are four times more likely to have used marijuana than students who have higher grade-point averages.
3. True. The brain produces endorphins—natural opiates that produce pleasure and hide pain.
4. False. Cannabis, or marijuana, is not classified as a hallucinogen. It contains nearly 400 chemicals and produces a variety of responses. It sometimes acts as a stimulant, sometimes a depressant, and only occasionally as a hallucinogen. It is not classified with any one group of drugs.
5. True. Between 30 percent and 50 percent of drug treatment patients remain drug free—rates comparable for people with chronic, relapsing health conditions such as asthma, diabetes, and hypertension.

CHAPTER

9

The Health Threats of Unintentional Injuries and Violence

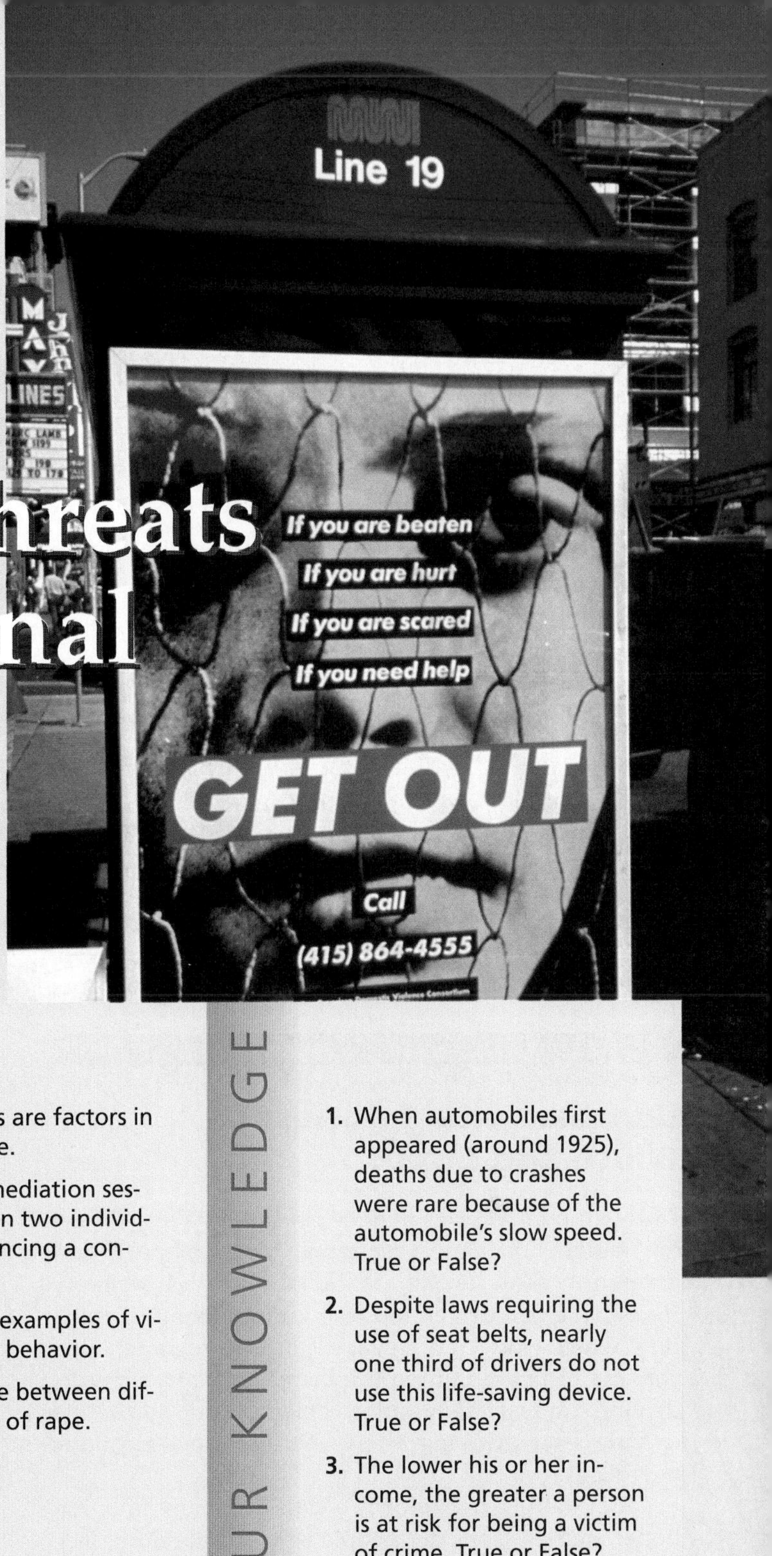
Line 19
LINES
If you are beaten
If you are hurt
If you are scared
If you need help
GET OUT
Call
(415) 864-4555

OBJECTIVES

When you finish reading this chapter, you will be able to:

1. Differentiate between an unintentional and an intentional injury (violence) and recognize that both are public health threats.
2. Describe a person at risk for an unintentional injury.
3. Recognize motor vehicle crashes as the primary cause of unintentional injuries in the United States.
4. Recognize that alcohol consumption greatly enhances the potential of encountering an unintentional injury.
5. List causes of unintentional injuries that occur in the home.
6. List several characteristics of the typical victim of violent crime.
7. Describe how television, drugs, and the availability of handguns are factors in violent crime.
8. Conduct a mediation session between two individuals experiencing a conflict.
9. Cite several examples of violent sexual behavior.
10. Differentiate between different types of rape.

TEST YOUR KNOWLEDGE

1. When automobiles first appeared (around 1925), deaths due to crashes were rare because of the automobile's slow speed. True or False?
2. Despite laws requiring the use of seat belts, nearly one third of drivers do not use this life-saving device. True or False?
3. The lower his or her income, the greater a person is at risk for being a victim of crime. True or False?
4. Having a gun at home significantly reduces a person's chances of dying violently due to the self-defense capabilities that a gun provides. True or False?
5. Most college students who have been raped report having known the rapist before the incident occurred. True or False?

Answers found at end of chapter.

No one intends to have an injury or be a victim of **violence**. Nevertheless, nearly one hundred thousand people a year in the United States are killed because of an **unintentional injury,** and millions more are left with serious disabilities; about 50 million people a year are victims of violence, or an **intentional injury.** But until it happens to you or someone close to you, you probably give little thought to injury or violence. College students may not feel vulnerable to these acts, but among fifteen- to twenty-four-year-olds—the age group that covers most college students—unintentional injuries and homicide (an extreme manifestation of violence) are the leading and second leading causes of death in the United States (see Figure 9.1). Suicide, another form of intentional injury, was discussed in Chapter 2.

Crossing the street against the light, riding your bike without wearing a helmet, leaving your front door unlocked, staying in an abusive relationship—these are all potentially dangerous situations that can result in injuries or acts of violence.

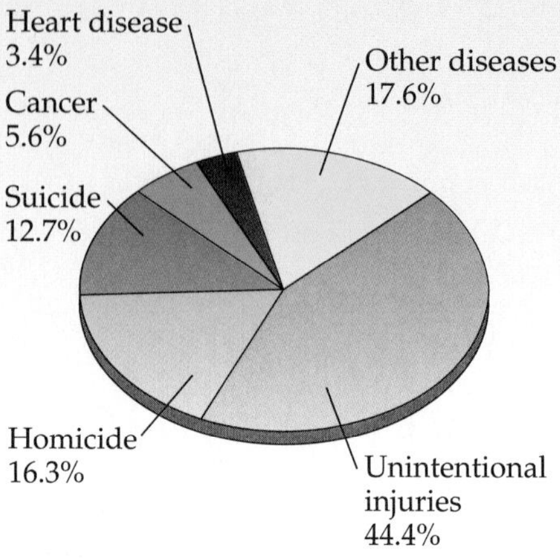

Figure 9.1 Unintentional Injuries and Violence Are the Leading Causes of Death in the College-Age Group

Accidents and homicide are responsible for more deaths for people aged fifteen to twenty-four than any other cause.

(*Source:* National Center for Health Statistics)

Unintentional Injuries: Cause and Effect

Unintentional injuries may be caused by many different factors. In some cases, one factor alone is not enough to cause an unintentional injury. How many times have you driven too fast without being injured? But when you add several factors together, the chances of being injured are increased—for example, driving too fast *and* failing to obey a traffic signal *and* driving after drinking a few beers or other alcoholic beverages.

Risk-taking behavior is a cause of many unintentional injuries. Consider people who, for the thrill of it, jump from a railroad bridge into a river. Drowning occurs more often as a result of such risky behavior than from accidents occurring in swimming areas patrolled by lifeguards.

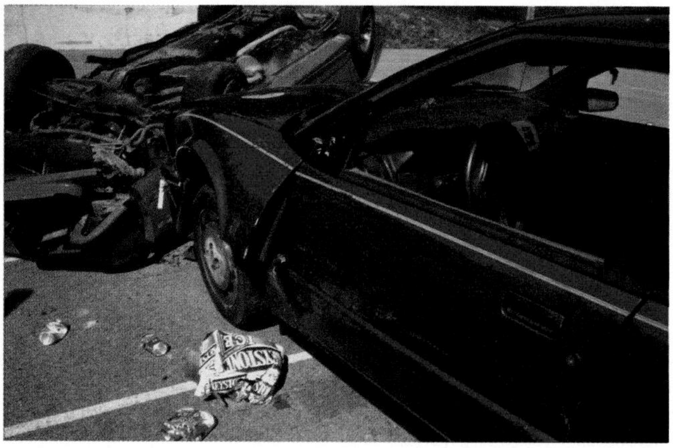

Alcohol is the number one cause of preventable traffic deaths.

Impaired functioning increases the likelihood of unintentional injuries. Alcohol is the number one cause of preventable traffic fatalities. Even moderate levels of alcohol in the blood have been found to impair judgment markedly. More than half a million college students experience an alcohol-related injury or death each year, frequently driving while under the influence of alcohol or riding in a car or on a motorcycle with an operator who has been drinking. Alcohol

violence The use of force with the intent to harm oneself or another person.

unintentional injuries Injuries that are caused by unplanned events, such as automobile crashes, falls, poisonings, fires, and drownings.

intentional injuries Injuries that result from planned events associated with suicide, homicide, and assault.

risk-taking behavior Actions that intentionally place an individual at risk for personal injury.

also is implicated in about one third of all fatal bicycle injuries and is a leading cause of drowning among young adult men.

Psychological factors are also related to unintentional injuries. Anger, for example, may be the cause of many fatal automobile injuries. The driver may be preoccupied with his or her anger about something unrelated to driving or may become angered by another driver's action on the road—a case of road rage.

Many unintentional injuries are caused by hazards in the environment. Some of these hazards are natural, such as ice on the road. Some are unavoidable or unrecognizable, such as being in or near a building during an earthquake or tornado. Natural events and unavoidable threats like these are difficult to predict, but much can be done to minimize the injuries that result. Studies show that people living in trailer parks have the highest risk of injury and death in a tornado. Seeking shelter in a school or other large public building when a tornado is predicted could significantly reduce these risks.

Profile of an At-Risk Person

Who is most at risk for unintentional injuries? In an attempt to answer this question, epidemiologists have studied people who have been injured.

- At all ages, men are at greater risk for unintentional injury than are women. Moreover, the injuries sustained by men are more serious than those of women. For example, men are twice as likely as women to die from injuries in car crashes.
- Deaths from unintentional injuries are more prevalent in rural areas, especially in the West. This may be due to greater distances to travel and more high-speed driving in these areas and to greater exposure to hazardous equipment, such as farm machinery.
- The poor in urban and rural areas are at greater risk because they tend to have older, less safe cars and to live in low-quality housing with hazardous products such as space heaters, which can cause fires.
- Native Americans often have multiple risk factors: They may be poor, live in rural areas, and consume a higher than average amount of alcohol. They have higher death rates from unintentional injuries than do other ethnic groups.
- High-risk jobs include mining, construction, agriculture, fire fighting, and working on oil rigs. Even in these risky jobs, the primary reason for on-the-job fatalities is a motor vehicle accident; second is a fall. Working for a bicycle messenger service and riding through downtown traffic and delivering pizza by car or truck are examples of jobs in which motor vehicle accidents might happen to college students.

Collectively, these factors characterize the individual prone to being injured, either by personal attributes or by environmental exposure. People who take care to reduce hazards to which they may be exposed may easily reduce risk and the chances of unintentional injury. Refer to the Assess Your Health box to explore your own risk level.

Safety on the Road and Waterfront

The rate of U.S. motor vehicle fatalities has dropped consistently and dramatically over the decades—from a high of 21.6 deaths per 100 million vehicle miles in 1925 to 1.6 deaths per 100 million vehicle miles in 2000. Even so, motor vehicles account for nearly half of all unintentional deaths in the country.

The decline in fatalities in recent years is associated with several factors, including the growing use of seat belts, air bags, and an increase in the drinking age to twenty-one. It is illegal in every state and the District of Columbia to sell alcoholic beverages to anyone under the age of twenty-one, and in some states, it is illegal for people in this age group to drive with any alcohol in their blood.

At the same time, increased use of cell phones while driving has led to more crashes. A recent study by the Harvard Center for Risk Analysis found that drivers talking on their phones are responsible for about 6 percent of U.S. automobile accidents each year. Cell phones, however, do have a safety side: Having a cell phone in your car can lead to quicker reporting of an accident or crime.

Seat Belts and Air Bags

All states except New Hampshire have mandatory seat belt use laws, but only about two thirds of the population use seat belts every time they ride in a car. It is clear that in an accident, seat belts can save lives and reduce injuries. To assess the impact of seat belt use on the extent of injuries sustained in automobile crashes, researchers retrospectively evaluated more than 1,300 patients who had been taken to one of four Chicago-area hospitals after an accident. Fifty-eight percent of the injured had been wearing a seat belt; 42 percent had not. Those wearing seat belts had a 60 percent reduction in the severity of injury and a 65 percent decrease in hospital admissions compared with injured patients not using a seat belt.

Assess Your Health

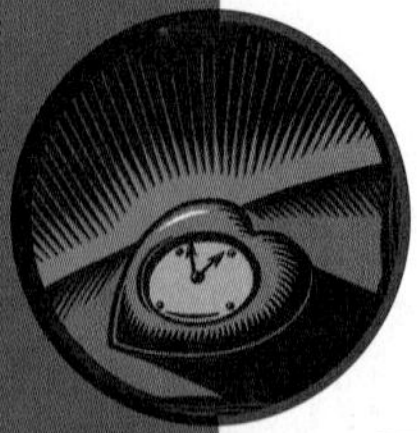

Are You at Risk for an Unintentional Injury?

Would you consider yourself an accident waiting to happen? Sometimes injuries can result from common, everyday behaviors such as those listed below. Often the injuries we experience can be avoided simply through better decision making. Take a look at the following list of behaviors and follow the three steps to evaluate your level of risk taking.

STEP 1: Rate your participation in the following behaviors.

1 = frequently 2 = sometimes 3 = never

Step #1		Step #2	Step #3
_____	1. Flying in a small private plane	_____	_____
_____	2. Flying in a commercial airliner	_____	_____
_____	3. Swimming alone	_____	_____
_____	4. Driving without seat belts on	_____	_____
_____	5. Living on an active earthquake fault	_____	_____
_____	6. Living in a "tornado belt" state	_____	_____
_____	7. Working in an underground coal mine	_____	_____
_____	8. Jaywalking across a street	_____	_____
_____	9. Exceeding the speed limit	_____	_____
_____	10. Waving away or swatting at a bee	_____	_____
_____	11. Tubing on a bumpy downhill course	_____	_____
_____	12. Riding double on a bicycle	_____	_____
_____	13. Petting or feeding a large stray dog	_____	_____
_____	14. Keeping guns and ammunition together	_____	_____
_____	15. Sleeping in a house without a smoke detector	_____	_____
_____	16. Driving a small compact car	_____	_____
_____	17. Taking pills or medicine in the dark	_____	_____
_____	18. Talking with food in your mouth	_____	_____
_____	19. Stopping incompletely at stop signs	_____	_____
_____	20. Driving/riding a motorcycle	_____	_____

STEP 2: For those statements that you marked as 1, try to identify one or more of the following reasons that explain why you participate.

a. Save time
b. Seek a thrill
c. Meet a dare
d. Perform a necessary function
e. Gain recognition, status, attention
f. Eliminate a hazard
g. Other reason

STEP 3: For those statements that you marked as 2 or 3 in Step 1, try to identify one or more of the following reasons that explain why you do not participate.

a. It is not economical for me. It might cost me more than the personal benefits derived.
b. It is too inconvenient. The time and hassle are not worth the benefits.
c. It is too dangerous. An injury could happen.
d. It does not provide enough psychological reward (i.e., thrill, recognition, etc.).
e. I do not have enough skill to participate.

Passive seat belts provide added protection to at-risk drivers who still do not want to buckle up. These belts automatically place a shoulder restraint around both driver and front seat passenger upon their entering the car. Unfortunately, these passive restraints are easy to disengage, making seat belt use still a matter of choice. Also, in some automobiles, passive restraints are not effective unless a lap belt is also used. Drivers and passengers may have a false sense of security if they rely only on the passive systems.

Air bags are another safety feature in cars used to protect the driver and front-seat passenger in case of an accident. Introduced as an optional feature in 1990, dual air bags are now required for all passenger cars and light trucks. Within one tenth of a second after impact, the bag concealed in the steering wheel or dashboard inflates, thus creating a protective cushion between the driver and the steering wheel or the front seat passenger and the dashboard and windshield. The bag quickly deflates after absorbing the shock of the forward force of the people in the front seat.

Seat belts and air bags are not without their problems, and drivers involved in crashes can be bruised in the chest, arms, and face. Short adults (under five feet two inches tall) are particularly at risk for air bag injuries since they tend to sit with their faces or chests close to the steering wheel, and they can sometimes get in the way of the inflating air bag. Small children, too, are at risk, and many of the children involved in air bag injuries are believed to have been riding without a safety belt, so they moved forward—into the path of the inflating air bag—during the braking just before the impact.

Bike and Motorcycle Helmets

As much fun and good exercise as biking is, more than half a million bikers are injured each year. Children are at particularly great risk of injury from bicycle use, and one child dies and about two hundred are treated every day in emergency rooms because of cycling-related head injuries. In fact, nearly one fourth of all significant brain injuries in children fourteen years or younger are bicycle related.

Studies show that bike helmets significantly reduce the risk of head and brain injury, and everyone—not just children—should wear a helmet when biking. Even experienced bikers crash every 4,500 miles on average, according to the Bicycle Helmet Safety Institute. Road rash and broken bones will heal; brain damage may be permanent.

States have had difficulty mandating safety helmet use among motorcyclists, even though data show that an unhelmeted motorcyclist is 40 percent more likely to suffer a fatal head injury than is a helmeted rider. In 1975, most states required helmet use, but under pressure from motorcyclists, many repealed their helmet laws. Presently, less than half the states require that all motorcycle operators wear helmets and 26 states require only motorcyclists under age eighteen to wear helmets.

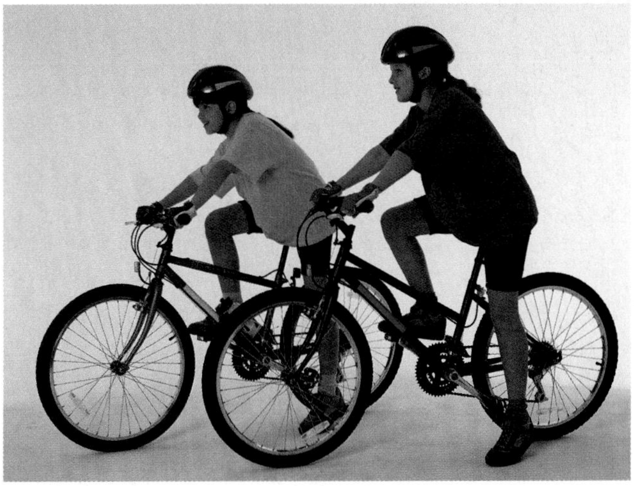

Helmets significantly reduce the risk of head and brain injury. You still may get hurt wearing a helmet, but broken bones and bruises will heal while brain damage might be permanent.

On the Waterfront

Going for a swim on a hot day sounds like a pleasant activity, whether it is at the beach, a public or private pool, or the old swimming hole in the country. Yet each year, about twenty-six hundred people drown while trying to cool off. Most vulnerable of all are children under age four and males aged fifteen to thirty-four.

The primary cause of drowning among young adult men is alcohol use in conjunction with boating and other water-related activities. It is against the law in every state to operate a boat while under the influence of alcohol, but enforcement is relatively weak. Restricting the sale of alcoholic beverages in boating and swimming areas might reduce the number of teenagers and adults drowning.

passive seat belts Seat belts that automatically place a shoulder restraint around the driver and the front seat passenger upon their entering the car.

air bags Safety devices located behind the steering wheel and/or the dashboard that automatically inflate on impact during a frontal or side crash.

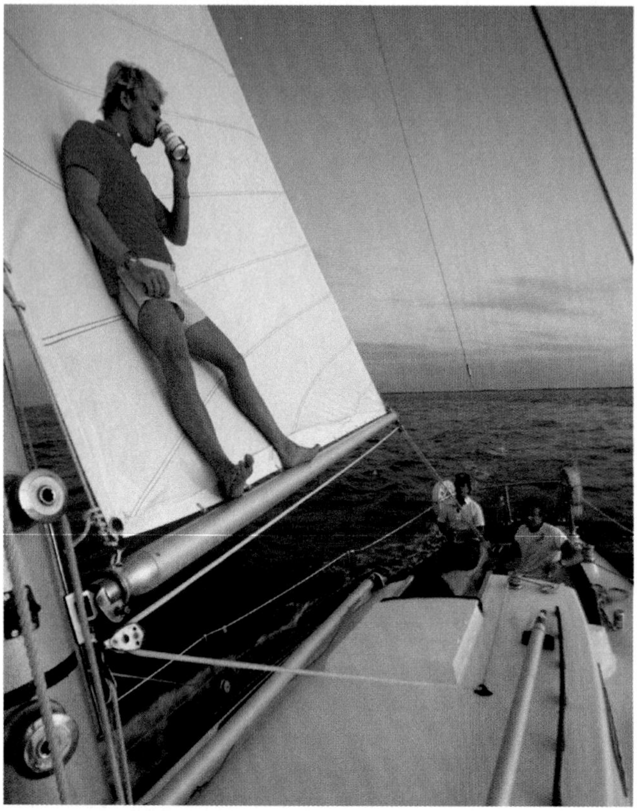

Alcohol in conjunction with boating and other water-related activities is the leading cause of drowning among college-age men.

Sometimes the setting itself causes the problem. It is estimated that 20 percent of drownings could be prevented by modifying the physical environment. Effective strategies include posting signs at the beach concerning depth and undertow and requiring fences, gates, and proper locking devices around home swimming pools.

Diving is another cause of water-related injury. An estimated five hundred to seven hundred swimmers are seriously injured each year by diving into shallow areas of swimming pools and other bodies of water. Diving injuries can damage the spinal cord and result in **quadriplegia**—paralysis from the neck down, affecting both arms and legs—to divers who hit the bottom or side of a pool. The typical victim of a diving injury is a male between the ages of thirteen and twenty-three. Almost 50 percent of all people with diving injuries have been drinking prior to being hurt.

quadriplegia Total paralysis of the body from the neck down, affecting arms and legs.

smoke detectors Smoke-sensitive devices designed to alert occupants of a room or space in the event of a fire.

Safety at Home

Many injuries occur at home, from falling down the stairs to falling asleep smoking and starting a fire. As with most unintentional injuries, many injuries at home can be avoided by changing the environment to make it safer.

When a Simple Fall Is Not Simple

When was the last time you fell? How badly were you injured? Most likely you had a scraped knee, a wrenched shoulder, perhaps a broken collar bone, but nothing life threatening. Unfortunately, this is not the case for everyone. Falls are the second leading cause of fatal injuries, after motor vehicle accidents, resulting in more than sixteen thousand deaths. With about 11 million fall-related injuries a year, most falls do not result in death, but they may result in a decrease in confidence, restriction of physical activity, or other reductions in independence—all of which can negatively affect the quality of life.

For example, one third of all elderly people fall each year, and most of these incidents take place at home during usual activities such as walking or using the bathroom. Falls are one of the primary reasons why an elderly person enters a nursing home. Much can be done in the home, however, to help prevent falls, including installing better lighting and handrails on stairs and in the bathroom, covering slippery floors with skid-free rugs, and wearing shoes with firm soles instead of slippers.

Up in Smoke

Reading in bed becomes a hazard when you are smoking as you read. Cigarettes are responsible for the largest percentage of home fires that kill or seriously injure children. Most cigarettes contain additives in both the tobacco and the surrounding paper that can cause them to burn for as long as twenty-eight minutes. Without these additives, a cigarette would self-extinguish after four minutes, which is rarely enough time for furniture to catch fire.

The number of fire deaths has been declining, in part because of greater use of **smoke detectors.** These electronic devices monitor the air in your home or dorm and sound an alarm at the first "sniff" of trouble. In most cases, this is before you even see the first trace of smoke. What the detector is responding to is the production of gases that precedes a full-blown fire. According to a recent study, smoke detectors can reduce the potential for death in 86 percent of fires and the potential for severe injuries in 88 percent.

Developing Health Skills

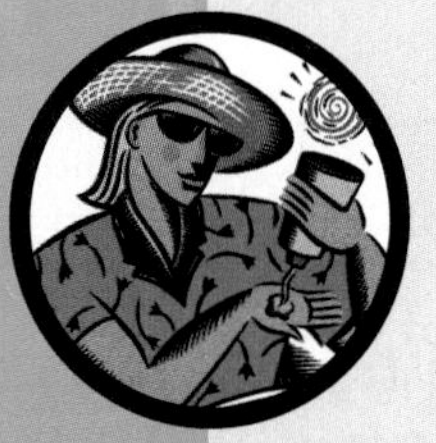

Be Prepared to Respond

The following are seven basic recommendations from the American Red Cross and the National Safety Council:

1. In an emergency situation, first protect yourself. Avoid approaching an automobile with downed electric power lines around it. Do not attempt to save a drowning person if you are not trained in water rescue. The situation can become worse if you become a victim, too.
2. Do not move the victim unless it is necessary to prevent further injury. Keep the victim in the position best suited to his or her condition or injury. Sometimes this means having the victim lie down; in other cases, he or she can sit.
3. Avoid or overcome chilling by using blankets or some other means of covering the victim's body. If the victim is exposed to cold or dampness, place blankets or additional clothing under him or her as well.
4. Find out what happened. Ask witnesses about the situation. Was there an incident that caused the injury? Did the victim suddenly get ill and fall down on the street? This information could reveal a great deal about the nature of the injuries.
5. Seek help immediately by calling 911 for emergency or 0 for the operator or by sending a bystander to call for medical assistance. When you call, talk clearly and directly, and tell the operator what happened in one sentence. For example, "I have just witnessed an automobile crash and someone is injured badly." The person on the other end of the phone will give you instructions on what to do. You will be asked where the incident happened. If you do not know the address, look for a street sign or landmark that will give the rescue team an idea of where to go. The operator might ask you for other information, including the extent of injuries. Answer these questions as best you can. When the operator has no more questions, he or she will tell you to hang up and go back to the scene of the accident to wait for assistance. Do not hang up until the operator tells you to.
6. If you are trained in **cardiopulmonary resuscitation (CPR),** start the procedure IF the victim is not breathing, has an open air passage, and no pulse. CPR involves rescue breathing (mouth-to-mouth resuscitation) as well as compressing the chest to get the victim breathing and blood circulating. Do not do CPR if you are not properly trained.
7. Check to see if the victim is bleeding severely. If so, control the bleeding by applying direct pressure over the wound and elevating it, if possible. Many people incorrectly believe that tourniquets—devices such as a handkerchief, neck tie, or scarf bound tightly above the wound to stop circulation—are necessary to stop severe bleeding.

Contact your local chapter of the American Red Cross, American Heart Association, or other groups for information on classes in first aid, CPR, and additional emergency techniques.

Other Burns

Burns aren't caused just by fire. Another kind of burn that occurs in the home and frequently seriously injures both children and the elderly are burns from hot—actually, scalding—water from the faucet. The culprits are water heaters that are adjusted to heat water as high as 150° to 160° Fahrenheit. It takes only a one-second exposure to 160° water to develop a burn. A similar burn would take 30 seconds to develop from direct exposure to 130° water.

For all their patriotic associations, fireworks present another very serious hazard, particularly to children. About nine thousand people are treated each year in emergency rooms for injuries associated with fireworks. More than half of these injuries are burns, many of them involving the head and face. Fireworks may also cause the victim to be permanently blinded or to lose fingers, arms, and legs.

Laws restricting the sale and use of fireworks are among the strongest ways to prevent fireworks-related injuries. Most cities have restrictions on fireworks, and many have mandatory fines if the regulations are violated.

Taking Prompt Action

Not all injuries can be prevented, but their impact can be minimized by proper and prompt action taken by men and women like yourself who come to the aid of injury victims. Although there is no substitute for complete first aid training through an accredited course of study, everyone—even the untrained—needs to understand a few basic principles of first aid and emergency medicine (see the Developing Health Skills box).

cardiopulmonary resuscitation (CPR) A combination of mouth-to-mouth breathing and chest compression used during cardiac arrest to keep blood flowing to the heart muscle and brain; an emergency procedure.

Violence: A Public Health Problem

Hardly a day goes by that a violent act is not reported on the front page of a newspaper or at the top of the local and even national television news. With thousands of lives lost in the attacks on the World Trade Center and the Pentagon, the events of September 11, 2001, changed the way most Americans think about violence. Violence in the United States is a public health emergency. Some possible reasons for violence are drugs, availability of firearms, urban poverty, and a variety of sociological factors.

Violence is often viewed as a law enforcement problem and, in this context, is associated with questions about gun control, policing, sentencing, and parole policy. In this textbook, however, we discuss violence as a personal and public health problem. It is a major cause of death for adolescents and young adults and a source of mental anguish, stress, and anxiety among the population as a whole. Statistically, you have a good chance of being a victim of some crime or act of violence at least once in your lifetime. Being a victim can be traumatizing and can affect the quality of life, even though not all crimes are life threatening or even require medical attention—for example, having your car stolen.

By definition, violence is the use of force with the intent to harm oneself or another person. Each year, according to the National Institute of Justice, about 50 million people are victims of violence in the United States. This includes homicide, child abuse, rape, arson, and other assaults.

Who Is at Risk for Being Assaulted?

Overall, crime is a male experience: Far more men than women commit and are victimized by violent crimes (see Table 9.1). Women are victims more often than men in only two categories: rape and personal larceny. (Purse snatching is an example of personal larceny.)

- African Americans are victims of crimes at a higher rate than whites, particularly for robbery and burglary. For instance, an African American's risk for being robbed is three times higher than a white person's. In part, this is because African Americans live in high-crime neighborhoods to a greater extent than do whites.
- The lower his or her income, the greater a person is at risk for being a victim of crime. Poorer people are more likely to be raped, robbed, or assaulted seriously. As annual family income increases, the incidence of violent crime generally decreases. There is one exception to this: Higher-income households are more likely to be robbed than are lower-income households.
- Teenagers and young adults are more likely to be victims of crime than are older people. However, the elderly are a particularly vulnerable crime tar-

Table 9.1 Who Are Victims of Crime?

Characteristic of victim	Rate of violent crime* and personal theft per 1,000 persons
Sex	
Male	32.9
Female	23.2
Age	
12–15	60.1
16–19	64.3
20–24	49.4
25–34	34.8
35–49	21.8
50–64	13.7
65 or older	3.7
Race	
White	27.1
Black	35.3
Other	20.7
Household income	
Less than $7,500	60.3
$7,500–14,999	37.8
$15,000–24,999	31.8
$25,000–34,999	29.8
$35,000–49,999	28.5
$50,000–74,999	23.7
$75,000 or more	22.3
Region	
Northeast	23.5
Midwest	30.4
South	24.9
West	33.9
Residence	
Urban	35.1
Suburban	25.8
Rural	23.6

*Violent crime includes rape, assault, and robbery

Source: Bureau of Justice Statistics

get. They tend to live alone; eyesight and hearing losses reduce their alertness to danger signs; physical weakness and chronic conditions such as osteoporosis or arthritis reduce the chance that they will fight back aggressively; and they are lonely and more likely to trust someone, thus making them more susceptible to fraud.

- Violence against gay people has increased significantly, according to a study by the National Gay and Lesbian Task Force. Incidents of victimization include verbal harassment and threats, physical assault, and police abuse.
- Nearly half of all victims know, or have seen, the person who has committed the crime against them. According to the Bureau of Justice Statistics, 38 percent of violent crimes were committed by acquaintances and friends and 9 percent by relatives.

As with all health threats, prevention is the key to avoiding becoming a victim of crime. Examine the Developing Health Skills box for pointers on crime prevention.

Homicide: Dying in America

"It's a jungle out there," said a political leader of one of the largest cities in the United States. What he was referring to is the number of **homicides** taking place. While the rate of homicide per 100,000 population has been dropping since 1993, it remains the third leading external (that is, not natural) cause of death after unintentional injuries and suicide. Criminologists do not have an adequate theory to explain why the homicide rate has fallen, but many experts point to more aggressive police tactics and tougher gun control laws.

Several factors prevalent in U.S. society are linked with violence. Three of the most widely discussed and debated factors are: the availability of handguns, drug and alcohol consumption, and viewing violence on TV.

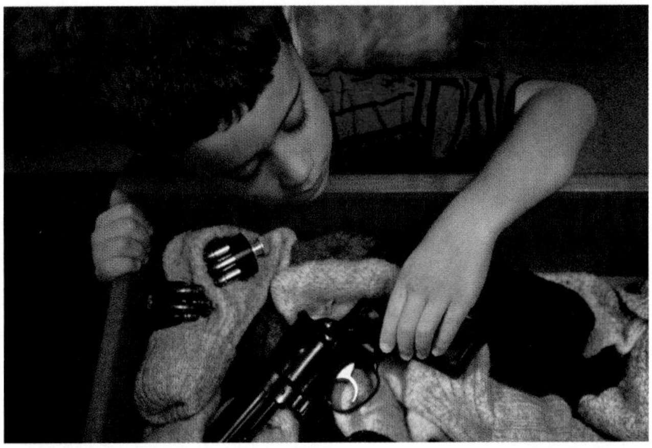

One of three American households has a gun. If you have a gun at home, you are eight times more likely to be involved in a homicide—as victim or murderer—than if you don't have a gun.

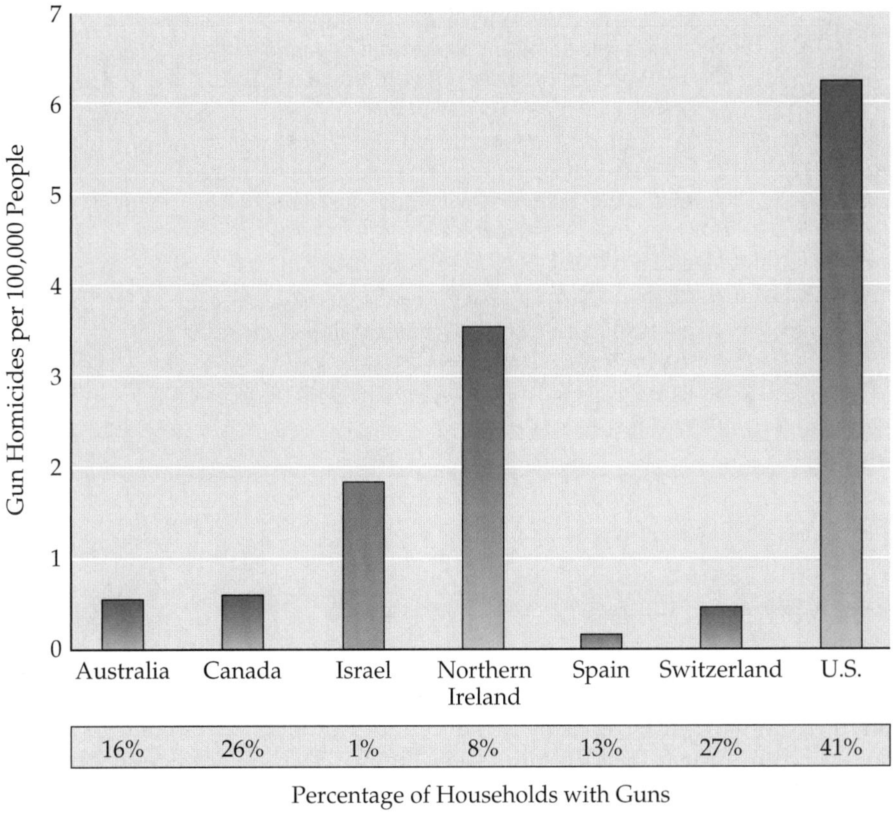

Figure 9.2 Homicide Rate and Gun Ownership

The homicide rate and percentage of homes with guns are highest in the United States than in any other country.

(*Source:* Coalition for Gun Control, Canada)

homicide The killing of one human being by another.

Developing Health Skills

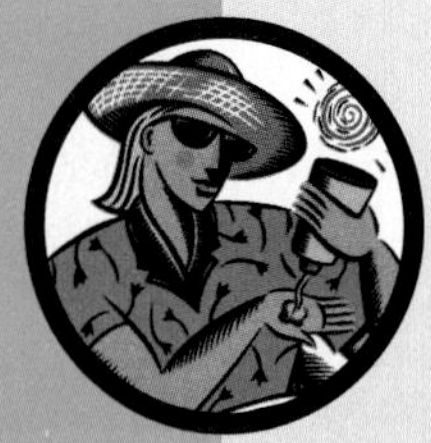

How to Avoid Being a Victim of Crime

Many preventive measures can be taken so that you can avoid being a victim of crime. The following tips come from various police departments.

At Home or in a College Residence

- Lock the windows and doors—including sliding glass doors—when you go out.
- Make your home or dorm room appear occupied when you go out by using a timer to turn on lights and a radio.
- Do not keep large sums of money at home or in your room or leave valuables such as jewelry in open view.
- Never let a stranger in without checking his or her identification. Install a peephole in your door and use it.
- Do not give the impression that you are alone if strangers telephone or come to the door.
- If you live in an apartment building, avoid being in the laundry room or garage by yourself, especially at night.
- If you come home and find a door or window open or other signs of forced entry, do not go in. Go to the nearest phone and call the police.
- Take care of your keys. Do not give anyone the chance to duplicate them. Do not hide extra house keys under a doormat or in other obvious spots.

On the Street

- Walk purposefully and look confident. Walk close to the curb. Avoid doorways, bushes, and alleys. Be alert to your surroundings.
- Use well-lighted, well-traveled routes and try to walk with friends.
- Avoid shortcuts through isolated areas, including parking lots and underground garages.
- Be careful when people stop to ask you for directions. Always reply from a distance and never get too close to the car.
- If you believe you are being followed, walk into a store or knock on a house door.
- If you are in trouble, attract help any way you can. Scream, yell for help, or yell, "Fire!"
- Have your house key in your hand as you approach your home.
- Carry change for emergency telephone and transportation use.

In Your Car

- Lock all doors and close all windows when leaving your car.
- Park in well-lighted areas and try not to walk alone in parking areas at night.
- Have your keys ready when you approach your car. Check the inside for intruders before entering and lock the door immediately after getting in your car.
- Always keep your gas tank at least half full.
- If you have a flat tire, drive on it until you reach a safe, well-lighted, and well-traveled area.
- If your car breaks down in an isolated area, raise the hood and then get back in the car. Stay in the locked car. If you have a cell phone, call the police. If not and someone stops to help, ask them to call. Sound your horn if you are threatened.
- Never pick up strangers.

Gun Killings

Guns are widely available in the United States, where more than one of every three households has a gun, according to a Justice Department survey. No other country comes near this record (see Figure 9.2). Researchers have calculated just how risky having a gun at home in the United States can be:

- If you have a gun at home, you are eight times more likely to be killed by or to kill a family member or close acquaintance.
- If you get involved in a fight with a family member or close acquaintance and one of you has a gun in the home, you are twelve times more likely to kill or to be killed.

The Influence of Drugs

A major factor contributing to homicides is the use of alcohol and illicit drugs. About 60 percent of people arrested for homicide tested positive for drugs at the time of arrest. The consumption (in contrast to the sale) of drugs and alcohol has a link to violent behavior. Classic studies of homicides show that the killer, the victim, or both were drunk in more than half the cases studied.

Although a close relationship between substance abuse and homicide does exist, studies do not prove conclusively that drugs and alcohol cause crime. In a report on drinking and crime prepared for the National Institute of Justice, researchers note that people may first decide to commit their crimes and then get drunk to muster courage or allay fears.

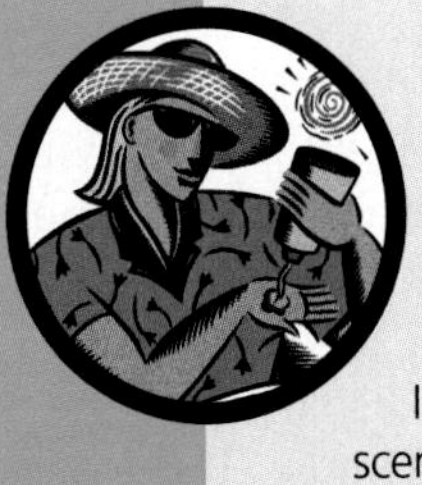

Developing Health Skills

Conflict Resolution

Many forms of violence begin as simple conflicts between two individuals but escalate into violent encounters. This is the case with fights that begin with an indirect insult, such as, "You took my chair; I was here first," or a more direct one, such as an obscene gesture made by one driver to another who passed improperly. Road rage—the term to describe this anger—can escalate to a car chase and result in serious injury to the drivers and people in nearby cars. Insults may also arise from racial or religious prejudices, feelings of unfair treatment, learned hatred, and simple miscommunication. Regardless of the source of insult, the outcome does not have to become violent.

One method of ensuring that conflicts do not escalate into violent encounters is a process known as conflict resolution. Conflict resolution is a process of negotiation between two individuals. It is facilitated by a third party. The goal of conflict resolution is, as the term suggests, to resolve the conflict.

You might want to use conflict resolution to handle a difficult encounter in your dorm or your community. Here are some guidelines for conducting a mediation session, the actual meeting between the two individuals in conflict:

1. **Emphasize your neutrality.** Introduce the mediation session by establishing your neutrality. Make it clear to each party that you do not have a personal interest in the outcome. Say, "I am neutral. I will not take sides or decide who is right or wrong. My role is to help you find a solution that is acceptable to both of you."
2. **Establish guidelines.** It is important to agree upon some rules that must be followed throughout the mediation session. Both parties must agree to:
   - Keep everything that is said confidential.
   - Be as honest as possible.
   - Avoid name calling and swearing.
   - Refrain from interrupting the other person.
   - Participate in proposing solutions that they can agree to.
   - Follow through on any agreed-upon solution.
3. **Allow each person to state his or her views.** Give each person a chance to state his or her view of the situation. Listen carefully and ask questions to clarify anything that is unclear. To make sure you understood what was said, restate something and ask, "Is that what you mean?"

   Do not go on to the next person until you really understand the first person's viewpoint. While you are listening and asking questions, try to get at the principle behind each person's position. That is, you should try to gain a deeper understanding of what each person truly cares about, not just what the person is saying.
4. **Explore possible solutions.** If participants seem relaxed, ask them to brainstorm a list of possible solutions together. Remind them that, during brainstorming, they should not judge the other person's proposed solution. Encourage the participants to invent new and different solutions and to use the other's suggestions to spark ideas in their minds.
5. **Do not give up.** It is not always easy to find a win–win solution, but it can be done. It is important to keep the focus on the common principle or goal that is behind the two different positions. Also, try to keep the participants actively involved in the process of proposing solutions. The more involved they are, the greater interest they will have in resolving the problem.

If, however, you are unable to find an agreeable solution, it may be necessary to ask for help. You may want to encourage the two individuals to seek counseling from a trained mediator.

The Role of Television

The average child in the United States watches 8,000 murders and 100,000 other acts of violence on television by the time he or she leaves elementary school. Children most likely to be aggressive are the ones who usually view violent programs when they air, who believe that the shows portray life just as it is, and who identify strongly with the aggressive characters in the shows.

For most television watchers, however, research does not fully support the view that watching violence on television causes an increase in violence in the real world. On the other hand, the relationship between watching violent shows and committing violent acts cannot be entirely dismissed. Several studies suggest that repeated exposure to violent acts in films and on television "desensitizes" people to violence, making an experience that would at first be repulsive seem commonplace or even acceptable.

Fortunately, there are nonviolent ways of dealing with violence. See the Developing Health Skills box to learn about **conflict resolution** techniques.

conflict resolution A process of negotiation between two individuals, facilitated by a third party, with the goal of resolving differences.

Sexual Violence

Many people do not find refuge from violence even in their own homes. Researchers estimate that some form of violence occurs in 25 percent of all marriages. It is also possible that some of the couples you see around the college campus are "battling it out," because the rate of violence among nonmarried couples may approach that found within marriage. This discussion of sexual violence focuses on **domestic violence,** sexual harassment, and rape.

Domestic Violence

Domestic violence is defined as a range of abusive behaviors perpetrated by one person against another within the domestic sphere. This can be interpreted to mean one member of the family against another or one partner against another. Although men suffer from domestic violence, the incidence and severity of victimization of men are substantially lower than for women.

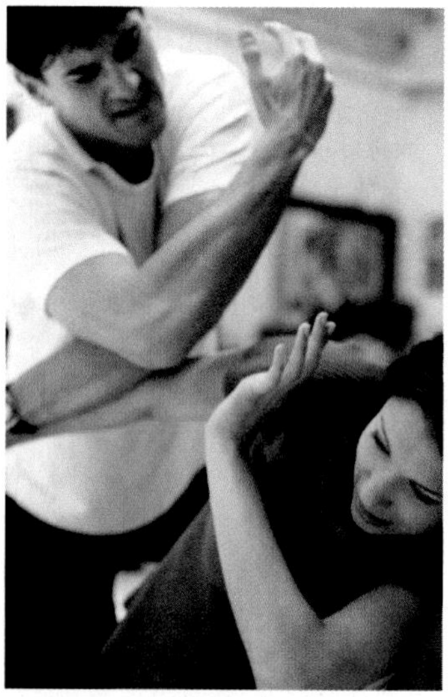

Left unchecked, a heated argument can escalate to domestic violence. Statistics from recent years indicate a rise in the incidence of domestic violence. This rise includes couples dating at college as well as married couples.

Kicks, punches, and chokings are typical examples of the **physical abuse** to which men and women are subjected in cases of domestic violence. These abuses often result in black eyes, split lips, broken noses, fractured jaws, damaged vocal cords, permanent eye damage, broken ribs, internal bleeding, ruptured spleens, lacerated livers, sexual organ damage, and numerous other injuries.

Another form of battering is **psychological abuse.** A spouse or partner can verbally batter the abused person with insults and threats, which can severely damage the victim's self-esteem. Victims are often required to perform demanding, demeaning, and unreasonable tasks. One abused woman reported that her husband was the only one permitted to wear shoes in the house. If she or their children forgot to take off their shoes, she risked being beaten. As one wife abuser said: "Violence is the way to keep control and maintain your identity. It is a way to lay down the law."

There is a big difference between laying down the law and taking the law into your own hands. Beating up someone, or **battery,** is a crime. Although laws exist to protect an abused person, the courts have often ruled in favor of the sanctity of the family. Even without a court ruling, most people stay in the abusive household because, typically, women are afraid of angering their husbands and of the consequences of that anger being directed against them or their children. They are also afraid because most abused women are financially dependent on their husbands.

All large cities and an increasing number of smaller ones have emergency shelters, places where an abused woman (and her children) can go. Recognizing the problem of abuse among young people in dating situations, colleges have begun to operate shelters for battered women students. See the Developing Health Skills box for some suggestions on how to detect an abusive relationship.

domestic violence A range of abusive behaviors perpetrated by one person against another within the domestic sphere.

physical abuse The infliction of physical injury that causes substantial harm over a period of time.

psychological abuse Acts such as threats, insults, and unreasonable demands that lead to mental anguish and that damage the victim's self-esteem over time.

battery Any illegal beating or touching of another person.

Sexual Harassment

Although seldom a violent crime, sexual harassment is a criminal offense involving the abuse of power. It is found on the job, in the classroom, and, in some cases, at home. It may be obvious, as in the case of a boss or professor imposing unwanted sexual attention or requests for sexual favors. It may also be less direct, such as the creation of a hostile, intimidating, or offensive work or class environment by actions or speech of a sexual nature based on gender. On the college campus, sexual harassment might take the form of offers of a good grade in a course or special treatment in exchange for sexual favors, repeated staring in a suggestive way, or unwanted touching. Even sexual comments, jokes, or personal questions that are offensive or distracting to the person who feels harassed may constitute sexual harassment.

Most commonly, it is women who are harassed, usually by men in a position of power or authority over them. However, men may be harassed by women, and either men or women may be harassed by persons of the same sex. If harassers are left unchallenged, others may become victims because harassers are usually repeat offenders.

The following recommended actions were developed by a university panel addressing sexual harassment on campus:

Speak up. Ignoring sexual harassment does not make it go away. Express your objections clearly, firmly, and in a timely way. There is a chance that the harasser did not realize the behavior was offensive. Also, if you should file charges at a later date, it is sometimes helpful (but not essential) to have objected to the behavior.

Keep records. Include in your records any notes or letters received from the harasser. Write down dates, times, places, witnesses, what happened or what was said, and what you said or did in response.

Tell someone. You may get a clearer perspective on what is happening, or you may find out whether the harasser is a previous offender. You may also establish witnesses who can vouch for your distress.

Take it seriously. A sexual harassment allegation has a considerable impact on the individual accused. Do not make allegations that are without foundation, as disciplinary action may result.

Developing Health Skills

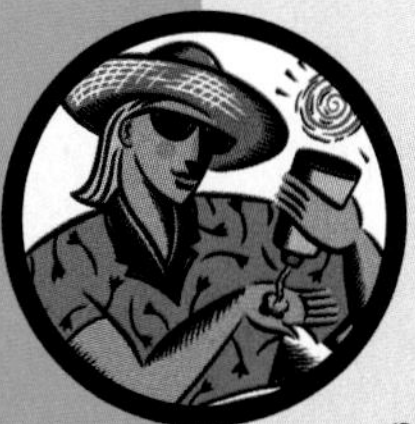

Detecting an Abusive Relationship

You probably know someone who has experienced an abusive relationship. Perhaps a friend's boyfriend behaved in a manner that made you suspect a problem. Or perhaps a friend shared anxiety or fear with you about a relationship. Getting out of an abusive relationship begins with recognizing that abuse exists. This is sometimes more evident to those on the outside than to the person in the relationship.

How can you detect an abusive relationship? Consider the following questions:

- Does one person often yell and scream at the other?
- Is one person occasionally frightened of the other?
- Does one person stop the other from seeing family or friends?
- Does one person force the other to have sex?
- Does one person occasionally hurt or threaten the other?

An answer of yes to any one of these questions is an indication that the relationship is not fair, that is, that one person expresses more power within the relationship than the other. An abusive relationship may exist.

An answer of yes to more than one of these questions is an indication that an abusive relationship does exist and outside help, in the form of counseling or legal aid, may be needed to end the abuse.

An answer of yes to all five questions is an indication that this may be a dangerous relationship and that the well-being of one of the partners may be at risk.

If you suspect that abuse is part of a friend's relationship, the most important action you can take is to talk to him or her about it and to suggest that he or she seek professional help from a mental health counselor, a lawyer, or a physician.

Rape

Rape—sexual intercourse through physical force or the threat of physical force—is one of the most misunderstood of violent crimes. Many women think, "It could never happen to me." But a recent survey indicates that about one in every eight women has been raped.

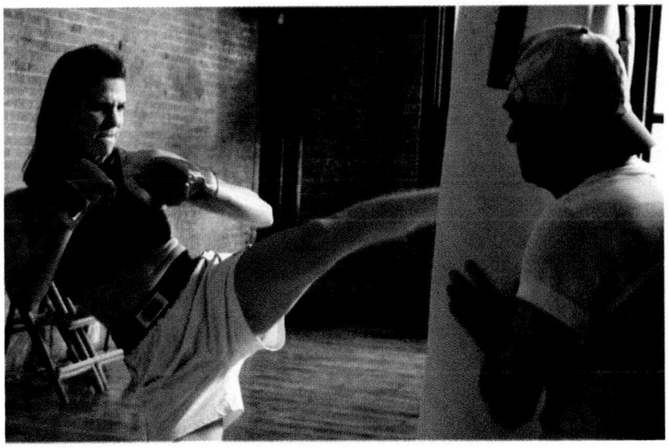

As a measure of self-protection, a growing number of women are signing up for karate or other self-defense techniques.

It is also popularly believed that women are "asking for it" with their dress and actions. Research shows that rapists look for targets they perceive as vulnerable, not for women who dress in a particular way. No one asks to be raped, just as no one asks to be robbed. Perhaps the most misunderstood aspect of rape is the myth that it is driven by sexual desire, when, in reality, it is driven more by the compulsion to control.

Rape is widely believed to happen only to young women. Although many rape victims are young, rape victims range in age from four months to ninety-two years. It can happen to women of all ages and to boys

rape An act of violence in which a person is forced to engage in unwanted sexual intercourse.

and men. Males are victims of about 5 percent of all sexual assault cases.

Two thirds of all rapes and rape attempts take place at night, mostly between 6 P.M. and midnight. Most rapes take place at or near where the victim—or a friend, relative, or neighbor of the victim—lives (see Figure 9.3).

Most rape victims offer some kind of resistance. The most common response is to try to yell for help; to resist physically; to threaten, argue, or reason with the offender; or to resist without force by running away or hiding. However, yelling works only if someone is around to hear. Running away makes sense only if there is a safe place to go to. And active resistance is a good option only when the person being attacked is trained in karate or another self-defense technique. What you should do to try to protect yourself when you feel threatened depends in great part on your assessment of the circumstances before you.

Acquaintance rape. About two thirds of all rapists are acquainted with the victim in one way or another. They may be the victim's spouse, former spouse, relative, date, neighbor, or co-worker. **Acquaintance rape** is the most common and most underreported form of rape.

One form of acquaintance rape is **date rape.** It is committed while on a date. The real problem leading to date rape begins with miscommunication. A male might say, "It wasn't rape. She really wanted me to do it." A female might say, "I didn't want to, but he forced me to have sex with him."

Studies show that date rape occurs more frequently among college students, particularly freshmen, than among any other group. One factor contributing to date rape is the so-called date-rape drug, Rohypnol, or Roofies, discussed in Chapter 8. In one survey, one in four college women reported being victims of rape or attempted rape. In 84 percent of the cases, the assailant was someone the women knew.

Another form of unwanted sexual act by an acquaintance is **marital rape.** This takes place when a spouse forces himself or herself on his or her spouse or estranged spouse. It often takes place in an atmosphere of anger, violence, and fear.

Characteristics of incident	Rape/sexual assault
Total	100%
Victim/offender relationship	
Relatives	11
Well-known	35
Casual acquaintance	21
Stranger	33
Time of day	
6 A.M. to 6 P.M.	31
6 P.M. to midnight	37
Midnight to 6 A.M.	32
Location of crime	
At or near victim's home or lodging	37
Friend's/relative's/neighbor's home	21
Commercial places	7
Parking lots/garages	6
School	3
Streets other than near victim's home	8
Other	17
Victim's activity	
At work or traveling to or from work	8
School	5
Activities at home	38
Shopping/errands	2
Leisure activities away from home	32
Traveling	6
Other	8
Distance from victim's home	
Inside home or lodging	34
Near victim's home	10
1 mile or less	12
5 miles or less	14
50 miles or less	23
More than 50 miles	6
Weapons	
No weapons present	84
Weapons present	16
Firearm	6
Other type of weapon	10

Figure 9.3 Rape: Who Does It, Where, and When?
Most rapes take place at night at or near the victim's home. The rapist is usually known by the victim.
(*Source:* Bureau of Justice Statistics)

acquaintance rape Sexual assault committed by a person known to the victim.

date rape Unwanted sexual contact that is committed on or by a date.

marital rape A rape that occurs when an individual forces unwanted sexual contact on his or her spouse or estranged spouse.

stranger rape A rape committed by a total stranger.

Attacks by strangers. Assault by a total stranger is the most commonly reported form of rape. However, it represents only about one third of all rapes; acquaintance rapes far outnumber **stranger rapes.** This is because a woman is twice as likely to report being attacked by a stranger as by someone she knows, according to the Bureau of Justice Statistics.

Gang rape is rape committed by a group. This is usually a group of males, but gang rape is also done by females. Closely related, **sadistic rape** occurs when the rapist is driven to torture or mutilate his victim. This form of rape comprises a very small percentage of reported rapes, less than 1 percent, but obviously is the most dangerous and threatening.

A rape can be over in minutes, but its traumatic effects can last for months, years, or even a lifetime. At a minimum, a person who is raped should go to a physician, clinic, or hospital to deal with the medical problems that may arise, including tissue injury, the potential for HIV and other sexually transmitted infections, and pregnancy. A victim may or may not wish to prosecute. Rape crisis centers are available in almost every city and county—and also on many college campuses—where women can get help in realizing—and dealing with—the impact the rape has had on them.

A Few Final Words on Unintentional Injuries and Violence

A strong probability exists that you will have a close involvement with unintentional injuries and violence in your lifetime. For some, this means being hurt directly. For others, it means helping a friend who has been injured in an automobile or diving accident—or has been mugged or raped—or grieving with the family of a victim of homicide. To help reduce your exposure to unintentional injuries and violence, as well as to assist people in need of help, periodically review the skills that you have learned in this chapter. Prevention of injuries and violence generally involves precaution and can be incorporated relatively easily into your lifestyle.

gang rape A rape committed by a group.

sadistic rape A rape that involves torture or mutilation of the victim.

CASE STUDY 9: Living with the Fear of Violence

After graduating from college in her small hometown, Faye moved to the city for better job opportunities and more excitement. She knew that big cities offer dangers along with the excitement. But she felt that the trade-off was worth it.

When actually confronted with big-city living, Faye found herself too frightened to enjoy it. Instead of taking advantage of the numerous social, cultural, and educational activities, she went straight home after work to her apartment. Although it was boring, she felt safe there. When she ventured out, even in the daytime, she looked at everyone as a possible mugger, rapist, or robber. After several months of living in fear and anxiety and seeing her quality of life diminish, Faye returned to her hometown.

When LaVerne moved to the city after graduating from college in a rural community, she was ready for some excitement, but she also wanted safety. She had taken karate in college, and she practiced it regularly. Now she took a course at the Y in women's assertiveness training so that she would be less intimidated if someone confronted her on the street.

LaVerne evaluated her environment and figured out what was safe, and unsafe, to do. For example, at school she had jogged in the evenings after studying. In the city, she switched to a lunchtime run, in daylight and with lots of other people on the streets. She also went out a lot at night—to listen to live jazz and to go to the latest movies—but she always went with friends and stayed on well-lit blocks.

In Your Opinion

To protect herself from crime on the streets, Faye stayed at home. In contrast, LaVerne took positive steps to protect herself against some of the dangers of living in a big city.

- What steps could Faye have taken to make her life more manageable yet at the same time safe?
- Both Faye and LaVerne take measures to insure their safety. Whose measures of prevention are better? Why? Does Faye's behavior protect her from violent crime?
- What would you do to protect yourself if you moved to a high-crime city?
- How would living in a big city enhance or compromise the quality of your life?

KEY CONCEPTS

1. Unintentional injuries include trauma associated with automobile crashes, falls, fires, and drownings. They are different from intentional injuries (violence) associated with homicide, rape, and battery.
2. Men are by far at greater risk for unintentional injury than are women.
3. The single largest cause of unintentional injuries is automobile crashes.
4. Even moderate levels of alcohol in the blood have been found to impair judgment markedly. Alcohol is the number one cause of traffic fatalities and of swimming and boating deaths.
5. Proper and prompt first aid can help injury victims.
6. Violence is the use of force with the intent to harm oneself or another person.
7. The homicide rate is believed to be related to the availability of handguns, the use of drugs, and the portrayal of violence on television.
8. One method of assuring that conflicts do not escalate into violent encounters is a process known as conflict resolution—negotiation between two individuals facilitated by a third party.
9. Some form of violence occurs in 25 percent of all marriages.
10. Rape is a crime of violence, not a sexual act. It can be committed by a stranger, an acquaintance, a date, or a spouse.

REVIEW QUESTIONS

1. Explain why unintentional and intentional injuries represent a significant public health concern.
2. How would you characterize a person at risk for an unintentional injury?
3. What is the primary cause of unintentional injuries in the United States? List secondary causes.
4. Explain how alcohol consumption greatly enhances the potential of encountering unintentional injuries.
5. List unintentional injuries that result from recreational activities and day-to-day living in the home and on the road.
6. Describe how the availability of handguns, the viewing of violence on television, and drugs are thought to contribute to the occurrence of violent crime.
7. Define homicide and describe its significance to public health.
8. List and describe three forms of sexual abuse. Compare the motives of the abuser in each case.
9. List five guidelines for conducting a conflict resolution session.
10. Name four types of rape and compare each according to (1) by whom, (2) where, and (3) how the crime is committed.

CRITICAL THINKING QUESTIONS

1. The *Healthy People 2010* objectives include the following: "Increase the number of states that have adopted a graduated driver licensing model law." An example of a graduated driver licensing law is one that requires six months in the learner stage and six months in the intermediate driving stage with night-driving restrictions. Such a law might also require drivers to have no seat belt violations. What is the target population of this law? Would the law be effective in reducing unintentional injuries? Would you support it if you were in a position to do so?
2. Have you noticed something about injuries discussed in this chapter? The risk of encountering virtually all unintentional injuries seems to be increased by the consumption of alcohol. Car injuries, bicycle injuries, motorcycle injuries, drowning, and diving injuries all occur more often when alcohol is present. If alcohol is such a critical risk factor, why is it so difficult to encourage people not to drink when driving an automobile or when taking part in potentially dangerous recreational activities such as biking, swimming, or boating?
3. It has been said that "guns don't kill people, people kill people." If this is the case, can the rate of handgun violence in the United States be reduced by restrictions on the sale of handguns? Is there a better way to get at the problem of handgun violence? Given the staggering amount of handgun violence in the United States, what are the chances that a ban on the sale of handguns will become law?
4. One *Healthy People 2010* objective states: "Reduce the rate of physical assault by current or former intimate partners." Such assaults (wife abuse, date rape, etc.) are not uncommon. Why do you believe that two people who care enough for each other to become intimate wind up experiencing violent encounters? Can such violent encounters be prevented? What can be done to assure that relationships do not turn violent?

JOURNAL ACTIVITIES

1. Conduct an inspection of your home, apartment, or dorm room. Make a list of safety hazards that you find. Be sure to include personal safety factors (proximity of neighbors, dead bolt locks) as well as physical safety

factors (temperature of hot water, nonslip stairways). Make another list of safety precautions in the design of your residence. Do you live in a safe place? Are there simple steps you can take to make it safer?

2. Interview someone at the emergency room in the hospital or a local rescue squad about their experiences relating to accidents (in contrast to heart attacks or other acute medical situations). You might want to ask questions particularly relating to seat belt use and drinking and driving. What accident prevention message(s) did you learn from these interviews?
3. An abusive relationship often goes unnoticed until the abuse becomes physically violent. Interview several of your friends and ask them, "How would you recognize an abusive relationship if no violence has occurred?" Compare and contrast your friends' ideas with the list of questions presented in the Developing Health Skills box on page 143.
4. Find out how many guns are registered in the city or county where you live, and correlate the number with the incidence of gun-related crime in the area. Do these figures surprise you? Would you have expected more or fewer guns to be registered? Would you have expected a greater or lesser degree of gun-related crime?

SELECTED BIBLIOGRAPHY

Criminal Victimization, 2000. Washington, DC: U.S. Department of Justice, Bureau of Justice Statistics, 2001.

Injury Facts (formerly *Accident Facts*). Itasca, IL: National Safety Council, (updated annually).

Injury Mortality Reports, 1999. Atlanta, GA: National Center for Injury Prevention and Control, Centers for Disease Control and Prevention.

Journal of Safety Research. Itasca, IL: National Safety Council (published quarterly).

Lack, R.W. *Safety, Health, and Asset Protection* (2nd ed.). Boca Raton, FL: Lewis Publishers (2002).

Rennison, C.M., and S. Welchans. *Intimate Partner Violence*. Washington, DC: U.S. Department of Justice, Bureau of Justice Statistics, 2000.

Report to the Nation on Crime and Justice (2nd ed.). Washington, DC: U.S. Department of Justice, Bureau of Justice Statistics, 1988.

Simon T., J. Mercy, and C. Perkins. *Injuries from Violent Crime, 1992–98*. Washington, DC: Bureau of Justice Statistics, U.S. Department of Justice, 2001.

Understanding and Preventing Violence. Washington, DC: National Research Council, National Academy Press, 1993.

HEALTHLINKS

Websites for the Health Threats of Unintentional Injuries and Violence

You can access better health as it relates to this chapter by checking out some of the following sites on the Internet. These sites can be accessed directly from the *Decisions for Healthy Living* Website located at www.aw.com/pruitt.

CDC National Center for Injury Prevention and Control (NCIPC)

Home page for the lead federal agency for unintentional injuries and violence prevention. It provides a link to statistical data, information on publications and resources, and links to related Websites.

National Criminal Justice Reference Service

A collection of clearinghouses providing extensive information, documents, and links about violence and criminal justice

National Highway Transportation Safety Administration

Through this site you can access information on motor vehicle safety, compliance testing, buying a safer car, recalls, technical service bulletins, and consumer complaints.

National Safety Council

Access to resources, statistics, and publications related to public safety and unintentional injuries.

HEALTH HOTLINES

The Health Threats of Unintentional Injuries and Violence

Foundation for Aquatic Injury Prevention (FAIP)
(800) 342-0330
12230 White Lake Road
Fenton, MI 48430

National Criminal Justice Reference Service
(800) 851-3420
P. O. Box 6000
Rockville, MD 20849-6000

National Domestic Violence Hotline
(800) 799-SAFE (799-7233)
P. O. Box 161810
Austin, TX 78716

Brain Injury Association of America
(800) 444-6443
105 North Alfred Street
Alexandria, VA 22314

National Highway Traffic Safety Administration, Auto Safety Hotline
(800) 424-9393
400 7th Street SW, Room 5319
Washington, DC 20590

Office for Victims of Crime Resource Center
(800) 627-6872
P.O. Box 6000
Rockville, MD 20849-6000

TEST YOUR KNOWLEDGE ANSWERS

1. False. In 1925, the number of deaths per 100 million vehicle miles driven was 12.6. By the year 2000, the number of deaths per 100 million vehicle miles driven had dropped to 1.6. Thus, the modern automobile is far safer than the earlier automobiles despite the higher speed of travel.
2. True. Even though seat belts are proven to save lives, a significant number of drivers do not use them.
3. True. Poorer people are more likely to be raped, robbed, or assaulted seriously. As annual family income increases, the incidence of violent crime generally decreases. There is one exception to this: Higher-income households are more likely to be robbed than are lower-income households.
4. False. If you have a gun at home, you are eight times more likely to be killed by or to kill a family member or close acquaintance.
5. True. Approximately two thirds of all rapists are acquainted with their victims.

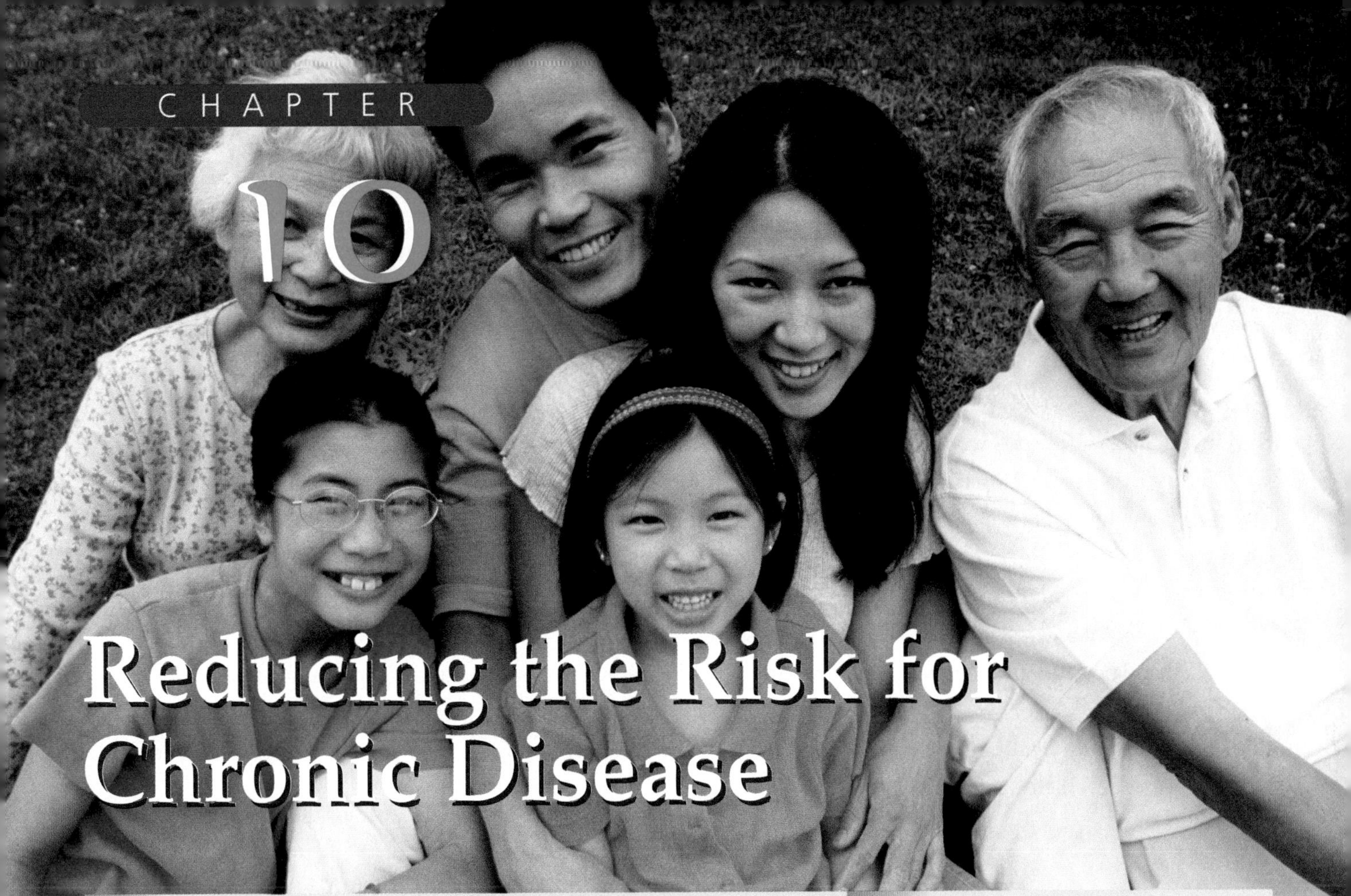

CHAPTER 10

Reducing the Risk for Chronic Disease

OBJECTIVES

When you finish reading this chapter, you will be able to:

1. Differentiate between chronic illness and infectious illness.
2. Explain the natural history of a chronic illness, including the asymptomatic and symptomatic periods.
3. Relate lifestyle choices to the occurrence of chronic illness.
4. Describe the risk factors associated with cardiovascular disease and determine your personal risk for cardiovascular disease.
5. Name several cardiovascular diseases and describe the symptoms and treatment modalities for each.
6. Describe the risk factors associated with cancer.
7. Name several types of cancer and describe the prevalence of each.
8. Explain the importance of early detection of cancer and name several screening procedures that can lead to early detection.
9. Name and describe at least three chronic diseases other than heart disease and cancer.
10. Examine ways of helping individuals who have chronic illness, including psychological support.

TEST YOUR KNOWLEDGE

1. Cardiovascular disease accounts for more deaths in the United States than any other disease. True or False?
2. The American Heart Association recommends that an electrocardiogram (ECG) test be taken annually after age forty in order to detect heart disease at an early stage. True or False?
3. Early detection of cancer is successful because if tumors are detected when benign, they can be removed before they become malignant and spread. True or False?
4. In the United States, lung cancer rates are in decline due to decreased tobacco use among men. True or False?
5. The most prevalent chronic diseases affecting both children and adults are cancers. True or False?

Answers found at end of chapter.

A chronic problem is one that is marked by long duration or frequent recurrence. In fact, the term chronic comes from the Greek word chronos, which means "time." In a social sense, think of chronic unemployment, chronic homelessness, or chronic urban decay. It is not a pretty picture. So, too, it is not pleasant to think of **chronic illnesses** with their accompanying progressive pain and increasing disability. In some cases, however, there are ways to interrupt and even reverse the course of a chronic disease.

Everyone knows someone who suffers from heart disease, cancer, diabetes, arthritis, asthma, tooth decay and gum disease, or a host of other chronic conditions. Chronic diseases are the leading cause of death and disability in the United States and a major source of pain and discomfort (see Figure 10.1).

Chronic diseases develop over a long period of time, in part as a result of lifestyle choices. Smoking alone is associated with an increased incidence of the leading chronic diseases—heart disease, cancer, and lung disease. Still other chronic diseases develop through the process of living in a highly industrialized country in the twenty-first century. Certain cancers and lung diseases, for example, are associated with polluted air and chemicals in the workplace. Another important factor associated with chronic diseases is that people are living longer and so are subject to diseases that usually do not present themselves until the later years of life, such as osteoporosis and Alzheimer's disease.

It may be difficult for young adults to appreciate the relevance of chronic diseases in their life because they may think it will be many years before they have symptoms of one. However, people of all ages are at risk for chronic conditions that can affect their quality of life.

Characteristics of Chronic Illness

Chronic illness is a generic term for diseases such as atherosclerosis, cancer, asthma, diabetes, multiple sclerosis, schizophrenia, or arthritis. Chronic illness may result from a genetic condition, such as cystic fibrosis, or from poor hygiene, such as tooth decay. A chronic illness can affect the individual physically, mentally, or both. Sometimes, a chronic illness only minimally interferes with daily functioning; at other times, it requires round-the-clock medical attention.

Even given these differences, chronic illnesses have several common characteristics:

- They involve some degree of permanence.
- They result in some form of disability.
- They are progressive—that is, they get increasingly worse or become more debilitating.
- They require a long period of care or supervision.

Chronic Versus Infectious Diseases

Chronic diseases differ from infectious diseases in three key ways. First, the two disease groups differ in their causes. For the most part, infectious or communicable diseases are a result of microorganisms and are contagious. (Infectious diseases are covered in Chapter 11.) Chronic diseases, in contrast, are generally not contagious. They are mostly a result of inherited factors or lifestyle factors, such as diet, personal hygiene, tobacco use, or exposure to toxic chemicals. (Recent research shows that microorganisms may play a role in some chronic conditions, for example stomach ulcers.)

Second, infectious diseases usually develop quickly and last for a comparatively brief period—sometimes only a matter of hours or days. Chronic diseases develop over a period of years and usually linger for a lifetime.

Third, chronic and infectious diseases differ concerning outcome. Persons who have infectious diseases may recover completely. Healthy people generally do not die of the common cold. As with many infectious diseases, they may feel miserable for a while, but in time, they usually recover completely. (There are exceptions to this rule, including malaria, hepatitis, HIV, and other virulent infectious diseases.) It is just the opposite with chronic diseases. People who have chronic diseases tend to remain ill for a long period of time. Again, there are exceptions. People have recovered from cancer, heart disease, and other chronic conditions.

Changing Patterns of Mortality

At the beginning of the twentieth century, infectious diseases were the leading cause of death. Now at the beginning of the twenty-first century, with thanks to

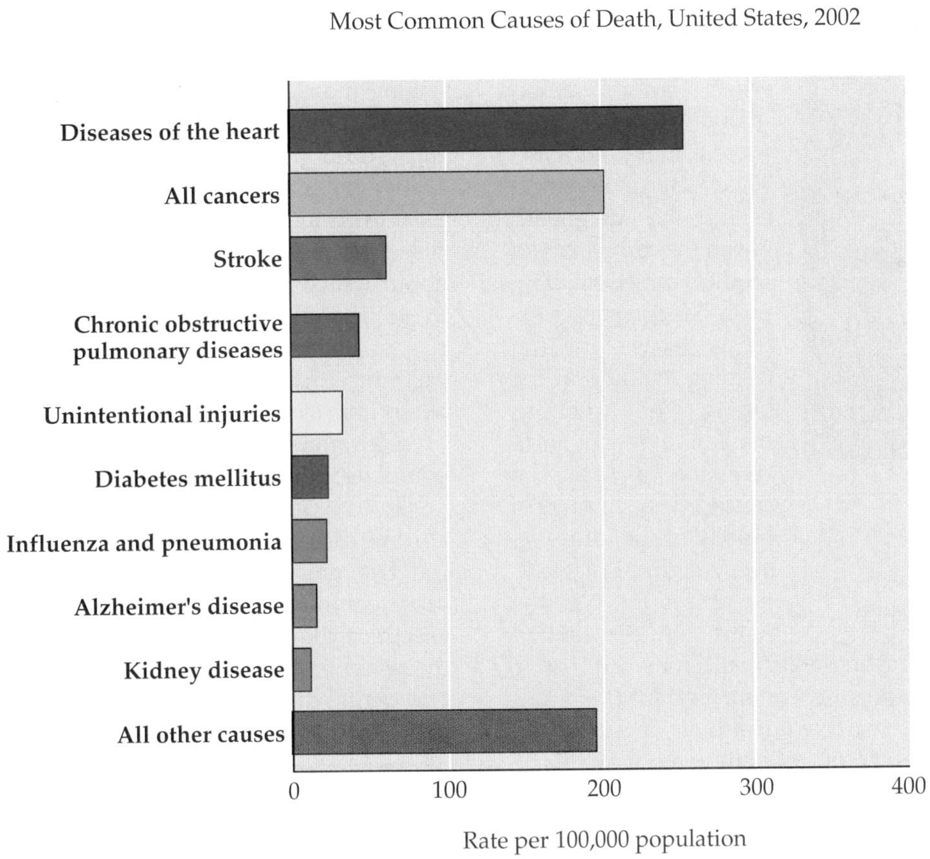

Figure 10.1 Most Common Causes of Death, United States, 2002
Chronic diseases are the leading cause of death in the United States, and are a major source of disability, pain, and discomfort. (*Source:* National Center for Health Statistics)

medical interventions and healthier lifestyles, infants, children, and young adults now survive what once were fatal illnesses and often live long enough to incur chronic illnesses. At a time when adults could anticipate living only about fifty or sixty years, chronic diseases were proportionately less common. But the proportion of population over age sixty-five is growing. In 1900, one out of every twenty-five Americans was sixty-five years old or older. As of 2000, one out of every eight Americans had celebrated his or her sixty-fifth birthday. And, according to the U.S. Administration on Aging, most older persons have at least one chronic condition and many have multiple conditions (see Chapter 14).

Natural History of Chronic Diseases

Chronic diseases occur over a long period of time, sometimes without initial outward signs or clinical symptoms. This is called the **asymptomatic period.** In most cases, people with asymptomatic chronic conditions live normal lives without knowing that they have a chronic disease.

In the case of cardiovascular disease, for example, the presence of **plaque,** or fatty deposits, in the arteries is a clear signal of disease. Yet until the symptoms of disease appear, most people do not know that they have been accumulating plaque in their arteries.

More dramatically, a college basketball player might not know that he or she has an enlarged heart until collapsing during a game, or an elderly woman might not know she has osteoporosis until she falls, compresses her spine, and is left crippled and in chronic pain.

At some point during the course of a disease, clinical symptoms appear. This is called the **symptomatic period.** These signs, such as a lump, lesion, or other abnormal growth, may be apparent to the trained eye or touch. But many of the symptoms of chronic diseases are nonvisual, such as an increase in blood pressure.

asymptomatic period A period in which a disease exists without outward signs or clinical symptoms.

plaque A deposit of fatty material in a blood vessel wall.

symptomatic period A period during the course of a disease in which symptoms appear.

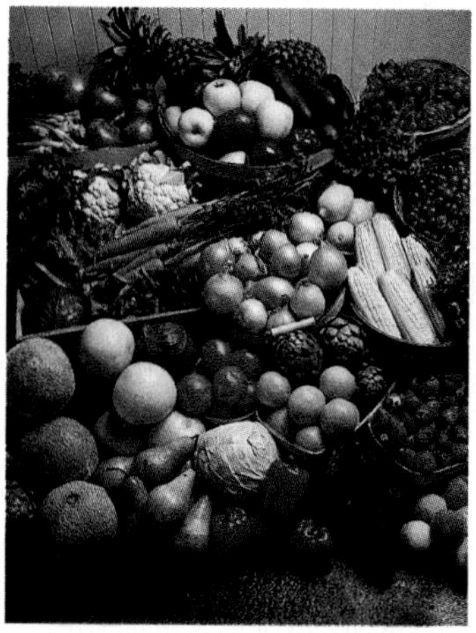

Eating a healthy diet is an important factor in preventing chronic diseases such as heart disease and some cancers. (*Source:* FPG International/© Ralph Pleasant)

It is usually up to a physician to determine when signs and abnormalities suggest the presence of a disease. This determination is called the **diagnosis.** Given the complexity of medical practice, diagnosis has become an extensive focus of medical training. A lump in the breast, for example, may or may not indicate the presence of cancer. Only through a **biopsy** of the lump tissue, a medical diagnostic procedure, can the lump be evaluated properly to determine whether it is cancerous.

Most chronic diseases, if left unrecognized and untreated, eventually lead to major impairment or even death. For this reason, early detection is highly important. Early signs, although not proof, should be taken as serious warnings and reasons to see your physician. One consistent fact concerning nearly all chronic diseases is that early detection through recognition of signs and symptoms leads to an increased chance of survival and a higher quality of life.

Lifestyle Choices and Disease

Lifestyle choices are important factors not only in chronic disease but also in overall personal health. Many such behaviors are presented in greater detail in other chapters of this book. The most common lifestyle causes of chronic diseases are smoking, poor diet, failure to exercise, and heavy consumption of alcohol.

Other factors contribute to the occurrence of chronic disease: not taking advantage of available health screening techniques, such as **mammography** to detect breast cancer and **sigmoidoscopy** or **colonoscopy** to detect colon cancer, or not taking medication for hypertension. Genetic predisposition, gender, and advancing age are recognized factors that contribute to chronic and degenerative diseases over which you have little control.

Given the current state of knowledge about chronic diseases, it is important to control the modifiable factors about which you are aware, monitor those you cannot avoid, and take steps to minimize the negative health impact of all lifestyle choices. Although prevention does not guarantee that you will not develop a chronic disease, it could improve your odds in favor of better health.

Chronic diseases are far too numerous to provide complete information about each one in this chapter. Table 10.1 provides a brief overview of the common chronic diseases.

The remainder of this chapter focuses on two of the most common and most life-threatening chronic diseases: cardiovascular disease and cancer. Three other diseases are presented briefly: Type II diabetes, asthma, and dental disease.

diagnosis A physician's opinion of the nature or cause of a disease based on observation and laboratory tests.

biopsy The removal of bits of living tissue and fluid from the body for diagnostic examination.

mammography A screening technique used to detect breast cancer.

sigmoidoscopy A screening procedure in which a physician uses a hollow lighted tube to inspect the rectum and lower colon.

colonoscopy A screening procedure in which a physician uses a hollow lighted tube to inspect the entire bowel and some portions of the small intestines.

cardiovascular disease Disease of the heart and blood vessels.

hypertension High blood pressure; generally means the heart is working harder than normal.

Cardiovascular Disease: The Nation's Leading Cause of Death

Diseases of the heart and blood vessels—collectively called **cardiovascular diseases**—are the leading cause of death in the United States. They claimed the lives of nearly one million Americans in 1999, and nearly 62 million more have some form of cardiovascular disease, according to the American Heart Association. To illustrate how great a toll cardiovascular diseases take, the National Center for Health Statistics estimates that if all forms of cardiovascular disease were eliminated, life expectancy would rise by almost ten years. In contrast, if all forms of cancer were eliminated, the gain would be three years.

Heart disease remains the number one killer despite the fact that the death rate from cardiovascular disease has declined dramatically over the past several decades (see Figure 10.2). This decline is due in great part to better surgical techniques, improved drugs, more effective medical management, and a better understanding of the risk factors for heart disease.

Who Is at Risk?

The major risk factors associated with cardiovascular disease are related to lifestyle and include smoking, **hypertension,** elevated cholesterol, elevated iron in the blood, obesity or being overweight, adult-onset diabetes, and sedentary lifestyle. Risk factors for cardio-

Table 10.1 Common Chronic Diseases and Risk Factors

Disease	Nonbehavioral risk factors	Behavioral risk factors	Symptoms	Preventive measures
Asthma	Allergies; family history; young age; viral infections; bronchitis	An attack may be triggered by cigarette smoking; perfumes; exercise; aspirin; industrial/occupational exposures to air pollution; emotional anxiety	Coughing; shortness of breath; tightness in chest; wheezing; itchy or sore throat; increased breathing rate	Stay away from triggers; take allergy medications; exercise; recognize and treat symptoms early
Breast cancer	Genetic predisposition; cancer in one breast; uterine cancer; age; Caucasian race; early menstruation—late menopause	Women who have delayed child-bearing; women over 35; increased use of alcohol; increased fat content in diet; never having given birth	Lump in breast, armpit; breast pain; nipple discharge; itching, enlargement, retraction of nipple; change in breast contour or symmetry	Self-examination of breast every month; mammography; physical examination by gynecologist annually
Cervical cancer	Genetic predisposition; age	Intercourse at early age; multiple partners; smoking; papilloma virus infection	Abnormal vaginal bleeding; abnormal Pap smear	Avoid early sexual intercourse; avoid multiple partners; avoid cigarette smoking; annual gynecological exam
Cirrhosis of the liver	Genetic predisposition	Heavy alcohol/drug consumption; hepatitis	Weakness, fatigue; weight loss; nausea; abdominal pain; jaundice; amenorrhea; impotence; male breast increase	Discontinue use of alcohol/drugs
Dental disease	Age; fluoride-deficient drinking water; poverty	Fear of professional care; excessive between-meal snacks; failure to brush and floss regularly	Stained teeth; bad breath; tooth cavities; tooth loss; painful gums and tongue	Well-balanced nutritious diet; limit between-meal snacks; brush and floss regularly; have regular professional dental care
Diabetes	Genetic predisposition	Obesity or being overweight; trauma to trigger onset	Increased urination; excessive thirst; rapid weight loss; high blood glucose levels; increased ketones in blood glucose	Well-balanced nutritious diet; maintain proper weight; exercise
Heart disease	Genetic predisposition; age; high blood pressure; diabetes	Poor physical exercise; cigarette smoking; obesity; poor stress management	Chest pain; breathing difficulty; spitting up blood; weight loss; lung collapse	Discontinuance of smoking; maintain low cholesterol levels; healthy diet (low in saturated fat, low amounts of junk food); regular exercise program; medical checkup
Lung cancer	Genetic predisposition; age	Cigarette smoking; environment (air, industrial pollution)	Cough; breathing difficulty; spitting up blood; weight loss; lung collapse	Discontinuance of smoking; elimination of environmental risks; education; medical checkup
Lung disease	Genetic predisposition; age	Environment (air, industrial pollution); cigarette smoking	Breathlessness; persistent cough; crowing sound during breathing; wheezing; spitting up blood; weight loss; lung collapse	Discontinuance of smoking; elimination of environmental risks; education; medical checkup
Stroke	Genetic predisposition; previous stroke; heart attack; age; high blood pressure	Cigarette smoking; heavy alcohol consumption; high-fat diet	Brief loss of vision; slurred speech; nausea; vomiting; sensory loss; weakness or paralysis	Discontinuance of smoking; control blood pressure; maintain low cholesterol levels; healthy diet (low in saturated fat, low amounts of junk food); regular exercise program; medical checkup

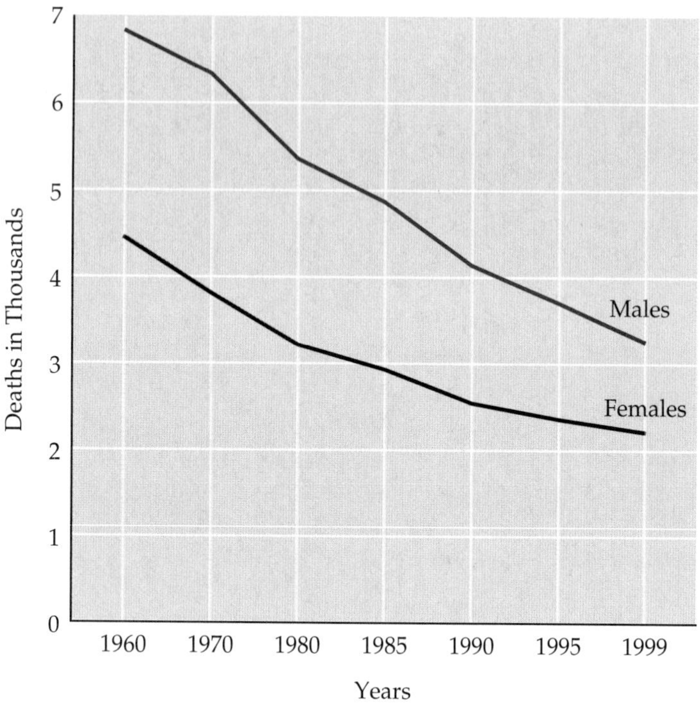

Figure 10.2 Cardiovascular Mortality Trends for Men and Women

Even though the death rate from cardiovascular disease has dropped dramatically for decades, it is the number one killer in the United States. (*Source:* National Center for Health Statistics)

vascular disease that are not related to lifestyle include family history of the disease, age, and sex.

Smoking is the single most important risk factor associated with heart disease. It is estimated that smoking accounts for more than 20 percent of all coronary heart disease deaths. The good news in this regard, however, is that smoking cessation can substantially reduce this death rate. According to the World Health Organization, after one year of not smoking, the risk of coronary heart disease drops by 50 percent. Quitting can also significantly reduce the risk for stroke.

Data from the Framingham Heart Study—the longest ongoing study in the United States of heart disease—show that people who have high blood pressure have three to four times the risk for developing coronary heart disease and as much as seven times the risk for a stroke as do those who have normal blood pressure. Obesity is a risk factor by itself, but it also contributes to high blood pressure levels. Even a 10 percent weight loss in an overweight, hypertensive person can significantly reduce his or her blood pressure. Obesity also contributes to adult-onset diabetes, which in turn is a risk factor for heart disease because it may speed the rate at which fat is deposited on the artery wall, thus clogging the flow of blood to the heart.

The Framingham Study has also found that the incidence of heart disease increases as blood cholesterol levels rise. The Centers for Disease Control and Prevention (CDC), however, has found that a 10 percent decrease in total cholesterol levels may result in an estimated 30 percent reduction in the incidence of coronary heart disease.

Sedentary lifestyle is another major contributor to heart disease, and recent data from the CDC show that people who are not physically active are twice as likely as physically active people to die of coronary heart disease. Less active, less fit individuals have a 30 percent to 50 percent greater risk of developing high blood pressure. Much has been written about athletes who drop dead from heart disease while competing, but it is important to note that healthy people usually do not die while exercising. The athletes in the news tend to have either serious heart defects (which are usually present from birth) or advanced but undetected coronary artery disease.

Diagnosing Heart Disease

Heart disease is diagnosed in two ways: **screening** and **detection.** Screening for heart disease involves an analysis of risk factors associated with the disease. Such procedures are done on individuals assumed to be healthy. Although screening tests do not provide absolute proof of the existence of an abnormal heart condition, so much is known about the relationship of specific risk factors to the incidence of heart disease that by identifying them early, a physician can prescribe the appropriate behavior change—for example, stop smoking, adjust your diet, or begin blood pressure medication. Should a screening test or a combination of apparent risk factors raise suspicion of the existence of heart disease, a physician is more likely to detect heart disease at a very early stage.

Detection of heart disease is done on individuals suspected of having some form of cardiovascular abnormality. In many cases, detection involves the same procedure as screening; the difference is mainly in the physician's purpose.

An **electrocardiogram (ECG)** is used for both screening for and detecting heart disease. To perform an ECG, a medical technician attaches electrodes to the body. As the heart beats, these electrodes transmit the

screening Analysis of risk factors done on a person thought to be well, for the purpose of preventing disease or making an early diagnosis.

detection Medical procedures (tests) done on individuals suspected of having a disease, for the purpose of confirming the presence of the disease and, if present, determining the progress of the disease.

electrocardiogram (ECG) A screening procedure used to detect heart disease; a graphic record of the heart's action obtained from an instrument that records heart activity.

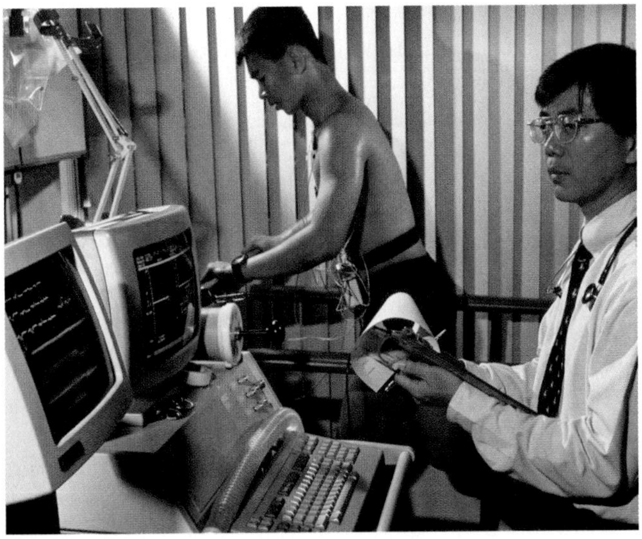

An electrocardiogram (ECG) can detect abnormalities in the heart at an early stage of disease. You should have a baseline ECG at age twenty and again at age forty to forty-five.

electrical impulses that cause the heart to contract to a device that records them. After a series of impulses is recorded, a trained technician or physician interprets the ECG and can identify any abnormalities.

An ECG is the principal test for screening asymptomatic individuals, that is, those who have yet to experience chest pains or have a heart attack. The American Heart Association recommends that a baseline ECG be taken at age twenty, again at age forty to forty-five, and then only as suggested by other risk factors. An ECG can also detect heart disease at an early stage. When used for detecting heart disease, an ECG should not be the only diagnostic tool used.

Some people, in addition, undergo a stress electrocardiogram (stress ECG). A stress ECG is also known as a maximal exercise tolerance test or treadmill test, because a treadmill is used to produce an elevated heart rate. Reliable testing protocols have also been developed using walking, running, a stationary bicycle, or going up and down steps. The stress ECG might be compared with a high-speed road test of a car. The results reveal how the heart performs under pressure—more precisely, under high-intensity exercise. A stress ECG is a better diagnostic procedure than a resting ECG. It is also an effective means of determining fitness level.

Stress tests are recommended for people who have a history of cardiac risk factors and for sedentary individuals who wish to begin an exercise program. This is because strenuous exercise may result in severe heart problems and even death for at-risk persons. Stress tests are also required in certain occupations that involve unusual endurance and strength and that affect public safety, such as police work and fire fighting.

Forms of Heart Disease

The term *cardiovascular disease* actually refers to many diseases. Some are directly related to the heart; others are related to the circulatory system, including veins and arteries. **Atherosclerosis,** the most common form of hardening of the arteries (also called arteriosclerosis), is the single biggest cause of heart and blood vessel disease. It is a slow, progressive disease that may start in early life. Atherosclerosis is characterized by thick deposits of fatty substances (plaque) such as cholesterol on the inner walls of the arteries. As a result of these deposits, the internal channels of the arteries become narrow, and blood moves through them with great difficulty. This makes it easier for a clot to form, which can block the artery and thus deprive the heart, brain, or other organs of blood.

Heart attack (myocardial infarction), the number one killer in the nation (about 500,000 deaths a year), usually results from atherosclerosis. Heart attacks are fatal for about 36 percent of the people who have them, so there are far more people who have had a heart attack and lived to tell the story than there are people who have died of them. However, those who survive a heart attack are at a significantly increased risk of having a second heart attack and of developing angina and other heart-related conditions.

Angina pectoris, a condition that results in a temporary reduction in the blood supply to the heart, can cause feelings of discomfort similar to but not as strong as those of a heart attack. Although an angina attack is not a heart attack, its symptoms should be taken seriously because they could be a forewarning of other heart problems. An angina attack usually takes place during physical activity or periods of emotional upset. Nitroglycerin or some other medication can prevent or reduce the pain of angina.

Arrhythmia is an erratic beating of the heart that can cause a heart attack. Nearly everyone experiences an occasional skip of a heartbeat due to too much excitement, too much caffeine, or for no reason at all. There is nothing dangerous about this. Arrhythmia becomes life threatening when a chain of beats is missed so that the heart muscle does not contract effectively. As a result of this, the brain does not get enough oxygen-

atherosclerosis A thickening and loss of elasticity of the inner walls of the arteries.

heart attack (myocardial infarction) A condition that occurs when the blood supply to part of the heart muscle (the myocardium) is severely reduced or stopped. Normally circulating blood brings oxygen and other nutrients to the heart.

angina pectoris Chest pain; a symptom of a condition in which the heart does not get as much blood as it needs.

arrhythmia An erratic heartbeat.

containing blood and the victim loses consciousness and can go into cardiac arrest and die. Arrhythmias may be caused by a damaged heart muscle or by extreme emotional distress. Common forms of arrhythmia include **tachycardia** (excessively rapid heart rate), **bradycardia** (abnormally slow heart rate), and **fibrillation** (irregular, convulsive movements of the heart muscle resulting in a failure to pump blood).

Stroke, also called a cerebrovascular accident (CVA), is the third leading cause of death in the country. Each year, according to the American Stroke Association, about 600,000 Americans have a stroke and more than 160,000 die from it. A stroke results when the supply of blood pumped by the heart to the brain is cut off or when bleeding occurs in the brain. When the damage takes place in the right side of the brain, sensory and motor function is lost on the left side of the body. This is known as left **hemiplegia.** When the damage occurs on the left side of the brain, loss of function occurs on the right side of the body, affecting communication skills, including speaking, writing, reading, and listening. This condition is known as right hemiplegia.

Transient ischemic attacks (TIAs) are little strokes that cause minimal damage but are warning signals of the possibility of a more severe stroke. Men are more likely to suffer all kinds of strokes than are women and African Americans are more likely to suffer strokes than are whites. Women who take oral contraceptives are more at risk for stroke than are those who do not. The risk for stroke increases with age for both sexes.

Hypertension (high blood pressure) is called the silent killer because it has few symptoms but affects about 50 million Americans and can lead to heart attack, stroke, and heart and kidney failure. High blood pressure adds to the workload of the heart and arteries and can cause them not to function as well as they should. Approximately 25 percent of adults have high blood pressure, defined as blood pressure greater than a **systolic pressure,** (contraction of the heart muscle) of 140 or a **diastolic pressure** (relaxation of the heart muscle) of 90. This is written as 140/90, and is referred to as 140 over 90. Normal blood pressure is about 120/80 for young adults.

Hypertension occurs more frequently after age thirty-five and among African Americans more often than among whites. It is associated with obesity, high-sodium diets, and other controllable risk factors, but by far the most important factor predicting hypertension is genetic predisposition. If one of your parents has or had hypertension, you have a 50 percent chance of having it too. This risk rises to 90 percent if both parents are or were affected. Blood pressure can be lowered successfully through salt restriction, weight control, and exercise. If these treatments fail to lower blood pressure, medication is indicated.

Repairing the Heart

From a good pair of walking shoes to a coronary artery bypass or a heart transplant, there are many ways to prevent and treat heart disease. Regular aerobic exercise, the kind that raises the heart rate and is done for 20 minutes three or more times a week, can help prevent and correct high blood pressure. As little as a five- to ten-pound weight loss can also help decrease blood volume and the amount of blood pumped by the heart, which in turn reduces pressure in the arteries.

Medications have proven successful in lowering blood pressure, stabilizing mild to moderate heartbeat irregularities, relieving angina, raising cardiac output, and lowering the heart's demand for blood. A class of cholesterol-lowering drugs called statins can reduce the risk of a heart attack or stroke by one third if taken daily. The cost: $2.50 a day. Another drug can reduce heart attack deaths by more than 25 percent if administered within the first few hours after the onset of heart attack symptoms and can cost more than $2,000 per dose.

Far cheaper is common aspirin. Extensive studies show that healthy men and women can cut their risk of a heart attack nearly in half by taking one low-dose or baby aspirin every day, a regimen recommended by the U.S. Prevention Services Task Force.

Drugs usually have side effects, and heart drugs are no different. Some side effects of heart drugs include fatigue, nausea, impotence in men, and depression. Even aspirin can cause stomach ulcers and internal bleeding when taken on a regular basis. If medications are successful in reducing the cardiac problem, however, more risky surgery can be avoided.

A low-cost lifesaving technique for heart attack victims is **cardiopulmonary resuscitation (CPR).** CPR, which involves rescue breathing (mouth-to-mouth resuscitation) alternating with pressure applied to the chest, is a basic life skill that is used in emergency situations. It has been estimated that if one of every three

tachycardia Excessively rapid beating of the heart.

bradycardia Abnormally slow beating of the heart.

fibrillation Irregular convulsive movement of the heart muscle.

stroke A clot or break in a blood vessel in the brain that disrupts blood flow to the brain.

hemiplegia The loss of sensory and motor function on one side of the body.

transient ischemic attack (TIA) A stroke that causes minimal damage but signals the possibility of a more severe stroke.

systolic pressure The pressure measured in the arteries when the heart contracts.

diastolic pressure The pressure measured in the arteries when the heart relaxes.

cardiopulmonary resuscitation (CPR) A combination of mouth-to-mouth breathing and chest compression used during cardiac arrest to keep blood flowing to the heart muscle and brain; an emergency procedure.

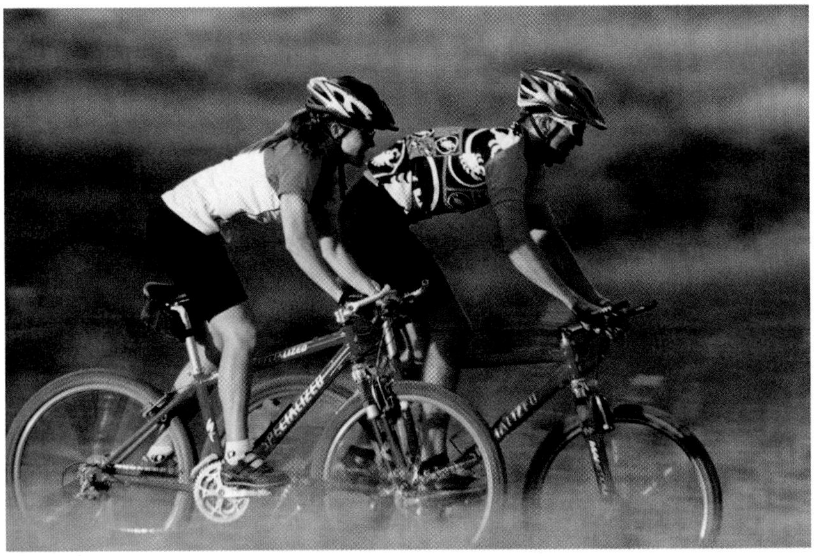

Exercise is a good way to maintain a healthy heart. It is also cost-effective: You can buy a good bike for a couple hundred dollars; a heart transplant costs several hundred thousand.

Americans were trained in CPR, more than one hundred thousand lives a year could be saved.

For people who have severely clogged arteries, surgical options include **coronary angioplasty,** in which the coronary artery is widened with an inflated balloon catheter; **coronary artery bypass,** in which the blood flow is rerouted from the blocked part of the artery using a length of vein taken from another part of the body; and a **heart transplant,** in which a normally functioning heart from a person who has recently died is implanted in place of the diseased one. Each of these procedures has limited success, but collectively, they have improved the quality of life and in many cases have extended the lives of millions of heart patients.

Artificial hearts have been used to extend the lives of otherwise terminal patients until transplant donors can be found. The artificial heart gets its power to operate from a source outside the body, so it is not an effective long-term replacement for the original organ. Even with incredible advances such as an artificial heart, the best advice is to take care of the organs you have and not count on medicine to provide replacement parts when they malfunction.

Cancer: The Nation's Second Leading Cause of Death

One of the most feared of all diseases, cancer, strikes people of all ages—in childhood, adolescence, the prime of life, and old age. Cancer is the second leading cause of death in the United States. It accounts for about one of every four deaths from all causes in the United States, and it kills more children than any other disease. It is estimated that in 2002, 1.3 million Americans were diagnosed with cancer and approximately 555,500 died of it. Because of exposure to **carcinogens** (cancer-causing substances) in the environment, the longer a person lives, the greater the chance of developing cancer.

The incidence of cancer in the population is increasing, mainly because of increases in lung cancer. To illustrate this point, lung cancer recently replaced breast cancer as the leading cause of cancer death among women.

The Basics of Cancer

Cancer is not actually one disease. It is a group of more than 100 diseases, all characterized by uncontrolled growth and spread of abnormal cells. Normally, cells reproduce in an orderly manner following the genetic rules of growth. But some cells become abnormal and fail to follow these rules. They continue to divide and grow and eventually band together into **tumors,** or masses of tissue.

Not all tumors are cancerous. In fact, most are **benign,** or harmless. **Benign tumors** do not invade other cells or spread to other parts of the body. They are different from cancerous tumors in their very structure, and they cannot change into cancerous tumors. Benign tumors, however, can cause problems if they block some crucial part of the body and prevent it from functioning.

Only **malignant tumors** are cancerous. If left untreated, malignant tumors spread into nearby tissues and organs, crowding out healthy cells and replacing them with cancer cells. The most dangerous characteristic of

coronary angioplasty A surgical procedure to widen the coronary artery with an inflated balloon catheter.

coronary artery bypass A surgical procedure to reroute blood flow from the blocked part of an artery by using a length of vein taken from another part of the body.

heart transplant A surgical procedure in which a normally functioning heart from a person who has recently died is implanted into a person with a diseased heart.

carcinogen A cancer-causing agent or factor.

tumor A mass of tissue that accumulates in the body.

benign Not harmful.

benign tumor A noncancerous tumor that is usually harmless and does not invade other cells or spread to other parts of the body.

malignant tumor A cancerous tumor that spreads to nearby tissues and organs, crowding out healthy cells and replacing them with cancer cells.

malignant tumors is that they **metastasize,** or spread to other parts of the body through the bloodstream or lymph system. In this way, a single cancer cell can spread the disease throughout the entire body.

No one knows exactly what causes a normal cell to become a cancer cell. Scientists believe that most cancers develop through repeated or long-term contact with cancer-causing agents. There are two basic kinds of carcinogens: **initiators** and **promoters.** Initiators start the cell damage that can lead to cancer. Examples of initiators are cigarette smoking, X rays, and certain chemicals. Promoters do not actually cause cancers, but they help them to grow. Alcohol, for example, promotes mouth, throat, and possibly liver cancer when combined with an initiator such as tobacco.

Who Is at Risk?

Although the basic causes of cancer are unknown, scientists have discovered several conditions often connected with abnormal cell growth. In some—but not all—cases, you can do something to reduce your risk for getting cancer.

The single behavior that most often results in death from cancer is smoking. People who smoke two or more packs of cigarettes a day are fifteen to twenty-five times more likely to die of cancer than are nonsmokers. Smoking also increases the risk for developing other cancers, particularly those of the mouth, pharynx, larynx, esophagus, pancreas, and bladder. Studies also show that cancer can be caused by passive smoking in healthy nonsmokers, by smokeless tobacco, and by the tar produced by smoking marijuana.

Repeated exposure to sunlight over a long period of time is a major cause of skin cancer. The sun's ultraviolet rays harm the skin. Fair-skinned people have less of a pigment called **melanin** in their skin to block some of the sun's damaging rays, and they are at greater risk of getting skin cancer than are dark-skinned people. The amount of time spent in the sun or in a tanning booth determines the extent of damage.

Large doses of X rays or ionizing radiation can cause cancer, depending on both the dose and the duration of exposure. The most common sources of ionizing radiation for medical reasons are diagnostic procedures and radiation therapy. Medical equipment is now designed to deliver the lowest possible dose without sacrificing the beneficial effects. Most of the information about the effects of radiation comes from studies of survivors of the atomic bombs dropped in Japan in 1945. The studies show increased rates among survivors of several types of cancer, including breast, thyroid, lung, and stomach cancer and acute leukemia.

Excessive amounts of alcohol are linked to a number of cancers. Heavy drinking is associated with cancers of the mouth, throat, esophagus, and liver. The cancer risks of alcohol are increased even more in drinkers who also smoke cigarettes.

Foods are linked to the risk of certain cancers, both positively and negatively. On the down side, cancers of the esophagus and stomach are common where large quantities of smoked, salt-cured, and nitrite-cured foods are eaten. Salami, bologna, and ham are examples of these foods. A high-fat diet not only is full of calories but also increases your risk for developing breast, colon, and prostate cancer. On the protective side, foods high in fiber—whole-grain breads, rice, broccoli, carrots, apples—appear to dilute intestinal contents and reduce the amount of time carcinogens spend in the intestine. A high-fiber diet may reduce your risk for developing colon cancer. Vitamin A protects against cancers of the esophagus, larynx, and lung, and vitamin C protects against cancer of the esophagus and stomach. Fresh fruits and vegetables are good sources of both of these vitamins.

Many occupations expose workers to toxic fumes, gases, airborne particles, and liquids. Occupational carcinogens include asbestos, vinyl chloride, formaldehyde, and arsenic. In addition to the worker being at risk, his or her family may also be in jeopardy. Some carcinogens such as asbestos attach themselves to workers' clothing, thus exposing family members who either wash the work clothes or include their own clothes in the same wash. Exposed workers and family members significantly multiply their risks if they smoke.

Certain families are no doubt cancer-prone, and up to 10 percent of all cancers may be hereditary. Specific examples of genetically linked cancers are retinoblastoma (an eye cancer that causes blindness) and familial polyps of the colon (which lead to colon cancer). Breast cancer in the family accounts for about 5 percent to 10 percent of all breast cancer.

metastasize To spread to other parts of the body through the bloodstream or lymph system.

initiator A carcinogen that starts cell damage that leads to cancer.

promoter A carcinogen that helps cancer to grow.

melanin Brownish-black skin pigment.

Types of Cancer

Cancer comes in many shapes and forms. It can affect your lungs or your limbs. It can affect your bones or your skin. All of the body's tissues and organs are susceptible to cancer (see Table 10.2). The following descriptions of several common cancers include statistics on incidence, risk factors, symptoms, and survival rates.

Lung cancer. Lung cancer is responsible for 28 percent of all deaths due to cancer. Since 1992, the number of new cases diagnosed has been declining, so eventually the rate of deaths will decline as well. The reduced rate of lung cancer is primarily a result of decreased tobacco use among men. Unfortunately, the rate of lung cancer in women continues to rise. The main risk factors for lung cancer are cigarette smoking, exposure to sidestream smoke, and occupational exposures to asbestos and other agents.

Symptoms include excessive coughing, chest pain, shortness of breath, chronic bronchitis, sputum containing blood, and difficulty in swallowing. Early detection may be difficult because these symptoms do not usually appear until the disease is at an advanced stage and has metastasized or spread.

The outlook for lung cancer patients is bleak: Most die within a year, and only 15 percent survive for five years after diagnosis.

Table 10.2 Where Cancer Strikes

Leading Sites of New Cancer Cases and Deaths—2002 Estimates*

	Cancer in Males			Cancer in Females	
	New Cases	Deaths		New Cases	Deaths
Prostate	189,000	30,200	Breast	203,500	39,600
Lung	90,200	89,200	Lung	79,200	65,700
Colon & rectum	72,600	27,800	Colon & rectum	75,700	28,800
Urinary bladder	41,500	8,600	Uterine corpus	39,300	6,600
Melanoma of the skin	30,100	4,700	Non-Hodgkin's lymphoma	25,700	11,700
Non-Hodgkin's lymphoma	28,200	12,700	Melanoma of the skin	23,500	
Kidney	19,100	7,200	Ovary	23,300	13,900
Oral cavity	18,900		Thyroid	15,800	
Leukemia	17,600	12,100	Pancreas	15,600	15,200
Pancreas	14,700	14,500	Urinary bladder	15,000	4,000
Liver	11,000	8,900	Leukemia	13,200	9,600
Esophagus	9,800	9,600	Brain	7,400	5,900
All sites	637,500	288,100	All sites	647,400	267,300

*Excluding basal and squamous cell skin cancer and in situ carcinomas except bladder. American Cancer Society Inc., Surveillance Research, 2002.

Source: Reprinted with the permission of the American Cancer Society, Inc., from *Cancer Facts and Figures* 2002.

Breast cancer. Breast cancer is the second leading cause of death from cancer for women (after lung cancer). The incidence of breast cancer increased about 4.5 percent a year between 1982 and 1998 and has recently leveled off. The increase is due in great part to screening programs that can detect tumors before they become clinically apparent. (A small percentage of men get breast cancer, and about four hundred of them a year die from it.)

The main risk factors for women are being over age fifty, a family history of breast cancer, never being pregnant, or having a first pregnancy after age thirty and estrogen therapy. (Estrogen is taken by some postmenopausal women to treat discomforts sometimes associated with the cessation of menstruation. Studies suggest that it can protect against heart disease and osteoporosis but also that it can promote the growth of existing breast cancer and contribute to cancer of the uterus.)

Symptoms of breast cancer include a lump, thickening or swelling of the breast, discharge from the nipple, or retraction of the nipple. Early detection by breast self-examination or mammography can significantly increase survival rates.

When the disease is localized at the time of diagnosis, five-year survival rates are as high as 96 percent. If the cancer has spread regionally to adjacent lymph nodes, survival rates drop to 76 percent, and for distant metastases, to 20 percent.

Prostate cancer. Prostate cancer is the second most common cause of cancer death in men (after lung cancer). The prostate is a small gland that surrounds the urethra and produces much of the liquid in semen. Risk factors are being over age fifty, workplace exposures to cadmium and other carcinogens, and a high-fat diet. The rate of prostate cancer in African American men is significantly higher than in whites. The increased incidence is thought to be due to lifestyle rather than to genetics, because this high rate developed in African Americans only in recent decades.

Symptoms include problems with urination, blood in the urine, and persistent pain in the back, hips, and pelvis. Prostate cancer grows slowly, and in the early

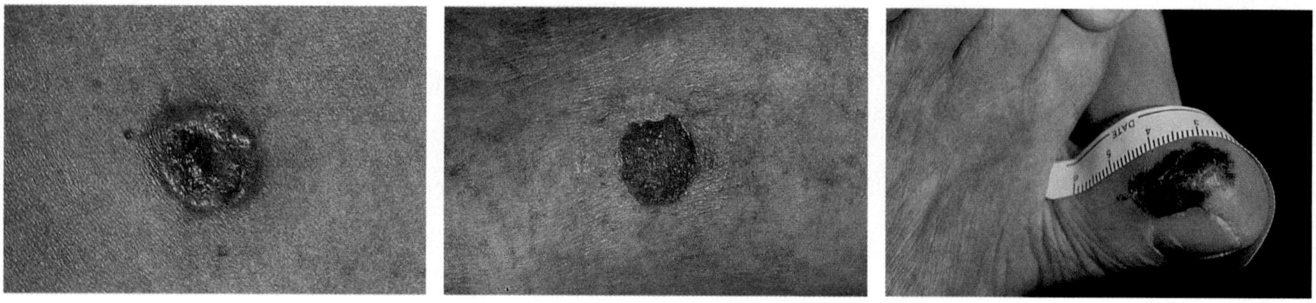

(a) **(b)** **(c)**

Photographs of skin cancers: (a) basal cell carcinoma, (b) squamous cell carcinoma, (c) melanoma.

stages, there are often no symptoms. Early detection can increase survival rates.

The outlook is excellent when the disease is confined within the prostate. These men are just as likely to be alive fifteen years later as men in the general population. If the disease is still localized, the five-year survival rate approaches 100 percent.

Colon and rectum (colorectal) cancers. Colon and rectum (colorectal) cancers have declined in recent years, probably because of increased sigmoidoscopic and colonoscopic screening and polyp removal (which helps prevent progression of polyps to invasive cancers). This decline is seen largely among whites; the incidence rates for African Americans have stabilized but have not yet begun to decline. The colon is the last five or six feet of the digestive tract. Major risk factors are being over age forty, family history of polyps of the colon, inflammatory bowel disease, and a high-fat diet.

Symptoms include rectal bleeding, blood in the stool, change in bowel habits (constipation or diarrhea), and general abdominal discomfort. When colorectal cancer is detected at an early localized stage, the five-year survival rate is 81 percent for colon cancer and 61 percent for rectal cancer. However, only about one third of cases are discovered at this stage.

Skin cancer. Skin cancer falls into two broad classes: **basal cell** and **squamous cell** cancers, which are more common and highly curable, and **melanomas,** which are relatively rare but more serious. The epidermis, or outer layer of the skin, contains both basal and squamous cells. Basal cells are small, round cells found in the lower part, or base, of the epidermis; squamous cells are flat cells that look like fish scales and make up most of the epidermis. More than 900,000 cases of basal and squamous cell cancers are diagnosed each year. Most are discovered so early and are so readily cured that few people die from basal or squamous cell cancers. Melanomas, in contrast, are far more fatal.

General risk factors associated with skin cancer are extensive exposure to the sun, fair complexion, and freckling (see the Developing Health Skills box). The incidence of skin cancer is very low among African Americans because of heavy skin pigmentation. For basal and squamous cell cancers specifically, additional risk factors include X-ray treatments for skin conditions, burn scars, occupational exposure to certain chemicals, and a precancerous change of the skin known as actinic **keratosis.** For melanomas, additional risk factors are brown moles and three or more blistering sunburns during adolescence.

Symptoms of skin cancer include a mole, birthmark, or beauty mark that changes color, size, or texture or an open sore that does not heal correctly. Early diagnosis is critical. For basal and squamous cell cancers, cure is likely if they are detected and treated early. Catching melanomas before they spread can result in an 89 percent five-year survival rate. About 80 percent of melanomas are diagnosed at the early stage.

Other common sites of cancer are the cervix, testicles, colon, and stomach. Some cancers are clearly linked to specific behaviors, such as oral cancer to smokeless tobacco use. Other cancers, such as leukemia (a cancer of the white blood cells), arise from unknown origins.

Screening for Cancer

As the statistics clearly illustrate, the best line of defense against a cancer spreading is early detection. Studies show that screening for cancer of the breast, cervix,

basal cell A small, round cell in the lower part (base) of the epidermis.

squamous cell A flat cell that makes up most of the epidermis.

melanoma A skin cancer that often starts as a mole-like growth and grows in size and changes color; the most serious of the various types of skin cancer.

keratosis A rough patch or horny growth of the skin.

Developing Health Skills

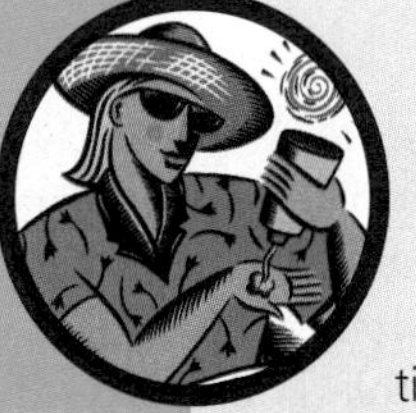

The Sun and Skin Cancer

The sun is the leading cause of cancer in the United States. One in six Americans can expect to develop some form of skin cancer, and for those who live in the Sunbelt states, the prediction is one in three. The most serious damage from overexposure to the sun occurs to children. Eighty percent of the skin damage that will eventually lead to cancer takes place when you are young. A bad burn before age eighteen heightens the chance of developing malignant melanoma later in life. But it is difficult to convince teenagers to wear sunscreen, and only one in five uses it.

The increased incidence of skin cancer is due in part to the gradual depletion of the ozone layer, which protects the earth from the sun's ultraviolet rays. As a result, the intensity of the sun's ultraviolet rays is greater than anything previous generations were exposed to.

Experts agree that the best way to combat the increased risk of cancer is to concentrate prevention efforts on the young. The good news is that nine out of ten women interviewed in a Gallup Poll said they were more careful with their children than they had been with themselves when they were younger. And in Hollywood, California, none of the celebrities has a tan, says a prominent dermatologist there. The same ultraviolet rays that cause skin cancer cause premature aging of the skin, and the actors and actresses know they will be ineligible for parts if they look old.

What Can You Do to Protect Yourself?

- Avoid peak sun hours whenever possible. Peak hours are 10 A.M. to 2 P.M., or 11 A.M. to 3 P.M. during daylight saving time.
- Wear a wide-brimmed hat and other protective clothing if sun exposure will be prolonged or occur during peak hours.
- Be aware that sand, snow, water, and even concrete can reflect up to 85 percent of the sun's rays—so you are getting a double dose!
- Do not assume that a tan protects against the sun. It is a sign of skin damage. Keep using sunscreen to avoid further damage.
- Keep babies under six months old out of direct exposure to the sun; their delicate skin is especially vulnerable to damage.
- Remember that it is never too late to be careful. Adults who stay out of the sun or use sun protection will reduce their risk of cancer and reverse existing skin damage; skin will become smoother, sunspots will begin to fade, and wrinkling will be less obvious.
- Examine yourself monthly for any changes in your skin, especially a mole or beauty mark, and make sure that a physician looks at any spot that has changed in color, texture, or size.
- Research about the benefits and possible side effects of sunscreen is still being done. Proponents of sunscreen advise liberal application 20 minutes before going into the sun, and they suggest that you use about one ounce per whole body application, that the sunscreen have a sun protection factor (SPF) of 15 or greater, and that if you live in the Sunbelt, use a sunscreen daily, year-round.

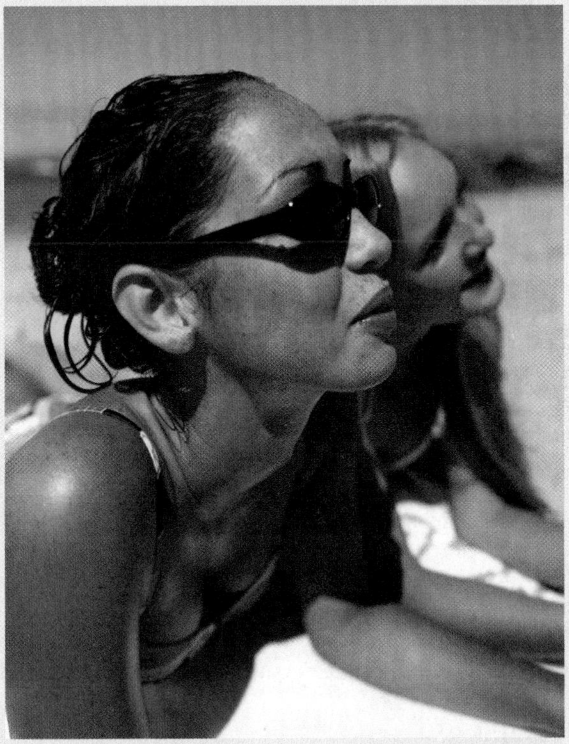

The sun is the leading cause of cancer in the United States. Don't bask in the sun, and when you go out wear a wide-brimmed hat and a sunscreen with a sun protection factor (SPF) of at least 15.

colon, rectum, uterus, and other areas can significantly reduce cancer mortality.

A **Pap test** involves scraping and analyzing some cells from the cervix and is effective in reducing death from cancer of the cervix. The American Cancer Society

Pap test A test for identifying cervical cancer that involves scraping and analyzing cells from the cervix.

recommends that women who are or have been sexually active or have reached age eighteen should have an annual Pap test and pelvic examination. After three consecutive normal annual examinations, the test may be performed less frequently.

Mammography, which is a low-dose breast X ray, along with a clinical breast examination can reduce death due to breast cancer. Women should get a baseline mammogram at age thirty-five to have for comparison, have a new one every year or every other year from age forty to age forty-nine, and then one every year thereafter. Based on studies reported in 2002, the U.S. Preventive Services Task Force found "fair evidence" that screening every 12 to 23 months significantly reduces mortality from breast cancer. Other studies, however, question the benefit of regular mammograms.

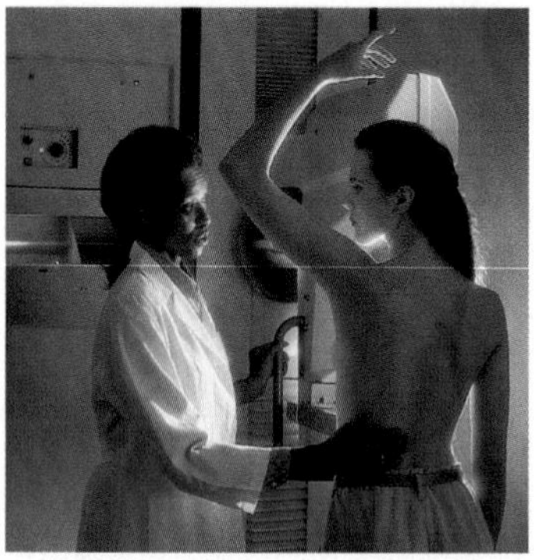

A mammogram—a low-dose breast X ray—and a clinical breast examination can detect breast cancer early and reduce death from this disease by 30 percent.

(*Source:* FPG International/© Jeff Kaufman)

A yearly **prostate-specific antigen (PSA) test** is recommended by the American Cancer Society for men over age fifty. A higher level of PSA in the blood can be a sign of prostate cancer. Men over age forty who have a family history of prostate cancer or who are African American should also have this test every year. The value of early detection of prostate cancer is controversial. Many prostate tumors are slow growing and no rigorous study has demonstrated that men who are treated early with surgery and radiation survive longer.

Self-Tests for Cancer

A free test, which is being done by a growing percentage of women, is **breast self-examination (BSE).** The American Cancer Society recommends that all women over age twenty do a BSE every month. Because BSE is not nearly as effective as mammography or examination by a physician, women are encouraged not to depend solely on it for early detection. See the Developing Health Skills box to learn how to do a breast self-exam.

Although testicular cancer is relatively rare—it accounts for only one percent of all cancers among men—the risk for dying from it can be reduced with a self-examination. Adult men—particularly young men—should conduct this **testicular self-examination** monthly. Testicular cancer is the most common form of cancer among men between the ages of twenty and thirty-five. This procedure is especially important for men who have a history of undescended testicles. A testicular examination by a trained physician is recommended as a routine part of all periodic health examinations. See the Developing Health Skills box to learn how to do a testicular self-exam.

To check for colon and rectum cancers, the American Cancer Society recommends a digital rectal examination every year after age forty, a stool blood test every year after age fifty, and sigmoidoscopy or colonoscopy every three to five years after age fifty. A digital rectal examination is also recommended each year for men over forty as a means of detecting prostate cancer. In sigmoidoscopy, a physician uses a hollow lighted tube to inspect the rectum and lower colon. In colonoscopy, the physician looks at the entire bowel, along with some portions of the small intestines.

In addition, a cancer-related checkup is recommended every three years for people twenty to forty years of age and every year after age forty. This checkup includes looking for cancer of the thyroid, mouth, skin, lymph nodes, testes, prostate, and ovaries. Your physician should also review good health habits, including tips on eating a healthy diet, quitting smoking, and other lifestyle choices that relate to cancer. This is because an unhealthy lifestyle is the cause of two thirds of all cancers. Your dentist, too, should check regularly for signs of oral cancer, most of which are associated with smoking and smokeless tobacco.

You should be aware of any changes in your own body and be alert to the American Cancer Society's seven caution signals:

- **C**hange in bowel or bladder habits
- **A** sore that does not heal
- **U**nusual bleeding or discharge
- **T**hickening or lump in breast or elsewhere
- **I**ndigestion or difficulty in swallowing
- **O**bvious change in wart or mole
- **N**agging cough or hoarseness

The American Cancer Society recommends that you see your physician if you have any of these warning signals.

prostate-specific antigen (PSA) test A blood test that can identify signs of prostate cancer.

breast self-examination (BSE) An examination done by a woman to herself to identify abnormal breast tissue; a screening exam for the presence of breast cancer.

testicular self-examination An examination done by a man to himself to identify abnormal testicular tissue; a screening exam for the presence of testicular cancer.

Developing Health Skills

How to Perform a Breast Self-Exam

The best time to do breast self-exam is right after your period, when breasts are not tender or swollen. If you do not have regular periods or sometimes skip a month, do it on the same day every month. Use the following procedure to perform your breast self-exam.

1. Lie down with a pillow under your right shoulder and place your right arm behind your head.
2. Use the finger pads of the three middle fingers on your left hand to feel for lumps in the right breast. Your finger pads are the top third of each finger.
3. Press firmly enough to know how your breast feels. A firm ridge in the lower curve of each breast is normal. If you're not sure how hard to press, ask your health care provider, or try to copy the way your health care provider uses the finger pads during a breast exam.

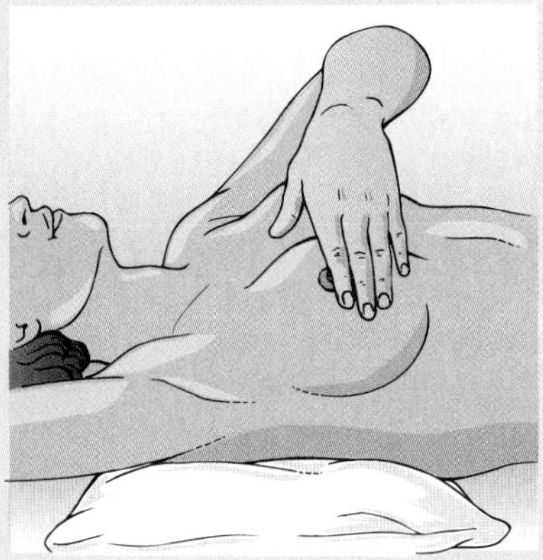

4. Move around the breast in a set way. You can choose either the up and down line, the circular pattern, or the wedge pattern. Do it the same way every time. It will help you to make sure that you've gone over the entire breast area, and to remember how your breast feels.

BSE Patterns

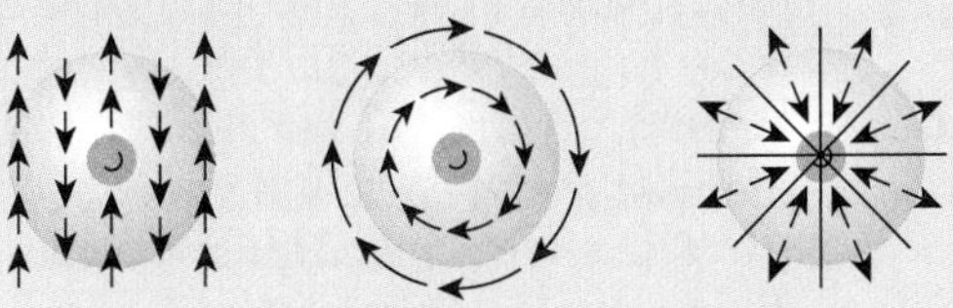

5. Now examine your left breast using the finger pads of your right hand. (Move the pillow to under your left shoulder.) If you find any changes, see your doctor right away.

For added safety, you should also visually check your breasts while standing in front of a mirror right after you do your breast self-exam each month. See if there are any changes in the way your breasts look: dimpling of the skin, changes in the nipple, or redness or swelling.

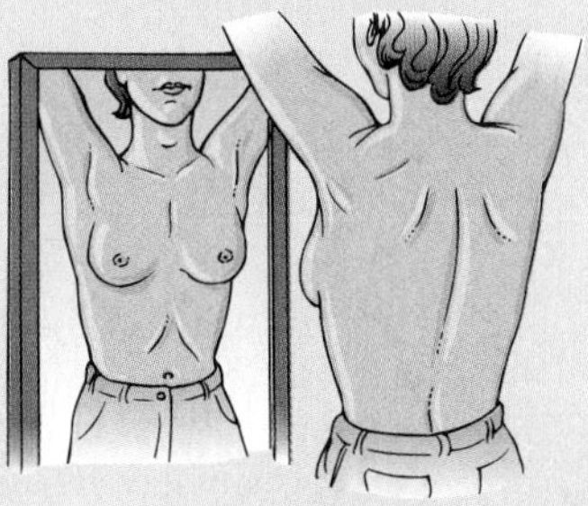

You might also want to do a breast self-exam while you're in the shower. Raise one arm above your head and press firmly in your preferred pattern. Then raise the other arm, and check your other breast. Your soapy hands will glide over wet skin, making it easy to check how your breasts feel.

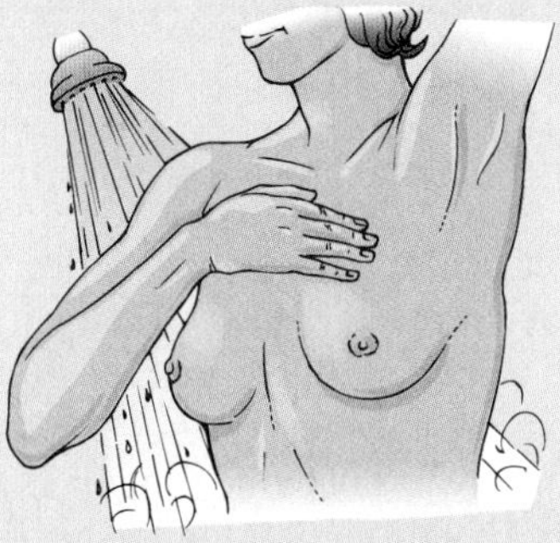

Source: Reprinted by the permission of the American Cancer Society, Inc.

Benefits and Risks of Treatment

Surgery, radiation, and chemotherapy are the principal forms of cancer treatment. Although each carries risks, the benefits—as documented in survival rates—more often outweigh them.

The primary treatment for cancer is surgical removal of the malignant growth. This is particularly effective when the cancer has not metastasized. Over the years, surgical techniques have improved so that removal causes less bodily disfigurement. For example, in 1970, most mastectomies done in the United States involved

Developing Health Skills

How to Perform a Testicular Self-Exam

The best time to do a testicular self-exam is during or after a shower or bath, when the skin of the scrotum is relaxed and the testicles descend. Some doctors recommend that all men do this once a month. Use the following procedure to perform your testicular self-exam.

Stand in front of a mirror and hold the penis out of the way. Check for any swelling.

Examine each testicle with both hands. Hold the testicle between the thumbs and index and middle fingers, and roll it gently between the fingers.

Look and feel for any hard lumps or nodules (smooth rounded masses) or any change in the size, shape, or consistency of the testes. Cancerous lumps usually are found on the sides of the testicle, but they can show up on the front.

You will also feel a soft tubelike structure behind the testicle. This is the epididymis, which contains the blood vessels, tissues, and tubes that conduct sperm. If you know what this feels like, you won't mistake it for a suspicious lump. Lumps on the epididymis are not cancerous.

If you feel a lump—or if you have any doubts—consult your doctor immediately.

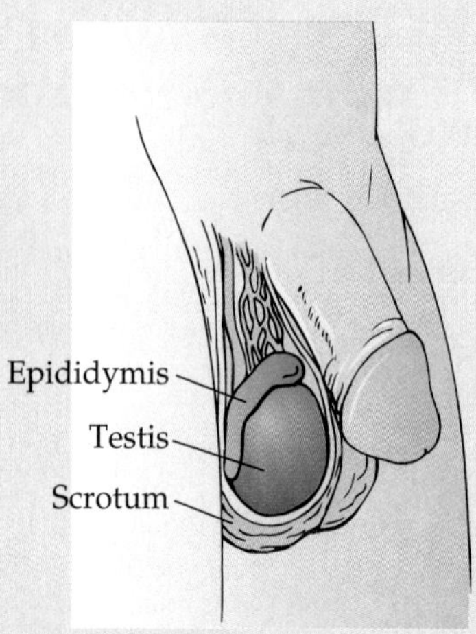

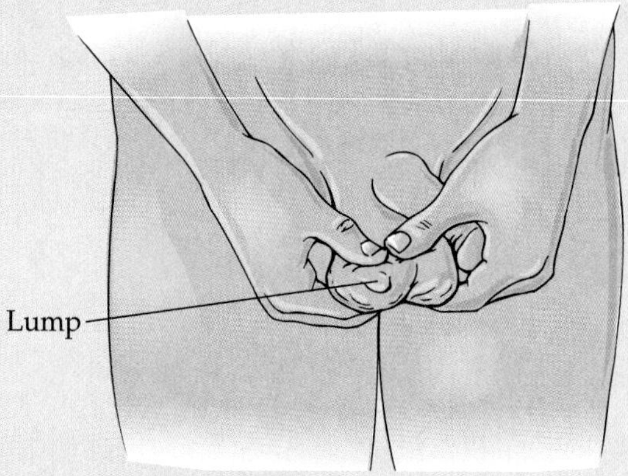

the complete removal of the breast and the surrounding tissue, particularly the lymph nodes. This is called a **radical mastectomy.** Today, such radical surgery is very seldom done. Alternatives include **lumpectomy,** a procedure that involves removal of the cancerous lump only; **partial mastectomy,** which involves removal of only the part of the breast containing the lump; and **modified radical mastectomy,** which involves selective removal of the breast and surrounding tissue.

For some kinds of cancer—notably cancers of the blood and lymph system—radiation and chemotherapy are the primary forms of treatment. With those treatments, the survival rates for patients who have the lymph node cancer known as Hodgkin's disease are around 83 percent. Men who have prostate cancer often choose radiation as the primary therapy because traditional prostate surgery can cause impotence.

For most other cancers, radiation and chemotherapy are used following surgery to prevent metastases, shrink growths that cannot be removed, and relieve pain. The side effects of radiation and chemotherapy are both dangerous and dramatic and may include anemia, severe nausea, uncontrollable infections, and baldness. In each case, the benefits of treatment, as documented in survival rates, need to be weighed against the risks and the resulting quality of life.

There are, in addition, alternative cancer treatments, most of which have proven to be ineffective. Alternative treatments include megavitamins, shark cartilage, and macrobiotic diets. These treatments may provide a ray of hope to the otherwise hopeless cancer patient, but a recent study by Harvard Medical School researchers found that these treatments had no effectiveness in delaying the effects of the disease, relief from the symptoms of cancer or treatments for it, and overall survival. Traditional medicine remains greatly concerned that patients who avail themselves of such

radical mastectomy The complete surgical removal of the breast and surrounding tissue, particularly the lymph nodes.

lumpectomy The surgical removal of only the cancerous lump from the breast.

partial mastectomy The surgical removal of only the part of the breast containing the cancerous lump.

modified radical mastectomy A selective removal of the breast and surrounding tissue.

ineffective approaches run the risk for greater suffering and may miss opportunities for treatment that could prolong life.

One form of alternative cancer treatment the Harvard researchers found to be beneficial is mind-body therapy, such as relaxation training, yoga, support groups and similar interventions that ease the stress of living with cancer. The field of mind-body therapy is officially called **psychoneuroimmunology**—*psycho* for the mind and emotions, *neuro* for the brain and central nervous system, and *immunology* for the body's natural defense against abnormal cells or external invaders such as bacteria or viruses. This chapter discusses mind–body treatments for cancer. Chapter 11 discusses their use in treating patients with infectious diseases.

In one study of people treated for the early stages of colon cancer or malignant melanoma whose cancers were in remission, thirty patients received an eight-week course in relaxation and cognitive therapy, a technique that focuses on changing a person's self-defeating beliefs. Researchers found that patients who took the course had more active natural killer cells, which protect the body against tumor growth, than did patients who did not take the course.

Another example of a mind–body treatment for cancer is imagery. Clinical studies show that cancer patients can reduce their level of pain through imagery—for example, thinking of something pleasant. This helps promote relaxation, which, in turn, can ease the pain. A more controversial use of imaging is to shrink a cancer by focusing the mind on an image of it being attacked by the body and visualizing the cancer getting smaller. To learn more about mind–body treatments and cancer, see the Cultural View box.

The Harvard study of alternative cancer therapies also endorsed moderate exercise, soy supplementation for prostate cancer, and acupuncture for chemotherapy-related nausea and vomiting.

Other Chronic Conditions

Type 2 Diabetes

More than seven million Americans have diabetes and the incidence rate for this chronic disease is rising at an alarming pace. **Type 2 diabetes** is the most common form of diabetes. It has sometimes been called adult-onset diabetes because most cases are diagnosed in adulthood. Some children, however, are diagnosed with Type 2 diabetes.

Type 2 diabetes has two possible causes: (1) either the body's cells ignore **insulin** that is produced (insulin resistance) or (2) the body does not produce enough insulin. Insulin is a substance produced by the pancreas that helps move glucose from the blood into the cells. Type 2 diabetes usually begins as insulin resistance. Then, as the need for insulin rises, the pancreas gradually loses its ability to produce insulin leading to an undersupply of insulin. If the body does not produce enough insulin, the body's cells may be starved for energy and, thus, fail to function. This condition, along with a build-up of glucose in the blood, may result in damage to the eyes, kidneys, nerves, or heart.

With a good treatment plan, however, a person with diabetes can maintain blood sugar levels within a normal range. Treatment includes careful meal planning, exercise, weight loss, and, when necessary, either diabetes pills, insulin shots, or both.

Asthma

Asthma is a serious, chronic lung disease characterized by wheezing, shortness of breath, chest tightness and coughing. Since about 1980, the prevalence of asthma has increased substantially, especially among children. Recent studies suggest that exposure to dust mites, cockroaches, mold, pet dander, tobacco smoke, and other biological and chemical pollutants influences the occurrence and severity of asthma.

Asthma is treated according to the severity of the disease and the persistence of symptoms. Long-term medications are used to control asthma and to limit the underlying airway inflammation that contributes to asthma attacks. Quick-relief medications such as inhalers are used to treat acute symptoms and to prevent exercise-induced asthma. Since there is no cure for asthma, the goal of asthma therapy is to successfully manage the disease. With proper management and care, a person with asthma can live a long, healthy life with few symptoms.

Dental Disease

Fortunately, the most prevalent of the chronic diseases affecting both children and adults is not life threaten-

psychoneuroimmunology A mind–body approach to treatment. It involves the mind and emotions (psycho), the brain and central nervous system (neuro), and the body's natural defense system (immunology).

type 2 diabetes The most common form of diabetes; also called adult-onset diabetes.

insulin A substance produced by the pancreas that helps move glucose from the blood into cells; without enough insulin, the body's cells do not function properly.

asthma A chronic lung disease characterized by wheezing, shortness of breath, chest tightness, and coughing.

Cultural View

Mind–Body Treatments for Chronic Conditions

Mainstream medicine is increasingly accepting some of the principles of mind–body treatment. Side by side with chemotherapy and radical surgery to remove tumors, doctors are "prescribing" meditation and mental exercises to breathe in good healthy air and exhale bad cancer cells. "The people who do the best are the people who say to themselves, 'I am going to beat this thing,'" says a California breast cancer patient who meditates, prays, and attends support groups.

Each year at just one Kaiser hospital in Sacramento, California, about eight hundred cancer and other patients listen to a tape while they are unconscious during surgery. What they hear is a soothing voice guiding their bodies through relaxation and then recovery. In addition to imagery, other techniques used in mind–body treatment include:

- Hypnosis: During a state that resembles sleep, the therapist can use the power of suggestion to help reduce perceptions of pain. Some studies show that hypnosis can prolong the lives of breast cancer patients; other studies do not confirm this.
- Meditation: Using this technique, a cancer patient can "breathe away" cancer, or "relax away" pain by relaxing all the muscles in the body, starting with the face and moving downward.
- Art therapy: Cancer patients use art therapy as a way to express themselves. The emotions that accompany a life-threatening disease such as cancer are sometimes difficult to express. Through art, however, a cancer patient can express emotions such as anger and fear without feeling that those expressions are a burden to his or her family, friends, and caregivers.
- Prayer: This is perhaps the oldest form of mind–body therapy. One study from a San Francisco hospital found that heart patients who knew they were being prayed for suffered fewer heart attacks and needed fewer drugs than did similar patients who were not being prayed for.

What is the science behind these treatments? Studies published in mainstream journals, including the *Journal of the American Medical Association* and the *Annals of Internal Medicine*, suggest that mind–body techniques reduce stress, which can hamper the response of the immune system. A more controversial theory considers mind–body techniques to be potent medicines in themselves. According to this theory, imagery, meditation, or prayer, for example, can trigger the body's endocrine or immune system to counterattack disease. Controlled clinical studies are under way to examine the effectiveness of several of the mind–body techniques being used.

So mind–body treatments may—or may not—cure cancer, but can they harm patients? Some doctors say yes. They are concerned that patients may rely more on their own healing powers and not seek traditional, proven treatments for cancer, such as chemotherapy.

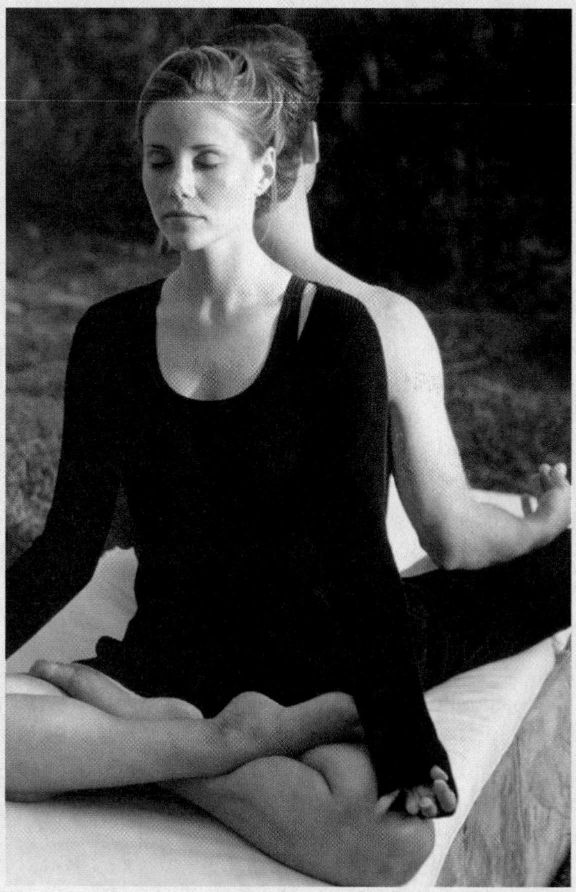

Mind–body treatments, which include meditation, can help patients boost their immune system.

ing, but it is often an overlooked source of discomfort, pain, and possible disfigurement: dental disease.

The two major families of dental disease are **dental caries,** or tooth decay, and **periodontal disease,** or gum disease. Tooth decay develops when the acids in plaque attack the teeth. **Dental plaque** is a colorless film of bac-

dental caries Tooth decay.

periodontal disease Gum disease.

dental plaque Noncalcified accumulation of microorganisms that attach to the teeth.

teria that forms on the teeth and gums. If not removed, dental plaque becomes concentrated colonies of bacteria. These colonies mix with sugars and starches to form acids that attack the enamel of the tooth, break it down, and lead to a cavity—a single location of decay in a tooth.

Plaque affects the gums as well, causing them to become red, tender, and swollen. This is called **gingivitis,** and it is the first stage of periodontal disease. If left untreated, periodontal disease can result in a degeneration of the gum tissue that holds the teeth in place. This is called **periodontitis,** or pyorrhea. Although this usually begins as a painless condition, it can result over time in painful loss of the supporting bone and ultimately in loss of teeth.

The good news about dental diseases is that they are preventable with routine brushing and flossing and regular professional dental care.

Living with a Chronic Disease

When you ask people how they feel, most respond, "Fine, thank you." But for people who have a chronic disease, and especially for those who have a degenerative disease such as arthritis, life can be difficult. Chronically ill people may never regain the full level of health they enjoyed before the onset of their illnesses, and they may face a continuing loss of function and the constant threat of even more serious medical problems as their illnesses progress. As medical advances help people who have chronic diseases live longer, they are left with the human challenge of coping with their disability. This may affect not only the person who has the disease but also his or her family and friends.

Psychological Adjustment

One of the most difficult adjustments for someone who has a chronic disease to make is modifying the view of him- or herself from a healthy, fully abled person to one who is not fully able. Think of how sick you view yourself when you are fighting a bout of influenza or are weak from mononucleosis. Yet your role as a sick person is likely to last only a few weeks at most. For people who have chronic diseases, being sick or in pain becomes a lifelong state. There is assault on self-esteem, and a period of depression is not uncommon. In fact, psychiatrists find that depression—not the threat of another attack—is one of the most formidable problems in getting heart attack patients through convalescence and rehabilitation.

Realistic adjustments in lifestyle often need to be made at school or work to accommodate a chronic disease. A college student recently diagnosed as a diabetic, for example, might have to allow some extra time during the day for monitoring blood glucose or administering insulin. With the same diagnosis, someone who has an extremely strenuous job—a police officer or firefighter, for example—might need to consider some job or career modifications.

Similarly, leisure activities might change as a result of chronic disease. An avid rock climber newly diagnosed with diabetes may find at some point that rock climbing carries too high a risk for foot injury. (People who have diabetes are at high risk for serious foot injuries because the disease compromises the body's circulatory system.) A safer alternative for exercise might be swimming or riding a stationary bike.

As with other health conditions, positive steps can be taken. For example, cancer patients who believe that they have some control over their health status are less likely to experience severe depression than are patients who give up. In addition to using basic coping skills (see Chapter 3), there are specific things that researchers have identified that chronically ill patients and their families can do to help themselves cope with the illness:

- Learn as much as possible about the disease and treatment options.
- Accept and adjust to physical changes in the body.
- Learn how to express feelings about having the disease.
- Express a personal sense of empowerment and control, particularly as related to health care decisions.
- Seek out support groups and other resources in the community.
- Develop meaningful relationships with family, friends, and members of the health care team (physician, nurse, social worker, and others).
- Maintain a sense of hope.

Concluding Thoughts

The best medical advice concerning chronic diseases is to keep them in the proper perspective for your life. For the most part, they tend to act slowly and provide years of warning. Preventive measures—most particularly, not smoking and following a healthy diet—along with early detection and medical intervention have proven effective in the treatment and cure of many chronic diseases that only a few years ago were considered death sentences.

gingivitis A condition in which the gums are red, tender, and swollen.

periodontitis Degeneration of the gum tissue that holds the teeth in place; also called pyorrhea.

CASE STUDY 10: Coping with Chronic Disease

Louise was in a state of panic. She had discovered what she thought could be a lump in her left breast. But her breasts were lumpy, so she wasn't sure. She had read a lot about breast cancer in the newspaper and in women's magazines, and the thought of it made her very anxious.

As the months went by, Louise's anxiety increased, and unfortunately, so did the size of the tumor. Eventually, she could no longer deny its existence. She went to a physician who, after running the proper tests, confirmed Louise's worst fears—the tumor was malignant. Because she had waited until the tumor had grown larger, Louise needed more extensive surgery than she might have had if she had seen her physician when she first detected the lump. In addition, there was concern that the cancer may have spread. Louise had a partial mastectomy, a course of chemotherapy, and a breast reconstruction. Five years later, she remains cancer-free and is happy to be alive.

When Mariana felt a lump in her breast, she, too, was in a state of panic. But she channeled that panic into swift action. She made an appointment to see her physician the next day, and her physician immediately ordered a mammogram and an ultrasound. When the results indicated the lump was malignant, she directed Mariana to a breast cancer specialist.

After a series of tests, including biopsies, and a second opinion from another breast cancer specialist, Mariana underwent a lumpectomy. Her doctors were confident that the cancer had been detected and treated early enough to prevent it from spreading to other tissue. Mariana's mental and physical scarring were minimal, but five years later, she remains vigilant and faithfully examines her breasts every month.

In Your Opinion

Louise avoided treatment; Mariana sought it immediately. Even so, both are living five years later.

- What health habits should Louise and Mariana have been practicing to detect breast cancer?
- Given that both women survived their breast cancer, how important is early detection and treatment?
- What advice would you give to a man or woman who had detected a lump or otherwise suspected that he or she had cancer?
- Would you respond differently if that person had early signs of heart disease?

KEY CONCEPTS

1. A chronic disease is marked by long duration or frequent recurrence.
2. A large percentage of the population has chronic diseases or disabilities, and the proportion of people who have to limit their activities due to chronic illness is increasing.
3. Over the past fifteen years, the death rate from diseases of the heart and blood vessels has declined dramatically due in great part to better surgical techniques, improved drugs, more effective medical management, and a better understanding of the risk factors for heart disease.
4. Smoking is the single most important risk factor associated with heart disease. Smokers have a 70 percent greater risk than nonsmokers for dying of heart disease.
5. Hypertension is called the silent killer because it has few symptoms but can lead to heart attack, stroke, and heart and kidney failure.
6. Cancer is a group of more than a hundred diseases, all characterized by uncontrolled growth and spread of abnormal cells.
7. Benign tumors do not invade other cells or spread to other parts of the body. Malignant tumors spread to nearby tissues and organs, crowding out healthy cells and replacing them with cancer cells.
8. Mammography, a low-dose breast X ray, and clinical breast examination reduce death from breast cancer by 30 percent.
9. The most prevalent chronic diseases are dental caries and periodontal disease—both preventable with brushing, flossing, and regular professional dental care.
10. Coping with a chronic illness includes making realistic adjustments in your lifestyle.

REVIEW QUESTIONS

1. Compare and contrast chronic illness and infectious illness.

2. List lifestyle choices that lead to chronic illness. List lifestyle choices that reduce the risk for chronic illness.
3. Describe controllable risk factors associated with cardiovascular disease. Describe noncontrollable risk factors that increase the potential for cardiovascular disease.
4. Identify the symptoms and treatment modalities for atherosclerosis, myocardial infarction, angina pectoris, arrhythmia, stroke, transient ischemic attacks, and hypertension.
5. Describe controllable risk factors associated with cancer. Describe noncontrollable risk factors that increase the potential for cancer.
6. Identify the symptoms and treatment modalities for lung cancer, breast cancer, prostate cancer, colon and rectum cancer, and skin cancer.
7. Explain the importance of early detection of cancer and name several screening procedures that can lead to early detection.
8. Explain the importance of good dental hygiene as a means of reducing the risk for dental disease.
9. List similarities and differences between cardiovascular disease, cancer, diabetes, asthma, and dental disease.
10. List specific strategies for coping with chronic illness and describe how you would help someone implement these strategies.

CRITICAL THINKING QUESTIONS

1. Two reasons cited for the rising mortality due to chronic disease are (1) medicine's success in dealing with infectious diseases and (2) medicine's success in extending life expectancy. Therefore, it could be said that successful medical intervention does not prevent death; it just changes the causes of death. Suppose cures for cardiovascular disease and cancer were discovered. What chronic disorder might then emerge as the next leading cause of death?
2. The *Healthy People 2010* objectives include the following: "Increase the proportion of adults who have had their blood cholesterol checked within the preceding 5 years." The relationship between high cholesterol and cardiovascular disease is well established, yet most Americans don't even know their blood cholesterol level. How might this situation be changed? Do you think the entire U.S. population should be required to have cholesterol screening? Would such an extensive program be cost-effective?
3. The *Healthy People 2010* objectives include the following: "Increase the proportion of persons who use at least one of the following protective measures that may reduce the risk of skin cancer: avoid the sun between 10 A.M. and 4 P.M., wear sun-protective clothing when exposed to sunlight, use sunscreen with a sun protective factor (SPF) of 15 or higher, and avoid artificial sources of ultraviolet light." Currently, only about 30 percent of the U.S. population take such precautions. Given the clear evidence that associates sun exposure with cancer, why do you think so few Americans use sunscreens and protective clothing? If it took more than forty years to change public opinion about the hazards of smoking, how long do you think it will take to change public opinion about sun exposure?
4. The most common chronic disease is not heart disease, cancer, or diabetes. It is dental disease. Even though dental disease does not cause death, it is similar in some ways to the major killers of our time. How is dental caries similar to heart disease and cancer? How is it different? What prevention strategies are effective in reducing the occurrence of all three?

JOURNAL ACTIVITIES

1. Carefully review your family's health history, going back as far as you can to grandparents and great-grandparents and including blood relatives such as aunts and uncles. Document risk factors for chronic diseases that you think might affect you. For example, is there a pattern of heart disease, breast cancer, or diabetes in your family? Given this information, what can you do to reduce your risks of developing a chronic disease?
2. Think about someone you know who has a chronic disease. This might be a classmate your age, an older relative, or a professor nearing retirement. Write down your feelings about this person and how he or she copes with the disease. How do you think you would handle living with a chronic illness?
3. Observe people in your community and try to identify those at risk for heart disease. A good place for watching might be a fast-food restaurant. Notice what people eat, whether they put salt on their food, whether they smoke and whether they have other noticeable risk factors. Do your habits mirror theirs?
4. Survey twenty students about their dental care. Ask how often they brush and floss their teeth, and when they last went to a dentist. Do you expect to find that college-age men and women take good—or poor—care of their teeth? Compare your expectations with your findings.

SELECTED BIBLIOGRAPHY

A Breast Cancer Journey: Your Personal Guidebook from the Experts at the American Cancer Society. Atlanta, GA: American Cancer Society, 2001.

The Burden of Chronic Diseases and Their Risk Factors. Atlanta, GA: Centers for Disease Control and Prevention, National Center for Chronic Disease Prevention and Health Promotion, 2002.

Burt, V., et al. "Prevalence of Hypertension in the U.S. Adult Population." *Hypertension* 25 (1995): 305–313.

Cancer Facts and Figures. Atlanta, GA: American Cancer Society (updated annually).

Heart and Stroke Statistical Update. Dallas, TX: American Heart Association (updated annually).

Hoffman, C., et al. "Persons with Chronic Conditions: Their Prevalence and Costs." *Journal of the American Medical Association* 276, no. 18 (1996): 1473–1479.

Lenfant, C. *Benefits of Exercise and Lifestyle Modification.* Rockville, MD: National Heart, Lung, and Blood Institute, August, 2000.

Peeters, A., et. al. "A Cardiovascular Life History: A Life-Course Analysis of the Original Framingham Heart Study Cohort." *European Heart Journal* 23, no. 6 (2002): 458–466.

Unrealized Prevention Opportunities: Reducing the Health and Economic Burden of Chronic Disease. Atlanta, GA: Centers for Disease Control and Prevention, National Center for Chronic Disease Prevention and Health Promotion, 2000.

Wilson, S., and Poulter, N. "Cardiovascular Risk: Its Assessment in Clinical Practice." *British Journal of Biomedical Science* 58, no. 4 (2001): 248–251.

HEALTHLINKS

Websites for Reducing the Risk of Chronic Diseases

You can access better health as it relates to this chapter by checking out some of the following sites on the Internet. These sites can be accessed directly from the *Decisions for Healthy Living* Website located at www.aw.com/pruitt.

CDC National Center for Chronic Disease Prevention and Health Promotion

The home page for the division of the Centers for Disease Control and Prevention dedicated to the prevention of chronic diseases and maternal and infant health. Access the latest information on cancer, cardiovascular disease, diabetes, oral diseases and conditions, and other serious chronic diseases and conditions and discover what is and can be done to prevent these disorders.

American Dental Association

A link with the leading private organization dedicated to dental health, containing pertinent information on research and clinical issues.

American Cancer Society

The leading private organization dedicated to cancer prevention, including information, statistics, and resources regarding cancer.

American Diabetes Association

Home page for the leading private organization on diabetes including patient and education information.

American Heart Association

The leading private organization dedicated to heart health, providing statistical data, and resources regarding cardiovascular care.

Asthma and Allergy Foundation of America

Home page for the leading private site for educational and clinical information on asthma and allergies, and links to other resources.

National Cancer Institute

Information about cancer diagnosis, treatment, and prevention, as well as trends related to the disease.

National Heart, Lung, and Blood Institute

Information about cardiovascular disease, lung and blood disorders, as well as the latest information on the Women's Health Initiative.

National Institute of Neurological Disorders and Stroke

Information about stroke and neurological disorders as well as trends related to them.

HEALTH HOTLINES

Reducing the Risk for Chronic Disease

American Cancer Society
(800) ACS-2345 (227-2345)
National Office
1599 Clifton Road NE
Atlanta, GA 30329

American Dental Association
(800) 621-8099
Public Information and Education
211 East Chicago Avenue
Chicago, IL 60611

American Diabetes Association
(800) 342-2383
1701 Beauregard Street
Alexandria, VA 22311

American Heart Association
(800) 242-8721
7272 Greenville Avenue
Dallas, TX 75231-4596

National Cancer Institute
Cancer Information Services
(800) 4-CANCER (422-6237)
6116 Executive Boulevard, MSC8322
Bethesda, MD 20892-8322

National Heart, Lung and Blood Institute
Education Programs Information Center
(800) 575-WELL (575-9355)
P.O. Box 30105
Bethesda, MD 20824-0105

National Institute of Neurological Disorders and Stroke
(800) 352-9424
P.O. Box 5801
Bethesda, MD 20892

TEST YOUR KNOWLEDGE ANSWERS

1. True. Heart disease takes such a toll that if it could be eliminated, life expectancy would increase by almost ten years.
2. False. The American Heart Association recommends that a baseline ECG be taken at age twenty, again at age forty to forty-five, and then only as suggested by other risk factors.
3. False. Benign tumors are not cancerous and cannot change into cancerous tumors. Thus, benign tumors cannot become malignant tumors. However, early detection of malignant tumors can help ensure that cancer is diagnosed at the earliest possible stage when there is the greatest chance of successful treatment.
4. True. Lung cancer rates among men are dropping because they are smoking less, but rates for women continue to rise.
5. False. Dental diseases are the most prevalent chronic diseases affecting both children and adults.

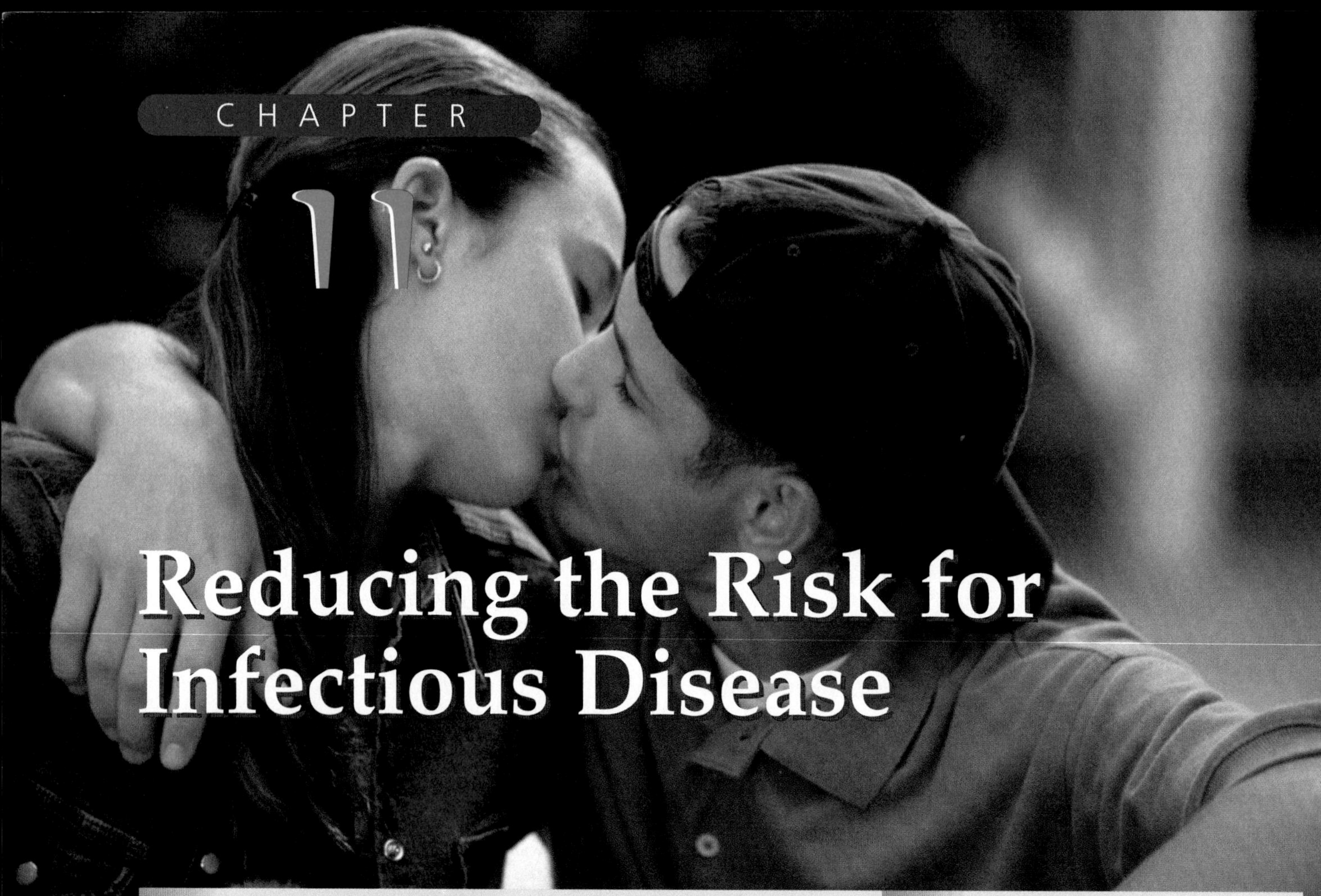

CHAPTER 11

Reducing the Risk for Infectious Disease

OBJECTIVES

When you finish reading this chapter, you will be able to:

1. Describe how infectious diseases spread from one person to another.
2. Understand the body's defenses against infections, including nonspecific and specific defense mechanisms.
3. Understand immunity and its function in the maintenance of good health.
4. Describe the progress of a disease once infection has occurred.
5. Differentiate between common infectious diseases and sexually transmitted infections (STIs).
6. Describe the significance of asymptomatic carriers to the overall STI epidemic.
7. List primary prevention measures that reduce the potential for contracting an STI.
8. Identify common infectious diseases and common STIs, and briefly describe the symptoms of each.
9. Explain why new infectious diseases appear to be emerging despite progress in the development of antibiotics and other therapies.
10. Suggest actions that an individual can take to reduce the risk for acquiring an infectious disease.

TEST YOUR KNOWLEDGE

1. Breast-fed infants have passive immunity to a number of diseases because of the antibodies they get from their mother's milk. True or False?
2. An antibiotic is the recommended treatment for colds and influenza, both caused by viruses. True or False?
3. Gonorrhea occurs fifty times more often in the United States than in any other industrialized country. True or False?
4. The human papilloma virus is associated with 90 percent of the cases of cervical cancer diagnosed in the United States. True or False?
5. Most men who have gonorrhea are asymptomatic and do not know that they have the disease. Women almost always have symptoms, and therefore are very aware when they have the disease. True or False?

Answers found at end of chapter.

Infectious diseases are a part of human history. In fourteenth-century Europe, bubonic plague, carried by infected rats, killed millions of people and decimated entire cities. The plague still exists and there are occasional outbreaks, but with **antibiotic** treatments, deaths from it are rare. Smallpox, a highly contagious, disfiguring, and much feared disease, dates back at least to ancient Egypt, with evidence of the typical scarring preserved on mummies. It lasted as a major health threat until 1977, when a worldwide effort to eradicate the disease was declared a success. In recent years, smallpox has emerged as a disease of concern because it is a possible agent of bioterror, and some people in the United States are being vaccinated against the disease as a precaution.

Over the centuries, medical scientists have developed a better understanding of how infectious diseases are spread and how to control them. In spite of these advances, infectious diseases remain a public health concern in the United States. Smallpox is just one example. The occurrence of **sexually transmitted infections** (STIs), such as chlamydia and gonorrhea, continues to rise. New **infectious diseases** continue to be discovered and new cures sought. Medical researchers are still debating the causes of chronic fatigue syndrome, and the search goes on for an acquired immune deficiency syndrome (AIDS) vaccine. In addition, the very young and the elderly are at higher risk of getting infectious diseases and dying. So it is that with infectious diseases we celebrate some of our most important health victories and face some of our most important medical challenges. See Table 11.1 for trends in selected infectious diseases.

How Diseases Are Spread

An infectious disease, also known as a contagious or communicable disease, is the result of an agent, such as a bacteria or a virus, that spreads through a variety of ways from someone who is infected to someone who is not yet infected. **Noninfectious diseases,** in contrast, are not contagious. You cannot contract cancer, heart disease, or hypertension from someone else.

Chain of Infection

Several factors influence the spread of disease within a population. These factors are best understood as links in a chain, each critical to the process of disease transmission, yet none alone is capable of causing disease. The six factors that make up the **chain of infection** provide insight not only into the spread of infection but also into ways the spread can be halted. Figure 11.1 shows the chain of infection using tuberculosis as the example.

- The first link in the chain of infection is the causative agent, a microorganism that causes the disease. This microorganism is also called a **pathogen.** There are six traditionally identified groups of pathogens: bacteria, viruses, protozoa, parasitic worms, fungi, and rickettsias. In addition, many researchers believe that there is another disease-causing agent, called a prion.
- The second link is the **reservoir of the pathogen,** the place where it resides. The reservoir, or source, is either a human or an animal. When the pathogen lives in a human, that person usually shows signs of the disease. Sometimes, however, that person is a carrier; that is, he or she carries the disease but does not have any symptoms or show any signs of it.
- The next link in the chain is called the **portal of exit.** This is how the pathogen moves from the source to

antibiotic A chemical substance that destroys or inhibits the growth of bacteria.

sexually transmitted infections (STIs) Infectious diseases and syndromes that are spread primarily through sexual activity.

infectious disease A disease caused by pathogens, such as bacteria or viruses, that spread from someone who is infected to someone who is not yet infected; also known as communicable or contagious disease.

noninfectious disease A disease caused by factors other than infectious microbial agents.

chain of infection A metaphor for infectious disease transmission in which each link in the chain represents a single factor necessary for disease to spread.

pathogen A microorganism, such as a bacterium, virus, protozoan, parasitic worm, fungus, or rickettsia, that causes disease.

reservoir of the pathogen A place (either a human or an animal) where a pathogen resides.

portal of exit The means by which the pathogen moves out of the source into a new host.

Table 11.1 Infectious Disease Trends: Reported Cases in the United States, 1950–2000

Disease	1950	1960	1970	1980	1990	2000
Acquired immune deficiency syndrome (AIDS)	–	–	–	–	41,595	40,758
Chlamydia	NA	NA	NA	NA	323,663	702,093
Diphtheria	5,796	918	435	3	4	1
Gonorrhea	286,746	258,933	600,072	1,004,029	690,042	358,995
Hepatitis A	NA	NA	56,797	29,087	31,441	13,397
Hepatitis B	NA	NA	8,310	19,015	21,102	8,036
Hepatitis C	–	–	–	–	2,553	3,197
Legionnaires' disease	–	–	–	475	1,370	1,127
Malaria	–	72	3,051	2,062	1,292	1,560
Measles	NA	NA	47,351	3,124	27,786	86
Mumps	NA	NA	104,963	8,576	5,292	338
Pertussis (whooping cough)	120,718	14,809	4,249	1,730	4,570	7,867
Polio	33,300	2,525	31	8	7	0
Smallpox	Last documented case occurred in 1949					
Syphilis (primary and secondary)	217,558	122,538	91,382	68,832	135,043	31,575
Toxic shock syndrome (TSS)	–	–	–	–	322	135
Tuberculosis	121,742	55,494	37,137	27,749	25,701	16,377

NA: Not Available (not previously nationally notifiable)
Note: AIDS, hepatitis C, and TSS data reflect post-1980 discoveries of an infectious agent. Legionellosis (legionnaires' disease) data reflect post-1970 discovery of an infectious agent. Polio data reflect reported cases in the wild only (not vaccine-induced cases).

Source: U.S. Centers for Disease Control and Prevention

a new host. It can move by means of mucus, spit, blood, semen, feces, or in many other ways.

- The means of transmission represents the next link. There are five main means of transmission of a pathogen: the air, direct physical contact, contaminated food and water, **vectors** (insects or animals), and pathogens existing in the body in a controlled state.
- In order for infection to spread, the pathogen must find a new home. This link in the chain of infection is called entry into new host. The pathogen can enter by many of the routes through which it left the reservoir—blood, semen, mucus, or through cuts or other open areas of the body.
- Finally, for the chain of infection to continue, the pathogen has to find a hospitable host. This link is called **host susceptibility.** The presence of a pathogen in the body does not necessarily mean that a person has to get sick from it. When conditions are right, the pathogens multiply and produce disease in the new host.

vectors Insects or animals that carry disease.

host susceptibility The ease with which a person is exposed to and becomes infected by a pathogen.

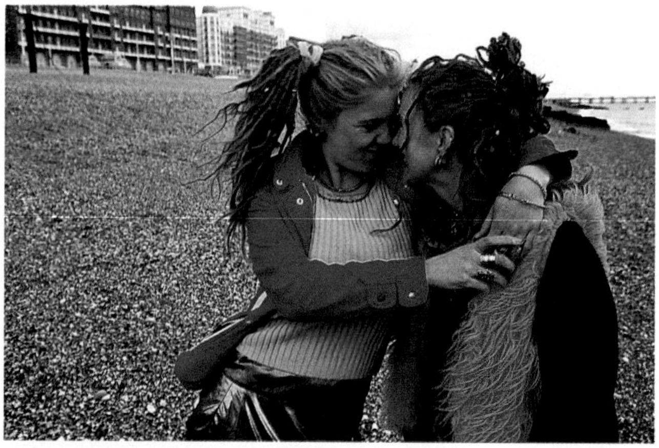

One of the links in spreading an infectious disease is when the infectious agent enters a new host. Body piercing can provide such an opportunity.

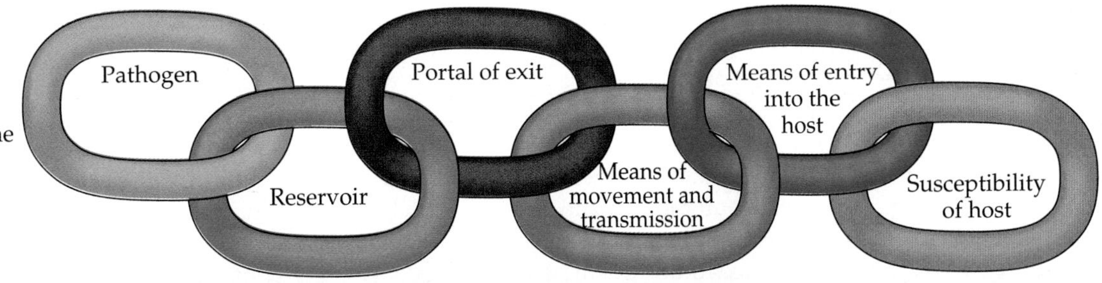

	Pathogen	Reservoir	Portal of exit	Means of movement and transmission	Means of entry into the host	Susceptibility of host
Description of the chain link:	The pathogen is *Mycobacterium tuberculosis.*	More than 16,000 cases of TB were reported in the U.S. in 2000.	The mouth and nose of an infected person carry droplets of moisture containing the pathogen.	TB is mainly transferred by droplets in the air.	Entry is usually via the lungs.	Individuals who have poor immunity and low resistance to infection.
Our best means of breaking the link in the chain of infection:		Test for the presence of the TB bacterium. Treat all individuals who test positive.	Cover mouth and nose when coughing or sneezing.	Avoid infected individuals.	Wear a mask.	Maintain overall health through diet, exercise, and plenty of rest.

Figure 11.1 **Chain of Infection**
Using tuberculosis as an example, the spread of infection can be stopped if any one of the links in this chain is broken or missing.

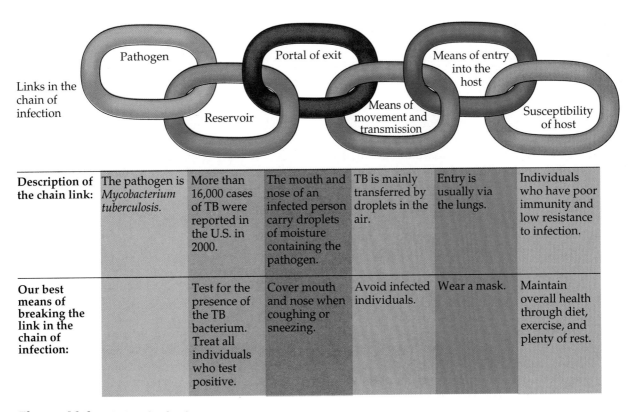

The chain of infection is a useful analogy for understanding how to prevent the spread of an infectious disease. Any link in the chain of infection represents a possible point of intervention. If any one of the links of the chain is broken or missing, the spread of infection can be stopped. For example, even before infectious diseases were fully understood, people used a method of quarantine to limit the spread of disease. By preventing uninfected persons from coming into contact with infected persons, the act of quarantine successfully cut the chain of infection by restricting the reservoir of the pathogen, one of the early links in the chain.

Most modern efforts at controlling infectious disease have been directed at breaking the last link in the chain, host susceptibility, through immunization. Scientists believe that through adequate immunization the pool of people who are susceptible to infection can be reduced and eventually eliminated. **Eradication** means that the first link in the chain, the pathogen, no longer exists in adequate amounts to cause disease. In the case of AIDS, vaccine research is still underway, so the focus of control is on the means of transmission—semen, vaginal secretions, and blood. By promoting abstinence, condom use for sexually active people, clean needles for injecting drug users, and a safe blood supply, the chain of infection can be broken.

Causes of Infection

Everything has to be caused by something, and infection is no different. There are six basic pathogens, or causative agents of infection.

Bacteria are single-celled microbes that act in a variety of ways to produce symptoms of infection. They produce **toxins,** or poisons, in the body. Although bacteria reproduce inside the body, they do so outside the human cell and thus can be killed or inhibited by antibiotics. Strep throat, tuberculosis, pneumonia, gonorrhea, cholera, and whooping cough are examples of infections caused by bacteria.

Viruses, chains of nucleic acid surrounded by a protein coat, are the most primitive form of life and cannot reproduce on their own. However, when they invade the

eradication The removal of a disease by the elimination of all reservoirs of the disease-causing pathogen.

bacteria Single-celled microbes that act to produce symptoms of infection.

toxin A poisonous substance produced by a microorganism; can cause certain infectious diseases.

virus A chain of nucleic acid surrounded by a protein coat that invades cells and uses the cells' reproductive capabilities.

human cell, they use the cell's reproductive capabilities. They are the tiniest and toughest of infectious pathogens. Antibiotics have no effect on viruses, and in most cases drugs that can kill them do not exist. Some physicians prescribe antibiotics for patients who have influenza to prevent **secondary infection,** but they have no effect on the flu itself. **Interferon,** a protective substance made by the body, is one of the main means of attacking viruses. Some viral infections have been successfully prevented with vaccines. Examples of infections caused by viruses include the common cold, influenza, measles, rabies, herpes, smallpox, and AIDS.

Protozoa are single-celled parasites that produce toxins and release enzymes that interrupt the body's ability to function normally. Protozoa-caused infections, such as malaria, sleeping sickness, and amoebic dysentery, are generally associated with a tropical environment and poor sanitation and are not a public health problem in the United States. The one major exception is giardiasis, which can be caught by drinking contaminated water. Hikers and travelers to countries where giardia is prevalent, such as Russia and other former Soviet bloc countries, are especially at risk for getting giardiasis. Protozoan infections can be treated with drugs.

As the name indicates, **parasitic worms** are multicelled animals usually shaped like flat or round worms. They release toxins inside the body and feed off blood and compete for food with the host. As a result, people infected with worms, for example, tapeworms, are often anemic and malnourished. Most worm infections can be treated successfully with drugs and can often be prevented with good hygiene and proper cooking of food. Trichinosis is an example of a parasitic infection caused by not cooking pork thoroughly.

Fungi are either single-celled or multicelled plant-like organisms that usually grow on the surface of the skin. They release enzymes that in turn digest cells. Antifungal topical ointments and drugs can kill fungi. Athlete's foot is an example of an infection caused by a fungus. Fungi are also **allergens** and in some parts of the country cause considerable discomfort.

A microorganism that is often described as somewhere between viruses and bacteria is **rickettsia.** It is much larger than a virus and is parasitic in nature (it requires living cells for growth). It is treated with antibiotics. Rickettsias are usually transmitted by insects, such as ticks. Common rickettsial diseases are Rocky Mountain spotted fever and typhus.

Prions are made of protein and do not contain any genes or genetic material. This feature distinguishes them from the other kinds of infectious agents discussed above. It is believed that these nonliving proteins can reproduce themselves, and thereby spread disease. Prions reside naturally in the brain cells of people and animals and normally do no harm. When they mutate into an abnormal shape, however, they change the surrounding prions into defective three-dimensional forms as well. These newly shaped prions multiply throughout the brain like a spreading infection, and pockets of the affected brain tissue gradually die. There is strong evidence that diseases characterized by poor muscle coordination and memory loss, such as mad cow disease and Creutzfeldt-Jakob disease, are caused by prions.

secondary infection An infection that occurs in conjunction with, or as a result of, another infection but which arises from a different pathogen.

interferon A chemical substance produced by white blood cells that "interferes" with growth of a virus and also inhibits the virus's ability to infect cells; also made synthetically.

protozoa Single-celled parasites that produce toxins and release enzymes that interrupt the body's ability to function normally.

parasitic worms Multicelled animals that release toxins inside the body, feed on blood, and compete with the host for food.

fungi Single-celled or multicelled plant-like organisms that usually grow on the surface of the skin.

allergen A substance that is perceived by the body as an irritant and induces an allergic reaction or hypersensitive state.

rickettsia A rod-shaped microorganism that is transmitted by vectors and causes a variety of diseases, such as typhus.

prion A mutated, three-dimensional protein that changes the shape of surrounding prions, causing pockets of diseased and dying brain cells.

How Infections Get into Your Body

When an infected person coughs or sneezes, microorganisms may be carried *through the air* on droplets of moisture and breathed in by another individual. Mumps, measles, and chickenpox are spread through the air. Until recently, it was thought that this was the primary means of spreading colds and influenza, but research now shows that they spread more *through direct physical contact,* such as through shaking hands, hugging, and kissing. Cold viruses can also be transmitted from inanimate objects through direct physical contact, for example, from a glass used by a person who has a cold. Examples of other infectious diseases carried through direct physical contact include STIs and leprosy.

Another means of transmission is *by contaminated food and water*. Hookworm can come from eating contaminated food, and giardiasis and cholera from drinking or swimming in contaminated water. Still other diseases are carried by *vectors* (insects or animals that carry diseases). Plague is carried by fleas that live on rats, malaria is carried by mosquitoes, and Lyme disease is carried by deer ticks.

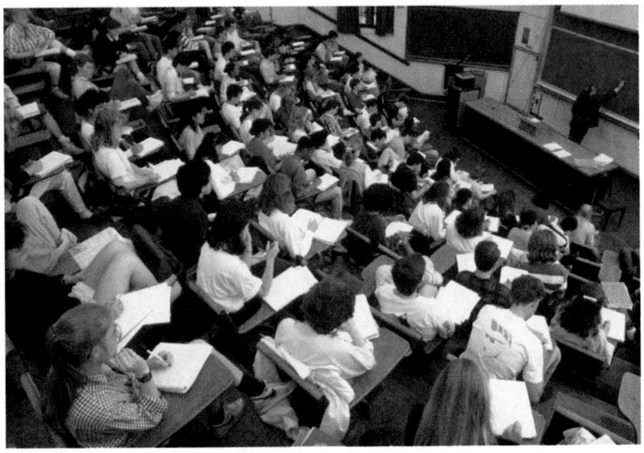

Infectious agents that can cause illnesses such as mumps and measles are spread through the air. This is why some diseases can quickly spread around a college campus.

Some diseases are not carried at all; they are simply *already there,* living in a controlled state within a person's body. That person develops symptoms of disease only when something upsets the body's normal state, which allows the infecting organism to begin reproducing. For example, women normally have yeast growing in their vaginas. Taking antibiotics, however, can change the environment of the vagina so that yeast growth takes place at a greater-than-normal pace, which in turn can result in yeast infection.

Why Doesn't Everyone Get Sick?

Not everyone gets sick when exposed to a disease-causing pathogen. This is because the conditions associated with getting sick can vary widely. First, the **virulence,** or strength, of the causative agent may vary even among pathogens causing the same disease. You might be exposed to a highly virulent strain of a virus, for example, while your neighbor is exposed to a weaker strain of the same virus. You would most likely show symptoms, but your neighbor might never know he or she had been exposed to an infectious disease.

Second, **dosages**—the amount of pathogens present during disease transmission—can vary widely. Your roommate might be exposed to a large dosage of the bacterium that causes strep throat, perhaps from kissing a person who is infected. Another classmate might be exposed to only a small dosage, perhaps from breathing the droplets of moisture exhaled by an infected person. Your roommate is more likely to become infected.

Finally, the **resistance** of individuals to infection varies. Resistance is the capacity of the immune system to handle the invasion of an organism. Some people have a strong resistance to disease; others have a low resistance. People who have a high resistance to disease are less likely to get sick even when exposed to infections. No one, however, goes through life infection-free, and even the hardiest of people have bouts of illness over a lifetime.

Nonspecific Lines of Defense

Given that we are constantly surrounded by disease-causing organisms, our bodies have developed highly successful ways to prevent pathogens from entering the body, and, in the event that they do, to prevent them from causing illness. **Nonspecific defense mechanisms** include the skin, the mucous membranes, cilia, and general chemical defense mechanisms such as interferon. The skin, for example, serves as a mechanical barrier as long as it remains intact. The **mucous membranes** that line most of the passageways leading into the body trap foreign material in their sticky secretions. And the cilia of the mucous membranes in the upper respiratory tract sweep impurities out of the body.

Body secretions, such as digestive juices and tears, may contain acids or enzymes that destroy invading organisms. Finally, certain reflexes aid in preventing foreign matter, including microorganisms, from entering the body; sneezing, vomiting, and diarrhea are reflexes that expel pathogens.

If a pathogen successfully passes these physical barriers, it will encounter one of the nonspecific defense mechanisms: **phagocytes,** interferon, and **inflammation.** Phagocytes are white blood cells that attack foreign invaders such as bacteria. For example, when an injury occurs, such as a cut in the skin, phagocytes are attracted to the area, where they surround invading bacterial cells and render them harmless. As the phagocytes do their work, large numbers of them are destroyed, so eventually the area around the cut becomes filled with dead white blood cells, a substance often referred to as pus.

virulence The strength of pathogens present during disease transmission.

dosage A specified amount of something; in infectious diseases, the amount of pathogens present during disease transmission.

resistance The capacity of the immune system to fight the invasion of an organism.

nonspecific defense mechanisms The body's various barriers to most disease, as opposed to those defense mechanisms intended to prevent one particular disease.

mucous membranes The moist, protective lining that covers most of the openings to the body and the air passages.

phagocytes White blood cells that attack and consume foreign cells.

inflammation The body's response to injury; it fights infection and promotes healing.

Interferon is a chemical substance produced by white cells that "interferes" with the growth of a virus and inhibits the viruses' ability to infect cells. Interferon works against all viruses, so it is considered a nonspecific defense mechanism. Synthetic versions of interferon, made by genetic engineering, have been used to treat viral infections and some types of cancer.

Throughout the time that phagocytes and interferon are fighting infection, inflammation occurs. Inflammation is the heat, redness, swelling, and discomfort that results from increased blood flow and secretions of histamine and other substances in the infected tissue. Often, inflammation is the first symptom of infection.

Specific Lines of Defense

Immunity is the most complex, most specific, and final line of defense against disease. Whereas the defenses against disease we have presented thus far are nonspecific (they act to prevent or reduce the harm of all invaders), immunity is specific not only to each disease, but also to each strain of organism that causes disease.

Active and passive immunity. Immunity is the body's ability to destroy pathogens that it has encountered in the past, before they are able to cause disease. It makes the body resistant to a particular organism that produces infection. There are two kinds of immunity: active and passive. In **active immunity,** the body develops its own resistance to disease. For example, once you've had measles, your body develops a lifelong immunity to the disease. In **passive immunity,** resistance to disease initially comes from an external source. Infants who are breast-fed carry passive immunity to certain diseases because they receive protective antibodies from their mothers' milk. This immunity usually lasts only about as long as the mother breast-feeds.

The key factor in both active and passive immunity is the presence of antibodies. **Antibodies** are specific proteins that are produced principally in the blood in response to foreign substances—called **antigens** (for antibody generators)—in the body. The antibodies react specifically with the antigen that produced them. Returning to the example of measles, if you are infected with the measles virus, your body first recognizes the measles antigen, then begins to produce antibodies unique to the measles virus. If you are exposed to measles a year later, the antibodies already in your blood protect you from getting the disease.

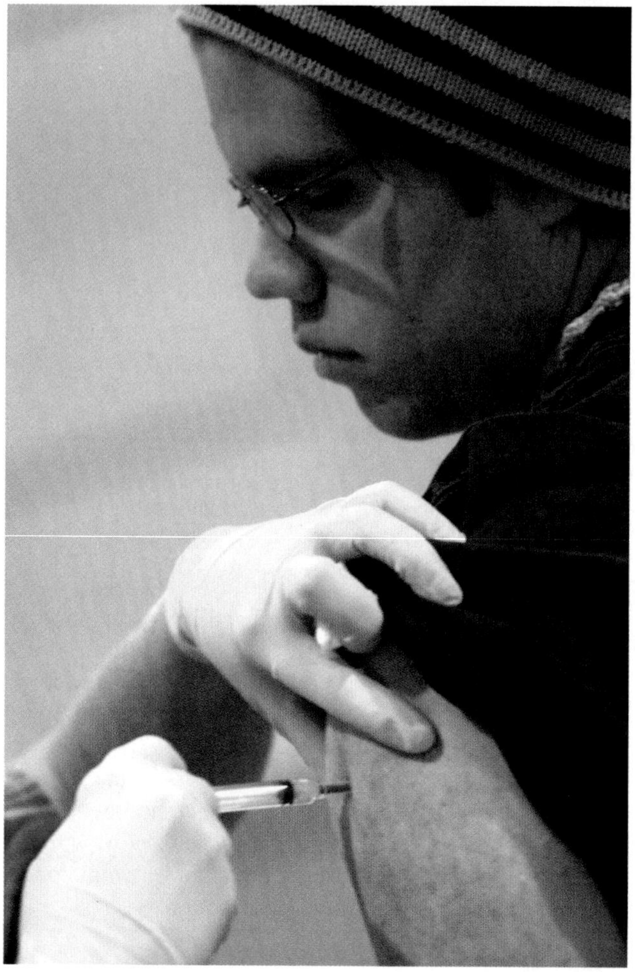

To make sure your immunizations are up to date, check with the college health service. A shot in the arm is good protection against infectious diseases.

Vaccinations. A single measles vaccine can provide the immunity you need to protect yourself from this potentially damaging disease. Once vaccinated against measles or a number of other diseases, the immune system is prepared to produce the appropriate antibodies. Thus, when exposed to measles, you do not get the disease. Some vaccinations provide lifetime immunity and others require periodic updates. For example, you need to get a vaccination against mumps only once in your life, but you need a new tetanus shot every ten years or when treated for a puncture wound if more

immunity The body's ability to destroy pathogens that it has once encountered, before they are able to cause disease.

active immunity The body's development of its own resistance to disease.

passive immunity Resistance to disease that initially comes from an external source.

antibodies Specific proteins that are produced principally in the blood in response to foreign substances in the body.

antigens Foreign substances in the body that cause the production of antibodies.

Assess Your Health

Keep Your Immunizations Up to Date

Keep a record of your immunization history. You will need this for enrollment in school and travel to exotic places, and to show another physician if you move or change physicians. The following list identifies the vaccinations that you may need as an adult.

Type of immunity	Frequency of booster doses	Your status
Cholera	Every 6 months while exposed	________
Diphtheria	Every 10 years	________
Hepatitis A	Only if traveling to a location where this disease is prevalent	________
Hepatitis B	Every 5 years for high-risk individuals	________
Influenza	Every year for people 65 or older and those with chronic illnesses	________
Measles	In late adolescence or early adulthood	________
Meningitis	Before starting college	________
Mumps	Lifetime immunity	________
Plague	Every 3 to 6 months while exposed	________
Pneumococcal pneumonia	Once for people 65 or older and those with chronic illnesses	________
Polio	Only when exposure is anticipated	________
Tetanus	Every 10 years or when treated for a puncture wound if more than 5 years have elapsed since last booster	________
Typhoid fever	Only if traveling to a location where this disease is prevalent	________
Typhus	Every year if exposed	________
Yellow fever	Only if traveling to a location where this disease is prevalent	________

than five years have elapsed since the last **booster** (see the Assess Your Health box).

Vaccinations are made in four different ways: with a live but weakened virus, with a dead virus, with a virus closely related to but weaker than that for which immunity is sought, or with a nonpoisonous version of a toxin produced by a bacterial agent. For example, the polio vaccine developed by Dr. Jonas Salk and approved for mass use in 1955 uses a killed virus, and the one developed by Dr. Albert Sabin and approved for mass use in 1961 uses live but weakened polio viruses. There are other differences between the two vaccines. The Salk vaccine is injected into the body; the Sabin vaccine is taken by mouth, usually on a lump of sugar. Prior to these vaccines, more than thirty thousand cases of polio a year occurred in the United States. When the polio virus attacks the spine, paralysis of the legs results; when the virus gets into the brain, it paralyzes muscles needed for breathing, swallowing, and other body functions. Because of the widespread use of the vaccine, the United States is nearly free of polio. The only recorded cases are related to the vaccine itself.

Protecting yourself or your family against an infectious disease by keeping immunizations up to date is only one aspect of immunity. Another is protecting the community by reducing the overall incidence through **herd immunity.** With herd immunity, a large proportion of the population is vaccinated against a particular disease, thus significantly reducing the chances of infection in any one individual. Widespread immunization against polio is an example of using the concept of herd immunity.

booster A dose of an immunization or vaccination given to renew or maintain the effect of a previous dose.

herd immunity The vaccination of a large proportion of a population against a particular disease to significantly reduce the chances of spread of infection.

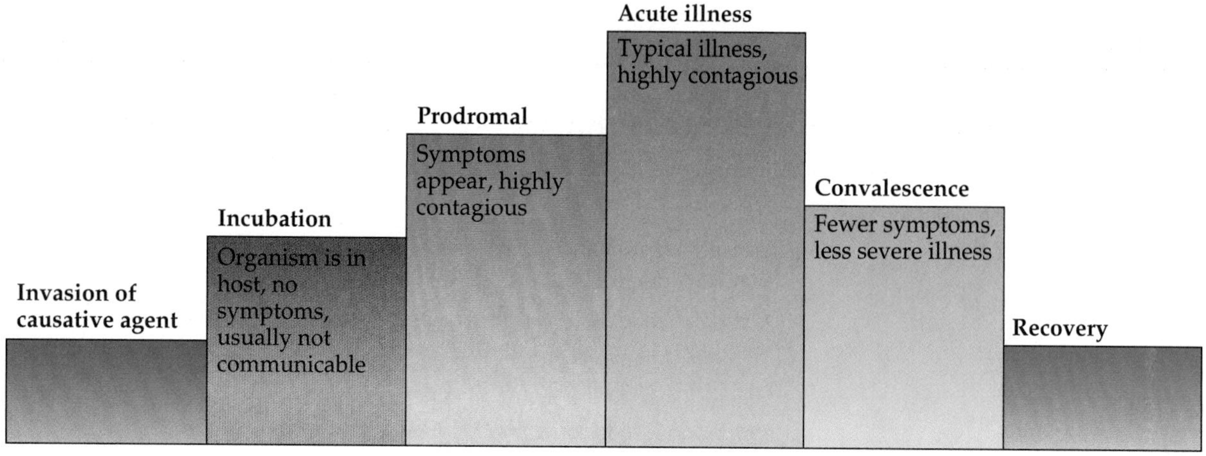

Figure 11.2 Stages of Disease
Infectious diseases follow a course of action beginning with incubation, progressing through the prodromal stage, acute illness, convalescence, and finally, recovery.

Stages of Infectious Disease

Although communicable diseases differ in how they are caused, there is a general pattern to the course of infectious diseases (see Figure 11.2). After the causative agent finds a hospitable host and begins multiplying, there is a period of **incubation.** During this time, there are no symptoms of disease, and in most cases, the infected person is not contagious. Incubation usually lasts a few days to two weeks.

Next comes the **prodromal** stage, which is a highly contagious period. Some symptoms are usually apparent, but the person does not feel sick enough to stay at home. Sometimes during the prodromal stage, an infected person has no symptoms and does not even know he or she is infected. Disease is easily and unknowingly spread during this time.

incubation The stage during which there are no symptoms of disease and, in most cases, the infected person is not contagious.

prodromal stage A highly contagious period in a disease in which some symptoms may be apparent but the infected person does not feel ill.

acute stage The stage at which symptoms of a disease are fully developed.

convalescence A state characterized by a decline in the severity of disease symptoms.

recovery A period in which infection is successfully defeated and the body returns to its healthy state.

The **acute** stage of illness occurs when symptoms are fully developed. Symptoms differ for each disease. During the acute stage, the infected person remains highly contagious.

The final stages of an infectious disease are **convalescence,** a decline in the severity of symptoms, and **recovery,** when the infection is successfully defeated and the body returns to its healthy state. During these stages, the infection leaves the body through mucus, pus, blood, feces, tears, sweat, and other flushing processes. A person is usually not contagious during these stages. In some infectious diseases, HIV for example, a person may remain in the acute stage, never reaching convalescence or recovery.

Common Infectious Diseases

Each year, Americans lose more than 2 billion days from school, work, and other major activities because of illnesses from infectious diseases other than sexually transmitted infections. Given the enormity of the problem, it is reassuring to know that most of us recover from these illnesses. The killer infectious diseases include AIDS, pneumonia, meningitis, and hepatitis B. Furthermore, because people who have AIDS have severely compromised immune systems, they are also more susceptible to infectious diseases such as pneumonia and tuberculosis. (For more on infectious diseases that are transmitted primarily through sexual means, see page 184.)

Table 11.2 provides an overview of several common infectious diseases. See Table 11.3 on page 188 for an overview of common sexually transmitted infections.

Table 11.2 Common Infectious Diseases

Disease name	Pathogen	How transmitted	Symptoms	Preventive measures	Treatment
Athlete's foot	Fungus	By contact with organism, usually on shower floors, towels, or by direct contact with infected person	Rash, peeling of skin; severe itching	Keep feet dry, change socks frequently, use antifungal foot powder	Antifungal creams/ powders
Chickenpox	Virus	By air, through inhalation of droplets exhaled from infected person	Rash develops 2–3 days after inhalation of virus; fever and itching of lesions over the body, perhaps mouth or throat	Immunization	Trim fingernails closely; oral acyclovir; calamine lotion, oral antihistamines for itching; acetaminophen or ibuprofen (not aspirin) for fever
Cold	Virus	By air, through inhalation of droplets exhaled from infected person; by direct contact	Runny nose; itchy eyes; generally uncomfortable feeling; nasal congestion; sore throat; cough	Avoid contact with infected individuals	Treat with bed rest, plenty of fluids, and aspirin, acetaminophen, or ibuprofen for relief of pain; pseudoephedrine for congestion
German measles (rubella)	Virus	By air, through inhalation of droplets exhaled from infected person; by direct contact	Rash; swelling of lymph nodes; fever (mild)	Immunization	Gamma globulin may block symptoms; fluids; rest
Influenza	Virus	By air, through inhalation of droplets exhaled from infected person; by direct contact	Fever for 1–7 days; nausea; sudden tiredness; vomiting; aching muscles; headache; sore throat; bronchitis	Immunization for high-risk persons (especially the elderly)	Fluids; aspirin (not young children), acetaminophen or ibuprofen to control fever; rest
Measles (rubeola)	Virus	By air, through inhalation of droplets exhaled from infected person; by direct contact	Red spotty rash; off-and-on high fever; unpleasant cough	Immunization	Aspirin, acetaminophen, or ibuprofen to avoid temperature variation; bland oral fluids
Mononucleosis	Virus	By direct contact	Severe sore throat; swollen lymph glands; tiredness; white spots on tonsils, tongue, and soft palate; enlarged spleen	Avoid contact with infected individuals	Confirm disease via blood count test for unusual white blood cells, positive monospot test; treat with bed rest; oral rinse for throat
Whooping cough (pertussis)	Bacterium	By air, through inhalation of droplets exhaled from infected person; by direct contact	Cough, sometimes creating a loud "whooping" sound; fever; vomiting	Immunization; antibiotic to household contacts of infected individuals	Antibiotics, corticosteroids in specific stages; frequent small feedings; cough medicines are of only slight benefit; careful observation

The Common Cold

The cold is indeed common. The average adult in the United States has at least two colds a year, and children have as many as twelve. Colds are caused by more than 120 rhinoviruses (*rhino* is the Greek word for "nose") as well as by adenoviruses, influenza viruses, and other viruses. Put them all together and you have more than one billion colds a year, which means a lot of runny noses, watery eyes, sore throats, headaches, fevers, aches, and pains.

Cold viruses are highly contagious. They contaminate the air and surfaces such as telephones and doorknobs and can survive in these environments for several hours or even days. You are likely to get a cold if you (1) breathe air filled with cold viruses, (2) shake hands with someone who has a cold virus on his or her hands, or (3) touch a virus-laden surface and then touch your own eyes or nose. Recent research indicates that more colds are spread by hand-to-hand contact than through the air and that families who wash hands frequently have significantly fewer colds.

Aspirin or acetaminophen can reduce fever and muscular aches, but there is no cure for a cold. The good news is that once you get a cold, it lasts for only about a week.

Influenza

Influenza, also called the flu, has many of the same symptoms as a cold—congestion, sore throat, fever, aches, and pains—but they are more severe and last longer. For example, it is not uncommon for adults who have the flu to have temperatures as high as 103° Fahrenheit or for temperatures to rise as high as 105° Fahrenheit in children.

Flu viruses are transmitted much the same way cold viruses are, except that flu viruses are more contagious. Moreover, the flu can be deadly, particularly for young children, the elderly, and those in poor health.

influenza A severe viral infection involving the respiratory tract; also called the flu.

pneumonia An inflammation of the lung tissue.

pneumocystis pneumonia A rare form of pneumonia that is often present in persons living with AIDS.

bacterial pneumonia The main type of pneumonia that follows an attack of influenza.

mycoplasma A tiny microorganism and causative agent of many diseases of the joints and lungs.

fungal pneumonia Inflammation of the lungs caused by a fungus.

tuberculosis An airborne bacterial disease spread by inhaling germs called tubercle bacilli; symptoms include fever, wasting, and cheesy formations in the lungs.

Vaccines are available against some flu viruses, but because strains mutate, or change, and new ones emerge, vaccination cannot provide full immunity. The flu vaccine, which must be taken annually, is recommended for the elderly, those with chronic illnesses, and other people at high risk. As with the common cold, aspirin and acetaminophen can reduce fever and muscular aches associated with flu.

Pneumonia

Pneumonia, an inflammation of the lung tissue, is among the leading causes of death in the United States. Pneumonia has more than fifty known causes, including viruses, bacteria, and chemical irritants. Although people over age sixty-five account for most of the deaths from pneumonia, the mortality rate is rising among young adults. This is due to an increase in the number and types of pneumonia-causing bacteria that are resistant to antibiotics; a worsening of air pollution, which can make the lungs more susceptible to bacterial infection; and a rise in the number of **pneumocystis pneumonia** cases, especially among people living with AIDS.

Bacterial pneumonia is the main type of pneumonia that follows an attack of influenza. The pneumonia bacteria normally live in the mouth or throat. One pneumonia-causing bacterium is *Legionella pneumophila,* also known as Legionnaires' disease because fifty-eight people became ill from it following a meeting of the American Legion in Philadelphia in 1976. A vaccine that protects against the most common pneumonia-causing bacterium (*Streptococcus pneumoniae*) lasts five years or longer and is recommended for people over age sixty-five and others with chronic illnesses.

Mycoplasmas and viruses, which are spread through droplets in the air or by contaminated hands, cause pneumonia primarily in children and young adults. The influenza virus can be deadly, particularly for pregnant women and people who have heart or pulmonary disease.

Fungal pneumonia is rare, but is occasionally found in isolated locations. For example, a pneumonia called valley fever, which is caused by fungi in the soil, is found in Southern California where smog in the air contributes to the sensitivity of people to the disease.

A chest Xray gives the clearest evidence of lung inflammation and pneumonia. Antibiotics are used for treating bacterial pneumonia; other forms are treated by rest and the body's natural healing capabilities.

Tuberculosis

An airborne bacterial disease, **tuberculosis** (TB) is spread by inhaling bacteria called tubercle bacilli that come from someone who has a contagious form of TB. It is most easily spread in a crowded, poorly ventilated environment, which is why it is often associated with poverty.

TB initially affects the lungs, but it can also settle in almost any organ in the body, including the kidneys, brain, heart, liver, and bones. It causes patients to lose weight and energy. In the nineteenth century, it was called consumption because of the way it ate away, or "consumed," its victims.

It was the leading killer at the beginning of the twentieth century, but mortality from it declined sharply in the United States with the introduction of antibiotics and improvements in sanitation, nutrition, and general standards of living. TB has reemerged as a public health problem, largely because many strains of TB have become resistant to the antibiotics used to treat the disease. Having more people infected with active TB contributes to the spread of the disease.

TB can be detected by a simple skin test, and most forms are effectively treated by taking antituberculosis drugs for a period of six months or longer.

Mononucleosis

A disease caused by the Epstein-Barr virus and transmitted in saliva by kissing or other person-to-person contact, **mononucleosis,** or "mono," strikes primarily adolescents and young adults. It is most common among fifteen- to nineteen-year-olds, followed by those in the twenty- to twenty-four-year-old range. Symptoms include fever, headache, nausea, extreme fatigue, and swollen spleen and lymph nodes. The disease is debilitating, and recovery requires several weeks and sometimes months. Although most of the symptoms usually last only two to three weeks, a person recovering from mononucleosis can expect to feel fatigued for several more weeks.

Mononucleosis can be detected by a blood test. The only treatment is rest and drinking plenty of liquids.

Chronic Fatigue Syndrome

Most people suffer from periods of fatigue, but people who have **chronic fatigue syndrome** suffer for prolonged periods—for six months and longer. In addition, they have several other symptoms, including muscle and joint pain, sore throat, impaired short-term memory or concentration, headaches, unrefreshing sleep, and lingering tiredness after exercise.

Chronic fatigue syndrome is a relatively new condition—it was first defined in 1988—and its cause is still unknown. A current hypothesis is that a virus, stress, or other transient traumatic condition may chronically activate the immune system. According to this hypothesis, the immune system, which ordinarily gears down after an infection has been eliminated, remains activated after the initiating condition has passed. The result is that unusually high concentrations of immune activating factors, some of which are known to cause fatigue at high doses, remain in the bloodstream.

Given that its causes are not known, treating chronic fatigue syndrome is difficult. General advice from physicians specializing in the disease include being as active as possible. Physicians sometimes prescribe low-dosage antidepressants to help patients sleep and feel better and other drugs to treat body pains. With these combined treatments, patients often improve.

Meningitis

Meningitis is an infectious disease of the fluid and membranes that surround the brain and spinal cord. It is caused by both bacteria and viruses. Viral meningitis is generally not very severe, while bacterial meningitis is much more serious. Early symptoms include a rash, headache, neckache, and confusion. The onset of bacterial meningitis is rapid and can be fatal in about 10 percent of all cases. Meningitis usually occurs during childhood. Because of close living conditions, college students who live in dormitories or residence halls have a slightly higher risk of bacterial meningitis than the general population. As a precaution, it is recommended that college students become immunized against meningitis. Such immunizations are safe and effective. Treatment for bacterial meningitis includes intravenous antibiotics. Viral meningitis is usually treated with bed rest.

Urinary Tract Infection (UTI)

A **urinary tract infection (UTI)** occurs when bacteria get into any part of the urinary system, including the kidneys, ureters, bladder, and urethra. Because of the structural differences between them, women experience urinary tract infections at a higher rate than men. As many as one in five women experience such an infection during their lifetime. Symptoms of a urinary tract infection for both sexes include a frequent urge to urinate, pain or burning during urination, and a greenish-yellow or white discharge from the penis or vagina.

mononucleosis A disease caused by the Epstein-Barr virus; symptoms include fever, headache, nausea, extreme fatigue, and swollen spleen and lymph nodes.

chronic fatigue syndrome A group of symptoms that result in a prolonged state of fatigue.

meningitis An infectious disease of the fluids and membranes that surround the brain and spinal cord; it can be viral or bacterial.

urinary tract infection (UTI) An infection that occurs when bacteria get into the urinary system.

When properly diagnosed, urinary tract infections are treatable with antibiotics.

To help prevent urinary tract infections, experts recommend the following:

- Drink plenty of fluids (8 to 10 cups of water daily).
- Urinate frequently to keep the fluids moving through the urinary tract.
- Wash your genitals daily (especially before and after sex if you are sexually active).
- Urinate after sex.
- Use a condom each time you have sex.
- Wipe from front to back after having a bowel movement.
- Avoid feminine hygiene products that contain deodorants.

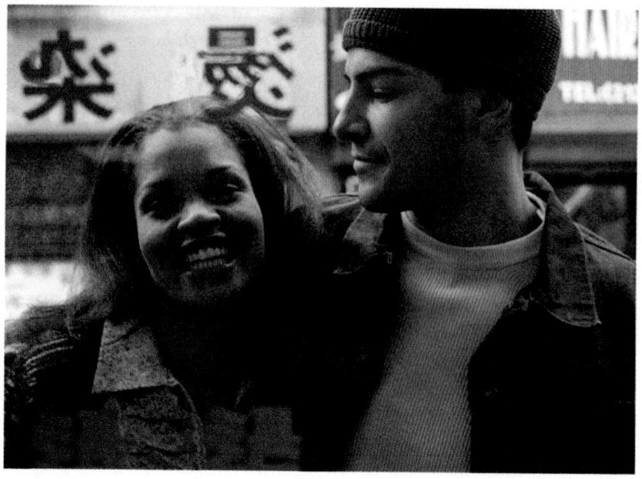

College students are at high risk of getting an STI, but this risk is significantly reduced among mutually monogamous couples.

Childhood Diseases

Although they can affect adults as well, several viral infectious diseases are called childhood diseases because they are usually contracted during childhood. These diseases include mumps, rubella (German measles), and measles. Mumps is generally a mild disease, causing some discomfort in children, but it may cause painful swelling of the testicles in men. Rubella, too, is a mild disease in childhood, but it can cause birth defects such as deafness, blindness, mental retardation, and behavioral problems if a woman contracts it during early pregnancy. Measles is a severe disease and can lead to inflammation of the brain. A combined measles, mumps, and rubella vaccine, the **MMR vaccine,** provides immunity from these diseases.

Sexually Transmitted Infections (STIs)

Sexually transmitted infections (STIs) are a major health concern for college-aged populations, which is why they deserve special consideration in this textbook. The United States leads among industrialized countries in rates of STI occurrence. For example, gonorrhea occurs in the United States 50 times more often than in Sweden. And secondary syphilis is reported 30 times more often in the United States than in Canada. Even though many STIs are treatable, the public health problems associated with them remain. There are effective treatments to combat many STIs, but these curable diseases continue to threaten the health of Americans largely because they go unrecognized and untreated.

MMR vaccine A vaccine that provides immunity to measles, mumps, and rubella.

What Are STIs?

Collectively, more than twenty-five infectious organisms that are transmitted through sexual activity are classified as STIs. These, along with the dozens of clinical syndromes that they cause, make up the group of infectious diseases and syndromes called STIs. Although STIs are caused by a variety of organisms, they all share one common factor: They have an affinity for the moist, warm genital areas.

STIs can result in mild discomfort, infertility, lifelong pain, or death. Some STIs facilitate the spread of other STIs and are highly correlated with serious chronic diseases such as cancer. Pregnant women who have STIs can pass along a range of disorders to their children, including mental retardation and blindness, as well as the disease itself. Women are more vulnerable than men to becoming infected with some STIs in part because the vaginal tract is subject to tears and abrasions. While not all college students are sexually active, those who are active are at an unusually high risk for STIs because they frequently have unprotected sexual intercourse and are often sexually involved with more than one partner.

The true incidence of STIs is difficult to pinpoint because physicians are required to report only a limited number of these diseases—including chlamydia, AIDS, gonorrhea, hepatitis B, and syphilis. The other STIs are more difficult to track precisely. See Figure 11.3 for an illustration of how STIs spread.

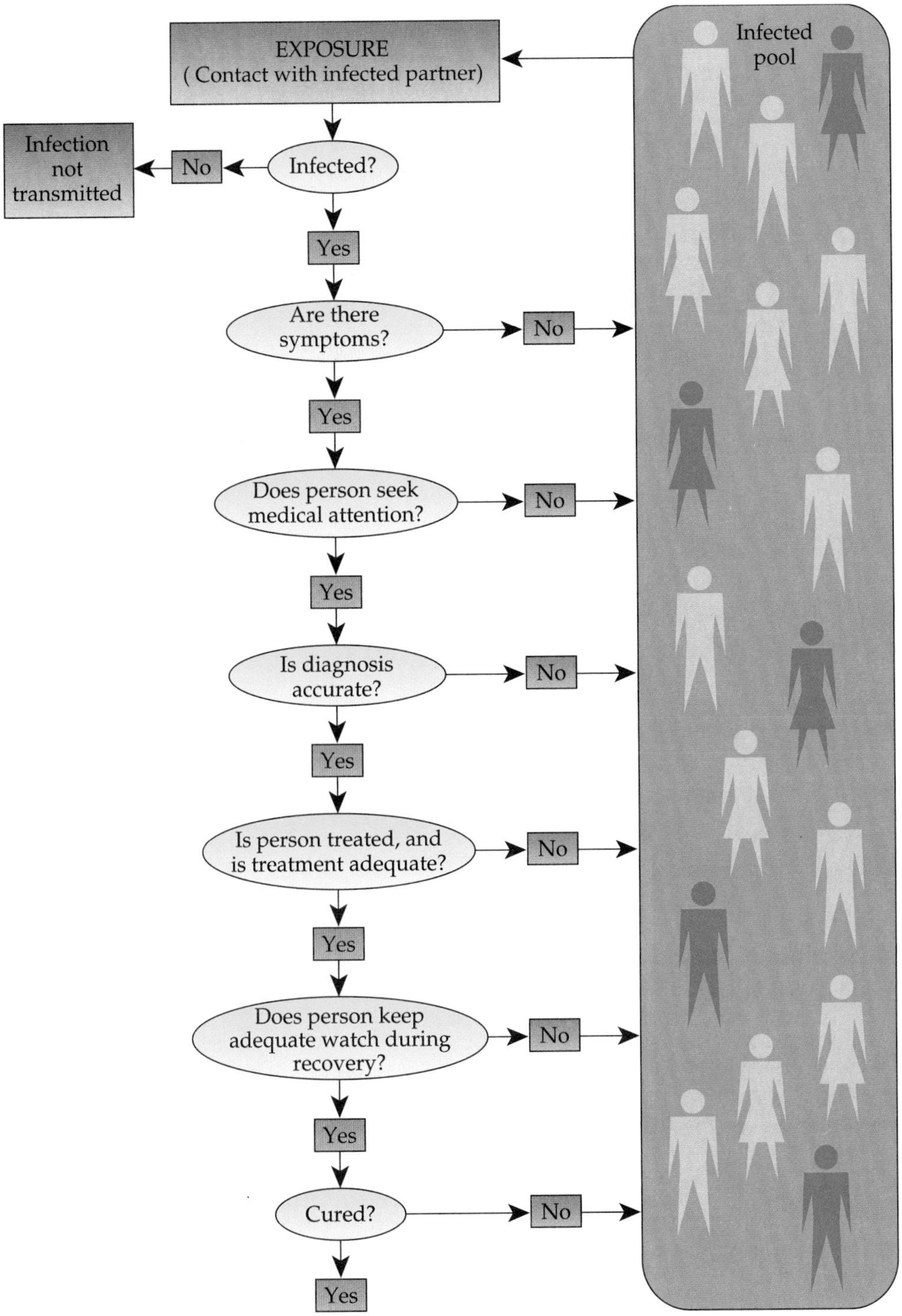

Figure 11.3 The Cycle of STI Transmission among Sexually Active Individuals
Asymptomatic carriers provide a constant pool that is a source of infection or reinfection for others. This diagram shows other sources that contribute to the pool of infected people.

related to STIs are reasonably well understood. No matter who you are—a teenager, a college student, a business executive—there are generally three ways to get one of these diseases.

First, in almost all cases, only sexually active people are exposed to STIs. Exceptions include congenital syphilis, yeast, pubic lice, and scabies. But, for the most part, to be exposed to an STI, a person must participate in an activity that allows the movement of pathogens from one individual to another through the genitalia or other tissue, such as the mouth or anus.

Second, to contract an STI, an individual must have sex with a person who is infected with the disease. (Remember, infection is not the same as having symptoms.) In a mutually monogamous relationship in which neither partner carries an STI, the risk for acquiring a disease is slight. When one or both members of the relationship have sexual contact with other partners, the risk rises.

Finally, the risk for being exposed to an STI increases when no prophylactics are used. The condom is not a guarantee of protection against STIs, but its use can greatly reduce the risk for transmitting or contracting most diseases. Until recently, only a male condom was available. A new condom designed for use by women provides protection similar to that of the male condom.

When an STI is suspected, what then? Steps can be taken to further prevent the spread of disease:

Prevention and Treatment

The best hope for controlling STIs rests in a combination of prevention and treatment. STI prevention is best accomplished by practices that reduce risk. The risk factors

- Have a medical examination as soon as signs of an STI appear so that the correct diagnosis is made and appropriate treatment begins in a timely fashion.
- Have follow-up examinations after treatment to confirm that the disease has been cured.

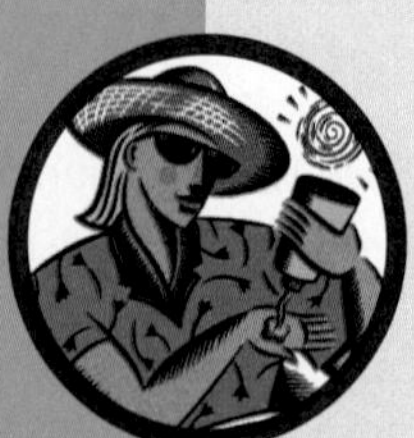

Developing Health Skills

Steps to Take for Primary Prevention of STIs

Before you decide to have sex:

- Assess your risk. What type of behavior are you interested in or willing to engage in? Does that behavior place you at risk? If so, what precautions can you take?
- Assess your potential partner's risk. If your partner has had sex with someone else, there is a possibility that he or she has contracted an STI. You cannot tell whether someone has an STI simply by looking at or even by asking him or her. Surveys show that both men and women lie about their previous sexual encounters.
- Communicate your feelings about safer sex to your potential partner. If he or she is not willing to respect your wishes to have safer sex, you should insist on postponing having sex.
- Have a checkup. If you suspect that you or your partner may be at risk for having an STI, postpone having sex until both of you have been checked by a physician. Although a checkup does not guarantee that a person is disease-free, it is the best means available for checking for the presence of STIs.

When you have sex:

- Use a condom. The proven method for reducing risk is to wear a condom during sexual activity. This does not guarantee protection against the transmission of all diseases, but it is the most important risk-reducing behavior for sexually active people.
- Select your sexual activity. Not only does the act of sexual intercourse place you at risk, so too does the type of activity in which you engage. For example, anal intercourse often results in tearing of tissues and some bleeding. People having anal intercourse are at high risk for contracting an STI. Vaginal intercourse carries risks as well, but not nearly as high.
- Visually examine your partner's genitals. Prior to engaging in sexual intercourse, take the time to look for a sore or any discharge. Any obvious sore is a warning sign. If you find such a sign, postpone sexual contact. Examining your partner's genitals can be difficult, but you can make it part of lovemaking and it can enhance open communication between the two of you.
- Wash your genitals before and after sexual contact. The risk of transmission can be reduced somewhat by simple hygiene. Washing the genitals with warm water and soap before and after intercourse can decrease risk of transmission of STIs.

- To prevent others from acquiring the disease, inform all sexual contacts of the problem. Their contacts should be notified as well.

See the Developing Health Skills box for suggestions for reducing the risk for getting an STI. Note that there are two phases—before you decide to have sex and when you have sex.

How Do You Know If You Have an STI?

Sometimes it is hard to tell if you have an STI or not. With some infections, a lot of people do not get symptoms. They may look and feel healthy but still have an STI. To take care of yourself properly, you need to know what the symptoms are of different STIs and when to see a physician for an accurate diagnosis.

If you are sexually active and suspect that you have been in contact with an infected person (or even if you have just changed sexual partners), it is important to have a checkup just in case, even when you feel fine.

If you have any of the following symptoms, a checkup is vital:

- Unusual discharge from the vagina or penis.
- Burning pain, stinging, or irritation when passing urine.
- A sore, blister, ulcer, warts, breaks in the skin, or rash in the genital area.
- A low abdominal pain or pain during intercourse.

Do not make the mistake of waiting to see if a rash or a pain "clears up." The fact that discomfort disappears does not mean you no longer have a disease. If you or your sexual partner has any of the above symptoms, discuss them together and do not have sex until you have seen a physician.

Safer Sex

The different STIs described in this chapter may threaten your health to a greater or lesser extent, depending on your sexual practices. Precautions are not guaranteed to result in total protection from STIs. But you can substantially reduce your risk by establishing a pattern of behavior that results in safer sex. This involves:

- **A willingness to prepare ahead for sex.** If you are considering having sex, preparation means knowing the facts and discussing them with your partner. Do not be embarrassed to talk about STIs. And do not be embarrassed to insist on protecting yourself.
- **A commitment to using condoms.** Condom use is the only proven risk-reducer other than abstinence. Although not perfect, a condom with spermicide is the best known protection against most STIs. Safer sex includes the use of a new condom every time you have sex.
- **An understanding that if you are sexually active you can get STIs.** One of the most dangerous attitudes relative to STIs is denial—to pretend that "it" will not happen to you. If you are sexually active, "it" can happen to you. If symptoms do appear, see a physician for early treatment.

Common Sexually Transmitted Infections

The following infections are either sometimes spread by sexual transmission (e.g., hepatitis and HIV/AIDS) or exclusively by sexual transmission (e.g., genital herpes, chlamydia, and gonorrhea). They are discussed below by type of infection. See Table 11.3 for an overview of common STIs.

Viral Infections

Hepatitis. **Hepatitis** is an inflammation of the liver usually caused by a virus. It is most often identified as three distinct diseases: hepatitis A, hepatitis B, and hepatitis C. The **hepatitis A** virus is shed in the bowel movements of infected persons and is often spread in child care centers and other places filled with young children, mostly because of poor hand-washing habits. The incubation period ranges from fifteen to fifty days. During this time, there are no signs of disease, and it is possible for an infected person to spread hepatitis unknowingly before he or she develops symptoms. Hepatitis A symptoms vary widely in severity, ranging from mild, flulike illnesses in young children to serious liver inflammation in the elderly. Some hepatitis patients become jaundiced (yellow). There is a vaccine against hepatitis A, which is recommended for people at risk and those traveling to areas with poor sanitation.

The **hepatitis B** virus circulates in the bloodstream and is excreted in the infected person's body fluids, including blood, saliva, semen, and vaginal secretions. It is seen mainly among men who have sex with men, injecting drug users, people with tattoos, dialysis patients, and health care workers. The incubation period is two to six months, and during the latter part of this period the infected person is contagious. Symptoms are fever, chills, nausea, loss of appetite, enlarged liver, jaundice, cirrhosis of the liver, and liver cancer. There is a vaccine against hepatitis B, which is recommended for people at risk. Employers must offer the vaccine to employees who might handle blood in their work. This includes all health care workers, firefighters, and police.

The **hepatitis C** virus is spread primarily by blood-to-blood contact. About 50 percent of all cases are related to injecting drugs. It is also seen among dialysis patients, people who have hemophilia and others receiving blood transfusions, and health care workers. There is also some concern that it may be spread through sexual contact.

Because of the way it attacks the body, hepatitis C is an infectious disease that results in a chronic disease. It causes an infection of the liver that is usually lifelong and incurable. This sets the stage for cirrhosis and liver cancer. The infection is most common among people aged thirty to forty-nine, most of whom contracted it at least a decade earlier. Because most infected people have few if any symptoms, they can carry the disease for years without knowing it. The recommended course of treatment is interferon injections three times a week for a year, but this defeats the virus in only 20 percent of the people treated.

HIV/AIDS. **Acquired immune deficiency syndrome (AIDS)** is caused by the **human immunodeficiency virus (HIV),** a virus that causes a lifelong infection that usually weakens the body's immune system. AIDS is a late manifestation of infection with HIV. AIDS was first reported in the United States in 1981, and since then, the number of cases has grown rapidly. Worldwide,

hepatitis An inflammation of the liver, usually caused by a virus.

hepatitis A A form of hepatitis transmitted in human wastes and contaminated food and water.

hepatitis B A form of hepatitis transmitted by blood and sexual contact.

hepatitis C A form of hepatitis, previously known as non-A, non-B hepatitis, that resembles the other forms of hepatitis but cannot be classified as either.

acquired immune deficiency syndrome (AIDS) A combination of symptoms caused by the human immunodeficiency virus (HIV).

human immunodeficiency virus (HIV) The virus that causes AIDS.

Table 11.3 Common Sexually Transmitted Infections

Disease name	Pathogen	How transmitted	Symptoms	Preventive measures	Treatment
AIDS	Virus (human immunodeficiency virus)	By contact with infected person, usually during sexual intercourse (anal, vaginal), and by exchange of blood	Often no symptoms exist; combination of weight loss, night sweats, cough, new skin rashes, changes in bowel function, unexplained chronic fever	Abstinence; avoid sexual contact and blood exchange with infected person; use a condom; do not share needles	No known cure; protease inhibitors, AZT, and other drugs taken orally can decrease symptoms; treat opportunistic diseases associated with AIDS
Chlamydia	Bacterium (*Chlamydia trachomatis*)	By contact with infected person, usually during sexual intercourse	Whitish pus discharge from the penis; frequent, painful urination; often no symptoms exist	Avoid sexual contact with infected person; use a condom	Azithromycin, tetracyclines, or erythromycin
Crabs	Parasite (pubic lice)	By contact with infected person, usually during sexual intercourse	Intense itching on genital area; nits on hair shafts	Avoid sexual contact with infected person; scrupulous cleaning after intercourse	Various topical ointments, shampoos, lotions prescribed by physician
Genital warts	Virus (papilloma virus)	By contact with infected person, usually during sexual intercourse	Pinky-brown raised areas with tendency to form a cauliflower-shaped mass on external genitalia	Avoid sexual contact with infected person; use a condom	Washing with soap and water twice daily; painting lesions with podophyllin; surgical removal
Gonorrhea	Bacterium (*Neisseria gonorrhoeae*)	By contact with infected person, usually during sexual intercourse	Burning on urination; milky discharge from penis; urgency to urinate; in women, inflammation of vagina; often no symptoms	Avoid sexual contact with infected person; use a condom; early diagnosis	One intramuscular dose of ceftriaxone plus seven days of oral doxycycline
Herpes simplex type 2	Virus (herpes virus)	By contact with infected person, usually during sexual intercourse	Small groups of blisters on a reddened base of external or internal genitalia; painful urination	Avoid sexual contact with infected person, especially during outbreaks; use a condom	No known cure; normal saline solution to help prevent infection; apply antiviral agents (e.g., acyclovir) to skin
Syphilis	Bacterium (*Treponema pallidum*)	By contact with infected person, usually during sexual intercourse	Primary—painless chancre on external genitals. Secondary—skin rash, achiness. Tertiary—lesion, problems with nervous system and cardiovascular system	Avoid sexual contact with infected person; use a condom	Penicillin or tetracycline
Yeast infection	Fungus (*Candida albicans*)	By direct contact with infected person or normal flora overgrowth with hormonal changes, diabetes, oral antibiotics, or immunodeficiencies	Vaginal discharge of thick, whitish, cheesy substance; skin may be bluish-red, scaly; intense vulval and vaginal itching	Identify early and treat early to reduce severity of symptoms	Nystatin suppositories in the vaginal canal for 2 weeks; axole antifungal creams in vaginal canal for 7–10 days; diflucan orally

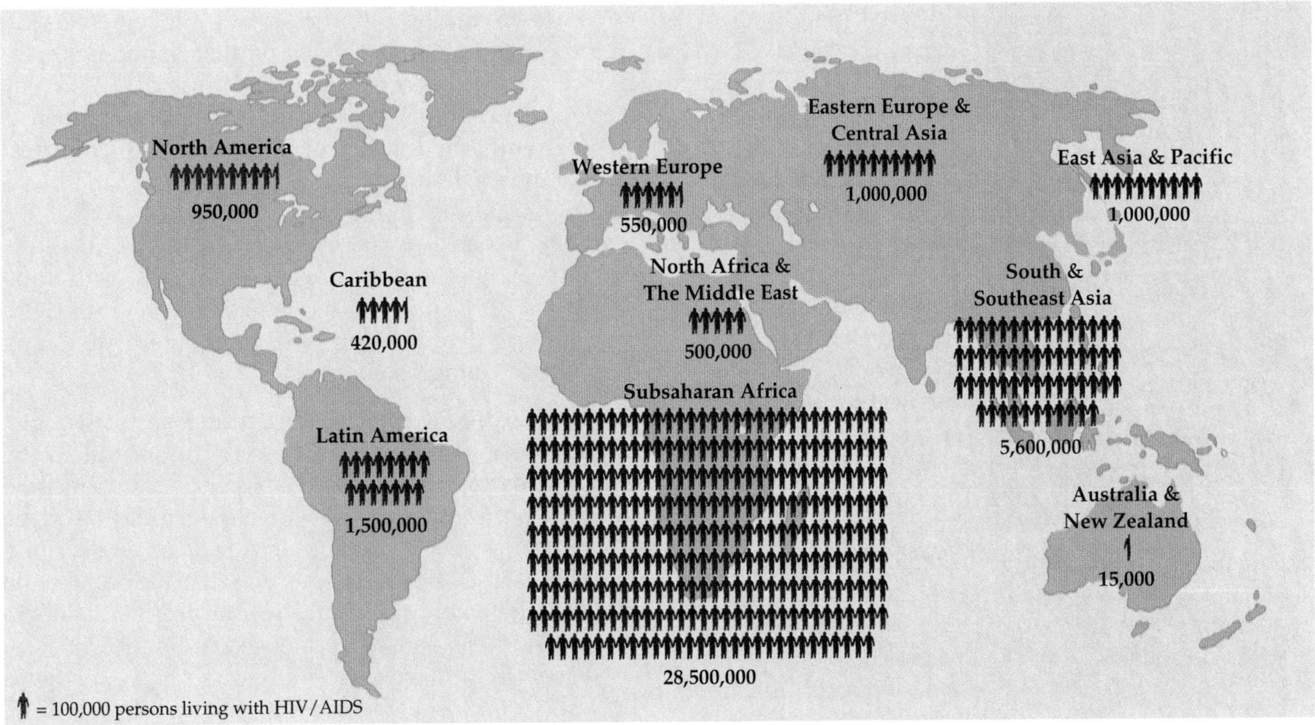

Figure 11.4 Distribution of HIV Infection and AIDS in Regions of the World
Each figure represents 100,000 persons living with HIV infection or AIDS.
(*Source: Report on the Global HIV/AIDS Epidemic 2002,* UNAIDS.

about 40 million people are infected with HIV, according to the 2002 global estimate from UNAIDS (see Figure 11.4). Furthermore, UNAIDS projects that 14,000 individuals became infected worldwide every day in 2001. In the United States alone, 40,000 people are infected each year, and African American women comprise the fastest growing group of infected people. More than fifty percent of U.S. infections are related to injecting drug use.

HIV kills a specific kind of white blood cell that is needed by the body's immune system to fight a variety of disease-causing organisms. Without these white blood cells (called **helper T-cells**), the body is vulnerable to infections. People with AIDS have a T-cell count of 200 or below. (Normal T-cell count is 1,000 to 1,200.) The early symptoms of AIDS, as well as the causes of death, are **opportunistic diseases,** or diseases that would otherwise be defeated by the body's immune system. The most common of such opportunistic diseases is *Pneumocystis carinii* pneumonia, which occurs in more than half of AIDS patients. **Kaposi's sarcoma,** an otherwise rare skin cancer, is also common among people living with AIDS.

HIV is transmitted during unprotected sexual contact with an infected person through body fluids such as blood, semen, and vaginal fluid. It is also spread in nonsexual ways, such as through needle sharing among injecting drug users and, less commonly and now very rarely, through transfusions of infected blood. The risk for getting HIV by receiving blood for medical reasons has been significantly reduced since donated blood began to be tested for the virus in 1985 in the United States and many other countries. Babies born to mothers who are HIV-infected may become infected themselves before birth, during the birth process, or through breast-feeding.

When HIV was first discovered, a positive diagnosis meant a prognosis of death within about ten years—and in most of the world, it still does. Today, there are several drug treatments, which focus on different stages of HIV and the biology of the disease. For example, passing HIV infection from mother to fetus can be greatly reduced by a course of azidothymidine (AZT).

helper T-cells White blood cells that are needed by the body's immune system to fight a variety of disease-causing organisms.

opportunistic diseases Diseases common to individuals infected with HIV that under normal conditions would be defeated by the body's immune system.

Kaposi's sarcoma A rare, deadly cancer characterized by reddish-purple blotches on the skin; one of the symptoms of AIDS.

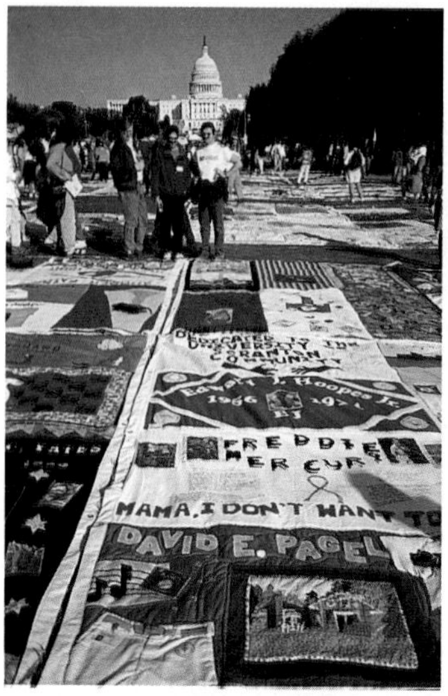

The AIDS Quilt, a personal memory of people who have died of AIDS, serves as a reminder of the serious consequences of unhealthy decisions. People with AIDS are living longer today, thanks to new combinations of drugs.

Most promising of drugs are protease inhibitors. These drugs stop—or inhibit—the replication of HIV by preventing the enzyme protease from making copies of itself and infecting cells. In effect, protease inhibitors lower the amount of HIV in a person's blood and can reduce the likelihood that the person will transmit the virus to others. Protease inhibitors also can substantially increase the life span of people living with AIDS. Another treatment, highly active antiretroviral therapy (HAART), has resulted in widespread reduction in HIV-related deaths in North America and Western Europe. Unfortunately, all of the successful drug treatments are very expensive.

Work is progressing on a vaccine to control HIV in already infected persons as well as to prevent uninfected persons from getting the disease.

Papilloma virus. The **human papilloma virus (HPV)** causes genital warts, or small bumps on the genitals. In men, these usually appear on the glans penis and in women on the labia or just inside the vagina.

The virus is highly contagious through direct contact with the warts. Thus, sexual intercourse, whether vaginal, oral, or anal, provides an ideal mode of transmission. Depending on the location of the warts, a condom may or may not provide protection against this disease. The most severe complication related to the incidence of genital warts is cervical cancer. Women who are infected or who have male partners who have genital warts are ten times more likely to develop cervical cancer. The papilloma virus is present in about 90 percent of cervical cancers tested. The virus may also play a role in cancer of the vagina, vulva, penis, and anus.

Currently, no test is available to determine the presence of the papilloma virus, so diagnosis is made by visual confirmation. Treatment involves removal of the warts by freezing or surgery. Because there is no cure, primary preventive measures are critical in controlling this virus. Preventive measures include bathing with warm soapy water before and after intercourse, and carefully selecting sexual partners.

Genital herpes. Genital herpes, a lifelong disease that has no cure, is a viral infection called **herpes simplex type 2.** Herpes sores, which resemble blisters, occur in men on the penis or near the anus. In women, sores may be on the labia majora, labia minora, inside the vagina, or around the anus. Genital herpes **lesions** may also be found in the mouth but are not to be confused with cold sores, a type of herpes simplex caused by a related pathogen.

When first infected, an individual may experience high fever and in some cases meningitis. In addition, the infected person may feel fatigued and achy and have enlarged lymph nodes. Herpes sores are often painful. An examination by a physician is the best means of diagnosing herpes simplex type 2.

About two weeks after the initial infection, the symptoms disappear. The disease is far from cured, however. The virus has simply retreated. It usually resides in nerve tissue and awaits some triggering mechanism that again causes it to produce symptoms. Recurrences are generally less severe than the initial herpes outbreak.

The most serious consequence of genital herpes infection involves its transfer from mother to baby, either across the placenta or during the birth process. Babies born with herpes infection suffer severe neurological and vision difficulties, and nearly half of those with **systemic infection** die.

There is no treatment that can cure herpes, but antiviral medications can shorten and prevent outbreaks during the period of time the person takes the medication. Research underway on a herpes vaccine looks promising as a way to protect women against one infection. But for now, prevention remains the best way to deal with an incurable disease like herpes.

Bacterial Infections

Chlamydia. The common bacterial infection **chlamydia** affects an estimated 10 percent of college students. Women are infected with chlamydia nearly six times more often than are men.

The symptoms of chlamydia infection in men include a whitish discharge from the penis and some dis-

human papilloma virus (HPV) The agent responsible for an STI characterized by warts, usually on the genitalia; also called genital warts.

herpes simplex type 2 A virus usually transmitted by sexual contact and causing open sores on the genitals.

lesions A localized change in tissue, or sores.

systemic infection An infection affecting the body as a whole.

chlamydia A common bacterial STI, which, if untreated, can cause serious, painful infections of the urinary tract in men and infection of the reproductive organs in women.

comfort. In women, there is some discomfort in the genitalia, itching, and burning. It is generally believed that 80 percent of women have no symptoms in the early stages of chlamydia infection and therefore do not seek treatment. Chlamydia is diagnosed through an examination by a physician using a swab from affected sites.

For pregnant women, the risk of premature delivery is much greater with chlamydia infection, and many babies of infected mothers develop the eye disease conjunctivitis. Because of this, some medical researchers believe that chlamydia infection is the greatest cause of preventable blindness throughout the world. HIV transmission is apparently aided by the presence of chlamydia infection.

If left untreated, chlamydia can cause irreparable damage to the reproductive organs. In men, inflammation from the infection can cause scar tissue on the vas deferens, which can result in sterility. In women, inflammation of the fallopian tubes can also result in sterility and, in some cases, an increased risk of tubal pregnancy.

A complication of chlamydia is **pelvic inflammatory disease (PID).** In the early stages of PID, chlamydia infection is generally located in the vagina. As the disease progresses, however, it spreads to the lining of the uterus, into the fallopian tubes and the pelvic cavity, and onto the ovaries. Symptoms of PID include severe abdominal pain and fever. Frequently, the tubes affected by PID are left partially or totally blocked by scar tissue. A partial block contributes to the increased risk of tubal pregnancy. A total block results in sterility. Early treatment may prevent permanent tube blockage but cannot repair damage already done.

Tetracycline and other antibiotics are used to treat chlamydia. Pregnant women should not use tetracycline because of its effects on the developing fetus.

Gonorrhea. Another widespread bacterial infection is **gonorrhea.** Symptoms in a man include a burning sensation when urinating and a whitish discharge from the penis. Because few men are asymptomatic, treatment for gonorrhea in men often begins in the early stages of the disease. Without treatment, the disease can cause urinary obstruction, inflammation and abscesses of the prostate, and sterility. Recent research has found that gonorrheal infection contributes to the transmission of HIV.

As with a chlamydia infection, 80 percent of women with gonorrhea are commonly believed to be **asymptomatic carriers** and therefore do not seek treatment early in the course of the disease. Those who do show symptoms often experience abnormal vaginal discharges, some discomfort in the vaginal area, and pain during urination. Unfortunately, these signs are unreliable indicators of gonorrhea because they may be caused by a range of other STIs as well as by other nonsexual related conditions. Diagnosis of gonorrhea is done by a test of secretions from the cervix, throat, rectum, or penis (depending on the kind of intercourse).

The most severe complications of gonorrheal infection in women include PID, blindness in infants, and gonococcal arthritis. Infantile blindness due to gonococcal infection was brought under control with the mandatory use of eye drops following birth.

Once diagnosed, gonorrhea is treated with antibiotic therapy, usually in the form of penicillin. In recent years, strains of gonorrhea have developed that are resistant to penicillin. In these cases, other antibiotic agents are used.

Syphilis. Once the most feared STI, the incidence of **syphilis** has been significantly reduced through prevention and treatment. It nonetheless remains a serious public health threat, with a recent rise in incidence among gay and bisexual men. In the United States, 31,575 cases of syphilis were reported by health officials in 2001.

Syphilis progresses through predictable stages. **Primary syphilis** is characterized by a painless sore at the site of the infection. The sore is usually round with raised edges and is called a **chancre.** Syphilis is highly contagious while a chancre is present. If left untreated, the chancre heals by itself, often leaving the infected person with the misconception that the disease is gone and there is no reason for concern.

Actually, the healing of the initial chancre is only an indication that the disease has progressed into **secondary syphilis,** which is characterized by a general rash on the body, sore throat, fever, and pains in the joints and muscles. As in primary syphilis, secondary syphilis is highly contagious.

A period of latency follows secondary syphilis, during which time no outward symptoms are present. This latent period can last from one to forty years and is usually not a period of contagion. Again, the infected individual may be fooled into thinking that the

pelvic inflammatory disease (PID) An infection in the pelvic area usually involving the uterus, fallopian tubes, and/or ovaries; half the cases are caused by chlamydia.

gonorrhea A sexually transmitted infection caused by *Neisseria gonorrhoeae,* a bacterium.

asymptomatic carrier A person who has a disease but no symptoms.

syphilis A bacterial STI that spreads through the bloodstream and causes a systemic infection.

primary syphilis A disease characterized by painless sores, called chancres, at the site of the infection.

chancre A painless, round sore with raised edges indicative of syphilis.

secondary syphilis A disease characterized by a general rash on the body, sore throat, fever, and pains in the joints and muscles.

syphilis infection is gone. In fact, the disease is spreading to other parts of the body, including the brain and spinal cord.

The final stage of the disease is referred to as **late syphilis,** or tertiary syphilis. This stage of generalized infection can produce heart failure, blindness, loss of muscle control, brain damage, and death.

At any stage, syphilis can be diagnosed by visual observation and/or confirmed with a blood test. Treatment is effective and involves a penicillin regimen. The body does not develop immunity to syphilis, so a person treated for the disease can contract it again and again. If a pregnant woman has syphilis, treatment is critical to avoid damage to both mother and fetus. The infection crosses the placenta and in most cases causes either a miscarriage or stillbirth or congenital syphilis, which often results in malformations of body parts and partial blindness and deafness.

Developing Health Skills

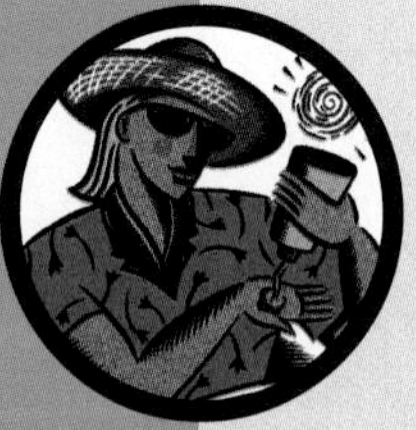

Preventing Vaginitis

Here are some suggestions for avoiding vaginitis:

- Wear loose cotton underwear and avoid tight pants or jeans. This is especially important when wearing panty hose or tights.
- Always wipe from the front (vagina) to the back (anus) after urinating.
- Use condoms, especially if having anal sex.
- If your sexual partner is an uncircumcised man, he should wash (with water only) and dry under his foreskin daily.
- Avoid excess soap, vaginal deodorants, deodorized panty shields, or bubble bath solutions.
- Minimize the use of antibiotics or request *Candida* treatment when antibiotics are prescribed.
- Keep healthy. When people are stressed or run down, they are more prone to infections.

Other STIs

Vaginitis. Virtually every woman experiences **vaginitis,** a vaginal infection, at some point in her life. In fact, vaginitis is a common reason for a woman to see a physician. It is usually caused by either a yeast or a protozoal infection.

One prevalent form of vaginitis is a **yeast** (fungus) **infection** caused by *Candida* (sometimes called *Monilia*). *Candida* is present in the vaginal area of many women. Under normal conditions, the presence of *Candida* causes no problems because the environment of the vagina is usually acidic enough to ward off infections. However, certain conditions can alter this, including antibiotic therapy, use of contraceptive pills, menstruation, wearing panty hose and nylon underwear, douching, and even lack of sleep. To avoid getting vaginitis, see the Developing Health Skills box.

Symptoms occur when the fungus grows fast enough to produce symptoms such as itching; burning during urination; a white, thick, odorless discharge; painful intercourse; and general discomfort. Diagnosis is through personal observations, which may be verified by a culture taken by a physician. Treatment is usually an antifungal drug in the form of suppositories or ointment. Antifungal drugs are now available over the counter, thus facilitating self-diagnosis and treatment.

One fact that is often overlooked by women who suffer from yeast infections is that their sexual partner can carry the infection without symptoms and reinfect them even after treatment is successful. This process of one partner infecting the other after treatment is called the ping-pong effect. It can be avoided simply by treating the male sexual partner with an antifungal cream regardless of whether any symptoms are present.

Protozoal vaginitis, unlike yeast infections, is transmitted primarily by sexual means. Sexually active women run an increased risk of this infection, which is called **trichomoniasis.** The symptoms include a foul or fishy odor, accompanied by itching, a burning sensation, and sometimes pain in the vaginal area. The most effective treatment involves the antiprotozoal drug metronidazole. There are no serious complications resulting from trichomoniasis. As with other forms of vaginitis, men can carry the disease organism and transmit it to a woman, so both partners should be treated at the same time.

Pubic lice and scabies. Another form of STIs, pubic lice (crabs) and scabies, is caused by spiderlike parasites that live in the genital area of both men and women. They are highly contagious and are common among

late syphilis A disease characterized by generalized infection that can produce heart failure, blindness, loss of muscle control, brain damage, and death; also called tertiary syphilis.

vaginitis A vaginal infection usually caused by yeast or protozoa.

yeast infection A condition characterized by itching; burning during urination; a white, thick, odorless discharge; painful intercourse; and general discomfort. Caused by *Candida*.

protozoal vaginitis A condition transmitted sexually and characterized by a foul or fishy odor, accompanied by itching, burning sensations and pain in the vaginal area.

trichomoniasis A protozoal vaginitis transmitted primarily through sexual means.

college students. Both are spread by close physical contact, and also by sheets, towels, and the infamous toilet seat. Diagnosis is usually a simple matter of checking pubic hair in a good light. The nits (eggs) or lice are visible to the naked eye. Symptoms include extreme itching and other skin discomfort. Because people who have lice and scabies tend to scratch their skin severely, secondary infection is a concern.

Treatment for lice and scabies usually involves an insecticide shampoo, topical creams, and overall good hygiene. Once diagnosis is confirmed, it is recommended that all bed linens, towels, and clothes be washed in hot water. What happens if these infestations are left untreated? Such a possibility is highly unlikely because the itching is so severe that help is almost always pursued. The presence of pubic lice or scabies may be a warning to have a complete STI checkup.

Emerging Diseases

The diseases presented in this chapter do not cover the infectious diseases that are about to face humankind. Concerning viruses alone, researchers have identified approximately one per year for the last several decades. And, because of the fact that microorganisms continue to mutate, the diseases known today may represent only a small fraction of those known tomorrow.

Excitement over what was once thought to be control of infectious diseases did not take into account the extraordinary resilience of pathogens, which have a remarkable ability to evolve, adapt, and develop resistance to drugs. Researchers also failed to take into account the fact that disease-carrying insects develop resistance to pesticides in a very short time. Other contributing factors to the increase in new or reemerging infectious diseases are population shifts, increased urbanization and crowding, environmental changes, and worldwide commerce, travel, and the threat of bioterrorism.

New or reemerging threats in the United States include multidrug-resistant TB; antibiotic-resistant staphylococcal, enterococcal, and pneumococcal infections; and diarrheal diseases caused by the parasite *Cryptosporidium parvum* and by certain strains of *Escherichia coli (E. coli)* bacteria.

Although salmonella, a bacteria found in poultry, eggs, meat, and milk, is a well-known cause of food poisoning, the Centers for Disease Control and Prevention now report that the number one cause of food-borne illness comes from a relatively obscure bacterium found in poultry, *Campylobacter jejuni.* Campylobacter causes bloody diarrhea and abdominal pain. Strains of it are emerging that are resistant to antibiotics. With an increase in antibiotic-resistant strains of bacteria and a decline in the number of new antibiotics introduced into the U.S. market, the resilient bacteria are winning the race between drug-resistant bacteria and new drugs.

West Nile virus has emerged in recent years in Europe and North America, presenting a new public health threat. Animal vectors, usually birds, carry this infectious disease. While getting infected with West Nile virus is usually not life threatening, in its most serious form, it can be fatal. Death is usually attributed to **encephalitis** (inflammation of the brain). This infectious disease threatens humans, horses, and certain domestic and wild birds. It was discovered, as the name suggests, in the West Nile District of Uganda in 1937, and the first reported case in North America was in 1999. By 2002, there were more than 150 reported human cases in the United States, including several deaths.

Perhaps the most frightening development in recent years regarding emerging infectious diseases is the threat by terrorists to use pathogens to create fear among large populations. Anthrax, for example, is an infectious agent that lends itself to such use. Anthrax is a disease caused by a spore-forming bacterium. It is common among cattle, goats, and other farm animals, but rare among humans. When found in humans, anthrax takes one of three forms: cutaneous, inhalation, and gastrointestinal. **Cutaneous anthrax** results when spores penetrate the skin, usually by means of a cut in the skin; **inhalation anthrax** is acquired through breathing in anthrax spores (a terrorist's likely choice); and **gastrointestinal anthrax,** a result of ingesting the spores in the process of eating or drinking.

Infectious diseases are reemerging despite advances by medical science to limit such diseases. The reasons for the resurgence of infectious diseases are complex and not fully understood. Perhaps most important, however, is the continual evolution of pathogenic microorganisms.

Protection Through Prevention

While medical researchers are continuing to expand the arsenal against infectious diseases, the best way to stop the spread of disease is prevention. And the best way to

encephalitis Inflammation of the brain.

cutaneous anthrax A form of anthrax that results when spores penetrate the skin, usually through a cut in the skin.

inhalation anthrax A form of anthrax acquired through breathing in anthrax spores.

gastrointestinal anthrax A form of anthrax acquired by ingesting the spores while eating or drinking.

prevent disease is through education and informed action taken by the public at large. Recent events have been encouraging.

Reducing Your Risk for an Infectious Disease

The ultimate responsibility for the prevention of infectious disease remains with you. There are some specific actions that you can take to reduce your risk. Here are several suggestions:

- Maintain overall good health. By eating right, exercising, and getting plenty of rest, you can boost your ability to fight off disease if and when you are exposed to an infectious disease. You can also boost your resistance by maintaining a positive mental attitude.
- Practice basic hygiene. Basic cleanliness is sometimes taken for granted, yet it is one of the most important aspects of disease prevention. Wash your hands frequently, bathe on a regular basis, and brush your teeth. All of these are effective ways to reduce the spread of infectious diseases.
- Keep your vaccinations up to date. Your immune system needs your help. By keeping up with all recommended vaccinations, you greatly reduce (prevent in most cases) the spread of specific diseases such as measles and mumps.
- Treat all minor infections seriously. A minor cut, a minor cold, or a minor boil presents little threat—until secondary complications set in. It is not uncommon, for example, for a boil to lead to generalized infection, resulting in a life-threatening situation. A minor case of influenza can lead to secondary infections, resulting in pneumonia, one of the most common causes of death.
- Support your local public health authority. The state and local public health departments are charged with health promotion and disease prevention. They need your cooperation to prevent disease. That support can be as simple as heeding the advice to get the latest flu shot. It can also mean volunteering to assist with a public education campaign to immunize children. Through working to reduce the threat of infectious disease in your community, you are actually reducing your own risk for disease.

CASE STUDY 11: Treating an Infectious Disease

Beth had a bad sore throat and went to the student health service to get some medicine. She had an important term paper to write and didn't want a "stupid" sore throat to get the better of her. The physician did a throat culture and when she found that Beth had strep throat, she gave her a prescription for an antibiotic medicine. Beth began as a compliant patient, taking her medicine as prescribed. But when the antibiotic made her feel better in two days, she stopped taking it. Unfortunately for Beth, treatment of bacterial infections with antibiotics requires a full course of treatment. Soon after she discontinued her medication, Beth had a relapse—and in fact felt even worse.

Kim lives down the hall from Beth, and she also paid a visit to the student health services to follow up on her flulike symptoms—achy joints and fatigue. Like Beth, she had a paper to write but was feeling so tired that she couldn't work on it. Kim's problem was diagnosed just as she feared it would be: the flu. She knew that the flu is caused by a virus, and that antibiotics cannot help a viral disease. Her best bet for recovery was to build up her health with plenty of rest, liquids, and a good diet. A weakened system would only lead to a relapse—and there were enough infectious diseases going around the dorm that she didn't want to take any chances on catching something else.

In Your Opinion

Both Beth and Kim had an infectious disease, but they followed different routes to recovery. They both started to do the right thing, seek medical attention, but only one followed through correctly.

- What do these two scenarios tell you about infectious diseases?
- Can you explain why Beth's behavior could contribute to the emergence of antibiotic-resistant bacteria?
- Why did Beth feel worse when she relapsed?
- What would you have done in either of their cases?

KEY CONCEPTS

1. An infectious disease is the result of infectious agents, such as bacteria or viruses that spread from someone who is infected to someone who is not infected.
2. Infectious diseases are caused by pathogenic microorganisms such as bacteria, viruses, protozoa, parasitic worms, fungi, rickettsias, and prions.
3. Infectious diseases follow a course of action beginning with incubation, and progressing through the prodromal stage, acute illness, convalescence, and, finally, recovery.
4. Asymptomatic carriers provide a consistent infected pool that is a source of infection or reinfection for others.
5. Immunity is resistance to infectious disease. In active immunity, the body develops its own resistance to disease. In passive immunity, resistance to disease initially comes from an external source.
6. Vaccines have been instrumental in wiping out epidemics of serious diseases such as polio and in eliminating smallpox.
7. STIs that are caused by bacteria are usually curable through antibiotic therapy, but few vaccines exist for such diseases.
8. For viral STIs, there are medical treatments, but none that "cure" the infected person. Thus, STIs caused by viruses result in a life-long infection.
9. The best hope for controlling STIs rests in prevention rather than treatment.
10. Public education campaigns resulting in informed action have proven to be effective in reducing the spread of infectious diseases, including sexually transmitted infections.

REVIEW QUESTIONS

1. List five links in the chain of infection and give one example of how each link can be cut.
2. Name the seven families of pathogens and give an example of a disease caused by each.
3. Describe four ways pathogens are carried.
4. Explain the importance of virulence and dosage to the spread of disease.
5. Describe the course of a disease beginning with infection through to recovery.
6. Explain the concept of immunity and how it protects the body against infection.
7. Identify two examples of successful public health campaigns to prevent disease and briefly describe each.
8. List common infectious diseases (not sexually transmitted) and briefly describe the symptoms and severity of each.
9. List common sexually transmitted infections and briefly describe the symptoms and severity of each.
10. List several actions that you can take to personally prevent the spread of infectious disease.

CRITICAL THINKING QUESTIONS

1. The *Healthy People 2010* objectives include the following: "Reduce or eliminate indigenous cases of vaccine-preventable diseases." Both diphtheria and polio are listed among the vaccine-preventable diseases, yet each has been virtually eliminated from the U.S. population. At what point can we declare a disease "eliminated?" Because vaccinations are not without risk, at what point does the vaccination become more risky than the disease?
2. One of the most common mistakes made when treating a bacterial disease is to take enough prescribed antibiotic to treat the symptoms of the disease, but not enough to fully treat the disease itself. This can "knock out" the least virulent strain of the bacteria and leave the harder-to-treat strains still in the body. Such a practice not only leads to a relapse but also can contribute to the development of a more virulent strain of the infectious agent. What kinds of implications can this practice have on public health? What might public health officials do to change such behaviors?
3. At present, HIV is a very delicate organism. It is not passed from one person to another through casual contact. Imagine for a moment that HIV mutates into a resilient virus that could be spread effectively through droplets in the air or through physical contact, much as the common cold is spread. What would be the threat to public health? How would public health authorities need to respond?
4. The *Healthy People 2010* objectives include the following: "Increase the proportion of sexually active persons who use condoms." Why has the use of condoms met with such resistance? Do you feel that the condom presents a barrier to sexual responsiveness? Or do you think the "it-couldn't-happen-to-me" attitude overrules the motive to use protection? Which reason do you think most represents the attitude of college students?

JOURNAL ACTIVITIES

1. Record your immunization history on a sheet of paper. You may need to call your parents or your

physician to get accurate, up-to-date information. Are there gaps?

2. Are you aware of an infectious disease on campus—for example, measles? How did the university respond? Were vaccines made available? Were special clinic hours provided? What else was done? Check with the student health service or campus administration.
3. Make a list of safer sex practices. Rate them from 1 to 10 as to their importance in reducing the risk of spreading or contracting an STI.
4. If someone asked you where to get a condom, could you help them? Survey your campus and surrounding community to get the answers to the following questions? Where is the nearest dispenser? Is there one in the women's bathroom in the student center? Where can you find free condoms? Where can you get condoms if you feel embarrassed?

SELECTED BIBLIOGRAPHY

Carpenter, C. "Antiretroviral Therapy in Adults: Updated Recommendations of the International AIDS Society—USA Panel." *Journal of the American Medical Association* 283, no. 3 (2000): 381–390.

Freed, G. L., et al. "Safety of Vaccinations." *Journal of the American Medical Association* 276, no. 23 (1996): 1869–1872.

Lederberg, J., et al. *Emerging Infections: Microbial Threats to Health in the United States.* Washington, DC: The National Academy Press, 1992.

Mikkelson, A. *Condoms Stop HIV Transmission Just as Well as They Do Pregnancy, Not Better.* University of Texas Medical Branch, 1999.

Report of the Global HIV/AIDS Epidemic 2002. Geneva: UNAIDS, 2002.

Rotheram-Borus, M. J., et. al. "HIV Risk Among Homosexual, Bisexual, and Heterosexual Male and Female Youths." *Archives of Sexual Behavior* 28, no. 2 (1999): 159–177.

"Summary of Notifiable Diseases, United States." *Morbidity and Mortality Weekly Report*. Published annually. See also ongoing weekly coverage of selected notifiable disease reports.

The Race Against Lethal Microbes. Chevy Chase, MD: Howard Hughes Medical Institute, 1996.

Tracking the Hidden Epidemics: Trends in STDs in the United States. Atlanta, GA: Centers for Disease Control and Prevention, 2000.

"What to Do About a Cold or Flu," *Consumer Reports*, January 1999.

Zenilman, J. "Chlamydia and Cervical Cancer." *Journal of the American Medical Association* 258, no. 1 (2001): 81–83.

HEALTHLINKS

Websites for Reducing the Risk for Infectious Disease

You can access better health as it relates to this chapter by checking out some of the following sites on the Internet. These sites can be accessed directly from the *Decisions for Healthy Living* Website located at www.aw.com/pruitt.

CDC National Immunization Program

The NIP provides leadership for the planning, coordination, and conduct of immunization activities nationwide. At this site, you can access the latest information on adult and child immunization needs, as well as press releases about emerging infectious diseases.

Immunization Action Coalition

This site provides information about vaccine-preventable diseases, including journal articles and other resources for the public and health professionals.

AIDS Info

AIDS Info provides information about federally approved treament guidelines for HIV and AIDS. AIDS Info is staffed by health information specialists who answer questions about HIV treatment options and refer individuals to an extensive network of federal information services and national and community-based organizations for treatment-related information.

National Center for Infectious Diseases

The NCID site provides the latest information on emerging and re-emerging infectious diseases in the United States and throughout the world.

HEALTH HOTLINES

Reducing the Risk for Infectious Disease

CDC National AIDS, HIV, and Sexually Transmitted Disease Hotline
(800) 342-AIDS (342-2437)
P. O. Box 13827
Research Triangle Park, NC 27709

Hepatitis Hotline
(800) GO LIVER (465-4837)
American Liver Foundation
75 Maiden Lane, Suite 603
New York, NY 10038

TEST YOUR KNOWLEDGE ANSWERS

1. True. Breast milk provides passive immunity to infants. However, this immunity usually lasts only about as long as the mother breast-feeds.
2. False. Antibiotics are ineffective in treating diseases caused by viruses, but are rather used to fight bacterial infections. If a physician prescribes an antibiotic to someone who has a cold or influenza, the purpose of the antibiotic is to reduce any infections that may accompany the cold or flu, not to treat the viral infection.
3. True. The United States leads among all industrialized countries in rates of STIs.
4. True. The human papilloma virus may also play a role in cancer of the vagina, vulva, penis, and anus.
5. False. Women who have gonorrhea are asymptomatic far more often than men. Nearly 80 percent of infected women are unaware of their infection.

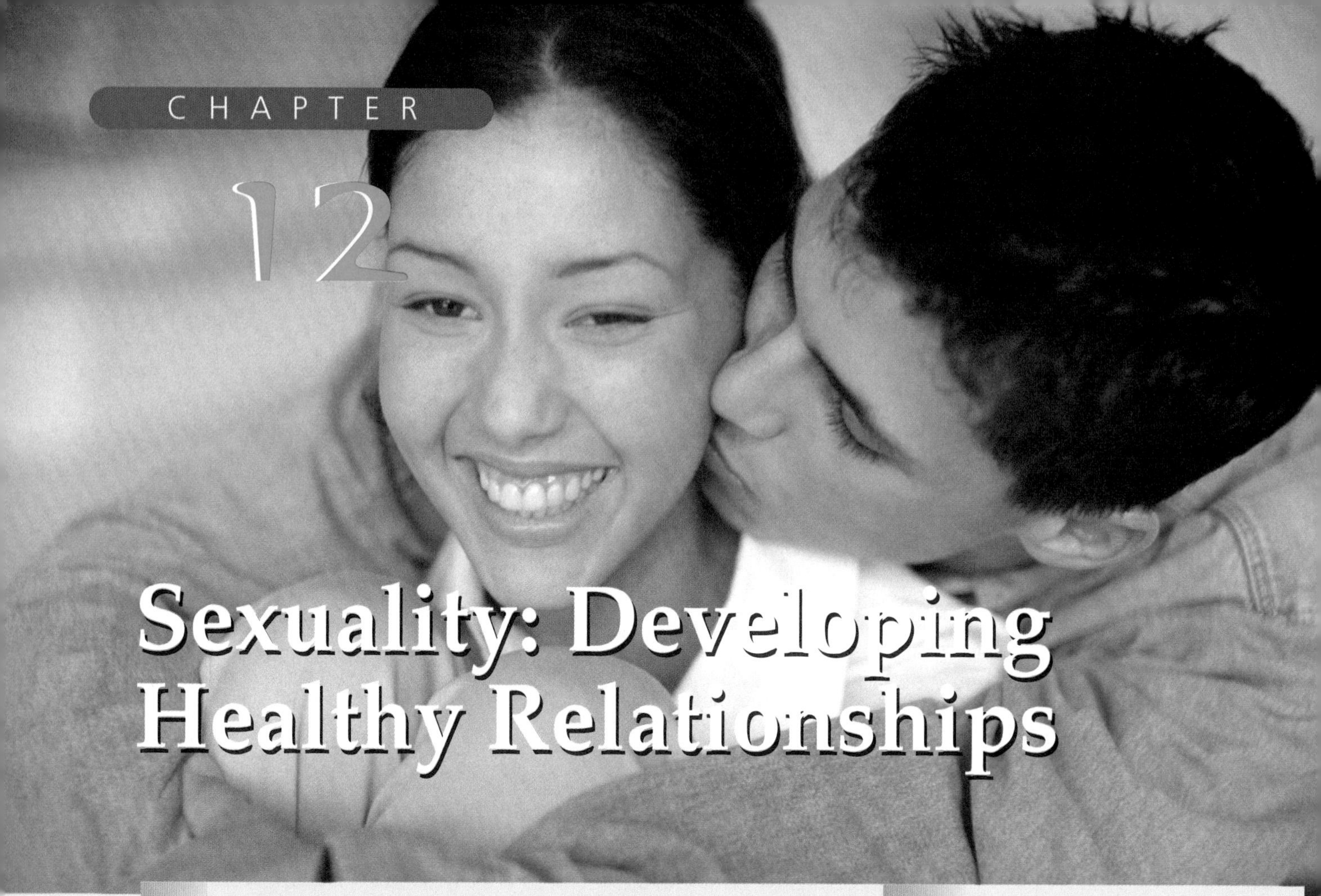

CHAPTER 12

Sexuality: Developing Healthy Relationships

OBJECTIVES

When you finish reading this chapter, you will be able to:

1. Recognize that sexuality is a complex collection of qualities that make up a person's sexual attitudes, influence a person's sexual behaviors, and affect relationships with others.
2. Recognize the four different perspectives—cultural, religious, personal, and biological—from which human sexuality is observed.
3. Explain the importance of gender identity and sex role relative to sexuality.
4. Recognize the hormones that most influence sexual development and secondary sex characteristics.
5. Differentiate between three sexual orientations: heterosexual, homosexual, and bisexual.
6. Recognize that when verbal and nonverbal languages conflict, miscommunication about sexual desires can result.
7. Define love in terms of intimacy, passion, and commitment.
8. Understand that sexual pleasure may take the form of masturbation, outercourse, or intercourse.
9. Understand the pattern of human sexual response, including its four phases: excitement, plateau, orgasm, and resolution.
10. Identify sexual dysfunctions that occur in both men and women, in men alone, and in women alone.

TEST YOUR KNOWLEDGE

1. After conception, the human fetus will develop sex characteristics as genetically directed regardless of hormonal signals. True or False?
2. The hormone testosterone affects sex drive in both men and women. True or False?
3. Androgen is a hormone unique to males that is produced mainly in a man's testicles. Estrogen is a hormone unique to females that is produced mainly in a woman's ovaries. True or False?
4. Vasocongestion, a condition where blood flow into the veins is increased by dilation of the arteries, is a normal response to sexual stimulation. True or False?
5. Most men experience a refractory (recovery) period after orgasm, during which no amount of stimulation can bring on another orgasm. True or False?

Answers found at end of chapter.

Sexuality means something different to almost every person. Over the course of time, it can also mean different things to the same person. Love, lust, intimacy, attraction, and infatuation are some of the feelings that are associated with sexuality. Just as personality is the embodiment of a collection of qualities that make up a person and his or her relationship with others, **sexuality** is the embodiment of a collection of qualities that make up a person's sexual attitudes and behaviors and influence his or her relationships with others.

The term *sexuality* is a broad term encompassing biological, psychological, sociocultural, and ethical components of behavior. Healthy sexuality suggests a number of conditions:

- A state of comfort with your gender and sex role.
- An ability to form positive interpersonal relationships.
- An ability to respond to erotic stimulation with pleasure.
- An ability to make mature judgments about sexuality.

A sense of comfort with your gender suggests an acceptance of your maleness or femaleness. This is sometimes referred to as **gender identity.** Your gender identity is evident in your **sex role** behavior—what you do to disclose yourself as male or female to others.

The ability to form positive interpersonal relationships (with persons of the same or opposite sex) suggests a desire to be close to someone else, the ability to empathize with another person's feelings, and the ability to commit to the importance of a relationship.

The ability to respond to erotic stimulation with pleasure suggests a healthy functioning sexual response, both biological and psychological.

Finally, the ability to make mature judgments about sexuality suggests a clear understanding of personal values and beliefs, the ability to make sex-related decisions that respect the dignity of others while acknowledging personal desires and drives, and the ability to restrain from sexual behavior when conditions suggest risk to personal health or to the health of others. Basic to all is honest and effective communication, particularly about sexual feelings.

Points of View about Sexuality

To further understand sexuality, it is helpful to consider different points of view. Consider the following four perspectives: cultural, religious, personal, and biological. These four points of view have shaped your sexuality to date and will continue to do so throughout your life (see Figure 12.1).

Your Culture

Sexual values, attitudes, and practices differ from culture to culture. Behaviors and attitudes can also differ and change within a culture over time. In the United States, for example, some of the pioneers in the birth control movement were jailed in the 1920s because of their beliefs. Today, various methods of birth control are widely available in drug stores, restrooms, and college health clinics; and most adult American women report using some form of birth control.

sexuality A collection of qualities that make up a person's sexual attitudes and behaviors and influence his or her relationships with others.

gender identity A sense of comfort with one's gender; an acceptance of one's maleness or femaleness.

sex role Overt behaviors that disclose ourselves as male or female to others.

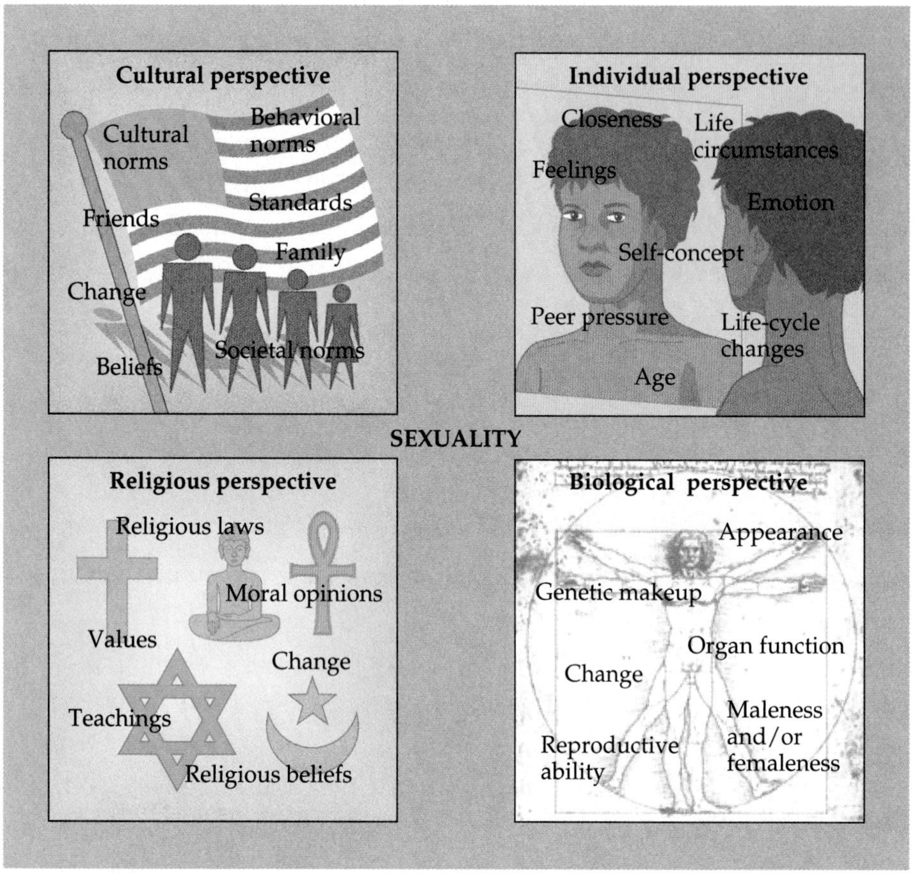

Figure 12.1 Cornerstones of Sexuality
Your sexuality has been shaped by at least four perspectives: biological, cultural, individual, and religious. These four cornerstones will continue to shape your sexuality throughout your life.

American attitudes about sex were strongly influenced by the Puritans, who considered sex a necessary evil. Again, sex was for procreation, not for pleasure. To reinforce this, rigid dress codes were developed to inhibit sexual thoughts or fantasies and temptations. Not all Puritans, however, were so sexually repressed. Early New England church records include the letters CF after a person's name, which refer to "confessing fornication." Another sign is readily seen in some cross-stitched family trees, where the birth date of the firstborn is well shy of nine months before marriage, indicating premarital sex.

Religion continues to affect society's view of sexual practices and behavior. Much of the controversy surrounding issues such as sex education, abortion rights, and sexual orientation has its roots in religion. Religion often plays a major role in the establishment of personal values, beliefs, and a moral and ethical code of conduct. Values, however, arise not only from religious mandates but also from an individual's interpretation of such teachings.

What has come to be known as the **sexual revolution** is a product of the last half of the twentieth century. Increased premarital and extramarital sexual activity and liberalized attitudes toward homosexuality, abortion, masturbation, and pornography are indications of change from earlier standards.

Your Religion

Teachings of all the major religions include standards for sexual conduct. As with cultural values, sexual values are subject to change and interpretation. The Old Testament, for example, endorsed sex for procreation. As it says in Genesis: "Be fruitful and multiply." Adultery, meanwhile, was forbidden and made part of the law in the Ten Commandments: "Thou shalt not commit adultery."

sexual revolution A period of time (thought to have begun in the 1960s) characterized by a significant liberalization of sexual behavior and attitudes.

You as an Individual

As important as culture and religion are to sexual attitudes and behavior, the primary determinant remains you, the individual. No two people are alike. Not only do you differ physically from your best friend but you also differ intellectually, emotionally, and sexually.

In sexual behavior, as in other behaviors, society pressures us to act like everyone else. Many people, both men and women, report that they become sexually active because of peer pressure. They want to appear "normal." Sometimes the desire for social acceptance conflicts with an individual's value system.

The individual perspective on sexuality may change throughout the life cycle. Our lives are made up of stages during which major changes and developments take place. Most broadly, these periods are: Childhood; adolescence; and early, middle, and late adulthood.

In childhood, the family has the most influence on a young person's ideas about sexuality. Sexuality within the family is evident in the sexual interactions of the adults. It is in childhood that sexual identity is estab-

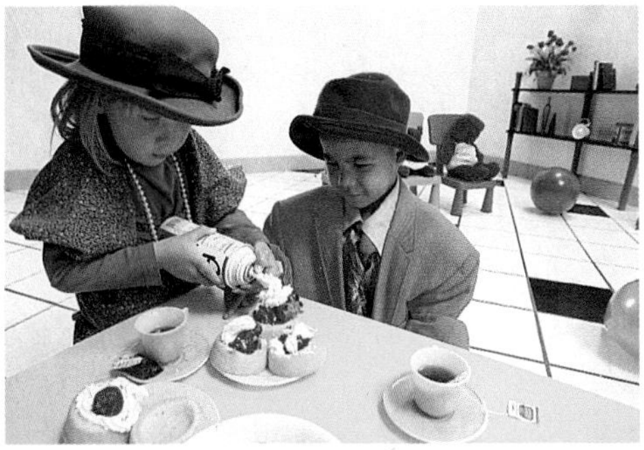
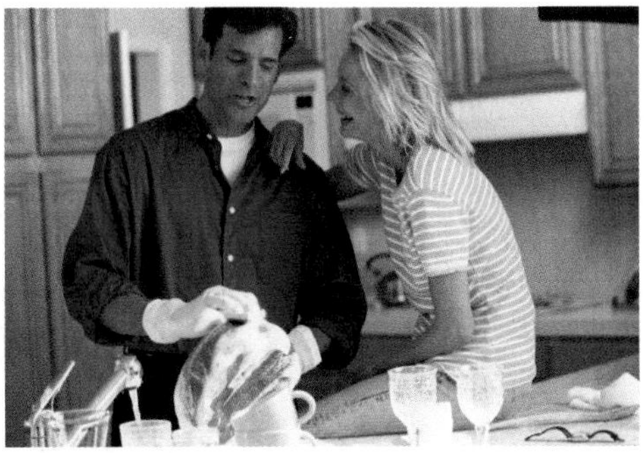

Children learn about sex roles from their family. They progress from playing house as youngsters to keeping house as adults.

lished, sex roles are learned, and beliefs and values about sex and sexuality are established.

Adolescent sexual development is marked by the development of secondary sex characteristics, those physical signs of maturity as one moves from being a child to being a woman or a man. Physical maturity is accompanied by an increased interest in engaging in sexual activity. The physical ability to engage in sexual activity, however, is not always accompanied by the cognitive development needed to understand and to act to prevent the health risks of sexual involvement.

For some people, the transition from **puberty** to adult sexuality is fairly smooth; for others it involves turmoil. Although the changes are predictable, much depends on how each individual perceives them. For example, the experience of pregnancy is significantly different for a married woman in her twenties or thirties who has always wanted to have children than for a teenager whose life is disrupted by the need to drop out of high school, at least temporarily, to deliver and care for her child.

Likewise, changes that take place in late adulthood can bring a renewed sense of intimacy to some people but threaten the sexuality of others. After menopause, some women see themselves as being past their sexual prime. For others, cessation of menstruation increases sexual interest because of the altered ratio of hormones and elimination of fear of pregnancy.

There is no correct, precise timetable for sexual life-cycle changes. Puberty usually takes place in the early teens, but individuals may mature early as well as late. The timing of first sexual intercourse experience likewise depends on physical as well as emotional maturity. Some sexual milestones are missed or are modified to fit a person's lifestyle.

Your Biology

Finally, there is a biological perspective to human sexuality. The functions of the genitalia have not changed for millions of years, yet our understanding of the biological aspects of sex and sexuality has definitely changed. For example, the seminal vesicle was so named because it was believed to be a storage site for sperm. Through scientific study, we now know that the seminal vesicle is a gland that secretes a portion of the semen, not a site for storage. (Sperm are stored for two to four weeks in the epididymis, a sac above the testes.) See *Your Sexual Body: A Primer on Reproductive Anatomy and Physiology* in the Appendix.

After conception, the human fetus has the potential to develop into either sex. After about the seventh week of development, the sex (male or female) is established under the influence of hormones. While genetics determine the genetic sex, hormones bring about differentiation of sexual organs and sexual characteristics. The normal female has two X (female) chromosomes (or XX), and the normal male has one X and one Y (male) chromosome (or XY). The sex chromosome is carried by the sperm. If an X-bearing sperm fertilizes an egg, the resulting XX combination produces a female. If the egg is fertilized by a Y-bearing sperm, the resulting XY combination produces a male. A fetus bearing an XY combination produces significant amounts of **androgens** during fetal development, thus male primary sex characteristics develop. A fetus bearing an XX combination does not produce androgens at a significant level, thus female primary sex characteristics develop.

The later development of physical and psychological sex characteristics is influenced by hormones that are secreted in response to genetic makeup. The hormones that most directly affect sexuality are androgens for men and **estrogens** for women. Androgens are produced chiefly in the testicles but are also produced by women. Estrogens are produced chiefly in the ovaries but are also present in men. Sexuality is adversely affected by a deficiency in these hormones. Men who have an androgen deficiency have a decrease in sexual responsiveness and sexual drive; for women, an estrogen deficiency can cause

puberty A period during early adolescence characterized by rapid physical change. A period during which sexual organs undergo maturation.

androgens Male sex hormones.

estrogens Female sex hormones.

infertility and atrophy of the genitalia. All men, whether they are **heterosexual, homosexual,** or **bisexual,** produce a small amount of estrogen. Homosexuals do not produce an increased estrogen level, nor can their orientation be changed by doses of androgens. Similarly, all women produce some androgens, and lesbians are no more likely to have increased levels of androgens than are heterosexual women.

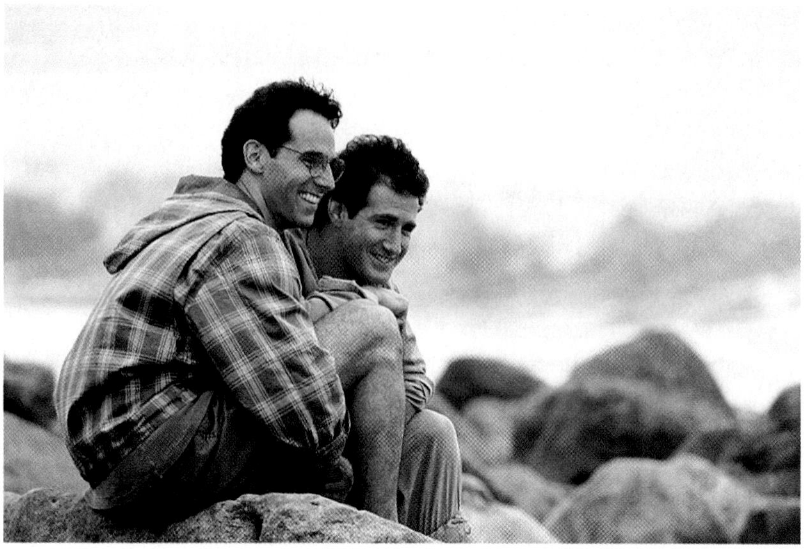

Scientists have not yet explained the origin of sexual orientation, but most do not consider it to be a conscious choice that can be voluntarily changed.

Your Sexual Orientation

Sexual orientation refers to a person's enduring attraction to individuals of a particular gender. Attraction can take many forms, emotional, romantic, or sexual. The word *enduring* is important, because a casual interest in the same or opposite gender is normal throughout life, and especially during early adolescence. Such a normal, but passing, attraction should not be considered a definitive sign of sexual orientation.

Three sexual orientations are commonly recognized: heterosexual, an attraction to individuals of a different sex; homosexual, an attraction to individuals of the same sex; and bisexual, an attraction to individuals of both sexes. Individuals who have a homosexual orientation are often referred to as **gay** (both men and women) or as **lesbian** (women only).

Despite extensive research, scientists have yet to explain the origin of sexual orientation. Some researchers suggest that genetic or inborn hormonal factors determine sexual orientation. Others believe that life experiences during early childhood are most important. Most scientists do agree, however, that sexual orientation is shaped for most people at an early age through the interaction of biological, psychological, and social factors, and sexual orientation is not a conscious choice that can be voluntarily changed.

Numerous false stereotypes and unwarranted prejudices exist toward individuals who have bisexual or homosexual orientations. As a result, the process of "coming out," or publicly confirming one's sexual orientation, can be difficult and may cause emotional pain. Lesbian and gay people often feel "different" and alone when they first become aware of same-sex attractions. They may also fear being rejected by family, friends, coworkers, and religious institutions if they do come out.

American society has traditionally discriminated against homosexual and bisexual individuals by declaring sexual acts between same-sex partners illegal, by not recognizing gay marriages as legal, and by denying custody or adoption of children to same-sex partners. After decades of gay rights activism, however, there has been some movement toward reducing the amount of discrimination based on sexual orientation, and an increasing number of gay couples have commitment services and legal partnerships and are raising families (see Chapter 13).

heterosexual A person who has a sexual attraction to people of a different sex.

homosexual A person who has a sexual attraction to people of the same sex.

bisexual A person who has a sexual attraction to people of both sexes.

sexual orientation A person's enduring attraction to individuals of a particular gender.

gay A homosexual orientation; a homosexual man or woman.

lesbian A homosexual woman.

Communicating about Sex

For many reasons, communicating about sex is difficult. For some college students, lessons learned as a child, such as "don't talk about sex," can create communication gaps between couples. For others, the language available to talk about sex is simply too limiting. For still others, sharing intimate thoughts and desires is psychologically threatening.

The fact is, we communicate about sex whether we know it or not. Our sexuality is communicated through the clothes we wear, the pattern of our speech, and even the way we walk. Our facial expressions and voice tones can communicate sexual attraction, or rejection, even when the subject "sex" is never broached. And we miscommunicate about sex. We may inadvertently send a signal of rejection that we do not really mean. Or we may inadvertently "turn on" someone when our intent is just the opposite.

To avoid the problems that miscommunication brings to a relationship, a couple should first acknowledge the importance of communicating openly about sex. Good communication can result in a more fulfilling relationship for both parties. In contrast, poor communication can result in dissatisfaction and tension and ultimately bring about the breakup of the relationship. Good communication is obviously important for couples who are sexually involved. It is just as important, however, to couples who practice sexual abstinence. **Sexual abstinence** is a behavioral choice to not engage in sexual intercourse. The choice to abstain from sex is not an indication of the absence of sexuality. Individuals or couples who abstain from sexual intercourse may express sexual feelings in a variety of other ways. The most important way that healthy couples who abstain express their sexual feelings is through verbal communications.

Nonverbal communication is a very powerful means of telling a sexual partner about desires, needs, and feelings. Facial expressions such as smiles or frowns clearly communicate pleasure or displeasure. Posture, such as sitting with legs and arms crossed and leaning away from a person, can signal that it is time to stop sexual advances. At the same time, posture that is open, such as two people facing each other with open arms and leaning toward each other, may be seen as an invitation to "go ahead." Moans of pleasure also serve to communicate a go-ahead; no sound or sounds of frustration can signal at least one partner's wish to stop.

When nonverbal language and verbal language conflict, an individual sends a mixed message. For example, when one sexual partner says no but his or her nonverbal responses signal pleasure and encouragement, the other sexual partner has a problem deciding what to do. Does he or she continue sexual activity and honor the nonverbal signals, or stop and honor the verbal signals? How well do you communicate about sex? See the Developing Health Skills box to learn how to say no and yes.

Developing Health Skills

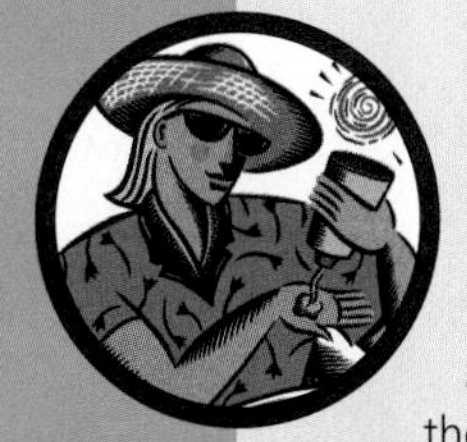

Learning How to Say No and Yes

The following three steps for saying no represent good advice for the person wanting to either avoid or delay sexual contact. By considering these, you can avoid being caught off guard and not knowing how to handle a situation.

1. Express appreciation for the invitation ("Thanks for thinking of me." "It's nice to know that you like me."). Perhaps you may also wish to validate the value of the other person ("You are a good person.").
2. Say no in a clear, unequivocal fashion ("I would prefer not to make love, get involved in a dating relationship," and so forth).
3. Offer an alternative, if applicable ("Perhaps we could have lunch sometime.").

Saying no can be difficult, particularly when sexual play has already started. Saying no should effectively bring sexual activity to a halt.

Saying yes can be more complex than saying no because rather than limiting alternatives, saying yes creates even more alternatives. Yes to what? For how long? Often people allow yes to be communicated through nonverbal means. Lovers often assume that they know what their partners want and need. Of course, it is not possible to literally read another person's mind, so nonverbal communication is open to misinterpretation.

Source: From *Our Sexuality* (with InfoTrac), 7th edition by Crooks/Baur.

Love: The Basis of Intimate Relationships

"How do I love thee? Let me count the ways," wrote Elizabeth Barrett Browning to her husband, Robert, in England in the mid 1800s. Indeed, there are numerous ways to love a person. Now, as then, love plays a major role in establishing a lifestyle as well as in the selection of a sexual partner.

Psychologist Robert Sternberg has identified three components of love:

1. **Intimacy**—the emotional component of love characterized by a desire to be close, to interact at the

sexual abstinence A behavioral choice not to engage in sexual intercourse.

intimacy The emotional component of love characterized by a desire to be close, to interact at the intellectual level, to share feelings, and to acknowledge each other's desires.

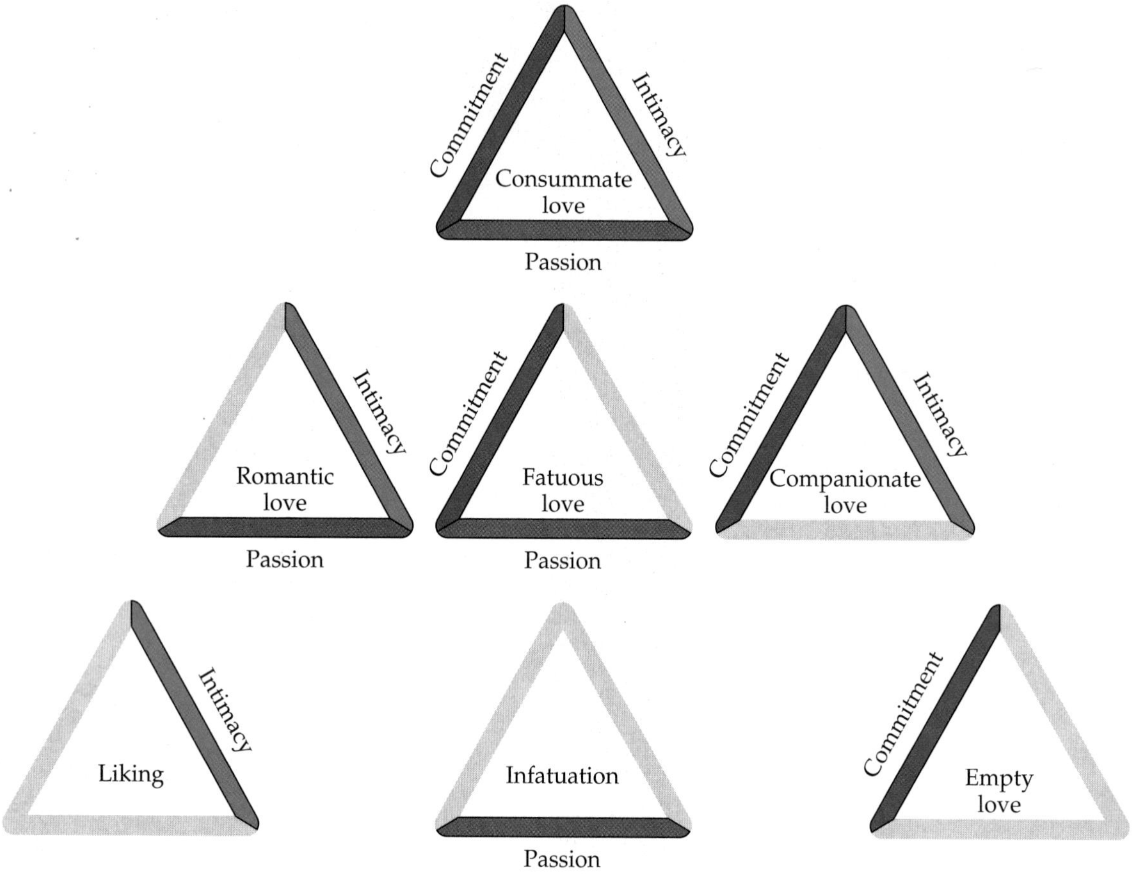

Figure 12.2 The Triangles of Love
The three components of love are intimacy, passion, and commitment. There are seven types of relationships that result from different combinations of these components.

intellectual level, to share feelings, and to acknowledge each other's desires.

2. **Passion**—the motivational component of love characterized by a desire to give and receive sexual pleasure and to achieve sexual gratification.
3. **Commitment**—the cognitive component of love characterized by a desire to maintain a highly valued relationship, even when self-sacrifice is required to do so.

Figure 12.2, the Triangles of Love, identifies the seven types of relationships that result from the different combinations of these three components.

passion The motivational component of love characterized by a desire to give and to receive sexual pleasure and to achieve sexual gratification.

commitment The cognitive component of love characterized by a desire to maintain a highly valued relationship, even when self-sacrifice is required to do so.

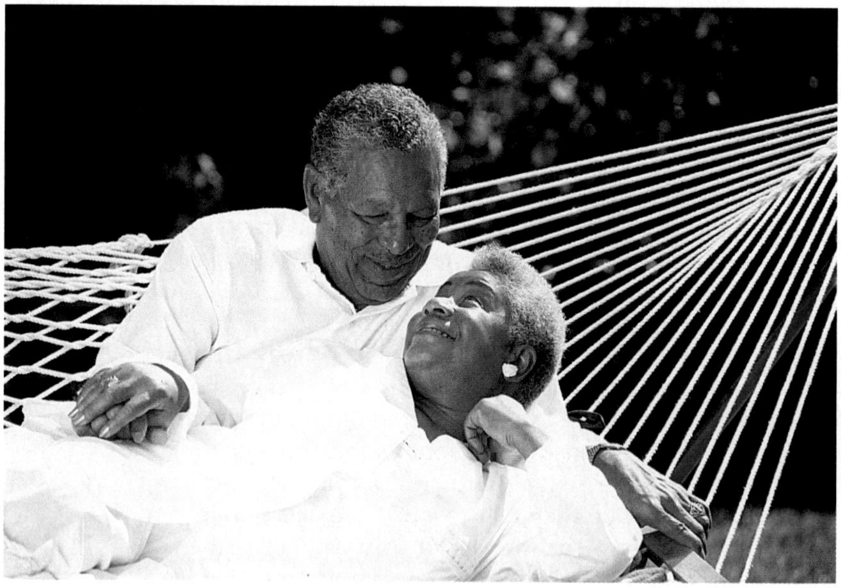

Commitment, along with intimacy and passion, are the three components of love. Commitment involves maintaining a highly valued relationship.
(Source: Stock, Boston)

The term *consummate love* is used for the very special relationships in which all three components of love—commitment, intimacy, and passion—are present. This complete love is the goal of many relationships, but it is difficult to achieve and even more difficult to maintain.

Romantic love involves intimacy and passion but no commitment. An example is the form of love experienced in a summer affair. It may be very romantic for the duration of the relationship, but it ends when the summer is over.

Fatuous love is exemplified by commitment and passion but no intimacy. Intimacy takes time to develop. Fatuous love usually develops very quickly, as in the case when two people meet, one week later are engaged, and two weeks later are married. Relationships based on this type of love usually do not work out.

Companionate love involves commitment and intimacy but no passion. Long-term friendship and the marriage in which physical attraction has died down are illustrations of this kind of love.

Liking involves only intimacy and refers to a relationship in which communication is possible. Friendship is apparent, there is warmth and closeness, but nothing more. Good friends like each other.

Infatuation involves only passion. This kind of love arrives very quickly and can be gone just as fast. You meet a person at a party and are sexually aroused. You go out together, have sex together and then the affair is over. Sometimes infatuation does not even involve an interpersonal relationship. A person can be infatuated with someone without having the nerve to speak to him or her.

Empty love involves only commitment. This kind of love may be seen in a long-term marriage in which the passion is gone and intimacy is only a memory. Habit replaces desire.

A healthy relationship exists when two individuals love each other with the same type of love and within an atmosphere of equality. An unhealthy relationship exists when two people don't "match," yet remain together. Add sex to the formula, and the complexity of relationships becomes greater. A healthy relationship may or may not involve sexual intercourse. When two sexual partners love each other, sexual intercourse may be an appropriate expression of that love. For religious, moral, and other reasons, such as wanting to avoid a pregnancy or a sexually transmitted infection, two people who love each other may choose to delay sexual intercourse. To see if you are ready for a mature sexual relationship, see the Assess Your Health box.

Assess Your Health

Are You Ready for a Mature Sexual Relationship?

There is no checklist that can determine when a person is ready to have a mature sexual relationship, but having certain personal characteristics can be an indication of readiness. Here are some questions that will help you determine if you are ready for a mature sexual relationship.

- **Commitment:** Is your relationship committed, mutually kind, and understanding?
- **Trust:** Do you trust and admire each other? Is your relationship honest? If you have intercourse, do you know what it will mean?
- **Motivation:** Is your motivation for this sexual relationship pleasure and intimacy? Have you experimented and found pleasure in nonpenetrative behaviors? Will a sexual relationship be mutually pleasurable? Have you enjoyed other sexual behaviors with your partner? Is your partner as committed to your pleasure as to her/his own?
- **Communication:** Have you talked about sexual behaviors before they occur? Is your relationship consensual? Have you talked about how far to go? Do you both agree?
- **Safety:** Is the setting for the sexual relationship safe and comfortable? Have you taken steps to protect yourself against pregnancy and/or disease? Have you obtained condoms and contraception (if penile/vaginal intercourse is planned)?

Source: Adapted SIECUS Fact Sheet (2002), *How do I Know if I'm Ready for Sex?* Reprinted by permission of SIECUS, 130 W. 42nd Street, New York, NY 10036-7802

Sexual Relationships

Once the decision is made to have sexual intercourse, it is important to understand both biological and psychological sex drives and responses. The sex drive, the practice of giving and receiving sexual pleasure, and physiological sexual response cycles are common to everyone, regardless of sexual orientation or practice.

Sex Drive

The **sex drive** is the biological urge or appetite for sexual activity. It usually arises in the mind and produces feelings of restlessness and an openness to sexual stimuli. The primary biological function of the sex drive is its contribution to human reproduction and continuation of the species. **Libido,** another term for the sex drive, changes according to a number of factors. The hormone testosterone, for example, affects the sex drive in both males and females. When levels of testosterone are relatively low, the drive for sexual activity is likewise low. As the level of testosterone rises, so does the sex drive. Other factors affecting the sex drive are sexual images, memories, and fantasies.

The sex drive is usually satisfied through physical stimulation. This can be achieved through sexual intercourse and/or **masturbation** (self-stimulation). Most studies on sexual behavior report that more than 90 percent of men and 60 percent of women have masturbated. No evidence supports the notion that masturbation causes any psychological or physical harm. Rather, there is reason to believe that it provides a safe and private outlet for sexual desires.

The sex drive serves much more than a biological purpose. It contributes to the development of interpersonal relationships as well. Specifically, it contributes to the initial attraction of one person to another and to the ultimate intimacy of a relationship by providing pleasure and fulfillment. Initial attraction is very important in our culture. Think about how much you deliberate about what to wear before you go out. Couples play out extensive scripts to make a positive impression on each other, including a positive sexual impression.

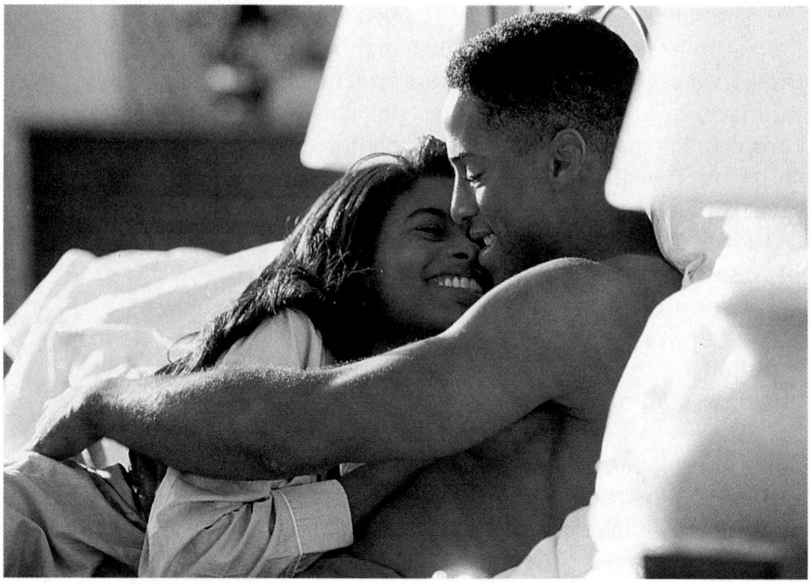

Physical stimulation can produce an elevated level of sexual excitement and pleasure. It can be as simple as hugging or more physically involved as stimulating certain erogenous zones.

sex drive The biological urge or appetite for sexual activity; also called libido.

libido The biological urge or appetite for sexual activity; also called sex drive.

masturbation Sexual self-stimulation.

erogenous zones Those areas of the body especially susceptible to sexual arousal such as the penis, vagina, clitoris, and nipples.

foreplay Sexual pleasuring.

outercourse Mutual masturbation; when two people manually stimulate one another's genitals to achieve sexual pleasure.

intercourse Sexual behavior involving penetration, usually of the penis of a man into the vagina of a woman; term applies to a variety of sexual behaviors, including anal, vaginal, and oral stimulation and/or penetration.

Sexual Pleasuring

Physical stimulation, particularly of certain **erogenous zones** (those areas of the body especially susceptible to sexual arousal, such as the penis, vagina, clitoris, and nipples), produces an elevated level of sexual excitement and pleasure. Sexual pleasure can be the result of interaction between two individuals, or it can be accomplished through masturbation. Sexual fantasy can also be very effective in stimulating a pleasurable response. Recent studies, however, point out that both positive and negative effects can result from sexual fantasy. Whereas some individuals find pleasure in it, others feel guilt and shame.

Foreplay is a term often used for sexual pleasuring. This can be as simple as touching or hugging. Kissing represents a more intimate form of sexual pleasuring. Manually stimulating each other's genitals represents even more intimate sexual pleasuring, and is sometimes referred to as **outercourse.** Because of the threat of sexually transmitted infections and unwanted pregnancy, many couples are choosing this as an alternative to intercourse.

The term **intercourse** literally means "running between." Other formal terms for intercourse include *copulation* (coupling or joining) and *coitus* (a coming together). Perhaps the most common term for sexual intercourse is *making love.*

Intercourse is traditionally defined in terms of heterosexual relations. When a man and a woman have sexual intercourse, the penis enters the vagina. Intercourse is also used for sexual activity between members of the same sex, for example in the phrase *anal intercourse*. Intercourse serves several functions, including achieving and giving physical gratification, expressing love, communicating, and reproducing.

The Body's Sexual Response

What happens to the body before, during, and after sexual activity? The human sexual response is highly individualized. If asked, each person is likely to describe different physical and emotional responses. However, common physiological changes take place in both men and women.

Physiological Changes

The two major processes that play a role in how the body responds to sexual stimulation are vasocongestion and myotonia. **Vasocongestion** refers to the pooling of blood in tissues that takes place during sexual excitement. Under normal circumstances, the inflow of blood through the arteries is balanced by an outflow through the veins. During sexual arousal, however, the flow of blood into the veins is increased by dilation of the arteries. This increase in blood results in engorgement of certain areas of the body, including the penis, testicles, clitoris, labia minora, and nipples.

Myotonia refers to muscle tension, a normal response to sexual stimulation. Some of these motions are voluntary, such as muscle flexing; others are involuntary, such as muscle spasms during orgasm.

Vasocongestion and myotonia each build up during sexual excitement and release afterwards.

Masters and Johnson's Four-Stage Model

In the 1960s, sex therapists William Masters and Virginia Johnson proposed their four-stage model of sexual response after studying hundreds of individuals during sexual activity. This model is widely accepted among sexologists today. The four stages are excitement, plateau, orgasm, and resolution. The stages may vary tremendously in length and intensity, and considerable variety in both may be expected even within individuals. The order of the stages, however, remains the same (see Figure 12.3).

Excitement is the period of time when the body initially responds to sexual stimulation. In the man, the first evidence of excitement is erection of the penis. In the woman, the first signs include vaginal lubrication and often nipple and clitoral erection. In both sexes, the heart rate increases, as does the rate of breathing. The excitement stage can last less than a minute or as long as several hours.

The **plateau** phase is the stage of sexual stimulation just prior to orgasm. The word plateau connotes a leveling off, but as a sexual response, it may be a period of increasing and decreasing sexual stimulation. The plateau phase varies in length from a very brief, undetectable period of seconds to a very lengthy period of an hour or more.

During the plateau phase, muscle tension remains evident and may increase, deep breathing continues, and the heart rate remains elevated. The clitoris often retracts during this phase of sexual excitement. This normal occurrence should not be misread as a sign of loss of sexual desire. In both sexes, a sex flush, a reddening of the skin due to surface circulation of blood, may spread, causing the sexually stimulated person to feel hot to the touch. The term *hot* has come to mean sexually stimulated.

The **orgasm** is perhaps the least understood phase of the sexual response cycle because each person experiences it in a different way. Scientists have been

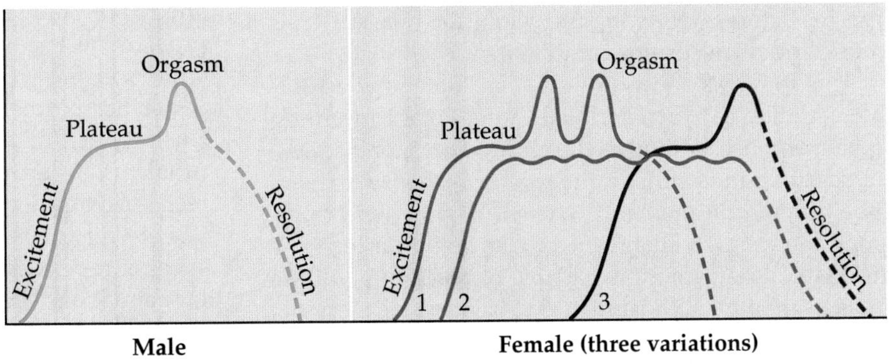

Figure 12.3 The Four Stages of Response
Masters and Johnson's four-stage model of sexual response includes excitement, plateau, orgasm, and resolution.

vasocongestion The pooling of blood in tissues during sexual excitement.

myotonia Muscle tension in response to sexual stimulation.

excitement The period of time when the body initially responds to sexual stimulation; includes erection of the penis in men and vaginal lubrication and clitoral erection in women.

plateau The stage of sexual stimulation just prior to orgasm consisting of increasing and decreasing sexual stimulation.

orgasm The climax phase of sexual excitement.

much more successful in learning what an orgasm is not than in learning what it is. For example, scientific study has shown that Sigmund Freud's theory about orgasm and masturbation is incorrect. He believed that there is a difference between orgasm reached during intercourse (mature orgasm) and that reached through masturbation (immature orgasm).

Physiologically, an orgasm is a reflex action usually elicited by tactile stimulation. It is the shortest phase of the sexual response cycle and typically lasts just a few seconds. Just prior to orgasm, the sexually stimulated person usually experiences a sensation of inevitability, a no-turning-back-now response. A tremendous buildup is followed by a rush, an explosion of feeling or a sense of euphoria. Following the orgasm, a great sense of relief from the tension that was building up is experienced.

In men, an orgasm is accompanied by ejaculation of semen. The semen is a milky fluid containing sperm from the testicles, sugars, bicarbonate buffers, and coagulators. These are all necessary to ensure that sperm have a chance to reach an unfertilized egg. In women, the orgasm is accompanied by quick rhythmic contractions of the uterus and vagina. In both men and women, orgasm does not necessarily happen in every sexual encounter.

Resolution follows orgasm, and the physiological responses reverse. Vasocongestion and myotonia subside. A sense of gratification is felt, and relaxation overcomes the body. Some individuals experience exhaustion and sleep. Women may experience multiple orgasms before completing the resolution phase. This is an uncommon occurrence among men.

It is important to point out that there is considerable variation between and within the sexes concerning sexual response. Although the ability to respond to sexual stimulation is similar, the rate of response appears to be different in men and women. Women tend to respond more slowly than men, but, as noted earlier, once stimulated, they are more capable of reaching multiple orgasms than men. Most men experience a recovery period, or a **refractory period,** after orgasm. This period can last from a few minutes to a few hours and even longer in older men. During the refractory period, no amount of stimulation can bring on another orgasm. There are other differences in sexual response between the sexes, but as more and more is learned, the similarities discovered far outnumber the differences.

resolution The stage of sexual response following orgasm in which physiological responses reverse and a sense of relaxation overcomes the body.

refractory period The recovery period experienced by most men after orgasm; during this period a man does not respond to sexual stimulation.

sexual dysfunctions Disorders that interfere with the ability to enjoy a healthy sexual experience.

inhibited sexual desire Persistent or recurrent deficiency (or absence) of desire for sexual activity.

Sexual Dysfunctions

Unfortunately, not everyone can respond normally to sexual stimulation. Collectively, the disorders that interfere with the ability to enjoy a healthy sexual experience are called **sexual dysfunctions.** They may be very mild and create only slight discomfort, or they may be so severe as to completely prevent a person from participating in sexual activities. *The Diagnostic and Statistical Manual of Mental Disorders, IV* identifies sexual dysfunction as a lack of sexual desire, lack of response to sexual stimulation, an inability to reach orgasm, or pain experienced during intercourse.

Some sexual dysfunctions have an organic cause and are due to structural problems or result from a disease involving the sexual organs. Others are the result of medications that interfere with normal sexual functioning. More commonly, sexual dysfunctions result from psychological causes, such as traumatic sexual experiences or simple ignorance about sexual practice.

Inhibited sexual desire is a sexual dysfunction that affects both men and women. It is difficult to define this problem because there is no normal level of desire. One criterion is how often a person's desire for sex matches his or her partner's. Frequent mismatches may lead to frustrations, misunderstandings, and communication problems. Severe desire problems may result from incorrect sex education (for example, believing that the genitals are dirty and should be avoided) or sexual trauma such as rape. Less severe problems result from temporary situations such as the birth of a baby or fatigue.

It is important to note that sexual problems may arise when the goal of sexual behavior is orgasm or mutual orgasm. It is not dysfunctional if one or both partners do not experience an orgasm during each sexual encounter. In fact, the expectation of orgasm can become a form of performance anxiety and actually lead to dysfunction.

Although the "I-have-a-headache" syndrome is a common means of communicating a disinterest in sex, it does not necessarily represent a sexual dysfunction. Each individual's desire for sex varies greatly. Only when the lack of desire persists and threatens the relationship can it be considered dysfunctional.

At the opposite end of the spectrum are people who are addicted to sex. As with all other addictions, sex addiction is an attempt to fill a vacuum resulting from in-

Developing Health Skills

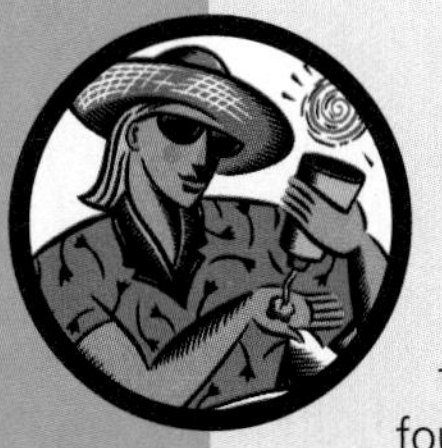

Consumer Health: New Treatments for Impotence

"I feel like I'm thirty years old," says one sixty-three-year-old man, who suffered from impotence after an operation for prostate cancer. His fountain of youth comes in the form of Viagra, a pill that he takes one hour before sex, which gives him the stimulation he needs to get an erection.

Once a taboo topic, advertisements for impotence now appear on prime-time television and in newspapers across the country. As a result, more and more men are seeking help. There are so many options on the market today that experts who specialize in sexual behavior are talking about a new sexual or Viagra revolution that could turn the estimated 20 to 30 million U.S. men who suffer from impotence into "virile teenagers" again. Sex researchers previously believed that nearly all impotence was psychological. Today, urologists (specialists in the genitourinary tract in males and urinary tract in females) believe that between 80 and 85 percent of impotence cases are caused by medical or physiological reasons. As one urologist says: "Really, it's all hydraulics."

Treatments available today include:

- A drug, such as Viagra, if taken about an hour before sex works in response to physical stimulation to cause an erection. Success rates for an erection range from 60 percent with few side effects to 80 percent with headaches and diarrhea. It should not be taken more than once a day.
- Oral testosterone can reduce impotence in some men with low levels of natural testosterone, but no scientific studies have proved its effectiveness. There are some observed improvements following use of testosterone, but this may be due to the placebo effect (a change that results simply from the patient's believing that an improvement will occur).
- A drug-laden pellet inserted about an inch into urethra can cause an erection within eight to ten minutes and may last 30 to 60 minutes. Common side effects include aching in the penis, testicles, and the area between the penis and rectum; a burning sensation in the urethra; redness of the penis due to increased blood flow; and minor urethral bleeding or spotting.
- An injection in the base of the penis 20 minutes before sex can cause an erection. It is effective in more than 50 percent of cases, but some of the injection therapies may be painful and cannot be used every day. It also can cause persistent erection and scarring.
- A pump placed around a sheathed penis just before sex causes an erection until the elastic ring at the base of the penis is taken off. While it is clumsy and sometimes makes ejaculation difficult, the pump has few physical side effects.
- Surgery that repairs arteries to boost the blood supply to the penis can restore the ability to have a normal erection. This procedure is effective only when the impotence problem is caused by a simple vascular injury.
- A penile implant, which is either malleable or inflatable and contains a pump and reservoir of saline solution, can cause an erection that lasts until the implant is unbent or drained. It can destroy erectile tissue.

Medical interventions will not solve all problems. For example, taking an impotence drug or injection to solve marital difficulties may not do the job. It might be better, says one sex therapist, for couples to learn how to accept each other's changing bodies. But one patient who had his prostate removed says, "If women can get face-lifts, why shouldn't men do this?"

adequacies and/or insecurities. For these individuals, sex is a consuming passion and overwhelming need that must be satisfied, even if it means risking their jobs, their families, or other relationships. Men and women who are addicted to sex usually have low self-esteem. After a sexual encounter, a sex addict is typically overcome with feelings of worthlessness, anxiety, agitation, guilt, depression, or shame and is driven to have sex once again in order to block out those feelings.

Male Problems

Among the many male sexual dysfunctions, two types appear more often than others: **premature ejaculation** and erectile dysfunction (also called **impotence**).

Rapid or premature ejaculation is considered the most prevalent sexual dysfunction in men. Ejaculation is considered too rapid only if the sexual partner is unable to achieve orgasm because of the premature ejaculation and subsequent loss of interest on the part of the man.

premature ejaculation Persistent or recurrent ejaculation occurring after minimal sexual stimulation or before, on, or shortly after penetration and before the person wishes it.

impotence Persistent or recurrent inability to attain erection or to maintain it until completion of the sexual activity.

Impotence is the inability to achieve and maintain an erection long enough to participate in sexual intercourse. Occasional erectile problems are very common and with an understanding partner present little or no difficulty for the relationship. When erectile problems occur in a chronic manner, over a long period of time, or repeatedly to the extent that the relationship is hurt, therapy is recommended. Prescription drugs are available that, in some cases, successfully treat erectile dysfunctions by increasing blood flow to the penis. With increased blood flow, a man is able to become sexually aroused, and maintain an erection longer (see the Developing Health Skills box).

Female Problems

Just as with men, many sexual dysfunctions occur among women. Two major ones are lack of orgasm and penetration problems.

The failure to reach orgasm by women is called **female orgasmic disorder.** It is attributed to a number of factors, including psychological inhibition and the fear of losing control. It may also result from limited sexual experience. Failure to experience orgasm during intercourse alone is not a sexual dysfunction. Repeated failure to the point of creating relationship problems, however, does suggest the need for some form of therapy.

A second and far more serious set of problems relates to penetration of the penis into the vagina. Vaginismus and dyspareunia are examples of two penetration-related conditions that cause serious interference with healthy sexual expression. **Vaginismus** is the involuntary constriction of the vagina. When this occurs, intercourse is impossible. Vaginismus usually has psychological origins, such as negative ideas about sex. Women who have been raped sometimes develop vaginismus. This condition requires therapy but is treatable.

Dyspareunia is a term that refers to painful intercourse. Pain and discomfort can be felt if lubrication is insufficient or if a disease is present. Lubrication problems that produce painful intercourse can sometimes be treated simply by extending the period of foreplay to allow adequate sexual excitement to occur. If adequate lubrication remains a problem, topical lubricants can be purchased at a pharmacy. Painful intercourse caused by diseases such as yeast infections or by allergic reactions to douches or birth control methods such as foam are relieved as soon as the disease causing the problem is cured or the source of allergic reaction is eliminated. In some cases, dyspareunia persists and requires more extensive therapy.

female orgasmic disorder Persistent or recurrent delay in, or absence of, orgasm in a female following a normal sexual excitement phase.

vaginismus Recurrent or persistent involuntary spasm of the musculature of the outer third of the vagina that interferes with sexual intercourse.

dyspareunia Painful intercourse.

sensate focus A therapeutic technique in which a couple is taught the nonverbal communication of touching in order to help alleviate difficulty having sexual intercourse or performance anxiety.

Therapeutic Interventions

Treatment of sexual dysfunctions involves medical, educational, and/or psychological interventions. A medical evaluation is necessary for many sexual dysfunctions in order to diagnose possible organic causes of the problem. A physician looks for structural problems and for diseases that may contribute to the sexual dysfunction.

Therapy may involve basic sex education, including instruction in methods of sexual technique and expression. Although sex is seen as a natural process that requires no instruction, evidence is clear that some knowledge of how the body responds to sexual stimulation can be beneficial.

Another form of therapy involves learning more about how to communicate sexual feelings. **Sensate focus** is a therapeutic technique in which a couple is taught the nonverbal communication of touching. It is used in treating couples who have difficulty having sexual intercourse or who experience performance anxiety.

The most complex problems related to sexual dysfunction require psychotherapy. For example, victims of rape or incest or individuals who have developed aversions to their genitalia may require extensive therapy.

To function well sexually, an individual must be able to abandon himself or herself to the erotic experience. A healthy sexual response is one that is unencumbered by guilt and anxiety.

CASE STUDY 12: Sexuality

Jorge was putting pressure on Marisa to have sex, but she wasn't sure she wanted to. She liked him, and they had a good time together going to the movies, but she felt the relationship was superficial. They laughed and had fun together, but they never had a serious discussion about how they felt about things that were important to each other. "Maybe he's immature," thought Marisa, "or maybe we just aren't right for each other." Whatever the reason, it was holding Marisa back from further involvement; and because communication between them was so poor, Marisa didn't think her feelings would change. Marisa decided that she was going to say no to Jorge—and to a relationship that never seemed to develop fully.

Alan and Nadia had been dating for a few months, and they both felt very comfortable with each other. They had so much in common, and they loved talking with each other and sharing ideas. When Nadia was upset over a poor grade on her English paper, Alan knew just what to say to make her feel better; and when either of them got an A, they celebrated together. Even though Alan was reluctant at first to talk about himself and what some of his dreams were for life after college, Nadia made him feel comfortable. Because of the trust they shared in each other, Nadia and Alan were able to discuss their fears and needs openly as their relationship grew and became more intimate.

In Your Opinion

Being able to communicate your feelings is an important component in the decision to say yes or no to having sex. Marisa and Nadia had different communication experiences—and different outcomes.

- Most people who are sexually active have said yes to sex sometimes and no on other occasions. What factors go into such a decision?
- What can a couple do to make sure that they are openly communicating with each other?
- How can a couple know when they are not communicating well? Identify specific signs of poor communication.
- What are the hazards of becoming sexually involved with someone who is difficult to talk with?

KEY CONCEPTS

1. Sexuality is the embodiment of a collection of qualities that make up a person's sexual attitudes and behaviors and his or her sexual relationships with others.
2. A specific individual's attitudes toward sexuality vary over time. Major sexual life-cycle changes include puberty, marriage, pregnancy, child rearing, menopause, and postmenopause.
3. Sexual orientation refers to the focus of a person's sexual interest—people of the opposite sex, the same sex, or both.
4. Good communication can result in a more fulfilling sexual relationship.
5. When nonverbal language and verbal language conflict, an individual is sending mixed messages.
6. Three components of love are intimacy (the emotional component), passion (the motivational component), and commitment (the cognitive component).
7. The sex drive, or libido, is the biological urge or appetite for sexual activity. It usually arises in the mind and produces feelings of restlessness and an openness to sexual stimuli.
8. Masters and Johnson's four-stage model of sexual response includes excitement, plateau, orgasm, and resolution.
9. Sexual dysfunctions can have an organic cause, due to structural problems or a disease, or a psychological basis, due to traumatic sexual experiences.
10. Treatment of sexual dysfunction involves medical, educational, and/or psychological interventions.

REVIEW QUESTIONS

1. Define the term *sexuality* by drawing a comparison between it and the concept of "personality."
2. Identify four perspectives from which human sexuality is observed.
3. Differentiate between gender identity and sex role relative to sexuality.

4. Explain the function of androgens and estrogens relative to sexual development and secondary sex characteristics.
5. Explain the similarities and differences between the heterosexual, homosexual, and bisexual sexual orientations.
6. Explain the importance of communication between two sexual partners and give an example of how verbal and nonverbal communication may conflict.
7. List the seven types of love according to Sternberg and explain the role of intimacy, passion, and commitment in each type.
8. Describe the difference between masturbation, outercourse, and intercourse.
9. Diagram and explain Masters and Johnson's four-stage model of human sexual response.
10. Identify two sexual dysfunctions common to men and two sexual dysfunctions common to women, and describe the symptoms and possible origin of each.

CRITICAL THINKING QUESTIONS

1. The sexual revolution of the 1960s was characterized by significant sexual behavioral changes. Based on what you know about it, what social impact do you think it has had on us today—positive and negative? What do you think the next sexual revolution will bring? Whereas the birth control pill played a major role in the last sexual revolution, what technology, drug, or social viewpoint might play the primary role in the next revolution?
2. The *Healthy People 2010* objectives include the following: "Increase the proportion of adolescents who abstain from sexual intercourse or use condoms if currently sexually active." In support of this objective, Congress has allocated large sums of money over the past several years to promote sexual abstinence. Will this initiative be effective? What accounts for an adolescent's decision to become sexually active? Will teenagers delay sexual involvement because the federal government, media campaigns, or their parents encourage them to do so?
3. Psychologists believe that negative attitudes toward homosexuals as a group do not result from actual experience with lesbians or gay men but rather from stereotypes and prejudices. What can be done to address prejudice and reduce the acts of violence against homosexuals?
4. The *Healthy People 2010* objectives include the following: "Increase the number of positive messages related to responsible sexual behavior during weekday and nightly prime-time television programming." Is it possible to know the effect of the media on the sexual behavior of the viewing public? Will the portrayal of "responsible" sexual behavior positively influence the sexual behavior of people watching TV? Should the media be restricted from portraying sexual themes or does freedom of speech extend to the freedom to explicitly show this?

JOURNAL ACTIVITIES

1. Make a list of your sexual turn-ons and turn-offs. Turn-ons are things that attract you to or excite you about another person. Turn-offs do just the opposite. Your class might want to compare the lists developed by women with those developed by men.
2. Identify as many ways as you can think of to express affection to another person in the absence of sexual intercourse. (This might include going for a walk together, holding hands, etc.)
3. Examine public expression of affection on your campus. Which behaviors do you feel are acceptable, and which offend you? Write a paragraph about your feelings.
4. With another member of your class, go to a movie or watch a television show. Afterwards, compare thoughts on the sexual relationships portrayed. Were they healthy or unhealthy? Positive or negative?

SELECTED BIBLIOGRAPHY

The Boston Women's Health Book Collective. *Our Bodies, Ourselves for the New Century.* Old Tappan, NJ: Simon & Schuster, 1998.

Browning, J. R., et al. "Power, Gender, and Sexual Behavior." *Journal of Sex Research* 36, no. 4 (1999): 342–347.

Eisenberg, M. "Differences in Sexual Risk Behaviors between College Students with Same-Sex and Opposite-Sex Experience: Results from a National Survey," *Archives of Sexual Behavior* 32, no. 6 (2001): 575–589.

Laumann, E. O., Paik, A., Rosen, R. C. "Sexual Dysfunction in the United States: Prevalence and Predictors." *Journal of the American Medical Association* 281, no. 6 (1999): 537–544.

Masters, W., and Johnson, V. *Human Sexual Response.* Boston: Little, Brown, 1996.

Rathus, S. A., Nevid, J. S., and Fichner-Rathus, L. *Human Sexuality in a World of Diversity*, 2nd ed. Boston: Allyn and Bacon, 2002.

Renaud, C. A., and Byers, E. S. "Positive and Negative Sexual Cognitions: Subjective Experience and Relationships to Sexual Adjustment." *Journal of Sex Research* 38, no. 3 (2001): 252–263.

Sternberg, R. *Love is a Story.* New York: Oxford University Press, 1998.

Surgeon General's Call to Action to Promote Sexual Health and Responsible Sexual Behavior. Rockville, MD: U.S. Office of the Surgeon General, 2001.

Thornton, A., and Young-DeMarco, L. "Four Decades of Trends in Attitudes Toward Family Issues in the United States: The 1960s Through the 1990s." *Journal of Marriage and Family,* 63. no. 4 (November 2001): 1009–1037.

White, K. *Sexual Liberation or Sexual License? The American Revolt Against Victorianism.* Chicago: Ivan Dee Publishers, 2000.

HEALTHLINKS

Websites for Developing Healthy Relationships

You can access better health as it relates to this chapter by checking out some of the following sites on the Internet. These sites can be accessed directly from the *Decisions for Healthy Living* Website located at www.aw.com/pruitt.

Alan Guttmacher Institute

A direct link with one of the top research institutes in the country dedicated to sexual behavior and human reproduction.

Planned Parenthood

An online source for sexual and reproductive health information.

Sexuality Information and Education Council of the United States (SIECUS)

Information, guidelines, and materials for advancement of healthy and proper sex education.

HEALTH HOTLINES

Developing Healthy Relationships

American Association for Marriage and Family Therapy (AAMFT)
(202) 452-0109
112 South Alfred Street
Alexandria, VA 22314-3061

Impotence Information Center
(800) 843-4315
10700 Bren Road West
Minnetonka, MN 55343

TEST YOUR KNOWLEDGE ANSWERS

1. False. Regardless of genetic predisposition, sex characteristics develop in response to hormones. Therefore, the human fetus has the potential of developing into either a male or female regardless of its chromosomal make-up.
2. True. For both men and women, when testosterone levels are low, the sex drive is low; when they are high, so is the sex drive.
3. False. Both androgen and estrogen are produced by both men and women.
4. True. The increase in blood results in engorgement of the penis, clitoris, labia minora, and nipples.
5. True. Men cannot be stimulated after an orgasm for a period lasting from a few minutes to a few hours. Women are able to have multiple orgasms.

CHAPTER

13

Planning a Family

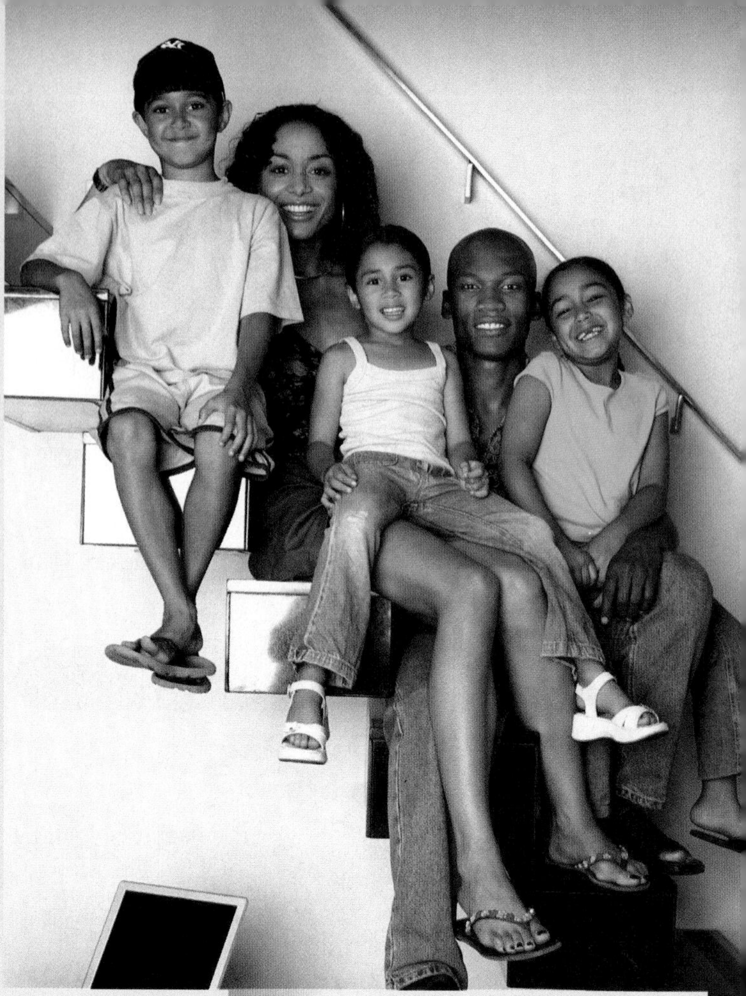

OBJECTIVES

When you finish reading this chapter, you will be able to:

1. Differentiate between family structures, including the nuclear family, the extended family, and the dual-career family and consider the place of traditional marriage in each family structure.
2. Define marriage as an institution and describe elements of marriage that contribute to a healthy life.
3. List issues that a couple should consider when deciding whether or not to have children.
4. Explain the concepts of and give support for preconception care and prenatal care as important health factors of a pregnancy.
5. Identify two means of studying fetal cells in order to test for the presence or absence of genetic abnormalities.
6. Describe fetal development, beginning with conception and carrying through each trimester to birth.
7. Understand the process of labor and delivery, including the three stages of labor.
8. Understand the place of birth control in overall family planning and identify several methods of birth control that men and women choose.
9. Understand the abortion controversy, including the political importance of this practice, along with characteristics of women who have abortions and why they do so.
10. Recognize that family planning is most effective when based on high-quality information.

TEST YOUR KNOWLEDGE

1. Approximately 2 million U.S. single-parent families are headed by a father. True or False?
2. Vermont, New York, and California are the only U.S. states to grant same-sex couples the same rights and protections as if they were married. True or False?
3. Pregnancy can be accurately detected soon after conception by the presence of the hormone *progesterone.* True or False?
4. The birth of a baby occurs in three stages. The baby is actually born in the third stage of delivery along with the placenta. True or False?
5. Women purchase nearly half of all condoms sold for use by males. True or False?

Answers found at end of chapter.

Much has been written about the demise of the American family, but the truth is that, as an institution, it is alive and for the most part well. From a statistical standpoint, the Census Bureau reports that 68 percent of the nation's 105 million households meet its definition of families—people bound by blood, adoption, or marriage.

A family can be defined in numerous ways. The immediate or **nuclear family** consists of parents and/or guardians and their children. It is best understood as those individuals living under the same roof, and it can include homosexual and lesbian couples. The **extended family** includes those who are connected by blood, marriage, or adoption. It consists of parents, grandparents, aunts, uncles, cousins, and other relatives.

The Beginnings of a Family

The concepts of nuclear and extended family go back to our earliest ancestors, who lived in small bands. The family then, as now, provided a structure for some of the most basic needs in life: psychological, physical, and economic security; sexual satisfaction; and procreation. It also fulfilled several social functions, particularly social support for its members.

Until relatively recently, the concept of family was represented—in the movies, on television, by artists, and to some extent in reality—as a working father or "breadwinner," a housewife who did not work outside the home, plus two children. This so-called traditional concept of family, although remaining firmly planted in the minds of the public, hardly represents the reality of today. In 1970, such a family structure accounted for 40 percent of all households. Today, married couples with children make up only a quarter of U.S. households.

Another change in the contemporary family structure is that often both parents work—so-called **dual-career families.** For economic reasons as well as for personal satisfaction, women are increasingly working outside the home. Today, more than 65 percent of all married women work outside the home versus 12 percent in 1940. This has had a profound effect on the structure of the family. Studies show that working women tend to have fewer children than do women who have no work experience outside the home. Dual-career families demand more of every member of the family. Unless a family assertively works at balancing the expectations of both home and work, problems can develop. For example, consider the woman who is employed full-time outside the home and at the same time is expected (perhaps for reasons of tradition only) to serve as a housekeeper, cook, and head of the family laundry service. Without the help of other family members, the demands of what amounts to two full-time jobs can result in excessive stress and burnout.

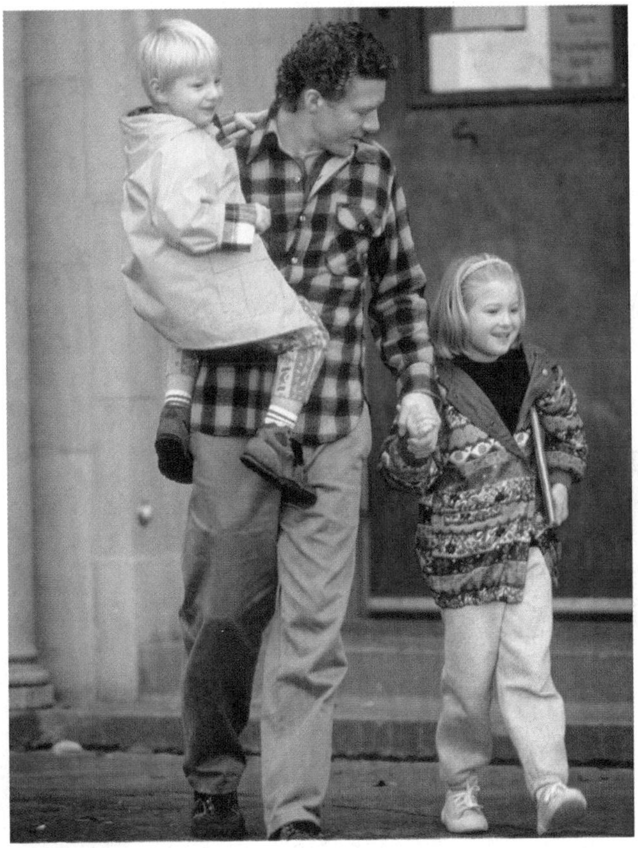

Single parenthood is often the result of divorce; but single women and men are also choosing to have children or to adopt them to have a family.

nuclear family The immediate family; parents and/or guardians and their children, usually living together.

extended family Family members connected by blood, marriage, or adoption.

dual-career families Families in which both parents work full time.

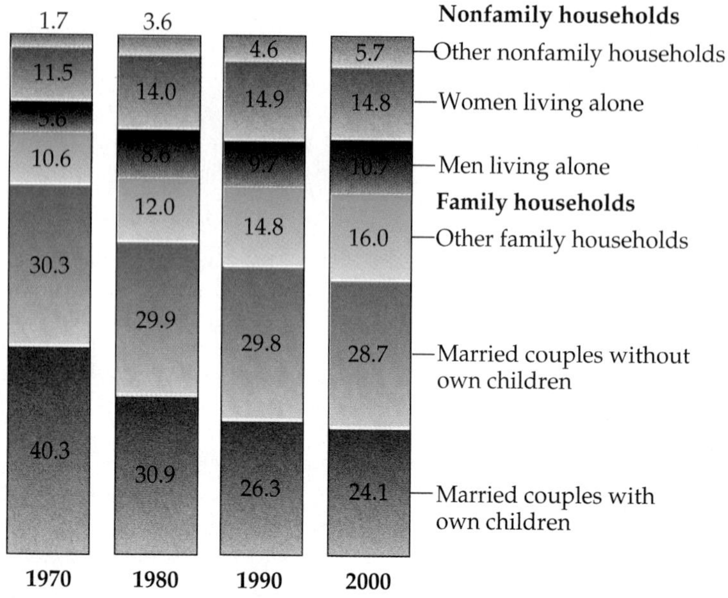

Figure 13.1 **The Changing American Household**
Over the past thirty years, there has been a decrease in the percent of households with married couples and an increase in other types of families.
(Source: U.S. Census Bureau)

Another variation of the nuclear family is the **single-parent family,** which usually consists of a mother and child or children. In the United States today, about 12 million families are headed by only one parent. Only about 2 million single-parent families are headed by a father. Increasingly, single women are choosing to have children or to adopt them so that they can have a family too. Single men—in much smaller numbers—are also adopting children. Because single parents must handle all family roles, they are particularly susceptible to the same stresses and burnout that occur in dual-career households when the burden of family responsibilities is not shared.

Living together is another lifestyle choice many unmarried couples make. What was once disapproved-of behavior is now a common practice. In 2000, more than 3 million unmarried couples were living together in the United States. While living together may seem to take the place of marriage, for many it just puts off the wedding date: More than half of all marriages today follow a period of **cohabitation.** See Figure 13.1 for a look at how family styles have changed over the years.

Marriage and Family

Marriage is the process of formalizing an interpersonal relationship and establishing a new family core. This makes marriage sound mechanistic, but, in fact, it involves elements of romance and psychological and sexual fulfillment and offers emotional support and security for both parties. A spouse can be a lifelong friend, a companion, and a buffer against loneliness.

Marriage is one of the strongest social and cultural traditions, and most people eventually get married. Statistically, about half of all U.S. marriages end in divorce, but most divorced people find new partners and marry again. Specifically, five out of six men and three out of four women remarry after divorce. Second marriages account for one third of all marriages today. Marriage counselors report that couples are working harder to hold their marriages together and an increasing number are turning to premarital counseling. What couples are looking for, and willing to work on developing, are commitment, bonding, and intimacy.

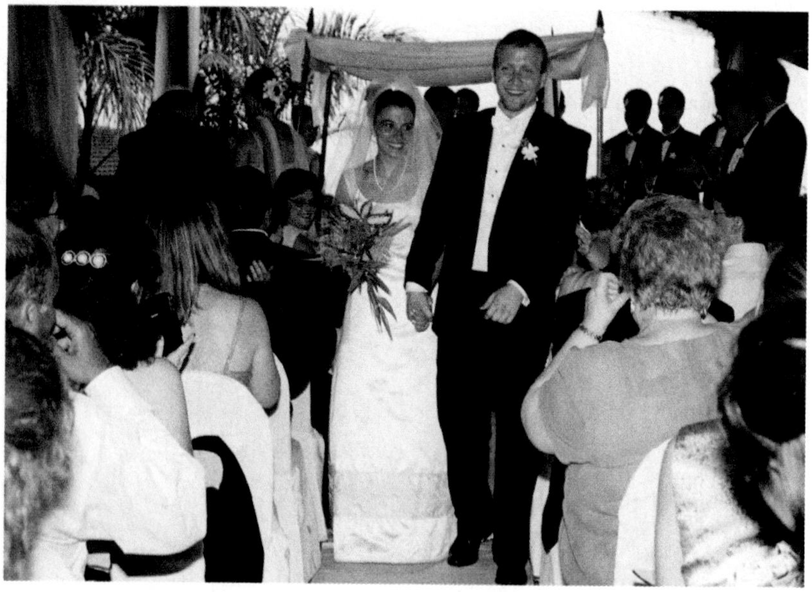

Marriage remains one of our strongest social and cultural traditions. Most people eventually get married.

single-parent family A family in which only one parent lives in the home and takes care of the children.

cohabitation A living arrangement in which two individuals live together in a sexual relationship without being married.

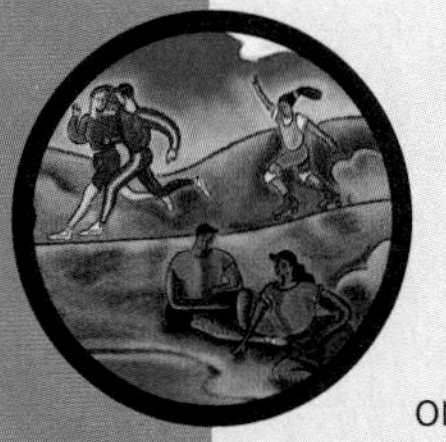

Cultural View

Domestic Partnership

When workers in Washington, D.C., were asked to define their families, they came up with 129 combinations including living alone, with a spouse, in a nuclear family, with minor children only, with unrelated children, and with a same-sex partner.

The changing demographics of the American household are prompting people to reexamine a basic question: What is a family?

Catching Up with Reality?

In cities across the nation, gay and lesbian groups are seeking to expand the traditional definition of a family to include couples of the same sex. The motivation is largely economic: homosexual couples want to get the same share of health and other fringe benefits that married couples get. These benefits can make up more than 30 percent of a worker's compensation package.

Scores of employers, cities, states, or counties in the United States have granted domestic partnership recognition to unmarried couples, including both heterosexual and homosexual pairs. For the supporters of such ordinances, the law is simply catching up with reality. Matt Coles, a San Francisco lawyer who was present at the creation of the family diversity movement, has pointed out, "This movement is not about changing society, because society has already changed. Large numbers of people already live in nontraditional households. History always teaches us that, sooner or later, government has to acknowledge where people are taking society."

Others disagree and see the family as the cornerstone of civilization and defined as people related by blood, marriage, or adoption.

Insurance and Legal Issues

Cities that already recognize unmarried relationships, including New York, Washington, San Francisco, and Seattle, have discovered that they face the worst resistance from insurers. The unspoken fear of some insurers is that they have to pay the catastrophic costs for the treatment of gay partners who have HIV/AIDS. Insurers also worry that a stampede of people will try to create sham partnerships to take advantage of the health benefits. But experience has shown that only a small percentage of employees—the majority of whom are heterosexual—sign up for the domestic partnership plan.

Establishing a domestic partnership is a serious step, and to qualify requires proof of a close and committed personal relationship. However, it is not legally the same as a marriage in several ways. Unless there is a will, a domestic partner does not have inheritance rights. Partners do not have a right to each other's pay or property. They cannot share Social Security benefits, immigration rights, veteran's benefits, or even frequent flier miles. And when a same-sex couple dissolves their domestic partnership, it is more difficult for them to get the same legal protections as a heterosexual couple that gets divorced.

A current controversy exists concerning whether homosexual and lesbian marriages should be recognized. Vermont is the only state to grant same-sex couples the same rights and protections as married heterosexual couples, including adopting a child, making medical decisions for each other, and transferring property upon death. While the law still defines marriage as the union of one man and one woman, Vermont has created a parallel to marriage for same-sex couples called a civil union that legally recognizes the lifelong commitment of a man to a man and a woman to a woman. Numerous cities have approved nonmarital domestic partnerships for same-sex as well as heterosexual couples. Read more about same-sex domestic partnerships in the Cultural View box.

Deciding to Have Children

Even though premarital sexual activity is common today, one reason why couples marry is to raise a family. Some couples want children right away while others want to wait until they settle into the new relationship. Having children is a serious decision, and not all couples choose to have them. No matter how long a couple waits to raise a family, there are certain issues to consider.

1. *Both partners should want to have a child.* Although some pregnancies result from contraceptive method failures, most unwanted pregnancies result from poor planning and poor decision making on the part of the parents. The obvious way to avoid unwanted pregnancy is through the proper use of effective contraceptive techniques.
2. *Both partners should be mature enough to accept the responsibility of childrearing.* Raising a child involves a lifelong commitment by both parents. There are periods of extensive nurturing of the very young, support during the often difficult years of adolescence, and guidance in gaining independence in the late teens and early twenties. In many cases, children continue to depend upon their parents well into their adult years.
3. *Both partners should be able to provide the economic support that the child will need to be healthy and properly nourished.*

The financial requirements of a young child range from adequate nutrition and quality medical care to day care. During the adolescent years, there are financial demands for social activities, clothing, and other day-to-day living expenses. Support for an older child can include expenses of college or job training.

What are the wrong reasons for wanting a child? Some parents think that having a child will add stability to their marriage. The presence of a child can seldom achieve this. In fact, a child often provides just the opposite by adding even more stress to an already unstable marriage. Another wrong reason to have a child is "because I need someone to love me." This response is often heard from pregnant teenagers who feel lonely and out of touch and believe that having a baby will solve their problems. Again, this seldom proves to be the case. Perhaps the greatest health threat related to unwanted childbearing is that it can result in little or no preconception and prenatal care.

Issues of Infertility

Not everyone who wants to become pregnant can easily do so. Each year about 3 million U.S. couples want to have a baby but cannot successfully conceive one. These couples are said to be infertile.

Infertility is generally defined as the inability of a couple to conceive after one year of intercourse without contraception. Infertility has many causes, including pelvic infections resulting from sexually transmitted infections, hormonal disturbances in women, and low sperm count in men. Stress, too much exercise, poor nutrition, smoking, and exposure to other environmental hazards can cause bodily changes that impair fertility. Knowing these problems, it is possible to prevent many of the causes of infertility.

Age is also a factor: the older the women, the higher the incidence of infertility. This is particularly important for women who want to establish their careers before having children. Only 2 percent of teenagers experience fertility problems whereas 27 percent of women over forty experience such problems. Overall, about 9 percent of people in their reproductive years experience fertility problems.

Perhaps the most common way for infertile couples to have children is adoption. But there are other options for women who want to have a birth experience or couples who want some genetic link to a child. One technique used for more than 100 years is **artificial insemination,** in which a woman is artificially impregnated by sperm from an unknown donor or by sperm collected from her partner. Artificial insemination from a sperm bank is also used today by some single women and lesbian couples who want to have children.

Medical and surgical interventions developed over the last thirty years are proving to be successful in the treatment of infertility. These interventions include microsurgery to repair damage to the ovaries, fallopian tubes, and testes, **assisted reproductive technology (ART),** including **in vitro fertilization** (literally "fertilization in a glass"), and **ovulation-inducing drugs** (hormones that bring about ovulation).

Assisted reproductive technology (ART) is defined as any procedure in which both eggs and sperm are handled outside the body. The breakthrough in ART took place in 1978 with the birth of Louise Brown, the world's first test-tube baby. In the process sperm and egg from the mother and father were combined in a glass container, and a fertilized embryo was implanted into the woman's uterus. Variations on this process include using a donor egg (not from the mother) or donor sperm (not from the father). These processes are controversial and costly and result in relatively few live births.

One of the most controversial developments is surrogate motherhood, which is when a woman contracts with a couple either to be artificially inseminated with a man's sperm or to have a fertilized embryo implanted in her uterus. The surrogate mother, who is typically well paid for her trouble, carries the pregnancy to term, delivers the child, and gives it to the couple for adoption. This is usually done anonymously—that is, the surrogate mother does not meet the adopting couple. Surrogate motherhood raises many ethical questions, including what to do if the surrogate mother does not give up the baby or, conversely, what to do if the baby is born with defects and the couple does not accept the baby.

Preconception Care

To help ensure a healthy pregnancy, care should begin before **conception.** Such health care is referred to as **preconception care** and includes an evaluation of a potential mother's health status and health behavior as well as environmental factors that may negatively affect the preg-

infertility The inability of a couple to conceive after one year of intercourse without contraception.

artificial insemination Introduction of semen into the vagina by artificial means.

assisted reproductive technology (ART) Any procedure in which both eggs and sperm are handled outside the body.

in vitro fertilization A procedure in which the sperm and egg from a man and a woman are combined in a glass container, and a fertilized embryo is implanted into the woman.

ovulation-inducing drugs Hormones that bring about ovulation.

conception The union of sperm and egg.

preconception care A health-promoting action taken prior to conception for the purpose of reducing health risks to mother and child.

nancy. Based on the outcome of such an evaluation, the mother-to-be can take positive steps to eliminate risk factors that may adversely affect her pregnancy. This is important because a large percentage of pregnancies in the United States are not planned—that is, the mother does not begin to think she is pregnant until there are telltale signs. By this point, the fertilized egg is developing very rapidly and the risks for harm to developing tissues are far greater than during the rest of pregnancy.

Preconception care has three basic components that, in part, overlap: a risk assessment, health promotion, and interventions for a healthy pregnancy.

Risk assessment. A risk assessment includes considering basic factors such as a woman's age, weight, and dietary habits. A woman who is underweight or overweight or who is a vegetarian might seek nutritional counseling to ensure that she is receiving the nutrients needed to sustain a healthy pregnancy. Other risk factors relate to adverse health behaviors, such as smoking, drinking, and taking drugs. As part of her preconception care, a woman may choose to stop smoking. By doing so, she reduces the risk for low infant birthweight related to tobacco use.

A risk assessment can also identify certain medical conditions that might need special attention during pregnancy. Through preconception care, a woman can learn whether she is at risk for getting rubella (German measles), which may cause severe birth defects if contracted during pregnancy. If so, she can be immunized against the disease and thus protect her child if she does become pregnant. Preconception is the ideal time for genetic counseling for families that have a history of genetic disease or a significant occupational or environmental exposure to toxic agents, or when maternal age is a factor. Genetic counseling helps couples better understand their risks and provides the opportunity for genetic testing if necessary. It could also be a determining factor in a couple's decision to adopt children.

Health promotion. Health promotion during the preconception stage includes practicing healthy behaviors, such as proper nutrition and exercise, and not smoking or drinking. It also involves counseling about family planning and spacing of pregnancies. During this stage, a couple should begin investigating resources in the community for good prenatal care so the woman can make appropriate arrangements once she knows she is pregnant. It also makes sense to know about your reproductive physiology. See the Your Sexual Body appendix of this textbook.

Interventions for a healthy pregnancy. There are a range of interventions that can be taken to promote a healthy pregnancy, such as getting appropriate immunizations and getting to the right weight.

A Healthy Pregnancy

When does life begin? This question prompts some of our culture's most heated debates. Some people believe that life begins at birth. Others believe that life begins when the fetal heartbeat is heard. Still others believe that it begins at the moment of conception. Although we cannot settle the "life" question, we can establish the point at which pregnancy begins. Pregnancy technically begins at the moment of conception. Conception is the point when sperm and egg unite. It takes place in the **fallopian tube,** and a few days later, the **blastocyst,** the multicelled descendant of the union of sperm and egg, implants in the uterine wall, where it will develop into the embryo and new fetus. The **uterus** expands to provide a home for the fetus to grow and serves as a muscular means of expelling the baby at birth (see Figure 13.2).

Early signs of pregnancy include a missed menstrual period, along with breast changes such as fullness and tenderness. Sometimes these symptoms are coupled with nausea (morning sickness) and increased urinary frequency. Because each of these symptoms also occurs in nonpregnant women, they should be considered an indication only that a pregnancy is possible, not that it is probable.

Pregnancy can be accurately detected soon after conception by the presence of a hormone, **human chorionic gonadotropin (HCG),** which is secreted into the urine from placental cells. The **placenta** is a structure that develops from the wall of the uterus and serves as an organ of interchange between the mother and the fetus. Pregnancy tests are available at college health services, family planning clinics, and physicians' offices. Over-the-counter pregnancy tests sold in drug stores have an effectiveness rate high enough to indicate, along with the signs described above, that pregnancy is probable. If you are using an over-the-counter test, positive signs of pregnancy should be confirmed by a physician.

fallopian tube A passageway (tube) that extends from the uterus into the abdominal cavity to a place near the ovary.

blastocyst The multicellular descendant of the united sperm and egg that will later develop into the embryo then the fetus.

uterus A hollow, pear-shaped muscular organ that functions to house the developing fetus.

human chorionic gonadotropin (HCG) A hormone secreted from placental cells; a pregnancy test looks for the presence of this hormone.

placenta The structure that develops from the wall of the uterus and serves as an organ of interchange between the mother and the fetus.

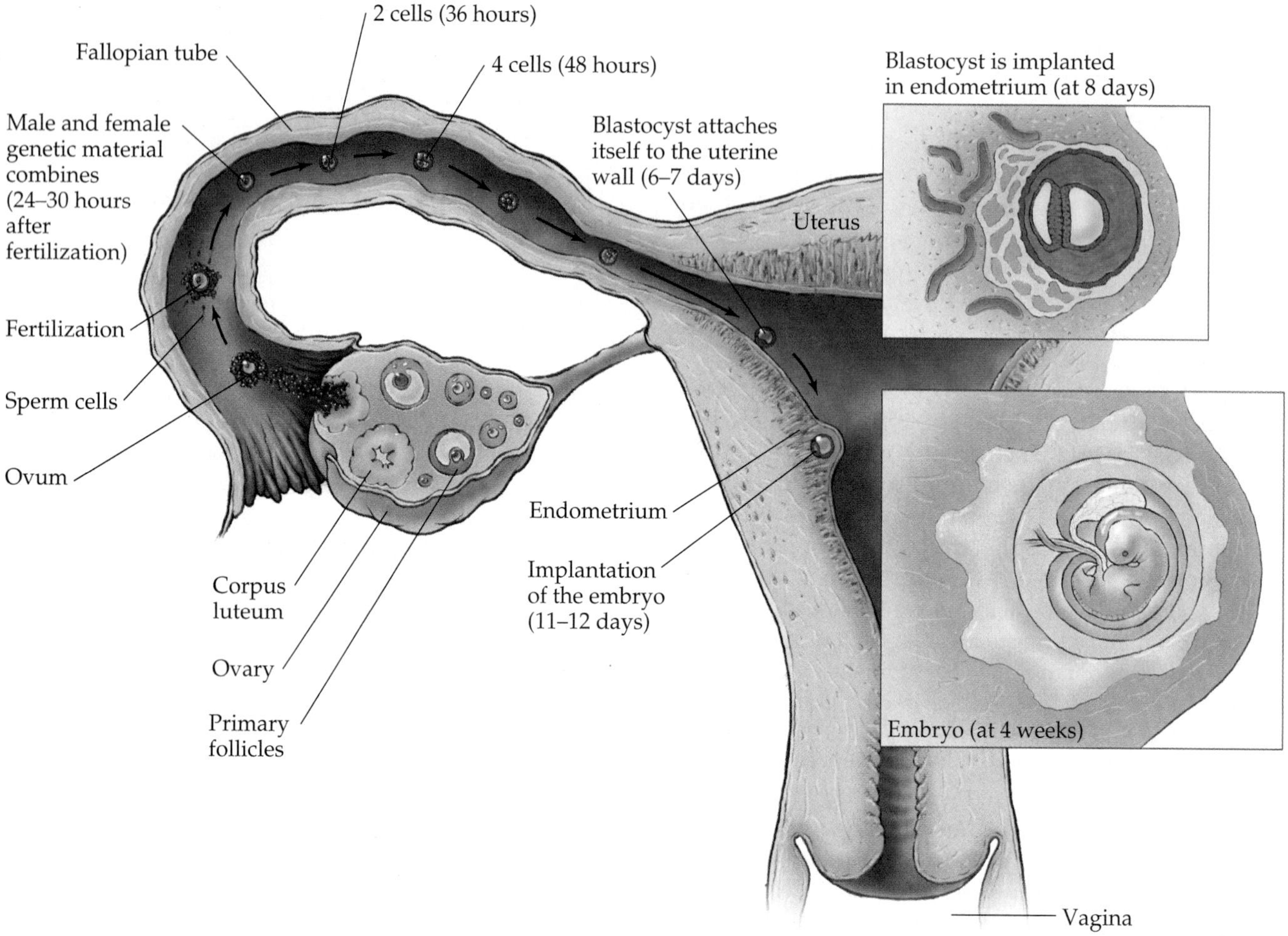

Figure 13.2 **The Process of Conception**

Conception takes place in the fallopian tube. About a week later, the blastocyst is implanted in the wall of the uterus.

The Importance of Prenatal Care

While the groundwork for a healthy pregnancy and birth begins before conception, it is important to take care during the pregnancy. Health care during pregnancy is called **prenatal care,** or care before birth. Good health care during this period can increase the chances of a healthy pregnancy and delivery.

During pregnancy, smoking, drinking, drug use, and exposure to sexually transmitted infections are critical health threats to the fetus (see Chapters 7, 8, and 11). Smoking during pregnancy is associated with higher infant mortality and **low birthweight babies.** Babies born to women who smoke during pregnancy are born weighing, on average, 6 ounces less than babies of nonsmoking women. The affects of alcohol can be so damaging that research indicates that no amount of drinking can be considered safe during pregnancy. Certain medications taken during

prenatal care A health-promoting action taken by the mother-to-be after conception and before birth for the purpose of reducing health risks to mother and child; medical care during pregnancy.

low birthweight babies Babies born weighing less than 2,500 grams, or five pounds eight ounces.

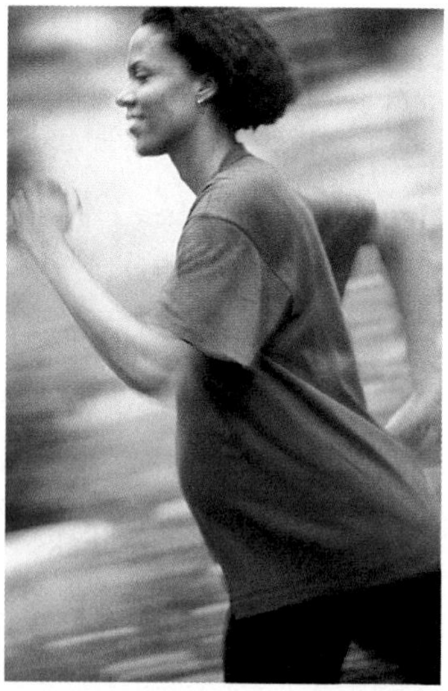

An important component of prenatal care is exercise. Being physically fit can help prepare a woman for the physical work involved in the delivery of a baby.

pregnancy can also harm the fetus. For example, the drug Accutane, used to treat severe acne, was found to cause fetal malformations.

Good prenatal care includes careful monitoring by a physician or certified nurse-midwife, proper diet, and appropriate exercise. The recommended weight gain during pregnancy is between 25 and 35 pounds for an infant weight between 6 pounds 8 ounces and 9 pounds, according to an Institute of Medicine report. Exercise helps prepare women for the physical work involved in delivering a baby and can result in an easier delivery. It also helps the mother's body return to its prepregnancy state after the baby is born. While most pregnant women should not start a highly strenuous exercise program, most physicians agree that healthy women can continue an exercise program through most of the pregnancy.

Diagnostic procedures that can be performed during pregnancy to test the health of the fetus are another component of prenatal care.

Testing the Health of the Fetus

The first picture in the baby book used to be the one taken at the hospital right after birth. This has now been replaced by the **sonogram,** a diagnostic tool that allows the physician to indirectly see the developing fetus and its individual organ systems. The sonogram is useful in determining fetal age, position, and size as well as in detecting certain abnormalities. This information can help a physician determine if the fetus is developing on schedule.

A growing number of other diagnostic procedures help physicians evaluate the health of the fetus. A test of the mother's blood, taken between the thirteenth and twentieth weeks of pregnancy, can detect levels of **alpha-fetoprotein (AFP),** a substance produced by the fetus's kidneys. High levels of AFP can indicate a neural tube defect, which could result in conditions such as **spina bifida;** low levels can be a sign of Down syndrome. The AFP blood test is a screening procedure. If a pregnant woman has a questionable level of AFP in her blood, she should speak with her physician about having further diagnostic tests.

Amniocentesis provides physicians with a reliable way to study fetal cells to test for the presence or absence of certain genetic conditions, such as **Down syndrome.** In this procedure, a needle is inserted through the uterus and into the **amniotic fluid** that surrounds the fetus. Some fluid, which contains cells shed by the fetus, is drawn out. The test is performed between the fifteenth and eighteenth weeks of pregnancy, when a sufficient number of fetal cells are available for study. It takes an additional two to three weeks to culture the cells and get results from the study. If the test results show a birth defect, the mother can consider whether to continue with the pregnancy or to terminate it.

As helpful as amniocentesis is, a woman is into her twentieth week of pregnancy—midway through it—before she gets the results of the test. A procedure that can be done earlier in the pregnancy is called **chorionic villus sampling (CVS).** The chorionic villi, hairlike projections on a membrane surrounding the interior of the uterus, contain the same information found in the amniotic fluid. The advantage of CVS is that it can be performed earlier in pregnancy—between the ninth and twelfth weeks—and results are available in six to twenty-four hours.

Both amniocentesis and CVS involve some risk to the mother and fetus, including miscarriage (spontaneous abortion) and infection. CVS carries slightly more risk for the fetus than amniocentesis, including missing or underdeveloped fingers or toes, and does not detect as many defects.

Growth by Trimesters

Pregnancy is divided into trimesters of thirteen weeks each. Most of the organs form, and much of the development of the fetus takes place during the first trimester. Sex, for example, is determined genetically at conception, but the physical differences between males and females are determined by hormonal influences on growth, and it takes about three months before these differences can be observed. The head, meanwhile, is disproportionately large (it accounts for nearly half of the fetus's size) at this stage because of the developing brain. The effects of drug use and infectious diseases on the fetus are particularly damaging during this trimester when so much development is occurring. By the end of three months, the fetus is approximately 4 inches long and weighs 1 ounce (see Figure 13.3).

sonogram A diagnostic tool that allows a physician to indirectly see the developing fetus and its individual organ systems.

alpha-fetoprotein A substance produced by fetal kidneys; high levels could indicate a neural tube defect.

spina bifida A birth defect in which the spinal cord or its covering is incomplete.

Down syndrome A birth defect in which the individual has extra genetic material (associated with the number 21 chromosome) that alters the course of development and causes specific physical and mental characteristics associated with the syndrome.

amniocentesis Means of testing amniotic fluid to indicate the presence or absence of certain genetic conditions, such as Down syndrome, in a fetus.

amniotic fluid The fluid in the amniotic sac surrounding the fetus during pregnancy.

chorionic villus sampling (CVS) A technique in which the chorionic villi, hairlike projections on a membrane surrounding the interior of the uterus, are tested to determine the presence or absence of certain genetic conditions.

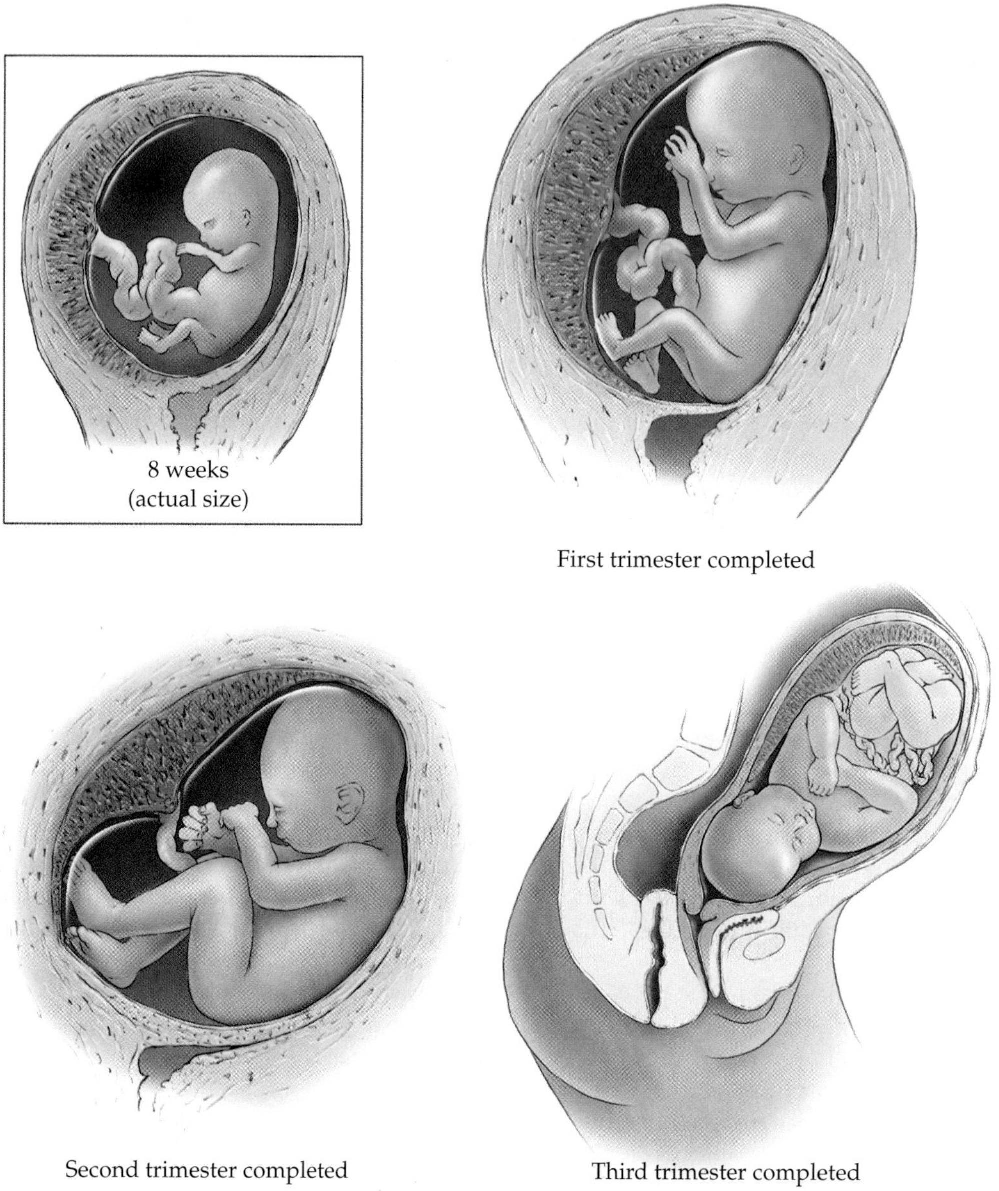

Figure 13.3 The Nine Months of Pregnancy
First trimester completed: By the end of month 3, the fetus is 4 inches long and weighs a little over 1 ounce. Second trimester completed: By the end of month 6, the fetus is 11 to 14 inches long and weighs 1 to 1 1/2 pounds. Third trimester completed: At 38 to 40 weeks, the baby is full term. The baby weighs 6 to 9 pounds and is 19 to 21 inches long.

During the second trimester, the fetus grows to approximately 1 foot in length and between 1 and 1.5 pounds in weight. Its eyes are open, but the lungs and intestinal canal are not yet completely developed. During this time, the mother begins to feel the fetus' movements, a sensation called **quickening.** The fetal heartbeat is also audible through a stethoscope. The mother's breasts grow, and the initial signs of pregnancy, such as morning sickness and frequent urination, usually subside.

quickening Fetal movements felt by the mother.

The third trimester is a time of growth and fine-tuning for the fetus. Fingernails start to grow and in many cases could use cutting—some babies are actually born with scratch marks from their own nails. More crucial to life, however, are the respiratory and digestive systems, which are the last systems to fully develop. The last trimester is a period of great weight gain and growth. A full-term baby, born thirty-nine weeks after conception, weighs between 6 and 9 pounds and is

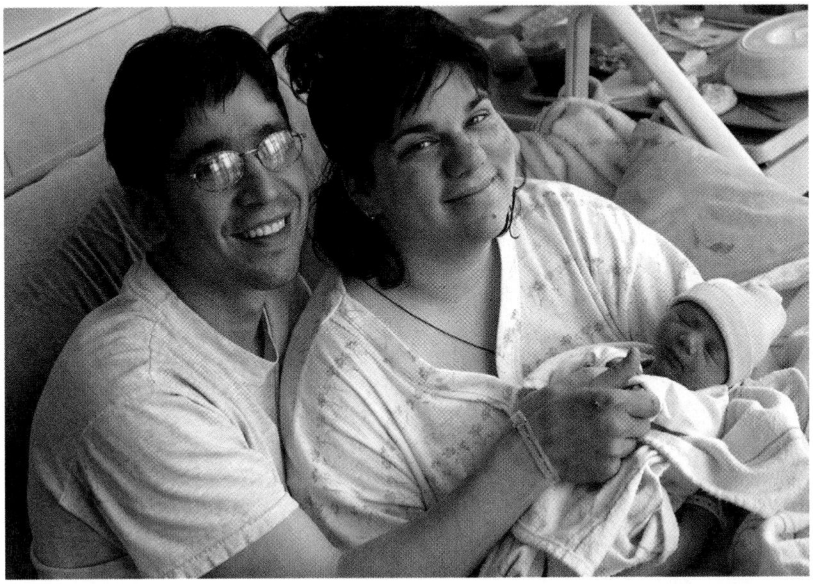

The first family portrait reflects the special bond that exists between parents and children.

about 20 inches long. At this time, the mother becomes somewhat uncomfortable with the weight gain associated with carrying a full-term baby, particularly with the crowding of her internal organs. She feels pressure on her bladder and can sometimes feel the fetus kicking and hiccuping. Between two and four weeks before birth, the baby "drops," or positions itself to be delivered through the **vaginal canal.**

Preparing for Childbirth

Most babies are born in a hospital where high-technology care is available if needed. Many women choose **natural childbirth,** and instead of relieving pain with drugs, they rely on a system of breathing and relaxation techniques based on the principles of Fernand Lamaze, a French obstetrician. In cases in which mothers receive pain medication, the effects are localized and the mothers are awake during the birth. Fathers are usually present at the time of delivery to give support to the mother and sometimes to assist the physician—for example, by cutting the umbilical cord. In recent years, hospitals have given much attention to making the birthing process feel more natural by providing homelike birthing rooms, and extensive and comfortable accommodations for family members. The advantage of such accommodations is that the birth process is carried out in a hospital with all of the advantages of high-technology medical care, but in an atmosphere that is warm and friendly.

An increasing number of women have their babies delivered by **nurse-midwives,** either in the hospital or in freestanding birthing centers located outside hospitals. These centers, which are usually homelike settings and staffed by certified nurse-midwives, offer a lower-technology alternative to a hospital delivery. Physicians are available as consultants in case a complication arises. Studies show that deliveries in birthing centers are as safe as hospital deliveries but cost about half as much money.

In addition, some women hire a **doula,** a person who is trained to work as an adjunct to the doctor or nurse-midwife, to provide emotional and physical support. Doulas suggest different positions and breathing techniques to help ease labor pain. Research shows that childbirth goes more smoothly with a doula, with labor time cut by 25 percent.

First-Stage Labor

During the first stage of **labor** (see Figure 13.4), the **cervix,** the opening to the uterus, gradually effaces (thins) and dilates (opens). **Effacement** can take place as much as three weeks in advance of labor. **Dilation** of the cervix is necessary to allow eventual passage of the baby through the birth canal. It is brought about by a series of contractions of the uterus, which are usually rhythmic in nature. The contractions of the uterus in the early part of the first stage of labor feel like a tightening of the lower abdomen. These contractions are spaced several minutes (perhaps twenty minutes) apart and are generally not uncomfortable. As the first stage of labor progresses, however, the tightening of the uterus during each contraction becomes more and more severe, and each contraction brings about a feeling of increasing pressure. At some point during the first stage of labor, the amniotic

vaginal canal The passage in females leading from the vulva (external orifice) to the uterus.

natural childbirth Delivery of a baby "naturally," without the aid of drugs.

nurse-midwife Registered nurse who has completed advanced training in gynecology and obstetrics.

doula A person trained to assist during delivery by providing emotional and physical support; does not deliver the baby.

labor The process of childbirth from the initial contractions of the uterus to the delivery of the baby and the placenta.

cervix The opening of the uterus into the vagina.

effacement The thinning of the cervix during the process of childbirth.

dilation Opening of the cervix either for examination or for delivery of a baby.

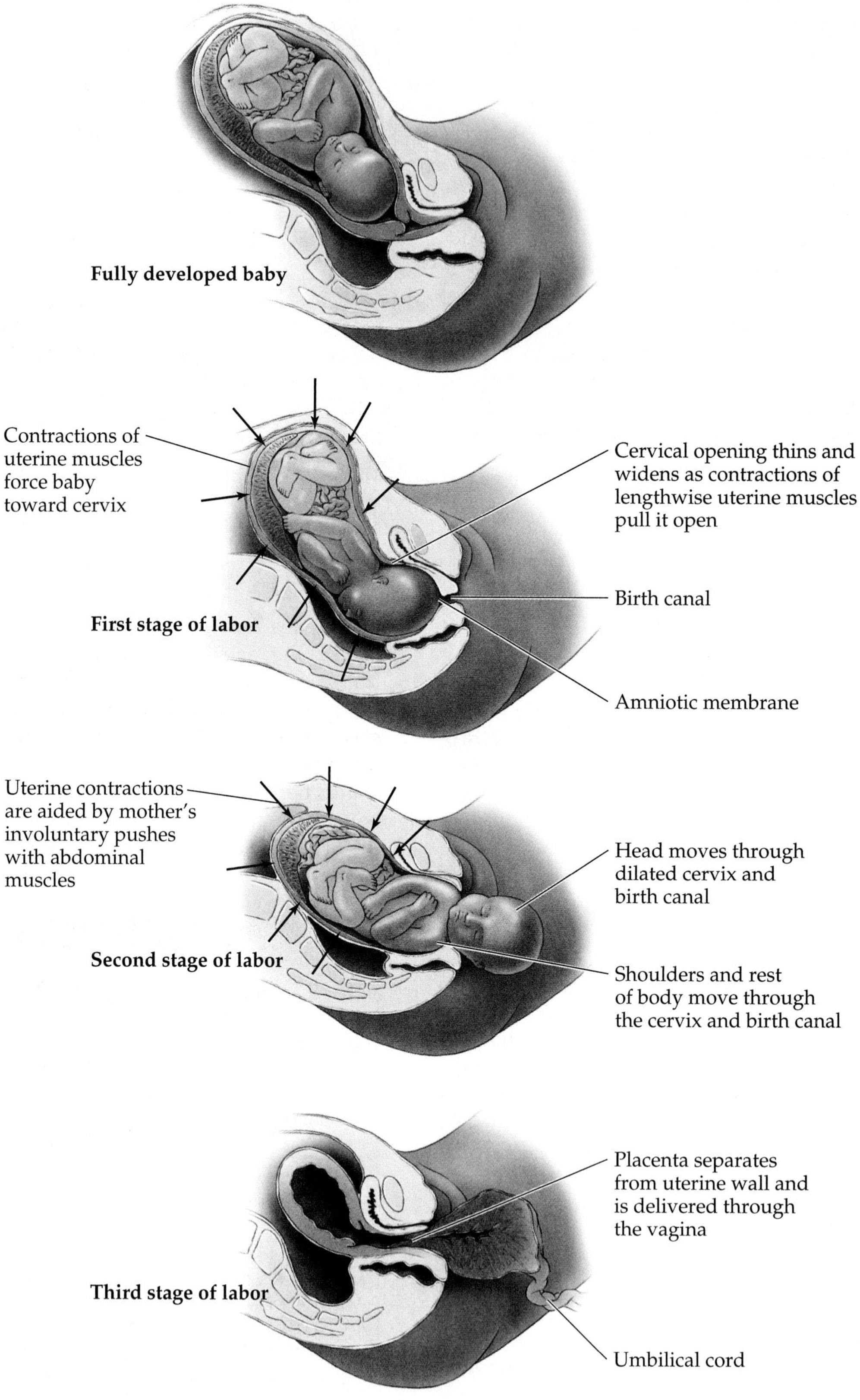
Fully developed baby
Contractions of uterine muscles force baby toward cervix
Cervical opening thins and widens as contractions of lengthwise uterine muscles pull it open
Birth canal
First stage of labor
Amniotic membrane
Uterine contractions are aided by mother's involuntary pushes with abdominal muscles
Head moves through dilated cervix and birth canal
Second stage of labor
Shoulders and rest of body move through the cervix and birth canal
Placenta separates from uterine wall and is delivered through the vagina
Third stage of labor
Umbilical cord

Figure 13.4 The First, Second, and Third Stages of Labor

fluid, which has surrounded and protected the fetus throughout the development process, is released. The release of the amniotic fluid is sometimes referred to as the "breaking of waters."

Dilation and effacement of the cervix usually occur within the first few hours of labor. In some cases, particularly in first births, the process may take much longer, perhaps even days or weeks. In the case of second and third births, the process may take only a few minutes. When the cervix is dilated between 2 and 3 inches (between 5 and 6 centimeters), the intensity of labor increases and the resting time between contractions is decreased as the body secretes a hormone that brings on the hard contractions needed to expel the baby. The first stage of labor is considered complete when the cervix is completely effaced and dilated to 10 centimeters and the baby's head can be seen. This is called **crowning.**

Second-Stage Labor

During the second stage of labor, the baby is born. The second stage of labor is usually much shorter than the first stage. It should never be allowed to last longer than one or two hours. Longer second-stage labor can be hazardous to the mother and child.

Several positions may be used for the delivery of the baby, including squatting or sitting, but the most common position for delivery is with the mother lying on her back with her legs apart (sometimes placed in stirrups), to provide the physician with easy access to the baby when birth takes place.

In the second stage of labor, the uterine contractions increase in frequency and intensity. At the same time, the mother uses her abdominal muscles to help push the baby out. The baby's head is normally the first part of the body to move through the cervix and out the birth canal. The physician may make a small incision from the vagina toward the anus called an **episiotomy** to ensure easier passage of the baby's head through the birth canal and to prevent tearing of the tissue. This procedure may cause discomfort to the mother during her recovery period due to the stitches needed to repair the incision. Some health professionals do not consider it necessary to do an episiotomy routinely believing that relaxation, pushing, manually stretching the area, and patience on the part of the physician can eliminate much of the need for one.

In some cases, the physician may recommend delivering the baby by **cesarean section (C-section),** that is, removal of the baby through an incision in the abdominal wall rather than through the birth canal. Cesarean sections are done in approximately one quarter of births in the United States. Physicians recommend cesarean sections for a number of reasons: The birth canal may be too small to accommodate delivery; the labor, for a variety of reasons, may not be progressing correctly; the position of the baby may be feet or bottom first, known as **breech presentation;** fetal distress may be evident; or natural delivery may be otherwise perceived as too risky.

While the lives of many mothers and infants have been saved through the use of cesarean sections, some physicians believe that many of these surgical births are unnecessary. For example, some women want a cesarean section because they can schedule the delivery date and make it more convenient for themselves and their family. It is believed that some physicians perform a cesarean section delivery because they are afraid of a malpractice suit if they wait to deliver the baby naturally and there is a problem. Women who are over thirty and/or have private health insurance are more likely to have cesarean section deliveries than are younger women and those who have no health insurance or who are receiving public health benefits such as Medicaid. Most women who have a cesarean birth deliver subsequent children the same way. Only one in four women deliver another child vaginally.

Third-Stage Labor

In the final stage of labor, the placenta separates from the uterine wall and is expelled. This is done naturally through a continuation of uterine contractions. The placenta is examined by the physician to determine if it is intact. The placenta must be completely removed from the woman or complications in recovery from childbirth can result. These complications include bleeding and infection.

This ends the long process of having a baby. The process began before conception, as plans were made about the timing of the pregnancy. Ahead lie years of parenting and decisions about future pregnancies.

Family Planning and Birth Control

Family planning is the process of establishing the preferred number and spacing of children in one's family

crowning The point of labor at which the cervix is completely effaced and dilated to ten centimeters and the baby's head can be seen.

episiotomy The small incision made between the opening of the vagina and the anus to ensure easier passage of the baby's head through the birth canal and to prevent tearing of the tissue.

cesarean section (C-section) Removal of the baby through an incision in the abdominal wall rather than through the birth canal.

breech presentation When the baby's feet or bottom are positioned first in the birth canal.

family planning A process of establishing the preferred number and spacing of children in one's family and choosing the means by which this is achieved.

and choosing the means by which this is achieved. The concept of family planning emphasizes the importance of both family and planning. It acknowledges that few events can be more treasured than the discovery of an intended pregnancy, and few events can be more potentially damaging to a family than the discovery of an unintended pregnancy.

Family planning is usually carried out through the application of one or more **birth control** methods or devices. Birth control is hardly a new idea. Many cultures have provided instruction on pregnancy prevention, including such recommendations as eating the genitalia of an animal prior to intercourse, squatting and attempting to sneeze following intercourse, and covering the penis prior to intercourse with a skin membrane of an animal (the first condom).

It wasn't until 1965, however, that the Supreme Court declared laws prohibiting the sale and use of contraceptives to be unconstitutional, calling them a violation of the right to privacy. Condoms are now sold openly in drug stores and on college campuses and are given away free in some high schools and other public settings. Women purchase nearly 50 percent of condoms sold for use by males. Condoms are now also available for women.

For some women, birth control provides the means to choose the number and spacing of children. Others have significant health reasons for using birth control. Teenage mothers, for example, face an increased risk for having low birthweight babies. Older mothers, meanwhile, face a higher risk for having children who have Down syndrome. In some situations, pregnancy might be harmful to the mother, particularly if she has other health problems, such as cancer or heart disease.

Birth Control Choices

When choosing from the wide range of birth control methods, it is important to become well informed about the various options. This can be done by visiting with a physician, college health professional, or birth control counselor who will review the various options and the advantages and disadvantages of each and discuss how each might or might not fit within your lifestyle.

A term that has become synonymous with birth control is **contraception.** Contraception is the intentional prevention of conception (the union of sperm and egg). Modern science has produced several means of contraception. Nontechnological methods also exist, such as the **rhythm method,** but they are relatively ineffective in preventing pregnancy.

The rhythm method relies on knowing when a woman ovulates (releases an egg) and then calculating when her fertile and infertile periods are. To use the rhythm method, a woman needs to calculate by calendar when she ovulates and to take her temperature regularly. Ovulation is often represented by a slight increase in temperature. Once the anticipated day of monthly ovulation is determined, abstinence from intercourse is necessary for the rhythm method to be effective. However, women often ovulate at unexpected times during the month, and even if all procedures are followed correctly, it is not uncommon for women who rely on the rhythm method of birth control to become pregnant. It has a failure rate of 24 percent. This means that 24 out of 100 women practicing the rhythm method for one year become pregnant during that year.

Another nontechnological method is **withdrawal,** in which the man withdraws his penis from the vagina before ejaculating so that sperm are not deposited at or near the birth canal. The failure rate for withdrawal is high, and it is considered to be ineffective in preventing pregnancy. The main reason for the failure of this method of birth control is that during intercourse, sperm are present even before ejaculation has taken place. Withdrawal, therefore, does not ensure that sperm are not placed in a position to bring about pregnancy.

The **birth control pill** consists of chemicals that are similar to hormones normally produced in a woman's body. When taken regularly for a full monthly series, this drug keeps the ovaries from releasing an egg. Hence, if there is no egg, conception cannot occur. The pill has a one percent failure rate with "perfect" use and a 6 percent failure rate with average use—which includes forgetting to take it on schedule. See Table 13.1 for failure rates of all contraceptives. The pill is prescribed by a physician and must be taken exactly as prescribed or it may not be effective. See the Developing Health Skills box for a discussion on why the pill is so popular.

An injectable birth control drug, **Depo-Provera,** provides three months of birth control with just one shot and has a very high level of effectiveness. As with the pill, it must be prescribed by a physician. Side effects of Depo-Provera include weight gain, some reports of depression or mood disorders, and irregular menstruating cycles with excessive bleeding between cycles.

birth control Prevention of pregnancy for the purpose of family planning.

contraception The intentional prevention of conception.

rhythm method The method of contraception that relies on knowing when a woman ovulates and then calculating when her fertile and infertile periods occur.

withdrawal The method of contraception in which the man withdraws his penis from the vagina before ejaculation.

birth control pill A pill, consisting of chemicals similar to hormones normally produced in a woman's body, that prevents pregnancy.

Depo-Provera An injectable method of birth control that lasts for approximately three months.

Another contraceptive, **Norplant,** is a surgically implanted hormone-releasing device. Once implanted, it protects against pregnancy for up to five years. Its success rate is extremely high. Fertility returns once the implant is removed or it has run its full course. This device provides all of the advantages of the birth control pill without the disadvantage of having to remember to take a pill every day at a prescribed time, and it is longer-lasting than the injectable drug Depo-Provera. The most common physical side effect of Norplant is menstrual irregularity, but that decreases after the first year of use.

There are two new contraceptives that contain hormones used in birth control pills. A patch emits low doses of the hormones through the skin. Women put on a new patch once a week for three weeks, and then go patch-free for a week for their menstrual period. About 5 percent of women had at least one patch slip off, which requires starting a new four-week cycle of patches and using a backup method of contraception for the first week. A **vaginal ring,** which is inserted for three weeks, provides a continuous low dose of birth control hormones as long as it remains in place. If the ring slips out of place for more than three hours, additional birth control must be used until it has been reinserted for seven days, giving the hormones time to rise to protective levels again.

There are several **barrier methods** of contraception that physically separate the sperm from the egg. Barrier methods also help prevent sexually transmitted infections. The **male condom** is a thin rubber sheath for the penis that collects semen ejaculated during intercourse. This inexpensive method of birth control also protects against most sexually transmitted infections (see Chapter 11). The condom, when used in conjunction with a **spermicide**—an acid substance that kills

Developing Health Skills

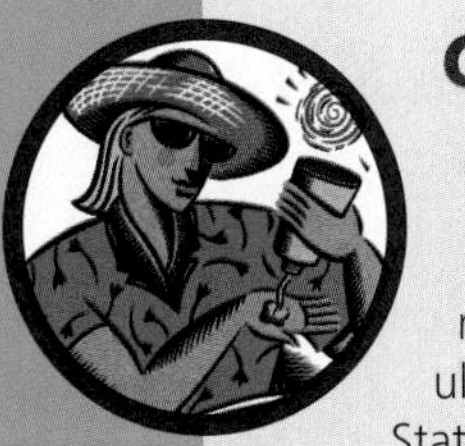

Consumer Health: Why the Pill Is So Popular

Oral contraceptives have been on the market for more than thirty-five years and are the most popular form of reversible birth control in the United States. The pill allows greater sexual spontaneity with a high rate of effectiveness, and has played a major role in the sexual freedom of women. This form of birth control suppresses ovulation (the monthly release of an egg from the ovaries) by the combined actions of the hormones estrogen and progestin. Besides preventing pregnancy, the pill offers additional benefits. For example, the pill can make periods more regular. It also has a protective effect against pelvic inflammatory disease, an infection of the fallopian tubes or uterus that is a major cause of infertility in women, and against ovarian and endometrial cancers.

If a woman remembers to take the pill every day as directed, she has an extremely low chance of becoming pregnant in a year. However, the pill's effectiveness may be reduced if the woman is taking certain medications, including some antibiotics. Birth control pills are safe for most women—statistically safer even than delivering a baby—but they carry some risks.

Source: National Women's Health Information Center, U.S. Department of Health and Human Services

Table 13.1 Birth Control: How Often Does It Fail?

Method	Average use	Perfect use
No method (chance)	85.0	85.0
Spermicides	30.0	6.0
Withdrawal	24.0	4.0
Periodic abstinence	19.0	9.0
Cervical cap	18.0	9.0*; 26.0**
Diaphragm	18.0	6.0
Condom	16.0	3.0
Pill	6.0	0.1
Intrauterine device (IUD)	4.0	0.8
Tubal ligation	0.5	0.5
Depo-Provera	0.4	0.3
Vasectomy	0.2	0.1
Norplant	0.05	0.09

*For women who have never given birth

**For women who have had two or more children

Source: Alan Guttmacher Institute, Contraceptive Use, *Facts in Brief,* New York: Alan Guttmacher Institute, 1999

Norplant A long-lasting method of contraception that consists of hormone-releasing silicon capsules surgically inserted under the skin, usually in a woman's upper arm.

vaginal ring A soft, flexible, transparent plastic that contains the hormones found in many birth control pills (oral contraceptives). The hormones are released slowly over 3 weeks in order to prevent ovulation.

barrier methods Methods of contraception that physically separate the sperm from the egg; include condoms and diaphragms.

male condom A thin rubber sheath for the penis that collects semen ejaculated during sexual intercourse; acts to prevent pregnancy and sexually transmitted infections.

spermicide An acidic substance that kills sperm.

Developing Health Skills

Correct Use of a Male Condom

For condoms to provide maximum protection, they must be used consistently and correctly. *Consistently* means using a condom from start to finish every time you have sex. *Correctly* means to:

1. Use a new latex condom for each act of intercourse—whether vaginal, anal, or oral.
2. Be careful when opening the condom. Do not use your teeth, fingernails, or other sharp objects to open the condom wrapper because you might tear the condom inside.

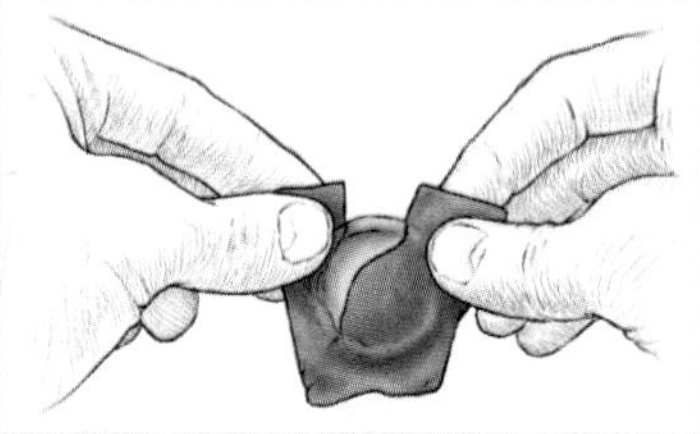

3. Put the condom on after the penis is erect and before any sexual contact.

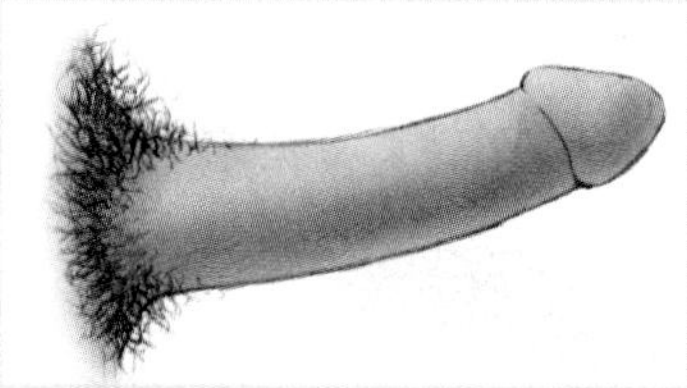

4. Hold the tip of the condom and unroll the condom all the way down the erect penis—the rolled rim should be on the outside. Leave space at the tip of the condom for semen, but make sure that no air is trapped in the condom's tip.

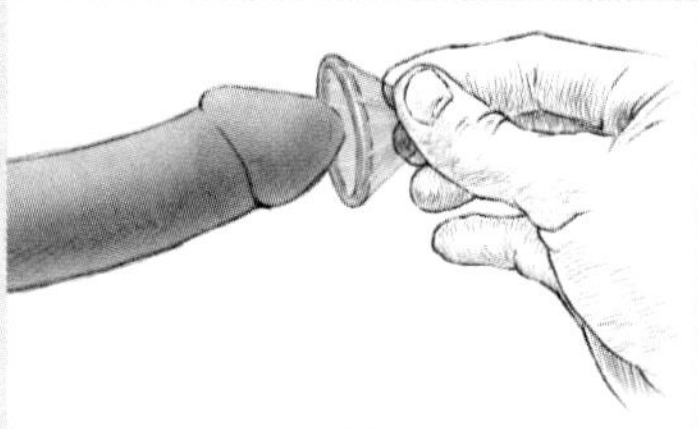

5. If additional lubrication is needed, lubricate the outside of the condom if it is not prelubricated. Use only water-based lubricants. You can purchase a lubricant at any pharmacy. Your pharmacist can tell you which lubricants are water-based. Oil-based lubricants, such as petroleum jelly, cold cream, hand lotion, cooking oil, or baby oil, weaken the condom. It is recommended that a spermicide be used in conjunction with the condom. This not only serves as a lubricant, but also enhances the condom's effectiveness in preventing unwanted pregnancy and disease.

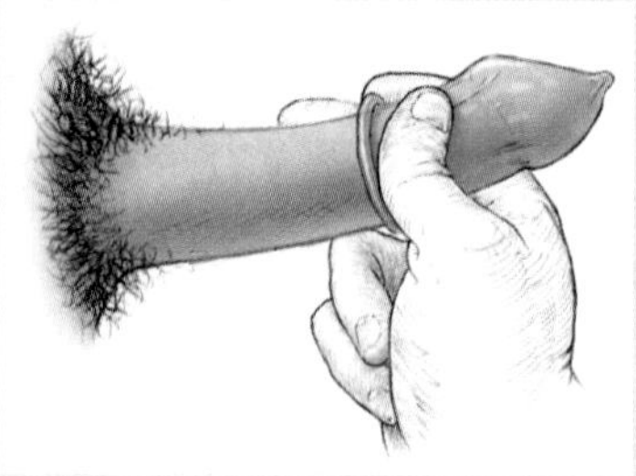

6. Withdraw from your partner while the penis is still erect. Hold the condom firmly to keep it from slipping off.

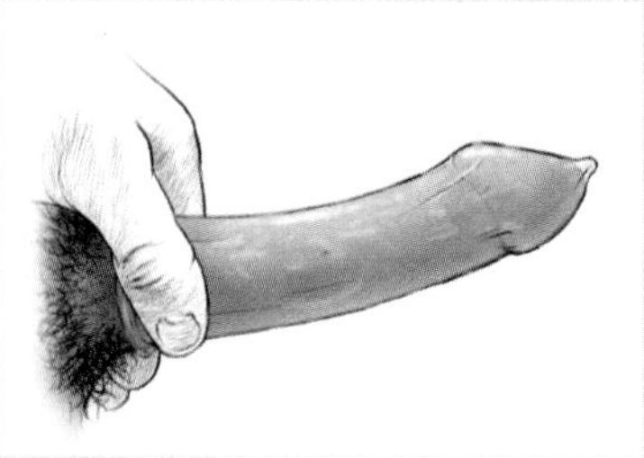

7. Throw the used condom away in the trash. Do not flush condoms down the toilet. They are not biodegradable.

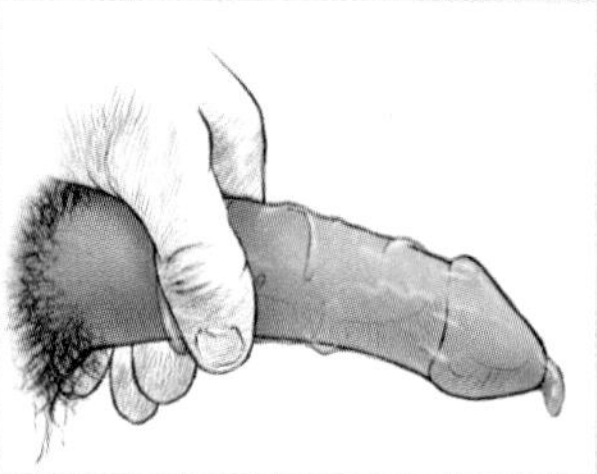

8. Never reuse a condom.
9. If the condom breaks during sex, withdraw from your partner and put on a new condom.

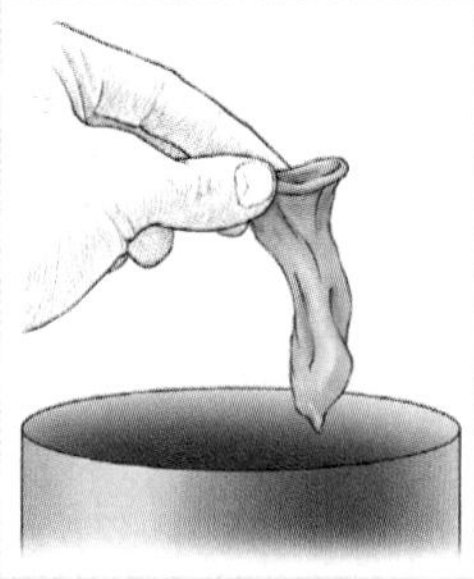

Source: Centers for Disease Control and Prevention

sperm—is considered a highly effective method of birth control. See the Developing Health Skills box for proper use of a condom. It is highly unusual for a condom to be manufactured with a defect. Failure of the condom can occur when a man does not hold the condom when withdrawing his penis. Condoms may also fail when used improperly—for example, if worn inside out or used more than one time. However, when used as directed, condoms are a reliable means of protection. Unfortunately, studies show that less than 50 percent of

Developing Health Skills

Correct Use of a Female Condom

1. Squeeze the inner ring for insertion.

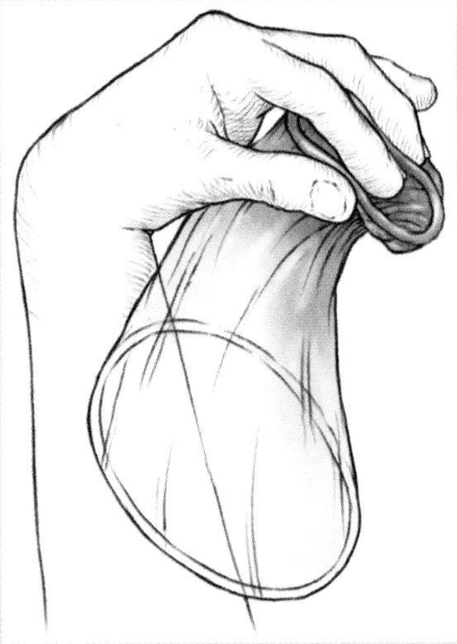

2. Insert the sheath as you would a tampon.

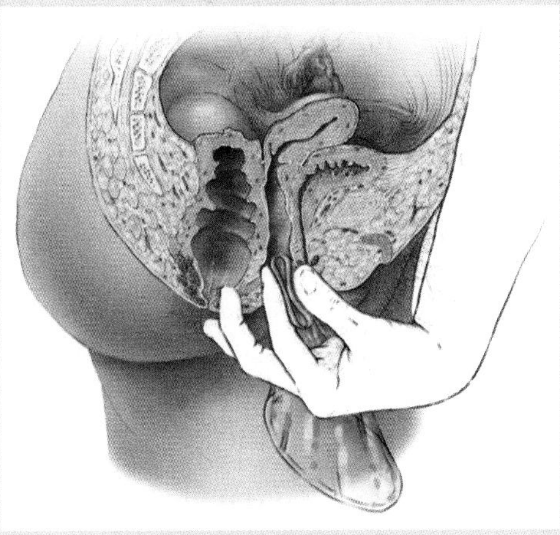

3. With your index finger, push the inner ring up as far as it will go.

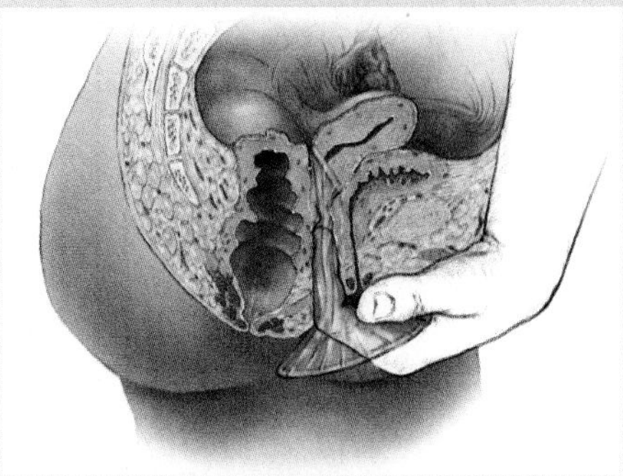

4. The condom is now in place.

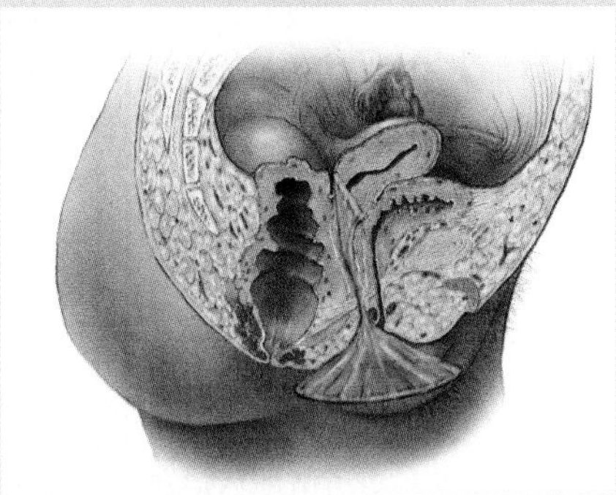

- Make sure the condom is in place and that your partner goes into the condom.
- Use enough lubricant.
- Never reuse a condom.
- Throw the used condom away in the trash. Do not flush condoms down the toilet. They are not biodegradable.

Source: Permission of The Female Health Company

U.S. college men always use condoms during sex, and almost 25 percent never use them at all.

Barrier methods for women include the **female condom, diaphragm,** and **cervical cap.** The female condom prevents sperm from reaching the cervix. It lines the inside of the vagina and keeps a barrier between the cervix and the penis, as the male condom does. It also provides protection against some sexually transmitted infections. The female condom has been sold in drugstores only since 1994. It is not widely used due to its awkward design. The effectiveness of the female condom remains somewhat unclear, although it is considered nearly as effective as the male condom. See the Developing Health Skills box for proper insertion.

female condom Lines the inside of the vagina and covers the cervix; acts to prevent pregnancy and sexually transmitted infections.

diaphragm A soft rubber cup that covers the entrance to the uterus.

cervical cap A thimble-shaped contraceptive device that fits snugly onto the cervix.

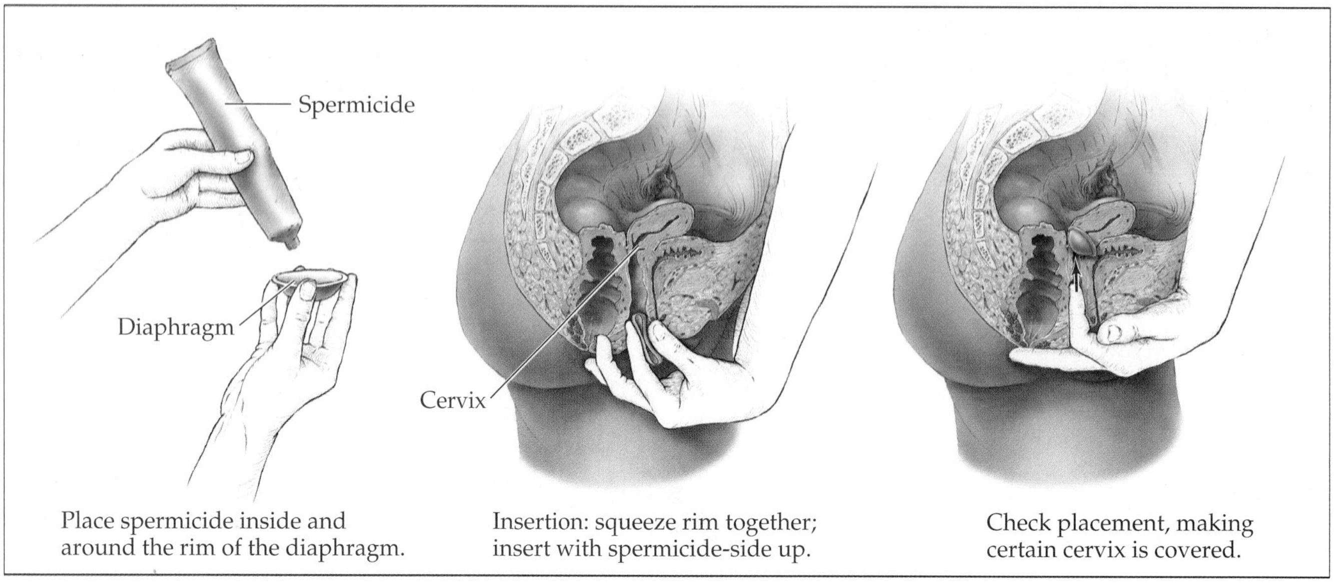

Spermicide
Diaphragm
Cervix
Place spermicide inside and around the rim of the diaphragm.
Insertion: squeeze rim together; insert with spermicide-side up.
Check placement, making certain cervix is covered.

Figure 13.5 The Correct Use and Placement of a Diaphragm
The diaphragm is the most popular barrier method used by women to prevent pregnancy.

Diaphragms and cervical caps are soft latex barriers that are intended to fit securely over the cervix. Both are used with a spermicide cream or jelly. The diaphragm is a dome-shaped cup with a flexible rim. It fits securely in the vagina to cover the cervix (see Figure 13.5). The cervical cap is thimble-shaped and smaller than the diaphragm. It fits snugly onto the cervix. Just before insertion, the diaphragm or cervical cap is coated with spermicide on the surface facing the cervix. It is then ready to be inserted into the vagina to cover the cervix before intercourse. The diaphragm blocks the entrance to the uterus, and the cream or jelly immobilizes sperm, preventing it from joining an egg. The diaphragm may be left in place for twenty-four hours. The cervical cap may be left in place for forty-eight hours. Both of these barrier methods are considered effective means of preventing pregnancy.

Spermicides also are available as foams, vaginal suppositories, and vaginal film. They form a chemical barrier that either kills sperm or makes them inactive and thus unable to pass through the cervix to the egg. Spermicides are available without a prescription and present no known risk to general health. They are less effective, however, than other contraceptive methods, but when they are used correctly with a male or female condom, their effectiveness increases significantly.

Contraimplantation refers to preventing implantation of the fertilized egg. The **intrauterine device (IUD)** is a small plastic object inserted by a physician into a woman's uterus. Some IUDs release tiny amounts of copper or a hormone. It is not fully understood why the IUD prevents implantation, but it changes the lining of the uterus in some way that prevents implantation and thus prevents pregnancy. One IUD, the Dalkon Shield, was taken off the market in the 1980s because it was associated with internal scarring, infertility, and, in some instances, death. As a result, the availability of all IUDs has fallen, and most companies have stopped producing them.

Sterilization is a form of birth control in which steps are taken to permanently end fertility. Sterilization, sometimes called voluntary surgical contraception, is by far the most popular method of birth control among married men and women. The most common forms of sterilization are vasectomy for men and tubal ligation for women (see Table 13.2).

Vasectomy involves surgically cutting and tying the man's **vas deferens,** thus preventing the passage of sperm. The vas deferens carries sperm from the testicles to the penis. A vasectomy does not interfere with normal sexual activity or the amount of semen

contraimplantation Preventing implantation of the fertilized egg.

intrauterine device (IUD) A small plastic birth control device that is inserted into the uterus by a physician.

sterilization A form of birth control in which steps are taken to permanently end fertility.

vasectomy Surgically cutting and tying the vas deferens of the man, thus preventing the passage of sperm.

vas deferens A tube that carries mature sperm from the testes to the ejaculatory ducts.

Table 13.2 Chosen Methods of Contraception

Method	Percentage of users
Tubal ligation	27.7
Pill	26.9
Male condom	20.4
Vasectomy	10.9
Withdrawal	3.0
Depo-Provera	3.0
Periodic abstinence	2.3
Diaphragm	1.9
Other methods	1.8
Norplant	1.3
Intrauterine device	0.8
Total	100.0

Note: Use of the female condom is too new to be reflected in these figures.

Source: Alan Guttmacher Institute, Contraceptive Use, *Facts in Brief,* New York: Alan Guttmacher Institute, 1999

ejaculated, but it does mean that no sperm are present in semen.

Tubal ligation is a surgical procedure in which the fallopian tubes are cut and tied in order to prevent the passage of the egg and the subsequent union of sperm and egg. Both procedures are considered permanent, although reconnecting the tubes or the vas deferens has been done with limited success.

Emergency Contraception

Occasionally an "emergency" form of birth control is needed. The **morning-after pill** is the nickname of one such emergency approach to contraception. It provides a backup if, for example, a condom breaks, a diaphragm becomes dislodged, or a woman forgets to take the pill. The morning-after pill is also used in cases of unplanned and unprotected sexual intercourse or unwanted sexual intercourse, as in rape or incest. A specific number of estrogen/progesterone birth control pills are taken within the first seventy-two hours following unprotected intercourse. This form of contraception, which can cause nausea and vomiting for a day or two, can prevent implantation. It is 75 percent effective in preventing pregnancy.

The morning-after pill is not widely used because most gynecologists prescribe it only if a patient asks for it, and most women do not know about it.

Deciding about Birth Control

There are pros and cons relating to safety, efficacy, and convenience associated with each form of birth control. Who is responsible for weighing the pros and cons? Who is responsible for birth control or for making the decisions about birth control? The best decisions are those made by both partners long before any sexual activity is initiated. Deciding what form of birth control to use, if any, is a highly personal one. Several criteria should be considered.

Safety. No one should consciously place his or her own health at risk in order to practice a form of birth control. The package inserts for the birth control pill identify specific conditions that indicate when the pill should not be used—for example, if a woman has diabetes or is over age forty and smokes.

Effectiveness. There are two types of effectiveness: theoretical and actual. Many methods of birth control are more effective theoretically than they are in actual use. The condom, for example, is theoretically 97 percent effective. Yet, because of improper use, its actual effectiveness is closer to only 84 percent. When choosing a birth control method, couples should find out the risk of pregnancy and take that risk into serious consideration. There is no perfect birth control method except total abstinence.

Acceptability. This represents the extent to which a birth control method fits within an individual's values and lifestyle. For example, sterilization is a more acceptable form of birth control for someone who has decided that he or she doesn't want to have any more children than for someone who has not made up his or her mind. Availability, ease of use, reversibility, and impact on sex drive are all considerations that can influence how acceptable a form of birth control is to an individual.

Because the choice of a contraceptive is a highly personal decision, it's important that the choice be made carefully and only after considering the range of complete information from a reliable source.

tubal ligation A surgical procedure in which the fallopian tubes are cut and tied in order to prevent the passage of the egg and the subsequent union of sperm and egg.

morning-after pill A form of hormonal contraception used within the first seventy-two hours after unprotected sexual intercourse; generally considered an emergency method of birth control that prevents implantation.

The Abortion Controversy

Abortion is one of the most controversial topics in U.S. society today. An **abortion** is the termination of pregnancy. Some abortions take place spontaneously in the form of a **miscarriage.** In fact, it is estimated that 33 percent of all pregnancies end in a miscarriage, or spontaneous abortion. The controversy arises over **elective abortions,** those that are medically induced for the purpose of ending unintended pregnancies.

According to the Alan Guttmacher Institute, 48 percent of pregnancies among U.S. women are unintended and half of these are terminated by abortion. The rest are carried to term. Each year, two out of every 100 women of reproductive age have an abortion; 47 percent of them have had at least one previous abortion and 55 percent have had a previous birth. At current rates, an estimated 43 percent of women will have had at least one abortion by the time they are forty-five years old. In addition:

- The majority of women getting abortions are young: 52 percent are under twenty-five, 32 percent are between twenty and twenty-four, and 20 percent are teenagers.
- Catholic women are 29 percent more likely than Protestants to have an abortion and are about as likely as all women nationally to do so.
- Black women are nearly three times as likely as white women to have an abortion, and Hispanic women are roughly two times as likely.

abortion The termination of pregnancy.

miscarriage Spontaneous abortion.

elective abortions Abortions that are medically induced.

vacuum aspiration A method of abortion performed in the first trimester, involving dilation of the cervix and removal of the contents of the uterus by suction; also called suction curettage.

suction curettage A method of abortion performed in the first trimester, involving dilation of the cervix and removal of the contents of the uterus by suction; also called vacuum aspiration.

RU-486 A drug that is taken after implantation to induce miscarriage. Also called a medical abortion.

dilation and evacuation A method of abortion performed in the second trimester of pregnancy in which the cervix is dilated and medical instruments are used to remove the contents of the uterus through a suction or vacuum procedure.

induction The method of abortion in which labor is artificially induced.

It is impossible to know the exact number of abortions that occur, but the Guttmacher Institute estimates that currently in the United States about 1.3 million abortions take place each year. The rate of abortion in the U.S. has declined steadily since 1980. There are several possible reasons for this drop in the abortion rate:

- Changes in attitudes about having an abortion
- Reduced access to abortion services
- Fewer unintended pregnancies
- Reduced fertility as the nation's population ages

Abortion became legal in 1973 with the *Roe v. Wade* Supreme Court decision. Since that decision, more than 30 million women in the United States have chosen to have an abortion rather than carry an unwanted child to term. Eighty-eight percent of elective abortions are performed during the first trimester of pregnancy. At this time, the fetus is very small, ranging in size from microscopic to approximately three inches long. Abortion is extremely safe during the first three months of pregnancy. In fact, at this stage, abortion presents fewer physical health risks than carrying a pregnancy to term.

The most common first-trimester surgical abortion method is **vacuum aspiration** or **suction curettage.** This technique is performed by a physician under local anesthesia on an outpatient basis. It involves dilation of the cervix (it is gradually opened) and insertion of a small tube into the uterus. The contents of the uterus are removed by a machine that creates a suction.

RU-486 is a pill that is taken after implantation to induce miscarriage. (This is in contrast to the morning-after pill, which prevents implantation.) The drug, a synthetic steroid called mifepristone, makes it difficult for the fertilized egg to adhere to the lining of the uterus. It triggers uterine contractions and the result is an abortion. RU-486 is also called a medical abortion. Unlike a surgical abortion, RU-486 is effective in producing abortions in the very early weeks of pregnancy—usually in the first forty-nine days, but it can be used safely up to the sixty-third day. Also unlike a surgical abortion, which is a one-step procedure, RU-486 requires three visits to a physician or clinic over a fifteen-day period to administer and monitor the drug. Side effects include bleeding, cramping, nausea, and vomiting.

Abortions that are performed in the second trimester are more complicated (because the fetus is much larger) and slightly more risky. About 10 percent of abortions are done in this period. The methods used for second-trimester abortion are **dilation and evacuation,** and **induction.** In the dilation and evacuation method, the cervix is dilated and suction is used to remove the contents of the uterus, much as in the first

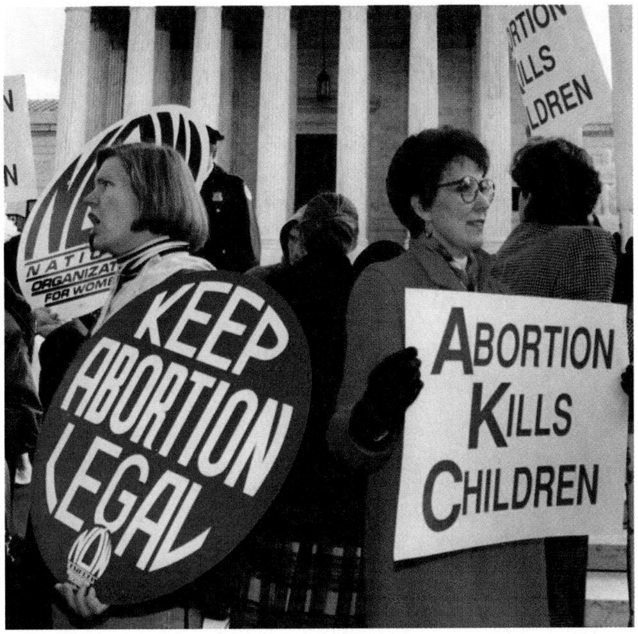

The two sides of the abortion issue make their position clear. Pro-choice advocates believe that a woman has the right to choose whether or not she wishes to continue a pregnancy, and pro-life advocates believe that the developing fetus has the right to live and needs someone to advocate for those rights.

trimester. Induction involves artificially inducing labor with the same hormone that causes uterine contractions during labor. Induction often involves a limited hospital stay. Fewer than 3 percent of women having an abortion in the United States choose this method.

Late-term abortions are probably the most controversial of all, even though only one percent of abortions are performed after more than twenty weeks of pregnancy. The procedure used is called intact dilation and extraction, and the fetus is vaginally delivered. Women seek late-term abortions because they face grave health risks or their fetuses have fatal abnormalities.

Regardless of the development stage of pregnancy, when a woman chooses to seek an abortion, counseling is offered. What to do about an unwanted pregnancy may be an easy decision for some women, but for others, there may be many factors that make abortion seem wrong.

The two sides of the abortion issue are politically represented by **pro-choice** and **pro-life** points of view. Pro-choice advocates support the idea that a woman has the right to choose whether or not she wishes to continue a pregnancy. Pro-life advocates believe that a pregnant woman must carry the pregnancy to term because the developing fetus is a human being and has a right to live. Both factions agree that an abortion represents a failure to control conception, whether intentional or unintentional.

The health risks of abortion remain widely debated. There is growing evidence, however, that abortion does not represent a major risk, either physically or psychologically. Less than one percent of all abortion patients experience a major complication such as serious pelvic infection, hemorrhage requiring a blood transfusion, or unintended major surgery. Proper counseling and follow-up normally keep psychological problems to a minimum.

A Final Word on Planning a Family

Decisions relating to family planning are among the most important that you will make. They not only affect your health but also the health of others in your family. With many of these decisions, you are likely to face controversies that are publicly debated. Information that you might need to make family planning decisions is constantly changing as new research is reported and other new developments take place. Your decisions should be based on the best information available.

pro-choice A political position that supports the idea that a woman has the right to choose whether or not she wishes to continue a pregnancy.

pro-life A political position that supports the idea that a pregnant woman must carry the pregnancy to term because the developing fetus is a human being and has a right to live.

CASE STUDY 13: Planning a Family

After Sheila and Arjun had been married for three years, they decided it was time to think seriously about having a family. They had talked about it before they were married, and both agreed that they wanted two children, but until now they were busy settling into married life and furthering their careers.

Sheila checked with her family physician to make sure she was in good health, and she began to watch what she ate and drank. Arjun did the same. After all, the consequences could be considerable. Sheila and Arjun were lucky. Within four months of deciding it was time to have a family, Sheila was happy, healthy, and pregnant.

Louise and Sam form quite a contrast. They, too, had been married for three years, but raising a family was far from what they wanted, at least for now. They were careless about using contraceptives, however, and Louise became pregnant. At first, she didn't know she was pregnant, even after she missed one period. But some other signs, including slightly swollen breasts, told her something was happening. Her physician confirmed that she was six weeks pregnant. Over the course of those six weeks, Louise had had a glass or two of wine several times a week and occasionally shared marijuana with Sam. There was still time to change her health behaviors for the rest of her pregnancy, but she had already compromised the first important weeks of her pregnancy.

In Your Opinion

If you were to look at them without knowing their case histories, Sheila and Arjun and Louise and Sam appear to be typical young married couples in the throes of raising a family. Both women are pregnant, one by decision, the other by default. Both wives have discussed the pregnancy with a physician, one in preparation of the event, the other weeks afterwards.

- What were the decisions that Sheila and Arjun made that could affect their baby?
- What actions did Louise and Sam take that ignored the implications of having a baby?
- Which couple made the healthiest decisions? for the mother? for the baby?
- How would you handle the decision to have a baby?

KEY CONCEPTS

1. The nuclear family consists of parents and their children, typically living under the same roof. Members of an extended family are connected by blood, marriage, or adoption.
2. Half of all marriages end in divorce, but most divorced people find new partners and marry again.
3. The early signs of pregnancy include a missed menstrual period, along with fullness and tenderness of the breasts.
4. Smoking, alcohol use, drug use, and some sexually transmitted infections during pregnancy are associated with higher infant mortality and babies having lower birthweights.
5. Good prenatal care includes careful monitoring by a physician or certified nurse-midwife, proper diet, and appropriate exercise.
6. During the first stage of labor, the cervix gradually opens or dilates to allow eventual passage of the baby through the birth canal. During the second stage of labor, the baby is born. In the final stage of labor, the placenta separates from the uterine wall and is expelled.
7. Contraception is the intentional prevention of the union of sperm and egg. Contraimplantation methods prevent implantation of the fertilized egg in the uterine wall.
8. An abortion is the termination of pregnancy. Ninety percent of elective abortions are performed during the first trimester of pregnancy.
9. Pro-choice advocates support the idea that a woman has the right to choose whether or not she wishes to continue a pregnancy. Pro-life advocates believe that a pregnant woman must carry the baby to term because the developing fetus is a human being and has a right to live.
10. Effective family planning requires extensive and objective information.

REVIEW QUESTIONS

1. Describe different family structures, including the nuclear family and the extended family. How have the dual-career family and the single-parent family changed our view of what constitutes a family?
2. Describe the controversy surrounding the marriage of homosexual couples. How does "marriage" differ from a nonmarital domestic partnership?
3. List three issues that a couple should consider when deciding whether or not to have children.
4. Differentiate between preconception care and prenatal care and establish a case for the importance of each.
5. Differentiate between amniocentesis and chorionic villus sampling. What is each test designed to do?

6. Divide a normal pregnancy into three trimesters. Identify significant developmental landmarks that should, under normal conditions, be complete during each trimester.
7. Explain the major events that take place during each of the three stages of labor.
8. List several methods of birth control that men and women choose and identify the advantages and disadvantages of each.
9. Differentiate between the pro-choice and pro-life positions on the abortion issue. What are the health implications of each proposed practice?
10. Describe the importance of high quality information to the process of planning a family.

CRITICAL THINKING QUESTIONS

1. Politicians are quick to blame many of the social and health problems that face our nation on the breakdown of the family. What argument might support this contention? How might you argue against such a claim? When might a single-parent structure be healthier than a traditional family structure?
2. Consider a situation in which a surrogate mother, who was well paid for carrying a pregnancy to term for another couple, delivers a child, but does not want to give up the baby for adoption. In effect, she has changed her mind. What recourse or legal action do you believe the couple should take in this situation? Conversely, what if the surrogate mother wants the couple to adopt the baby, but the couple changed their mind. This could happen if the baby was born with a birth defect. What recourse or legal action should the surrogate mother take?
3. The *Healthy People 2010* objectives include the following: "Increase the proportion of females at risk of unintended pregnancy (and their partners) who use contraception." Baseline data suggest that at the time of first intercourse, a significant percentage of women and men do not use contraception. If the prevention of unintended pregnancy is a simple matter using contraception, why is there such reluctance to use it? Could it be misconceptions about contraceptive methods? Or is it because those having sex for the first time deny the possibility an unintended pregnancy?
4. The *Healthy People 2010* objectives include the following: "Increase male involvement in pregnancy prevention and family planning efforts." Can you explain why males tend to be less involved in family planning than females? Is it because they are affected less? Or is family planning traditionally a responsibility of women?

JOURNAL ACTIVITIES

1. How do you define your family? Write a paragraph that identifies each person in your family and points out how each member depends on the others. Write another paragraph on how your family is different from other families.
2. Develop a personal checklist for choosing a birth control method. You may want to pick up brochures from the student heath center or a local family planning clinic.
3. Interview a local health official to learn more about family planning issues of concern to your community. This could be the incidence of teenage pregnancy or accessibility to birth control methods. Are public health efforts working or are they missing the mark?
4. Develop a position paper on one side of the abortion issue—pro-choice or pro-life. Identify why people have such strong feelings about this, and what they believe they must do to act on them.

SELECTED BIBLIOGRAPHY

American College of Obstetricians and Gynecologists. "Emergency Oral Contraception." *ACOG Practice Bulletin,* 25. Washington DC: The American College of Obstetrics and Gynecologists, 2001.

Facts in Brief. New York: The Alan Guttmacher Institute, 2002. The series includes "Contraceptive Use," "Induced Abortion," and other family planning-related topics.

Field, J. and L. M. Casper. "America's Families and Living Arrangements: Population Characteristics," *Current Population Reports.* U.S. Department of Commerce, 2001.

Ginty, M. M. "The New American Family." *Parenting* 14, 1: 32 (2000).

Grady, W. R., O. G. Billy, and D. H. Klepinger. "Contraceptive Method Switching in the United States." *Perspectives on Sexual and Reproductive Health* 34, no. 3 (2002).

Hatcher R. A., et al., *Contraceptive Technology,* 17th ed. New York: Irvington Publishers, 1998.

Journal of Marriage and Family (published monthly).

Medical Aspects of Human Sexuality (published monthly).

National Center for Health Statistics. "Births: Final Data for 2000." *National Vital Statistics Reports* 50, 5 (2002):1–104.

Profiles of General Demographic Characteristics: 2000. U.S. Census Bureau, 2001.

HEALTHLINKS

Websites for Planning a Family

You can access better health as it relates to this chapter by checking out some of the following sites on the Internet. These sites can be accessed directly when you visit the *Decisions for Healthy Living* Website located at www.aw.com/pruitt.

American College of Obstetricians and Gynecologists

A link into the nation's leading group of professionals providing health care for women. The site provides women with the latest information on women's health issues.

American Society of Reproductive Medicine

The ASRM is a voluntary nonprofit organization devoted to advancing knowledge and expertise in reproductive medicine and biology. The site provides the latest information on reproductive care, and current clinical trials.

Lamaze Association

Lamaze International promotes natural childbearing experiences for women and families through education, advocacy, and reform.

Office of Population Affairs

The OPA provides resources and policy advice on population, family planning, reproductive health, and adolescent pregnancy issues.

HEALTH HOTLINES

Planning a Family

Association of Women's Health, Obstetric, and Neonatal Nurses
(800) 673-8499
2000 L Street, NW, Suite 740
Washington, DC 20036

International Childbirth Education Association
(800) 624-4934
P.O. Box 20048
Minneapolis, MN 55420-0048

National Adoption Center
(800) 862-3678
1500 Walnut Street, Suite 701
Philadelphia, PA 19102

Planned Parenthood Federation of America
(800) 829-7732 (National Office)
(800) 230-7526 (for nearest local office)
434 West 33rd Street
New York, NY 10001

TEST YOUR KNOWLEDGE ANSWERS

1. True. Most single-parent families are headed by mothers, but fathers are starting to take on this responsibility too.
2. False. Only Vermont provides legal protections to same-sex couples that are comparable to those provided to heterosexual couples.
3. False. Progesterone is present in both nonpregnant and pregnant women, so detecting this hormone will not indicate pregnancy. However, the hormone human chorionic gonadotropin (HCG) is only found in pregnant women so its presence is an indication of pregnancy.
4. False. The baby is born in the second stage of the birth process. In stage three the placenta is delivered.
5. True. Both men and women are taking responsibility for safer sex.

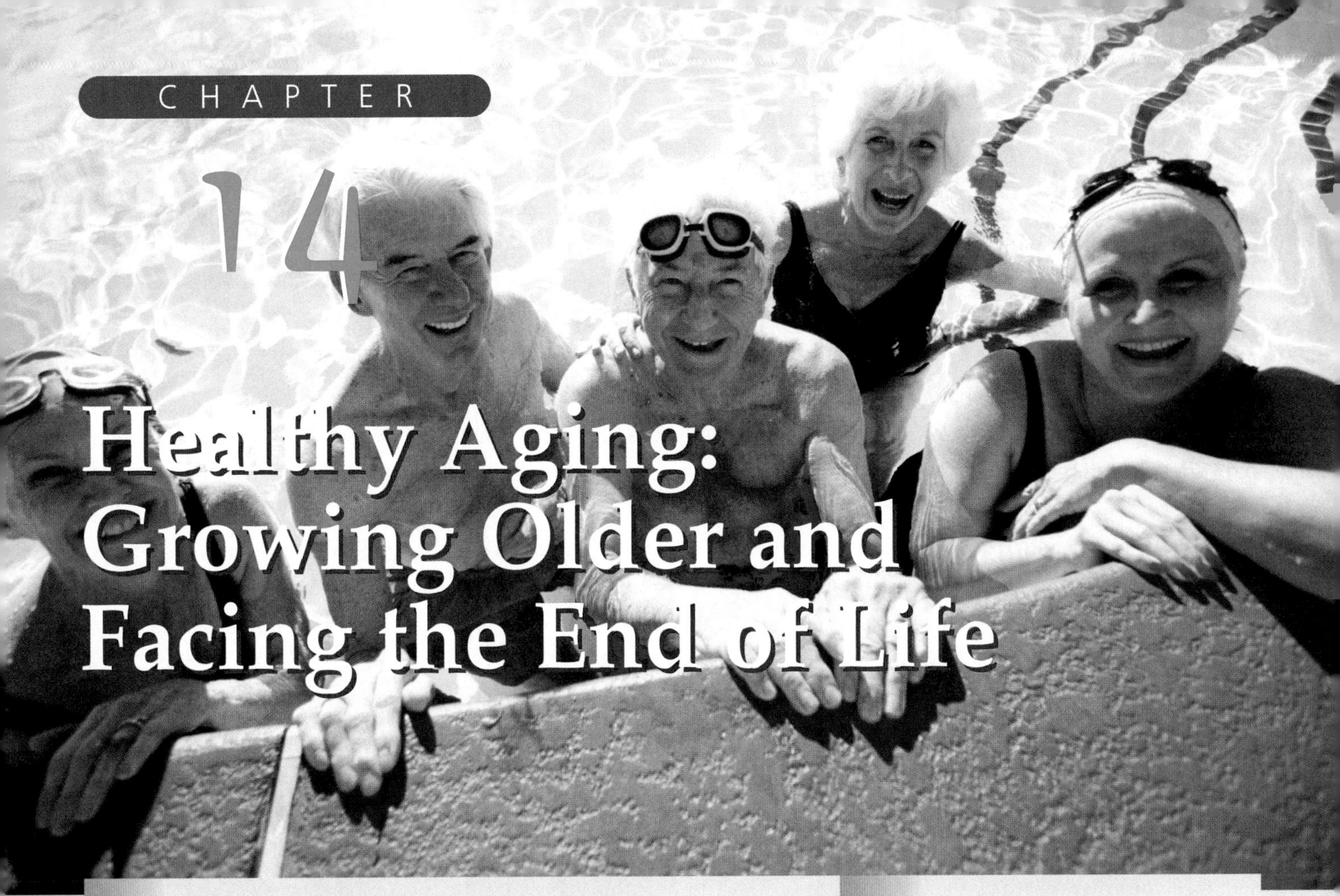

CHAPTER 14

Healthy Aging: Growing Older and Facing the End of Life

OBJECTIVES

When you finish reading this chapter, you will be able to:

1. Differentiate between chronological, functional, and psychological methods of measuring age.
2. Describe how aging influences health status.
3. Understand what happens to the bones, the senses, and the brain during the aging process.
4. Understand how to prevent some of the major health concerns of aging including depression, medicine abuse, and falls.
5. Recognize the importance of regular physical activity as a key element of healthy aging.
6. Understand the legal and biological perspectives on death.
7. Recognize Elizabeth Kübler-Ross' five psychological stages of dying: denial, anger, bargaining, depression, and acceptance.
8. Understand the importance of documents such as a will, a durable power of attorney for health care, and a uniform donor card.
9. Recognize the three stages of grieving: impact, recoil, and recovery.
10. Understand death and loss as inevitable elements of life and that grief can lead to an inspiration or a recommitment to life.

TEST YOUR KNOWLEDGE

1. Swimming is recommended for the prevention of osteoporosis, as it is not a weight-bearing exercise. True or False?
2. Ninety percent of women over sixty report that sex is as good or better than when they were younger. True or False?
3. Forty percent of all elderly people hospitalized for fall-related injuries do not go home, but are discharged directly into nursing homes. True or False?
4. The living-dying interval—that time between diagnosis and death—can last for years or be a matter of seconds. True or False?
5. Death, from a biological perspective, takes place when spontaneous cardiac or respiratory activity ceases. True or False?

Answers found at end of chapter.

When you think of yourself as "old," what age do you have in mind? For a twenty-one-year-old college student, being thirty can seem old because it carries an image of responsibilities far beyond what is expected of students—for example, having a full-time job or being a parent or a homeowner. Over the span of a lifetime, however, being thirty is not really very old because a person born today can expect to live for nearly seventy-seven years—up considerably from the beginning of the 20th century, when life expectancy was only about forty-seven years.

Given these statistics, what age do you now have in mind when you will think of yourself as old? What do you expect the quality of your life to be like when you are sixty-five years old? What about when you are eighty-five years old? These questions are often raised but seldom given serious consideration until the later years of life become a reality for you or your parents.

Although some elderly people are sickly or otherwise lead impaired lives, most people over age sixty-five are active and involved members of the community. They lead productive lives, have paid or volunteer jobs, take classes, get advanced degrees, engage in sports, and have sexual experiences. Growing older for these people is a testament to good health due to their genetic makeup, their health styles, and advances in medicine.

However, no person or living thing lives forever. A basic fact of life is that it will end in death. For most people, death is a natural stage at the end of life. Death, however, does not happen only to those who have led full lives. Children, teenagers, young adults, and the middle-aged can also die of disease and accidents. In fact, college students face the issue of death more often than you think. By age eighteen, one in twenty students has lost a parent. Suicide, AIDS, cancer, and automobile accidents have also taken the lives of classmates. There is no way to know how you will face your own death or the death of a loved one. In part this is because there is no one correct way to perceive death or prepare for it. It is a highly individual event.

Growing Older

If you think of aging as a numbers game, it starts at age sixty-five. The U.S. Census Bureau defines people aged sixty-five to seventy-four as elderly, people seventy-five to eighty-four as aged, and people eighty-five and more as very old. The number of older adults, of all ages, is growing. In the last hundred years, the number of Americans aged sixty-five or older has increased eleven-fold. In 1900, there were around 3 million Americans sixty-five years old or older. In 2002, that figure was nearly 35 million. By 2030, the number of older Americans is projected to more than double to 70 million. That means that soon one in every five Americans will be considered elderly, aged, or very old.

gerontologists Specialists who study the social, biological, behavioral, and psychological aspects of aging.

Gerontologists, specialists who study the social, biological, behavioral, and psychological aspects of aging, see enormous differences among people of these various age groups. Some of the so-called young-old—people in their sixties—might be in nursing homes, whereas some of the old-old—eighty-five and older—are still living independently.

Aging Theories

Several biological theories have surfaced concerning why and how people age:

- The *wear-and-tear theory* contends that simply as a consequence of living for many years, the effects of disease and damage over time produce aging. Running for thirty years, for example, can have a wear-and-tear effect on a person's knees.
- The *free radicals theory* suggests that foreign elements in the blood build up over time in the body and produce aging. Free radicals are highly reactive molecules that can cause damage or destroy cellular activity.

- The *biological clock theory* assumes a relationship between time lived and biological decline. Even younger people—for example, women in their thirties and forties who want to become pregnant—talk about the biological clock.

Several sociological and psychological theories have been proposed as well, including how active in or disengaged from society a person is. While gerontologists are not in agreement as to what causes aging, they do agree that aging is an inevitable element of living and is a process influenced by lifestyle decisions.

Measuring Age

There are three common measures of age. **Chronological age,** represented in the number of years since birth, provides markers to differentiate life stages. It is also used as a qualifier for certain privileges. For example, privileges for people age sixty-five years and older include Social Security payments and reduced senior citizen rates for buses and movie tickets.

Chronological age, however, can sometimes be misleading. **Functional age** is a better way to represent the physiological capacity of the body. An eighty-five-year-old tennis player, for example, may have a functional age of fifty-five in terms of cardiopulmonary output.

There is also **psychological age**—how old you feel you are. Upon turning fifty a shoe salesman who was in good health said he now "felt" old. He began taking naps in the middle of the afternoon and soon took early retirement because he found work too strenuous for "an old man like me." In contrast, a healthy and active eighty-four year old woman, who gardens and ice skates as the seasons dictate, says that she "helps the old people in the community by delivering food to them."

Aging Body and Mind: Changes That Occur over Time

Changes that occur with age take place over time. In fact, it may take years before the cumulative effect of aging is realized. For example, a gradual reduction in hearing may not be apparent at first. Slight deficits in memory or thought processes are often not noted immediately by the older person or even by family and friends.

Health Status

Are older people sicker than younger people? Asking such a question is like asking whether a glass is half full or half empty. The answer: It depends.

Surveys consistently show that the majority of elderly people say that their health is good or excellent even though they suffer from more illnesses than younger people. Clearly, older people have more chronic conditions. Although chronic and degenerative diseases are not usually the cause of death or disability in early adulthood or middle life, for many older people they are a serious threat. More people over age sixty-five die of heart disease than of any other cause. The second leading cause of death in this age group is cancer.

Older people also have more illnesses related to their weakened immune systems. Aging immune systems may become less adept at recognizing invaders. They may also become less resistant to infection. A common viral infection such as influenza or a bacterial infection such as pneumonia can be life threatening for an elderly person.

With age comes reduced energy. While this does not have much effect on normal day-to-day functioning, it could be a sign to slow down a bit. What is behind this loss of steam? Research on the heart and lungs illustrates some of the causes.

The heart of an older person, for example, might pump at the same pace as it did when he or she was younger, but now it pumps less efficiently and less powerfully. This means that in carrying out normal activities, an older person's vital organs receive less blood flow than those of a younger person having the same heart rate. During exercise, the differences are even greater. For example, a seventy-year-old circulates far less blood per minute than a thirty-year-old participating in the same activity.

The lungs are among the most resistant organs to change due to aging—provided they are cared for. Even so, as a person gets older, there is a natural reduction in the maximum amount of air they can exchange. This is due in part to the reduced effectiveness of the bronchial tubes' lining, which helps filter the air in the lungs.

Telltale Signs

One of the most visible signs of aging is a loss of the fatty and connective tissues that provide skin tone. The result is wrinkles. For many people, wrinkling begins in the early twenties and is usually first seen along the

chronological age A number representing the number of years a person has lived since birth.

functional age A number representing the ability to function; a tool for comparing actual age with ability to function.

psychological age A number representing a perceived age (how old you feel).

forehead. By age thirty, it is common to find "crow's feet" beside the eyes. Once a person reaches their forties and fifties, more pronounced aging lines develop, including radial and vertical mouth lines, baggy eyes, and jowls. Excess exposure to sunlight may also contribute to a more rapid wrinkling of the skin than would otherwise be the case.

Changes in hair color or amount provide another indication of aging. Although some people's hair turns prematurely gray in their early twenties, graying of hair usually begins in the late thirties and forties. The balding process is almost entirely determined by genetics and is seen mostly in males. If a man's father or grandfather lost his hair at a young age, that man is very likely to lose his hair at approximately the same age. Women can also have a genetic predisposition to thinning hair. This can develop in the forties but is more prominent in the seventies and eighties.

A change in body shape and weight often occurs with age. For example, the body of a twenty-year-old female is between 17 and 20 percent fat. As a woman ages, this percentage increases, and by age sixty, fat accounts for about 40 percent of a woman's total body weight.

With age, muscles undergo a loss of contractility and flexibility and become susceptible to strains, pulls, and cramps. As people grow older they also shrink in height as a result of muscle weakening, decreased space between the bones of the spine, and osteoporosis. It is not uncommon for a person to be two to three inches shorter in old age than in young adulthood.

Bone Density

In young people, living bone constantly renews itself and becomes harder and stronger. However, bones reach a peak mass—their maximum density and strength—around age thirty-five. After that, bone mass begins to diminish.

Thinning bones, a condition called **osteoporosis,** affects one in two women and one in three men over age seventy-five. It occurs less frequently in men in part because they have heavier bones than women. It is believed that estrogen, a female hormone secreted during the childbearing years, helps ensure a strong skeleton. After menopause, women are at significantly increased risk for osteoporosis. Estrogen replacement, also called hormone replacement therapy (HRT), can increase bone density, but it can also increase the risk of breast cancer, heart disease, and strokes for some women. The benefits and risks of HRT, or more importantly the decision to use or not to use it, should be discussed with a physician.

Osteoporosis can significantly affect a person's quality of life. For a person with osteoporosis, a simple stumble or fall can lead to a crippling fracture or compression of the vertebrae, which can result in severe back pain as well as a disfiguring stooped appearance.

Heredity plays a large role in osteoporosis: It is more prevalent among fair-skinned people, and a woman is more likely to develop this condition if her mother or grandmother had it. Other risk factors are cigarette smoking and heavy alcohol consumption because they can impair calcium absorption. The best time to prevent osteoporosis is during young adulthood. Having a good diet with adequate amounts of calcium, doing weight-bearing exercise (walking, playing tennis), and not smoking can help keep bones thick and strong.

osteoporosis A disorder in which bone density decreases, making the bones more likely to break.

presbyopia A difficulty in reading materials at close range; common in older people.

cataracts Clouding of the lens of the eye.

The Senses

Almost everyone's visual capacity declines with age. As people age, their eyes take longer to adjust to changes in light or to see darker colors. Another difficulty that begins in the late thirties but becomes very pronounced by age sixty—affecting nearly 100 percent of the elderly—is **presbyopia,** which involves difficulty in reading materials at close range. Presbyopia (*presby-* means "elders") is easily corrected with glasses or contact lenses.

Another eye condition common among older people is **cataracts,** which is a clouding of the lens. Fifty percent of all Americans between the ages sixty-five and seventy-four and 70 percent of those over age seventy-five have cataracts. Surgical removal of cataracts can help restore vision in many cases.

Hearing loss is also common among older people, particularly with high-frequency sounds such as those produced by the letters *s, z, t, f,* and *g.* One common cause of hearing loss over time is the damage of hair cells in the inner ear due to noise, illness, injury, or toxic medication. Hearing aids can help improve hearing.

Sexual Activity

Lovers at age seventy? Not only is it possible, it is happening to people who might be just like one of your grandparents—physically and mentally active, and "looking around." According to the Census Bureau, more than 112,000 older couples are living together.

With age, men often experience reduced sex drive and problems maintaining erections, while women may experience vaginal dryness or a decline in sexual responsiveness. Nonetheless, research studies show that 90 percent of women over sixty report sex to be as good as or better than when they were younger. Although many men think that by the time they reach sixty or seventy, they will be too old to have an erection, the truth is that impotence is due to factors that can happen at any age and not to the aging process alone (see Chapter 12). Overall, studies consistently show that sexual activity is possible among older people well into their eighties and nineties.

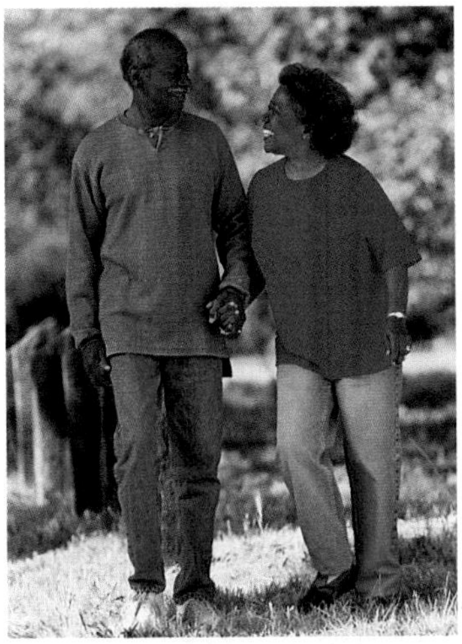

Contrary to popular belief, sexual interest is alive and well for senior citizens. For many people, living in a retirement home or community actually increases their chances of meeting someone.

Mental Ability

One of the greatest fears about getting old is the decline of mental faculties. The good news is that research shows that age alone does not necessarily cause a loss of brain function or reasoning ability. According to the National Institute on Aging, disease—not age in itself—may underlie many or even most cases of mental decline in the elderly.

People of all ages can learn new things. Older people, however, may not learn as rapidly as they did when they were younger. They are also not as quick to recall things from their long-term memory. This is a normal function of information retrieval, not memory loss. In effect, the older you are, the more information you have to sort through in your memory.

Short-term memory is a different issue. It is a complex process that involves the release of chemicals called **neurotransmitters,** which facilitate the passage of impulses in the brain. The aging brain produces smaller amounts of neurotransmitters, and unless steps are taken to keep brain **neurons** stimulated, short-term memory slows down considerably as people grow older. Studies show that mental exercise, much like physical exercise, can help keep you alert even late in life. Examples of memory tips, including mental exercises, are provided in the Developing Health Skills box.

Memory problems in the elderly can also be caused by poor nutrition, depression, **hypoglycemia** (low blood sugar), and adverse reactions to medication. In most cases, these problems are reversible with appropriate and timely treatment of the underlying condition. **Alzheimer's disease** and other forms of **dementia** are not curable.

Alzheimer's disease is not normal forgetfulness or a normal result of aging. It is a serious progressive and irreversible disease that affects the cerebral cortex and produces dementia in middle to late life. It is believed that up to 4 million Americans suffer from Alzheimer's disease. About 3 percent of the population between the ages of sixty-five and seventy-four have Alzheimer's, and nearly 50 percent of those eighty-five and older *may* have it. Alzheimer's disease starts with an inability to find the right word but progresses to misusing words, asking the same question over and over again, writing many reminder notes, wearing the same clothes every day, not paying bills, and not taking medicine. Personality changes include abusive behavior, disorientation, paranoia, depression, and other cognitive and behavioral deterioration.

At some point, people living with Alzheimer's disease cannot write or speak coherently, do not understand when people speak to them, and may not recognize themselves in a mirror. In time, they cannot feed themselves or even chew and swallow. They become bedridden and **incontinent** and eventually lose consciousness and die. On average, the course of the disease may last seven to nine years, but it can last as long as twenty years.

Autopsies show that people who have Alzheimer's disease often have tangles in their brain tissue and abnormally high amounts of some brain chemicals and deficiencies in others. One chemical that is deficient in Alzheimer's patients is acetylcholine, which is necessary for the transmission of messages from one part of the brain to another. Scientists do not know what causes this chemical abnormality, but taking acetylcholine supplements does not change the course of the disease. There are numerous theories concerning the cause of Alzheimer's disease. Possible causes include a slow virus, a malfunction of the immune system, and a genetic abnormality. None has been proven or rejected.

Without a known cause or treatment, Alzheimer's patients and their families are left to cope with the

neurotransmitters Chemicals that facilitate the passage of impulses in the brain.

neurons The basic cells of the nervous system.

hypoglycemia Low blood sugar.

Alzheimer's disease A degenerative disorder that causes dementia in middle to late life.

dementia A disorder characterized by the general and often slow decline of mental abilities.

incontinent Unable to control bowel or bladder function.

Developing Health Skills

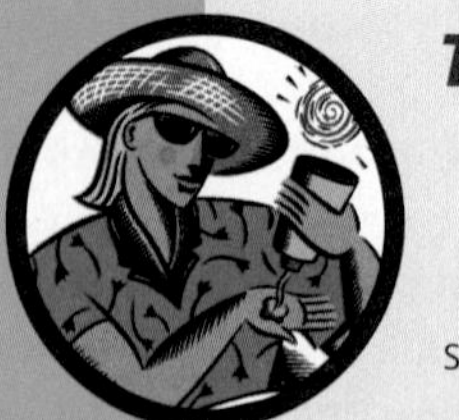

Tips for a Better Memory

All of us have problems recalling a stray fact or name at times, but some of us are so disorganized and forgetful that our brains sometimes seem more like a sieve.

No need to panic. Psychologists at Beth Israel Deaconess Medical Center in Boston have developed an innovative program called Memory 101 that's gaining attention from researchers around the nation. Here are some tips from Memory 101:

- *Make a memory notebook.* Use a notebook with a calendar in it to help you plan the minutiae of your life. Fill it with your to-do lists for the day, week, and month. Your notebook can become a portable filing cabinet for phone numbers, addresses, birthdays, medical information, phone messages—you name it. Carry it with you or carry a smaller notepad to jot down information that you will later transfer into your notebook. The act of writing something down reinforces it into your memory. Make sure to look at your notebook several times a day.
- *Talk aloud to yourself.* Say: "I'm walking up the stairs to get my glasses." "I'm putting my parking ticket in my pocket so I can get it validated." "I'm going to the store to buy milk and eggs." If a great idea strikes while you're in the shower, rehearse it out loud to help you remember it. Consider carrying a tape recorder to record things you need to remember.
- *Post reminder signs in your house, office, and car.* Write: "Remember to buy stamps!" "Remember to take out the garbage on Thursday!" "Take your pills!"
- *Get in the habit of keeping items where you will need them.* Keep your keys by the front door, an umbrella in the sleeve of your coat, and so on. Record these locations in your memory notebook.
- *Minimize distractions.* Do one thing at a time. Turn off the television or radio when you're talking with someone. At a restaurant, try to face the wall so you can easily focus on the conversation at your table.
- *Use mnemonic tricks.* Use acronyms, rhymes, and so on. When tightening or loosening lids, remember "righty-tighty, lefty-loosey." To recall the Great Lakes, remember "HOMES" (Huron, Ontario, Michigan, Erie, Superior).
- *Exercise your mind.* Reading, playing the piano, watching shows like Jeopardy, playing cards or chess—all these activities help keep your brain sharp and active.
- *Understand your own style of learning.* Most people are visual learners, remembering best what they see. They benefit the most from memory notebooks and signs. Others are auditory learners, remembering best what they hear. These people benefit from talking out loud or using a tape recorder. A few people are kinesthetic learners, remembering best what they experience. They benefit most from writing things down or acting them out. Knowing your strength will help your memory run at peak efficiency. To enhance your memory, try using all three learning modes.

Source: Adapted from WebMD, Aug. 5, 2002

disease at home and in nursing homes. About two thirds of people who have Alzheimer's disease are cared for at home, and more than 50 percent of all nursing home patients have either Alzheimer's disease or a related condition. Caring for someone who has Alzheimer's disease can involve feeding, dressing, bathing, diapering, watching to make sure the patient is not doing something unsafe, and dealing with his or her wanderings at all hours of the night.

Preventable Health Problems

Many of the health risks that the elderly face are preventable. Key among these are depression and other mental states, undermedication or overmedication, and falls. Exercising, good nutrition, and other healthy lifestyles can help prevent health problems among the elderly.

Sadness in Old Age

Depression is the most common psychological disorder among older people. It can be triggered by two very common situations for an elderly person: the loss of a loved one or the onset of a disease. Perhaps the elderly are right to be depressed and to feel lonely and abandoned. How do you think you would feel if your spouse died after fifty years of being together? How would you cope with living alone again—at age seventy-five? How would you respond to the onset of and increasing disability caused by not one or two, but four or even six different medical conditions? Other causes of depression in the elderly can be conditions that are treatable, including thyroid abnormalities, nutritional deficiencies, and infections. Suicidal thoughts often accompany depression for people of all ages, but the elderly have the highest suicide rate of any age group. Depression can be successfully treated in most older people with psychotherapy, antidepressants, or a combination of the two.

Medication Abuse

Older people are particularly sensitive to the effects of medicine and suffer reactions including confusion, decreased coordination, mental deterioration, and tremors. Even so, numerous studies show that the elderly lack knowledge about appropriate drug use. It is estimated that about 60 percent of the elderly do not comply correctly with medication directions. They might decrease the proper dosage (**undermedication**) to stretch out the prescription or take a larger dose (**overmedication**) thinking that if a little is good, more might be better. Either situation could result in an adverse reaction. Drug misuse is not limited to prescription drugs. It is common for older people to misuse over-the-counter drugs as well. Because many older individuals take several medications, problems related to drug interactions are common.

Although the following advice is important to people of all ages, it is particularly important for the elderly—and for their caretaking friends and relatives:

- Before leaving the physician's office or the pharmacy, make sure the instructions for taking your elderly relative's medicine are clear to you and your relative or another family member or friend.
- Make sure to notify your relative's physician of any symptoms that he or she develops after starting a new drug. They may be caused by the drug.
- Ask your relative's primary care physician or pharmacist to coordinate all drug use—both prescription and over-the-counter.

Falls

The elderly are at particularly high risk for unintentional injuries. Fall-related injuries send 8 percent of people over seventy to the emergency room each year. Forty percent of people hospitalized for fall-related injuries do not go home, but are discharged directly into nursing homes. Hip fractures are by far the most dangerous fractures associated with falls among the elderly, and are largely associated with osteoporosis.

Although some falls have a single, obvious cause, researchers believe that most falls are due to a combination of factors:

- Mental changes such as confusion, dementia, or mini-strokes
- Cardiovascular or circulatory problems, especially an inability to adjust blood pressure to sudden changes in posture, which can cause fainting
- Antianxiety drugs, antidepressants, and other sedating medications
- Effects of diseases, such as the pain of arthritis
- Osteoporosis, muscular weakness and overall decline in physical vigor
- Changes in vision, hearing, reflexes, and coordination
- Environmental hazards, such as loose rugs or torn carpeting, poor lighting on stairs, and trailing electrical cords

Carefully adjusted home environments and increased physical skill by the elderly can reduce the risks associated with falls.

Help from Exercise

No single group can benefit more from exercise than the elderly, according to gerontologists. Researchers report that simply walking four hours a week can decrease the risk for future hospitalization for heart disease. Another moderate exercise, T'ai chi (discussed in Chapter 3 as a way to reduce stress), is believed to improve balance, reduce the risk for falls, and increase strength. Regular physical activity by older people may also reduce risks

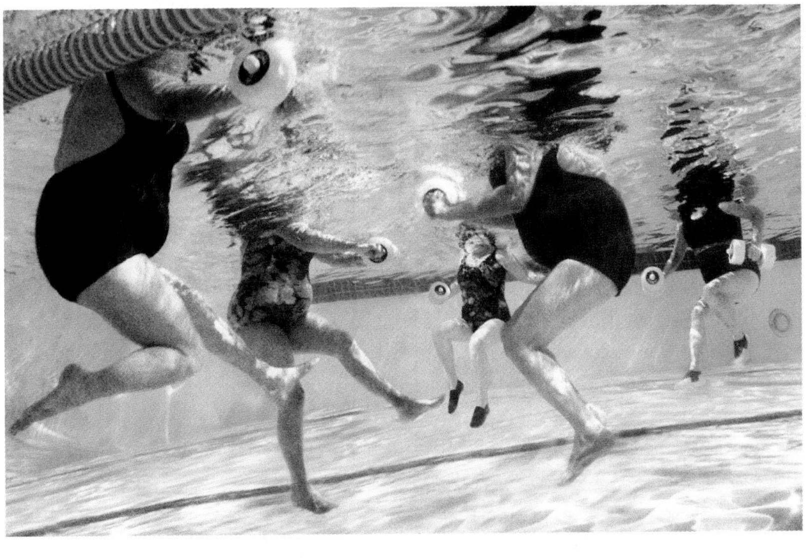

Maintaining an active lifestyle, which includes regular exercise, is a key component to healthy living throughout the lifespan and can be particularly beneficial in later adulthood.

undermedication Consuming a lower drug dosage than prescribed, which can compromise accurate medical care.

overmedication Consuming a higher drug dosage than prescribed, which can compromise accurate medical care.

Table 14.1 Benefits of Physical Activity for the Elderly

Health Issue	Health Benefits of Physical Activity
Cardiovascular health	Improves performance of heart muscle Increases heart muscle contractility Reduces premature ventricular contractions Increases aerobic capacity Reduces systolic blood pressure Improves diastolic blood pressure Improves endurance
Obesity	Decreases abdominal adipose tissue Increases lean muscle mass Reduces percentage of body fat
Osteoporosis	Slows decline in bone mineral density Increases bone density
Psychological well-being	Improves perceived well-being and happiness
Muscle weakness and functional capacity	Improves strength and flexibility Reduces risk of falls due to increased strength Reduces risk of fractures Increases reaction time Increases quadriceps strength Sustains cognition

Source: National Blueprint: Increasing Physical Activity Among Adults Age 50 and Older, The Robert Wood Johnson Foundation, 2001

for chronic disease by maintaining normal body weight, blood pressure, glucose tolerance, and lipoprotein lipid levels (see Table 14.1).

Health education and fitness programs for senior citizens are cropping up across the country, and participation in athletic events for older people is increasing. For example, the Over-the-Hill Gang, a national outdoor organization for people over age fifty, plans activities such as hiking, biking, and skiing, as well as social evenings.

Age sixty-five might be the point of retirement from the workplace for some people, but it can be the starting point for health promotion, community involvement, and what one psychiatrist calls a "psychic aliveness."

thanatology The study of death and the psychological and social problems associated with it.

brain dead A state that occurs when there is no longer brain activity.

electroencephalogram (EEG) A device that measures brain activity.

The Meaning of Death

By this time in your life, you have probably known at least one person who has died. For most college students, this usually means a grandparent or another elderly relative. To help students better understand the concepts of death and dying at any age, many colleges have instituted courses and other studies on the topic. The study of death and the psychological and social problems associated with it is called **thanatology.** In Greek mythology, Thanatos was death personified.

Death is a certainty, but defining it is not simple. For a friend, death can mean the tremendous loss of a close personal companion. For a relative, death can mean not only a crushing personal loss but also dealing with legal requirements such as a will. For a physician, death can mean following a set of criteria to determine when—or whether—death has actually occurred. The meaning of death changes as the point of view changes.

The Biological Perspective

From a biological perspective, death is a natural event that happens to all living things. In the past, death was traditionally defined as the moment when spontaneous cardiac or respiratory activity ceased—that is, when the heartbeat and breathing stopped. However, modern medical advances have made this definition obsolete because with the help of a respirator, or breathing machine, a person can "live" indefinitely. The brain controls breathing, so if a person no longer has brain activity, then he or she is called **brain dead.** Criteria for declaring someone brain dead include confirming—and reconfirming twenty-four hours later—total unresponsiveness in the patient, including a flat reading on an **electroencephalogram (EEG),** which measures brain activity. After such reconfirmation, family and hospital staff are notified and death may be declared. At that point, the respirator is removed and artificial breathing ceases.

To date, no consensus exists on the biological definition of death. It remains one of the great ethical controversies facing the nation.

The Legal Perspective

The difference between the biological and legal perspectives on death is a bit fuzzy because they both hinge on the same question, "When does death take place?" An estimated 5,000 to 10,000 Americans in a persistent vegetative state are kept alive with machinery that helps them breathe, eat, and remove bodily wastes. A person in a vegetative state is completely unresponsive and has no awareness of his or her environment. But is this living? Physicians, lawyers, judges, ethicists, and family members have debated the issue, but the legalities of the right to die are still unclear.

Withdrawing or withholding life-sustaining medical treatment is considered legal in the United States. For example, cancer patients unable to relieve the intense pain resulting from their terminal disease may want to discontinue the use of artificial feeding or a respirator.

However, **euthanasia,** or mercy killing, a practice that hastens a suffering person's death, is not legal in the United States. Euthanasia can be voluntary—when a mentally competent patient requests a physician to give him or her a lethal drug, injection, or other means to bring about death. It can also be involuntary—when a physician, nurse, or other health care worker engages in an act to end a patient's life without that patient's full consent.

A different practice of ending one's life is **physician-assisted suicide.** This is when the physician supplies the means, usually a prescription for a lethal dose of medication, which a terminally ill person can use to end his or her own life. Arguments in favor of physician-assisted suicide are that competent individuals should be able to exercise control over their own lives and deaths, and that since it may not always be possible to alleviate suffering, assistance in dying may be a compassionate act. Arguments against it are based on the sanctity of life and the potential for abuse of this option by family members or physicians.

A recent Harris Poll found that 65 percent of Americans think it should be legal for physicians to help terminally ill patients to end their lives. The U.S. Supreme Court has given the responsibility of legalizing or banning physician-assisted suicides to each state. Dr. Jack Kevorkian was convicted in Michigan of second-degree murder for this practice. In 1994, Oregon became the first state to make it legal for doctors to help competent, terminally ill patients die, but this law is being contested by federal regulators on the grounds that physicians are not permitted to prescribe certain lethal, controlled substances for the purpose of ending a person's life (see Chapter 9).

To help avoid confusion about the right to die, a federal law requires that every adult patient entering a hospital, nursing home, or hospice be told about the right to choose—and refuse—treatment in the event of terminal or incapacitating illness. Since then, patients are asked if they have a **living will** or other written declaration about what they want to happen if they are unable to make decisions about their own medical care (see Figure 14.1). A living will allows you to stipulate under what conditions you wish and no longer wish to have medical treatment, including artificial life supports, such as respirators or intravenous feeding, in the event that you cannot express these preferences to physicians or relatives. You can modify and add to the conditions of your living will in any way you choose as long as those conditions comply with the laws in your state.

Another way to let your end-of-life wishes be known is by giving decision-making authority to a relative or friend through a **durable power of attorney for health care** document. This document names a representative to speak for you about your health care if you are unable to do so. The representative does not have to be an attorney, but it should be someone who is aware of your wishes and understands what is and would be important to you if you were in a vegetative state or otherwise unable to make health-related decisions.

It is important to let your physician and family members know that you have a living will or durable power of attorney for health care document. Such documentation should be kept as part of your medical records.

euthanasia The hastening of a suffering person's death, also called mercy killing; illegal in the United States.

physician-assisted suicide A death that occurs when a physician supplies the means, usually a prescription for a lethal dose of medication, which a competent, terminally ill individual can use to end his or her life; also called physician-hastened death.

living will A legal document that stipulates which medical treatments are and are not to be used in the final days of life.

durable power of attorney for health care A legal document that identifies a representative to speak for a person about his or her health care if the person is unable to do so.

LIVING WILL

This Living Will has been prepared to conform to the law in the State of New York, as set forth in the case In re Westchester County Medical Center, 72 N.Y.2d 517 (1988). In that case the Court established the need for "clear and convincing" evidence of a patient's wishes and stated that the "ideal situation is one in which the patient's wishes were expressed in some form of writing, perhaps a 'living will.'"

I,________________________________, being of sound mind, make this statement as a directive to be followed if I become permanently unable to participate in decisions regarding my medical care. These instructions reflect my firm and settled commitment to decline medical treatment under the circumstances indicated below:

I direct my attending physician to withhold or withdraw treatment that merely prolongs my dying, if I should be in an **incurable or irreversible mental or physical condition with no reasonable expectation of recovery,** including but not limited to: (a) **a terminal condition**; (b) **a permanently unconscious condition**; or (c) **a minimally conscious condition in which I am permanently unable to make decisions or express my wishes.**

I direct that my treatment be limited to measures to keep me comfortable and to relieve pain, including any pain that might occur by withholding or withdrawing treatment.

While I understand that I am not legally required to be specific about future treatments **if I am in the condition(s) described above I feel especially strongly about the following forms of treatment:**

I do not want cardiac resuscitation.
I do not want mechanical respiration.
I do not want artificial nutrition and hydration.
I do not want antibiotics.

However, I **do want** maximum pain relief, even if it may hasten my death.

Other directions:

These directions express my legal right to refuse treatment, under the law of New York. I intend my instructions to be carried out, unless I have rescinded them in a new writing or by clearly indicating that I have changed my mind.

Signed________________________________ Date____________

Address____

I declare that the person who signed this document appeared to execute the living will willingly and free from duress. He or she signed (or asked another to sign for him or her) this document in my presence.

Witness 1____

Address____

Witness 2____

Address____

Figure 14.1 Living Will

This signed and witnessed declaration lets physicians and family members know your wishes about using life-sustaining procedures.
(*Source:* Reprinted by permission of Partnership for Caring, Washington DC 1-800-989-9455)

Dying as a Process

Death is a state. Dying, on the other hand, is a process. At what point in life do we begin the process of dying? Some people say that the process of dying begins at birth. A more functional understanding of the dying process suggests that dying begins with the diagnosis of a terminal disease or condition and continues until the point of death. The time between the diagnosis and death is called the **living–dying interval.**

A twenty-year-old person who is diagnosed with a brain tumor, for example, may be given two or three years to live. That person's living–dying interval begins when he or she is informed of the tumor and ends with his or her death. On the other hand, a twenty-year-old in a fatal automobile accident has a brief living–dying interval—perhaps lasting only a few hours or even seconds.

Stages of Dying

Although everyone would prefer to be healthy and not sick, studies show that more than 80 percent of the people asked say they would want to know if they were dying when they are very ill to enable them to better prepare for their own deaths. In her classic book, *On Death and Dying,* Elisabeth Kübler-Ross delineated five stages that terminal patients go through in accepting the fact that they are dying. Hope usually persists throughout all these stages.

The first stage is **denial**—"No, it can't be happening to me." In this period of denial, the patient is still in shock and cannot believe that he or she is going to die.

The second stage is **anger**—anger at almost everything. The patient is angry with the physician for giving him or her the diagnosis or for not having a cure. Sometimes, the patient is angry with God for giving him or her such an illness.

In the third stage, **bargaining,** the patient bargains for a little more time. "Let me live long enough to graduate from college," or, "Give me just a few days without pain."

Depression is the fourth stage of accepting death. The anger that had been experienced earlier is replaced with sadness and a sense of loss. This is also called a preparatory depression—preparatory for the final separation from this world.

The final stage is **acceptance,** when the patient finally understands that he or she is dying. When patients accept death, it is often a painful time for the survivors, who may misinterpret it as a rejection of their caring efforts. How could someone ever be ready to die and, at the same time, continue to hold onto meaningful relationships? With acceptance, the struggle is over and, as one patient put it, it is time for "the final rest before the long journey."

It is important to note that these stages are not universally experienced: Some people never accept the fact that they are dying. And, when the stages are experienced, they do not necessarily occur in order. Some individuals accept the fact that they are dying long before they bargain for more time.

Hospice: Comfort for the Dying

The three greatest fears of a dying person are pain, loss of control, and isolation/abandonment. **Hospice** care is designed to lessen these three fears and to help the dying person live as fully as possible. The goal of hospice care is not to treat or cure the terminal condition and thus save the life of the ill person. Rather, the goal is to relieve the pain and suffering associated with the dying process. (In the Middle Ages, a hospice was a way station for travelers.)

Most hospice care is received at home, but there are also special inpatient hospice facilities. Typically, a hospice program offers support services to patients and families through a team of professionals including physicians, registered nurses, therapists, home health aides, social workers, chaplains, and volunteers. This team effort addresses not only physical distress but also any emotional, social, financial, or spiritual problems that may be troubling the patient or family.

living–dying interval The time between the diagnosis of a terminal condition and death.

denial The stage of dying in which the person does not believe that death is going to happen to him or her.

anger The stage of dying in which the person is angry at almost everything.

bargaining The stage of dying in which the person bargains for more time.

depression The stage of dying in which anger is replaced with sadness and a sense of loss.

acceptance The stage of dying in which the person understands that death is inevitable.

hospice A specialized health care program, usually for the last weeks or months of life, emphasizing the management of pain and other symptoms associated with terminal illness, in contrast to treatment.

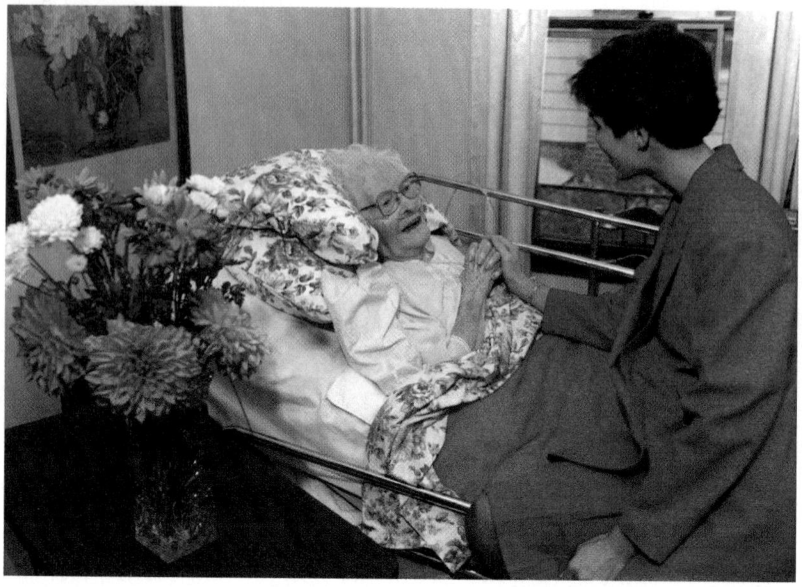

Hospice is a specialized health care program emphasizing the management of pain and other symptoms associated with terminal illness. Most hospice care is delivered at home surrounded by family and close friends.

For Survivors: A Time of Decisions and Bereavement

Coping with the death of a loved one does not stop with the death itself. The **bereaved,** or the survivors of the recently deceased person, are left to plan the funeral, handle financial matters, and, above all, work through the grieving process. Bereaved family members can be greatly aided if the deceased had a valid and up-to-date **will** that contained instructions about what to do with the body, what kind of funeral to have, and other personal issues surrounding death. Wills also contain information about how to dispose of the deceased person's property, money, and other possessions. If there is no valid will, the person's body is handled and property distributed according to rules established by the state in which the person lived.

bereaved Survivors of a recently deceased person who experience a sense of loss and grief.

will A legal declaration of a person's wishes about how to dispose of his or her body and personal property after death and other personal issues surrounding death.

uniform donor card A card signed by a person age eighteen or older that shows he or she has agreed to donate all or specified parts of his or her body upon death.

autopsy An examination and dissection of a dead body to discover the cause of death; usually conducted by a coroner.

embalming The use of chemicals, internally and externally, to temporarily preserve the body for open-casket viewing and/or transportation.

cremation The burning of a dead body into ashes.

columbarium A special vault for urns containing ashes of cremated bodies.

Decisions about the Body

Upon death, there are several decisions that have to be made right away about the physical remains of a body. Many body parts can be transplanted immediately following death and can give life to others. These organs and tissues include bone, bone marrow, eye, heart, kidney, liver, lung, pancreas, and skin. By signing a **uniform donor card,** a person over age eighteen can agree to donate all or specified parts of his or her body upon death (see Figure 14.2). If the deceased did not specifically state prior to death that he or she wanted to donate organs, family members can make this decision.

Depending upon the circumstances of death, some families may request an **autopsy,** a surgical postmortem examination of the body to determine cause of death. This information can be useful in learning more about sudden, unexplained deaths, in investigating infectious diseases that may be harmful to the public, as evidence in legal proceedings, and for insurance purposes.

Some people wish to have the body embalmed. **Embalming** is the use of chemicals, internally and externally, to temporarily preserve the body for open-casket viewing and/or if the body has to be sent to a distant destination for burial. Another option is **cremation,** or having the body burned. Cremated remains can be privately scattered, kept by the family in an urn at home, entombed in a special vault called a **columbarium,** or buried in a cemetery.

Planning a Funeral

A funeral provides family and friends with the opportunity to celebrate the life of the deceased and to offer support to the bereaved. It also brings a sense of closure to that person's life. A eulogy delivered by a close friend can be a meaningful way to express these feelings. (See the Cultural View box to learn more about religious traditions about death.)

Most people choose to be buried in a cemetery. Family members can select a wide array of caskets from a simple pine coffin to an ornate copper or bronze one.

National Kidney Foundation
Please detach and give this portion
of the card to your family.

This is to inform you that, should the occasion ever arise, I would like to be an organ and tissue donor. Please see that my wishes are carried out by informing the attending medical personnel that I have indicated my wishes to become a donor.
Thank you.

____
Signature Date

For further information write or call:
National Kidney Foundation
30 East 33rd Street, New York, NY 10016
(800) 622-9010

- -

Uniform Donor Card

of ______________________________
(print or type name of donor)

In the hope that I may help others, I hereby make this anatomical gift, if medically acceptable, to take effect upon my death. The words and marks below indicate my wishes.
I give: ☐ any needed organs or parts
☐ only the following organs or parts

____
specify the organ(s), tissue(s) or part(s)

for the purposes of transplantation, therapy, medical research or education;
☐ my body for anatomical study if needed.

Limitations or special wishes, if any: ____________

Figure 14.2 Uniform Donor Card
By signing a uniform donor card to donate body parts upon death, the gift of life can be a part of death.

Selecting a headstone and the epitaph to go on it is another decision that the family must make. This is usually done several months after the burial.

A Time of Bereavement

During this time, the most difficult issue at hand for loved ones of the deceased is dealing with **grief,** the deep sadness caused by a loss. **Mourning** is expressing grief at someone's death. **Bereavement** is the period during which a sense of loss is felt as a result of the death of a loved one. (Grief and mourning also can take place after exposure to a local or national tragedy, such as the fatal attacks of September 11, 2001.)

The length of time a family mourns and the behaviors they exhibit in this period are usually defined in cultural terms. Religious and cultural rituals—for example, an Irish wake or the Jewish seven-day mourning period of *shiva*—provide opportunities to share mourning.

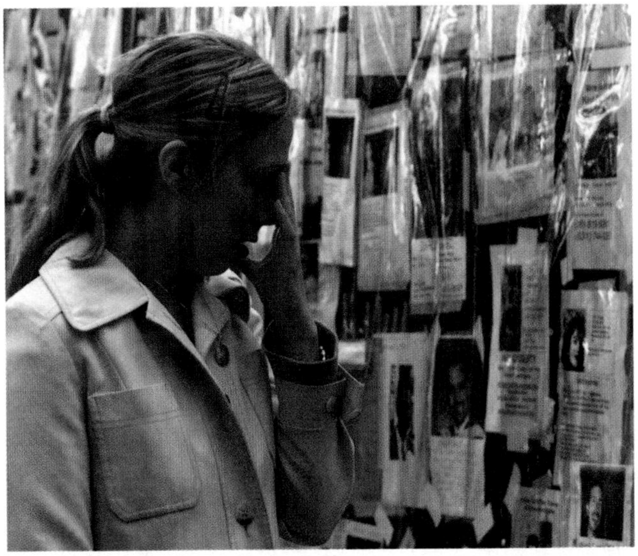

For survivors, there are emotional stages of grieving, starting with the impact of hearing the news to recovery to a more normal life without the person. During the early stages of grieving, family members and friends need support from each other.

The grieving process—like the dying process—involves stages of gradual adaptation to loss. There are three basic stages of bereavement: impact, recoil, and recovery. In actuality, these stages are not as sharply delineated. People handle these stages quite differently, and they frequently shift back and forth among stages to meet the needs of the moment.

The **impact** of the news of the death of a loved one is usually met with shock, disbelief, or denial, even when the person has been sick and was expected to die. Such reactions may last only a few minutes or may linger for several weeks. This period of shock provides the bereaved with a buffer from reality in order to start accepting the loss of a loved one.

The second stage of the grieving process is a period of **recoil,** during which the bereaved find themselves in a vacuum, superficially carrying on and trying to return

grief A deep sadness caused by a loss.

mourning Expressing grief at someone's death.

bereavement The period during which a sense of loss is felt due to the death of a loved one.

impact The stage of bereavement in which loved ones react with shock, disbelief, and denial.

recoil The stage of bereavement in which the bereaved superficially carry on and try to return to normal.

Cultural View

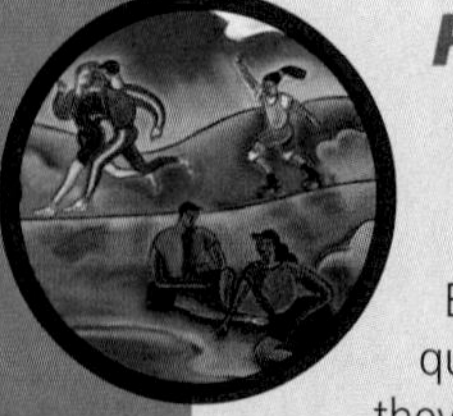

Religious Traditions about Death

What happens to human beings after death? Every religion has an answer to this important question. And while the answers are different, they all have this in common: the belief that there is some kind of life after death. It may be the Christian belief of death and resurrection or the Buddhist belief in the rebirth of the soul to another person.

The hope that life in some way goes on seems to be an almost instinctive response among people since human history began. Just as there are enduring beliefs about the afterlife, there are funeral rites in every culture that mark the transition between the two phases of existence.

Paying Respect

Until modern times, funerals in all known societies were religious rites. In the Western world, there is a small but growing trend toward secular rites. This trend emphasizes the universal human need to respond to the disruption caused by death, even among those who are not religious. Funerals are a means of showing respect for the dead, while at the same time providing an occasion for mourners to express their grief and find comfort from friends and family members.

The mourning period after death is well defined in several religions. It is set aside as a special time to express grief, so that the survivors can gradually disentangle themselves from the deceased and eventually continue with their lives unencumbered by unresolved relationships.

Thousands of years before the development of modern psychology, Judaism defined four phases of mourning that are very similar to the cycle of bereavement and the modern insights about the benefits of expressing grief rather than repressing it. At the end of the mourning period, Jews are expected to get back to business as usual, and Jewish tradition chides anyone who mourns beyond the prescribed period.

Burial Traditions

While Jews bury their dead as soon as possible, traditionally in a plain shroud and wooden coffin to level distinction of wealth at the time of the funeral, Christian burials in the United States have become expensive and elaborate, leading to a barrage of criticism.

The common practice of a wake, where the face is made up and the body is embalmed and viewed in a comfortable-looking coffin, is regarded as reinforcing the denial of death, because the corpse is made to appear as if it is only sleeping.

In the United States, burial is most common but cremation is gaining acceptance despite some prescriptions against it in the Jewish and Christian faiths. Hindus and Buddhists normally dispose of their dead through cremation. In the Hindu religion, all the relatives of a dead person are looked on as ritually impure, and the mourners are secluded from the rest of the world for ten days after the funeral. Daily ceremonies are performed to give the naked soul of the dead person a new spiritual body with which it may pass on to the next life. The soul is reborn after death to live in another body and continue an endless round of birth, death, and rebirth. There are some differences between Buddhist and Hindu beliefs about the transmigration of the soul, but essentially, both religions believe in rebirth.

Unlike Buddhists and Hindus, Muslims bury their dead. They believe in the promise of a paradise where they will be rewarded for faithfulness to Allah and for any suffering they endured in this life.

Among Native American Plains Indians, the most common forms of burial were scaffold and tree burials. In a traditional tree burial the body remained there until it decomposed. Burial grounds were usually avoided by Indians because they feared that the grounds were haunted by spirits of the deceased. At the time of the burial, close relatives would come to linger near the corpse, preparing food for the spirit's journey to the hereafter, which was described as a duplicate of the living world. The hereafter was the place where spirits were reunited with their dead relatives. To show their grief, mourners would often cut their hair short, gash their arms and legs, and blacken their faces. It was also customary for relatives of the dead to give away the deceased's belongings to the needy.

Modern Plains Indians, such as the Indians of the Lakota tribe, combine elements of Christian burial with ancient Indian customs. Although the tree or platform burials are no longer allowed, Indians still follow the custom of giving away the deceased's belongings either at the time of death or one year later. Indians still gather one year after the death of a loved one to honor the deceased and release his or her spirit to the hereafter.

Today in the United States and Western Europe, the elaborate apparel of mourning common in the nineteenth century, such as black buntings draped over buildings, arm bands, and widows' weeds (black clothing), have disappeared. This is seen by some as a sign that death has become taboo in our culture and that mourning is considered morbid. Without such outward signs, traditionalists worry that the bereaved will be left to suffer alone, aggravating their sense of loss. Traditions, however, are strongly rooted; those discussed here, and others, are likely to continue in some fashion.

Developing Health Skills

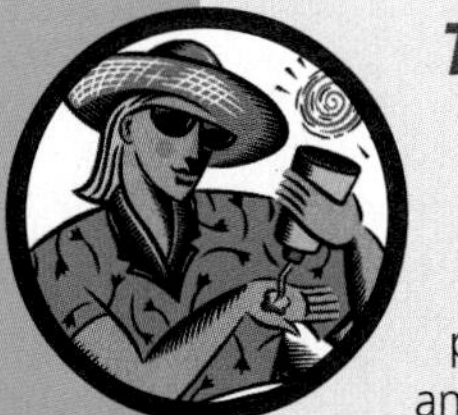

The Biology of Grief

Grieving following bereavement takes its toll on the body as well as on the mind. Physical symptoms of grief include stomach pain, loss of appetite, intestinal problems, sagging energy levels, and too much or too little sleep.

The relationship between bereavement and sleep has generated great interest among researchers as a factor in increased psychiatric and medical conditions and mortality. The strong link between sleep and the immune system suggests that disrupted sleep following bereavement can indirectly affect health by suppressing the immune system.

"Sleep is a vital element in overcoming grief," says Martica Hall, Ph.D., assistant professor of psychiatry at the University of Pittsburgh School of Medicine.

Grieving individuals experience more sick days and hospital admissions in the year following their loss than nonbereaved individuals, particularly where depression is a factor. In fact, depression is a significant contributor to disrupted sleep, whether the individual is bereaved or not. Intrusive thoughts and avoidance of reminders of the deceased that often accompany prolonged, more intense grief also impair the quality of sleep and health.

Younger people and those already showing symptoms of stress and depression are most at risk for health consequences following bereavement. Conversely, the most physiologically resilient individuals are those who have worked out effective coping strategies, have good social support networks, and maintain a healthy sleep profile.

While there are many variables based on age, expectations, and other factors, sound physical and mental health before loss predicts that a grieving individual will cope more easily when loss takes place. "Re-establishing and maintaining regular eating and sleeping patterns are important to maintaining overall health," says Hall.

Source: Grief: Coming to Terms With Loss Six Months After Sept. 11, *Facts of Life* 7, no. 3 (2002). Reprinted with permission from the Center for the Advancement of Health, Washington, DC

to normal. This can last for weeks for some people, for months for others. One mother, for example, set a place at the table for months after her teenage son died of leukemia.

During the **recovery** stage, which can last for as long as a year or two, grievers continue to feel sadness and despair and are usually preoccupied with thoughts about the deceased person. There is great variability at this time. Some grievers can become irritable, angry, restless, and depressed (see the Developing Health Skills box on the biology of grief).

This period is best described as a series of steps forward and backward. Only time appears to increase the steps forward and reduce the number of slides backward. Sliding backward is not bad, and, in fact, may be necessary for the bereaved to deal with many intense feelings. Gradually, the bereaved accepts the person's death, has fewer bouts with despair, and builds a new life (see the Developing Health Skills box about how to help a grieving friend).

Loss as a Creative Force

Facing death is seldom easy. With preparation, however, thanatologists believe that the loss experience of death can be a creative force for the living. They suggest that preparation for death involves attempting to answer several questions. They emphasize that it is not as important to reach concrete answers as it is to become involved in the process of seeking those answers. When facing death, the following questions may be important:

- What do I believe about life and about death?
- Is there purpose in my living? What is life all about?
- Is there more to life than what I have perceived thus far?
- What happens when I die?
- Is death something to be fought off and postponed for as long as possible?
- Are there circumstances in which death is something to be welcomed?
- How do I feel when I accept that someday I will die?

The answers to these questions, and the process of seeking answers to them, are influenced by our experiences, what we have learned from those around us, and

recovery The stage of bereavement in which the bereaved begin to show signs of returning to a more normal life.

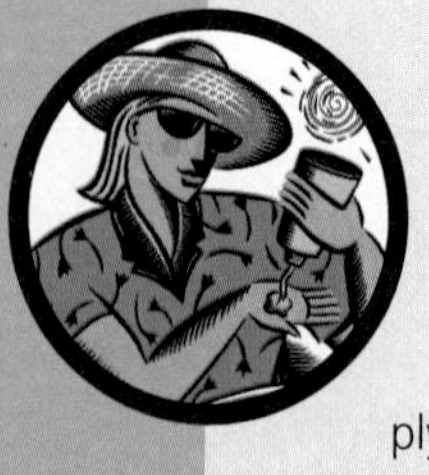

Developing Health Skills

How to Help a Grieving Friend

Many people feel uncomfortable and awkward calling or visiting a friend who is grieving. But if you really care for your friend, you can help by simply communicating your feelings of shared grief and concern.

- Get in touch. Call, write, or visit and let your friend know you care.
- Help your friend attend to practical matters. You might be needed to call people and let them know when the funeral will take place. This kind of help can create a special bond.
- Encourage others to visit or help. Call on your network of friends to help out. You may want to schedule their visits so everyone doesn't come at the same time. Ask people to prepare food.
- Be a good listener. Your friend might want to talk emotionally about the deceased. But don't force conversation. Be prepared to accept silence. It is better than aimless chatter.
- Don't tell the bereaved how he or she feels. Good friends mistakenly think they are helping by saying things like, "I know you must feel relieved now that your mother is out of pain."
- Do not probe for details about the death. If your friend offers information, listen with understanding.
- Encourage postponing major decisions. Wait until after the period of intense grief. Whatever can wait should wait. In time, draw your friend into quiet outside activities. Some people do not have the initiative to go out on their own.
- When your friend returns to activities, treat him or her as a normal person. Acknowledge your friend's loss, but don't dwell on it.

what we have come to understand about our existence from our cultural and religious heritage. The experience of death can have a positive side. When a loved one dies, grief cannot be avoided, but it can lead to an inspiration or recommitment to life. In this way, loss may actually become a creative and healthy force.

CASE STUDY 14: Facing the End of Life

George was a junior in high school when he was diagnosed with bone cancer and his left leg was removed above the knee. He was fitted with a prosthesis and got along well with his life. Unfortunately, when he was a junior in college, his cancer returned and spread to other parts of his body. This time, his condition was terminal, and George was having difficulty coping with this fact. He sank into a deep depression and gave up hope. In the final weeks of his life, George refused help, including an appropriate level of pain medication. He could have made many decisions concerning his medical care, his funeral, and his personal belongings, but George steadfastly refused to discuss these issues.

Several weeks before he died, George could no longer handle the pain and he was admitted to the hospital. He was placed on a life support system that involved numerous tubes inserted into his body—although his family had no idea whether this accorded with his wishes. Despite visiting often, his parents and sister were not in the hospital when he died.

Krista's fatal illness was leukemia. Like George, she thought she had beaten a childhood disease, but soon after she entered college, the symptoms began to reappear, beginning with weight loss and extreme fatigue. She managed to complete her freshman year, but by the summer, she was fading rapidly.

With support from her parents and brother, Krista chose to enter a hospice care program to enable her to lead as high-quality a life as possible in her final weeks and to die at home. With proper pain medication, Krista remained alert and involved. She read books, listened to music, and kept in touch with the people most important to her. Her hospice team helped her not only with pain management but also with planning her own funeral. Krista wanted her roommate to recite a poem that they both loved. She and her brother spent long hours talking about her impending death and gaining strength from each other. As she neared death, Krista was at home, where her surroundings were familiar and she could be at peace with herself.

In Your Opinion

George and Krista dealt with dying in different ways. George thought he was being brave by "fighting" death; Krista "fought" in another way.

- What could George have done to make his last weeks more manageable for himself and his family?
- Do you think he gave up by going to the hospital?
- What health skills did Krista have that helped her through this time?
- How would you compare the quality of the last few days of George and Krista's lives?
- Which would you choose for yourself, and why?

KEY CONCEPTS

1. The Census Bureau defines people aged sixty-five to seventy-four as elderly, people seventy-five to eighty-four as aged, and people eighty-five and more as very old.
2. The majority of elderly people say that their health is good or excellent even though they suffer from more illnesses than younger people.
3. One of the most visible signs of aging is a loss of the fatty and connective tissues that provide skin tone. The result is wrinkles.
4. Memory loss that is due to poor nutrition, depression, hypoglycemia (low blood sugar), and adverse reactions to medication is both preventable and reversible.
5. Regular physical activity by older people may reduce risks for chronic disease by helping them maintain normal body weight, blood pressure, glucose tolerance, and lipoprotein lipid levels.
6. A biological definition of death may address the irreversible loss of all bodily functions.
7. A living will stipulates under what conditions you wish and no longer wish to have medical treatments that will extend your life.
8. Most people say they would want to know if they were dying when they are very ill to enable them to better prepare for their own deaths.
9. Elisabeth Kübler-Ross delineated five stages that terminal patients go through in accepting the fact that they are dying: denial, anger, bargaining, depression, and acceptance.
10. The grieving process, much like the dying process, involves stages of gradual adaptation to loss, including impact, recoil, and recovery.

REVIEW QUESTIONS

1. Describe three methods of measuring age: chronological, functional, and psychological.
2. Identify the primary health concerns related to the bones, senses, and brain during the aging process.
3. Describe the symptoms of Alzheimer's disease.
4. List actions that can be taken to prevent depression, medicine abuse, and falls among the elderly.
5. Make a list of reasons why regular physical activity is important for healthy aging.
6. Write a definition of death from a biological and legal perspective.
7. Name several important written documents that should be completed by everyone in order to assure that personal end-of-life desires are known by medical providers and family members.
8. Briefly describe the five stages of dying according to Elisabeth Kübler-Ross.
9. Identify the significant tasks that survivors must undertake when a loved one dies.
10. Describe the impact, recoil, and recovery stages of grieving and estimate the time involved in each stage.

CRITICAL THINKING QUESTIONS

1. The *Healthy People 2010* objectives include the following: "Reduce the proportion of adults with osteoporosis." The degenerative disease osteoporosis presents a threat to the health and well-being of elderly people in the United States. The best-known means of reducing the disease's impact is weight-bearing exercise. How would you suggest that private sector and government health care organizations promote

exercise to seniors? What are the implications on the nation's health if this objective is met?

2. The perception of time changes as we age. From the perspective of a four-year-old, two years represents half a lifetime. The same two years, however, are viewed as only a brief period of time by an eighty-year-old. How can younger generations learn the value of time? Would such a value influence their health-related decisions? How might the development of health skills influence an appreciation of time?
3. In *Healthy People 2010,* about 40 objectives depend on "mortality" data to monitor outcomes. Should the objectives for the nation give such emphasis to measures of length of life? Or should the objectives give more attention to the quality of life, regardless of the length of life?
4. Are there any conditions under which you would support someone's choice to end life, either through physician-assisted suicide or through voluntary euthanasia? If so, what are those conditions? Do they relate to pain and suffering? If so, how much pain and how much suffering would be necessary before you supported euthanasia? How can you be sure that all conditions would be met?

JOURNAL ACTIVITIES

1. Compare and contrast your view of human aging with that of another object—a tree, a house, or a car. Be careful not to fall victim to stereotypes. An old car can be a rusty junk heap or a well-cared-for and highly valued possession.
2. Look at pictures of your parents and grandparents for hints of what you might look like later in life. Imagine what you will look like at age forty, sixty, or eighty, and what you will be doing. Write a description of your "older" self.
3. When you die, how do you want your family and friends to remember you? What do you think your best friend will say as a eulogy? Write an obituary of someone you admire—a historical figure, family member, friend, your religious leader. Now try writing your own obituary.
4. For a period of one week, monitor the obituary column of the newspaper. Record the age and cause of death of all persons listed. Does the average age at death compare to the national figures for life expectancy? Can you explain the differences?

SELECTED BIBLIOGRAPHY

Aging Research and Training News (published 22 times a year).

Approaching Death: Improving Care at the End of Life. Washington, DC: Institute of Medicine, National Academy Press, 1997.

Breslow, L., D. Reuben, and S. Wallace. Introduction: Health Promotion Among the Elderly. *American Journal of Health Promotion* 14, no. 6 (2000): 341–342.

Chernoff, R. Nutrition and Health Promotion in Older Adults. *Journal of Gerontology, Series A.* 56A (Special Issue II) (2001): 47–53.

Health after 50: The Johns Hopkins Medical Letter (published monthly).

"Healthy Aging: Preventing Disease and Improving Quality of Life Among Older Americans 2002." *CDC At A Glance,* Atlanta, GA: Centers for Disease Control and Prevention, 2002.

Kübler-Ross, E. *Death: The Final Stage of Growth.* Englewood Cliffs, NJ: Prentice-Hall, 1975.

Lynn, J., M.D., and J. Harrold, M.D. *Handbook for Mortals: Guidance for People Facing Serious Illness.* New York: Oxford University Press, Inc., 1999.

National Blueprint: Increasing Physical Activity Among Adults Age 50 and Older. Princeton, NJ: The Robert Wood Johnson Foundation, 2001.

Perkins, S. A. "Physical Activity and the Healthy Older Adult." *Health Education Monograph Series* 18, 2 (2000): 38–43.

Swanson, E. A., T. Tripp-Reimer, and K. Buckwalter (Eds.). *Health Promotion and Disease Prevention in the Older Adult: Interventions and Recommendations.* New York: Springer Publishing Company, 2001.

HEALTHLINKS

Websites for Healthy Aging: Growing Older and Facing the End of Life

You can access better health as it relates to this chapter by checking out some of the following sites on the Internet. These sites can be accessed directly from the *Decisions for Healthy Living* Website located at www.aw.com/pruitt.

AARP

The nation's leading organization for people age fifty and older, providing information and education, advocacy, and community services offered by a network of local chapters and experienced volunteers throughout the country. Explore back issues of *Modern Maturity* magazine and the monthly *AARP Bulletin,* and examine the latest information on tax and policy changes.

Administration on Aging

A link to the federal Health and Human Services agency dedicated to addressing the health needs of the elderly.

Hospice Web

A link to resources for and information about hospice care, including a listing of hospices around the country.

Last Acts

A coalition of more than 420 national and local organizations dedicated to improving end-of-life care.

National Institute on Aging

NIA, part of the National Institutes of Health, promotes healthy aging by conducting and supporting biomedical, social, and behavioral research and public education. The site includes recent announcements of significant findings from NIA-supported research and publications on health and aging for health professionals and the public.

Partnership for Caring

A national not-for-profit organization dedicated to helping patients and their families participate in decisions about end-of-life medical care. It provides living wills and advance directives by state and offers a range of publications and services, such as the Right-to-Die Law Digest, that summarize important developments in the field and describe changes in the law.

HEALTH HOTLINES

Healthy Aging: Growing Older and Facing the End of Life

Alzheimer's Association
(800) 272-3900
919 North Michigan Avenue, Suite 1100
Chicago, IL 60611

Grief Recovery Helpline
(800) 445-4808
P.O. Box 461659
Los Angeles, CA 90046

National Association of Area Agencies on Aging, Eldercare Locator
(800) 677-1116
927 Fifteenth Street NW, 6th Floor
Washington, DC 20005

National Council on the Aging
(202) 479-1200
300 D Street, SW, Suite 801
Washington, DC 20024

National Hospice and Palliative Care Organization
(800) 658-8898
1700 Diagonal Road, Suite 625
Alexandria, VA 22314

National Institute on Aging Information Center
(800) 222-2225
Building 31, Room 5C27
31 Center Drive, MSC 2292
Bethesda, MD 20892

United Network for Organ Sharing
(888) 894-6361
P.O. Box 2484
Richmond, VA 23218

TEST YOUR KNOWLEDGE ANSWERS

1. False. Weight-bearing exercises such as walking or jogging (not swimming) are recommended for the prevention of osteoporosis and to help keep bones strong.
2. True. Interest in sex does not stop for healthy adults. Studies consistently show that sexual activity is possible (and pleasurable) among older people well into their eighties and nineties.
3. True. The elderly are at particularly high risk for unintentional injuries. Fall-related injuries send 8 percent of people over seventy to the emergency room each year. Forty percent of those hospitalized are discharged directly into nursing homes.
4. True. In the case of an automobile crash, severe injuries can lead to a quick death, so that the living-dying interval for the crash victim is a matter of seconds. In the case of a cancer victim, however, the time between diagnosis and death can be years.
5. False. In the past, death was traditionally defined as the moment when spontaneous cardiac or respiratory activity ceased—that is, when the heartbeat and breathing stopped. However, modern medical advances have made this definition obsolete because with the help of a respirator, or breathing machine, a person can "live" indefinitely.

CHAPTER

15

Living in a Healthy Environment

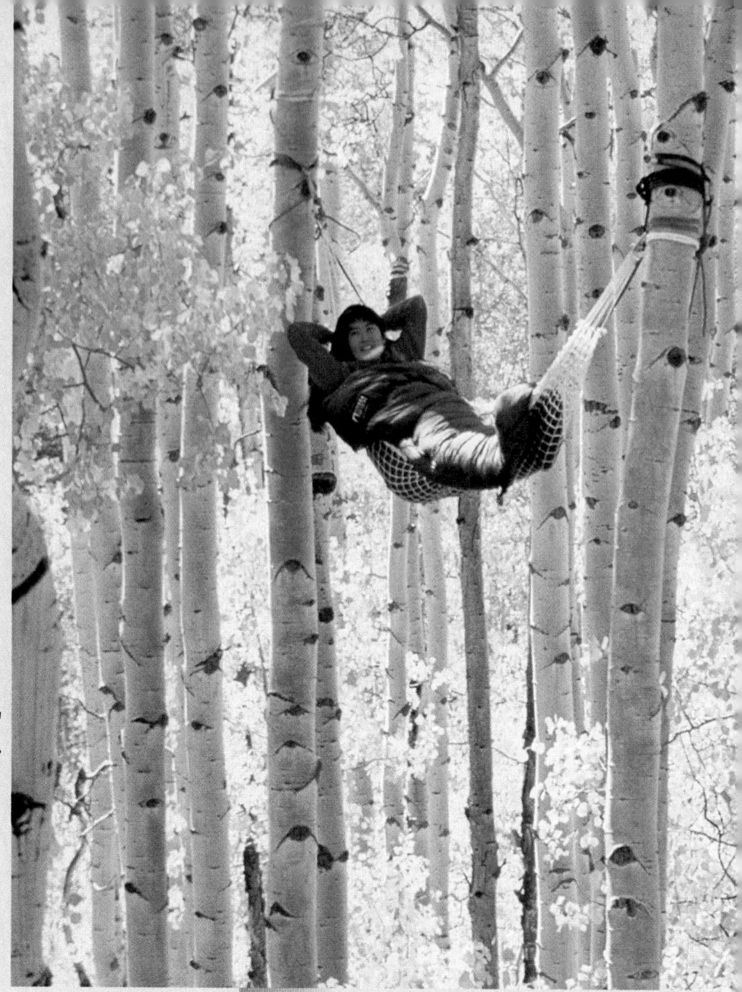

OBJECTIVES

When you finish reading this chapter, you will be able to:

1. Differentiate between serious environmental threats and those that are perceived to be serious but that actually present little risk to the global environment.
2. Recognize the difficulty of measuring environmental health threats.
3. Understand the meanings of carcinogen, teratogen, and mutagen.
4. Describe the health effects of air pollution and list the principal air pollutants along with the primary source of each.
5. List the principal water pollutants and identify the source of each.
6. Understand the health threat of solid waste.
7. Recognize the practices of precycling and recycling and their potential for reducing solid waste.
8. Understand the health hazards of toxic wastes in the environment.
9. Recognize noise as an environmental pollutant.
10. Recognize a range of opinion concerning environmental policy and action.

TEST YOUR KNOWLEDGE

1. Over the last forty years, the average number of children born to each woman in the world has fallen from five to fewer than three. True or False?
2. Smog results from natural elements in the environment such as fog and ozone. True or False?
3. The ozone layer filters ultraviolet rays from the sun and serves as a protection against the sun's radiation. True or False?
4. A major ecological advance was the development of the disposable diaper—a product that rapidly degrades. True or False?
5. Exposure to radio waves, microwaves, and infrared waves of radiation present a significantly greater health hazard than ionizing radiation such as ultraviolet rays. True or False?

Answers found at end of chapter.

From the air you breathe to the water you drink, the environment that you depend on for life sustenance can cause major health risks. This does not mean that you need to worry about your health every time you go outdoors or drink a glass of water. In fact, there is likely to be a wide difference in perception between what you think is risky and what scientists consider risky. Even health experts do not always agree about which environmental risks are most harmful to human health.

Part of the confusion about environmental health stems from the fact that the science of assessing environmental risks is still relatively young. Many health specialists believe that the public's concern about chemicals and cancer is out of proportion to the actual risk. This has given birth to the idea of **acceptable risk.** According to this idea, although exposure to a specific chemical or other hazardous material might be capable of causing disease, the likelihood of a person actually getting sick from it is very small. Other scientists argue against this idea because they believe that there have not been enough studies of the long-term effects of exposure to chemicals and other pollutants to be sure if any level of risk is acceptable.

Environmental Health: How Big Is the Problem?

Scientists cannot precisely determine the extent of environmental harm, particularly as it relates to health, for several reasons. First, the impact of pollution on the human body is often subtle and goes undetected for long periods of time. Due to this delay, when symptoms do appear, people tend to focus on them and not on their root cause.

Another reason is that pollutants come from many sources, making a cause-and-effect determination difficult. The compounding effects of **multiple hazards** further complicate the effort to determine the source of the problem accurately.

Finally, people react differently to pollutants and other health hazards and to different exposure levels. Sunbathing over a twenty-year period may cause **melanoma** in one person and nothing beyond a tan in another. Individual responses are due in part to your genetic composition, exposure to other pollutants, and lifestyle habits, such as cigarette smoking.

Identifying Health Effects

Three terms are becoming familiar to the public as awareness of environmental health hazards increases: carcinogens, teratogens, and mutagens.

A **carcinogen** is a substance that causes cancer. If the level of exposure to a carcinogen in the environment is sufficient, the effect of carcinogens on human tissue is generally irreversible. A diagnosis of cancer today may reflect an exposure to a carcinogen many years ago. Similarly, carcinogens added to the environment today may not reveal their damage until many years from now. In addition, substances that are not carcinogenic by themselves may interact with other substances to promote cancer.

Many environmental pollutants are not only carcinogenic but teratogenic and mutagenic as well. A **teratogen** causes birth defects. For example, children born to mothers who have eaten food contaminated by methylmercury frequently develop a disorder resembling cerebral palsy. A **mutagen** causes hereditary changes on the cellular level that may be passed from one generation to another. Although many chemicals are mutagenic in large doses, it is not known whether mutagenic risks also exist at the levels at which these chemicals currently appear in the environment.

Environmental pollutants have other serious health effects, including damage to the lungs and kidneys and to the nervous and immune systems. Exposure to high

acceptable risk A circumstance in which the benefits outweigh the risks; when the likelihood of ill effects is very small.

multiple hazards Simultaneous exposure to more than one health threat.

melanoma A skin cancer that often starts as a molelike growth and grows in size and changes color; the most serious of the various types of skin cancer.

carcinogen An agent that causes cancer.

teratogen An agent that causes birth defects.

mutagen An agent that causes hereditary changes on the cellular level that may be passed from one generation to another.

levels of lead, for example, can result in mental retardation and brain damage. Mercury poisoning also affects the brain as well as the kidneys and bowels.

Population and the Environment

Before addressing the more obvious threats to the environment (air, water, solid waste, and noise pollution), it is important to consider the changing nature of the world's population and how population growth (some would say overpopulation) impacts the environment. The United Nations projects that by 2050, the world's population will reach nearly 10 billion. This growth will take place despite the fact that for more than forty years the average number of children born to each woman in the world has fallen from five to less than three.

Falling population growth rates present a tempting opportunity to conclude that population size no longer presents the same threat it once did. However, from an environmental impact point of view, even a population sustained at the present level creates competition for our already limited natural resources. According to Population Action International, more than 400 million people in the world currently face water scarcity. Nearly 2 billion people live in countries where forest cover is critically low. In addition, most of the world's waters are being fished to their maximum capacities. How can we handle more people, even if the population growth rate is slowing?

Access to family planning is a critical variable influencing population growth. Use of family planning leads to lower fertility rates, later childbearing, and thus slower population growth. Family planning, however, is a source of much debate in the United States. For example, policies that call for the funding of and dissemination of information about contraception and abortion are controversial political issues.

Given this situation, what role can we play in reducing the threats to the environment brought on by overpopulation? Perhaps the most important contribution we can make is to control our own fertility (see Chapter 13 for information on birth control). The concept of zero population growth suggests that married couples should limit the number of children they have to no more than two—that is, a one-to-one replacement. When a couple has two (or fewer) children, then the population growth rate, at least on a very personal level, is not affected.

Many individuals, however, for religious or philosophical reasons, do not support the idea of zero population growth. For those individuals, a response to the population growth problem might be to support policies that develop existing natural resources in a more ecologically sound way so that they are available to support and feed more people, and thus sustain the planet for a longer period of time.

Despite successes in lowering the rate of population growth, much remains to be done. Without reducing the size of the world's population, natural resources such as fresh water and clean air will have to be shared with more and more people.

The Air You Breathe

People have known for centuries that the air we breathe can make us sick. Before the age of sophisticated air-quality monitoring, coal workers took caged canaries down into the mines with them. Since canaries are more sensitive to deadly gases than humans, if the birds died the miners knew that the air they were breathing contained deadly gases that they could not smell. The saying "mad as a hatter" referred to nineteenth-century hatmakers, who often became irrational—or "mad"—from breathing the fumes from the mercury they used in the making of felt hats. Today, the automobile is the single most significant cause of air pollution. See the Developing Health Skills box for tips on what you can do to reduce air pollution from your car.

Whether the pollutant is invisible, as is mercury, or as visible as smog's brownish haze, air pollution can cause serious ill health effects. Environmental scientists are increasingly concerned because, given that high levels of air pollution can cause adverse health effects, it is reasonable to assume that low levels over a long period of time can have negative health effects as well.

Table 15.1 presents a listing of major pollutants in the United States and the health concerns associated with each. "Criteria pollutants" are those for which the U.S. Environmental Protection Agency (EPA)—which regulates hazardous air pollutants—sets national standards. There are only six criteria air pollutants, but they are discharged in relatively large quantities by a variety of sources. The six criteria pollutants are: ozone, nitrogen dioxide, particulate matter, sulfur dioxide, lead, and carbon monoxide. These six are among the thousands of hazardous air pollutants that pose a danger to health.

Why Dirty Air Is Unhealthy

Toxic gases occur naturally in the environment, and under normal circumstances the body's excellent filtering system, which includes the nose, mucous membranes, and cilia (small, hairlike projections from cells lining air passages leading to the lungs), assures that we breathe in "safe" air.

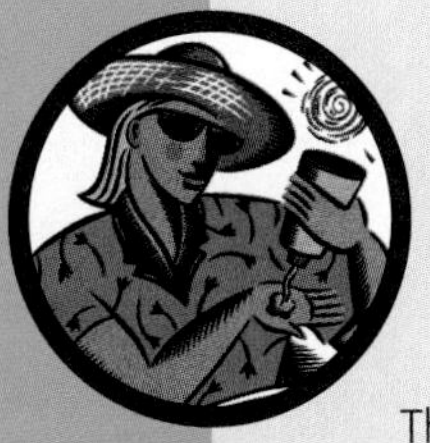

Developing Health Skills

Consumer Health: Your Car and Clean Air: What You Can Do to Reduce Pollution

There are three easy things you can do to help keep emissions as low as possible from your car.

Avoid unnecessary driving. The most effective way to reduce emissions from your car is to use it less.

- Consolidate your trips (plan to do several errands in one trip; drive to a central location, park, and walk between nearby destinations).
- Establish and make use of car pools.
- Use public transit whenever you can.
- Ride a bike or walk to school or work.

Maintain your car properly. By following the manufacturer's recommended maintenance guidelines, you will get the best fuel economy (gas mileage) as well as extend the life and value of your car.

- Do not tamper with your car's emission control system. Have it checked to make sure it is working properly.
- Do not use leaded gas in a car designed for unleaded. Doing so could irrevocably damage the emission control system.
- Premium- or super-grade gasoline contains additives to increase octane, a measure of how much a fuel can be compressed in an engine before it spontaneously combusts. It is not a measure of fuel power or quality. Unless your car needs high-octane gas, using it will not improve performance, but it will put additives into the air and also cost you more money.

Drive wisely. Your car's emission will be lower if you apply common sense to your driving.

- Don't idle. You will prevent pollution by avoiding long idles, such as warming up the car in cold weather. Today's cars need little warm-up (or idling) time.
- Using air conditioning in the car increases the load on the engine, which can increase emissions and decrease fuel economy. Open the windows or the fresh air vent to cool the inside of your car. Park in the shade if you can, to prevent the car from heating up in the sun.
- Spilled gas pollutes the air when it evaporates. When you fill up, try to avoid spills and "topping off."
- Your car burns more gas and emits more pollution when the engine is working especially hard. Try to limit extra load conditions such as running the air conditioning, high-speed driving, quick acceleration, revving the engine, and carrying extra weight.

Source: U.S. Environmental Protection Agency

Air pollution, however, is not normal. It overtaxes the filtering system of the body. The result is that we breathe in noxious particles and gases. Illnesses related to air pollution include diseases of the lung, throat, bronchial tubes, sinuses, and nose because these organs come in direct contact with the polluted air.

Asthma, for example, is a serious chronic lung disease that is increasing in prevalence, in part due to air pollution. People who have asthma have an allergic overreaction to airborne particulates such as dust as well as other air pollutants. As a result, a flood of antibodies causes lung inflammation, airway restriction, and a life-threatening shortness of breath. More than 15 million Americans suffer from asthma today. According to the Centers for Disease Control and Prevention (CDC), about two thirds of asthma sufferers live in areas where air quality is poor. Particulate matter inside homes may also play a role because cat dander and dust mites are asthma-triggering substances.

As the pollutants pass from the lungs into blood vessels and throughout the body, other organs are compromised, including the heart. Less life-threatening diseases related to air pollution include allergies, eye irritation, and **dermatitis** (skin reactions).

In some cases, an air pollutant can become even more hazardous when it is breathed along with another pollutant or when the same pollutant emanates from two different sources. The term **synergistic effect** is used when the simultaneous actions of two separate entities together have a greater total effect than would be expected from the sum of the individual effects. As you read in Chapter 8, this also can occur when two drugs are taken together.

air pollution The contamination of air by waste products.

asthma A breathing disorder that causes wheezing, coughing, and shortness of breath.

dermatitis A skin disorder in which an area of skin may become red, swollen, hot, and itchy.

synergistic effect When simultaneous actions of two separate entities together have a greater total effect than would be expected from the sum of the individual effects.

Table 15.1 Health Effects of Air Pollutants

Pollutants	Health concerns
Criteria pollutants	
Carbon monoxide	Ability of blood to carry oxygen impaired; cardiovascular, nervous, and pulmonary systems affected
Lead	Retardation and brain damage, especially in children
Nitrogen dioxide	Respiratory illness and lung damage
Ozone	Respiratory tract problems such as difficulty breathing and reduced lung function; also, asthma, eye irritation, nasal congestion, reduced resistance to infection, and possibly premature aging of lung tissue
Particulate matter	Eye and throat irritation, bronchitis, lung damage; also impaired visibility
Sulfur dioxide	Respiratory tract problems, permanent harm to lung tissue
Hazardous air pollutants	
Arsenic	Cancer
Asbestos	A variety of lung diseases, particularly lung cancer
Benzene	Leukemia
Beryllium	Primarily lung disease; also affects liver, spleen, kidneys, and lymph glands
Coke oven emissions	Respiratory cancer
Mercury	Several areas of the brain as well as the kidneys and bowels affected
Vinyl chloride	Lung and liver cancer
Radioactive Particles	Cancer

Source: U.S. Environmental Protection Agency

Benzene, a chemical that can cause leukemia in humans, is an example of the synergistic effect and air pollution. Benzene is a chemical widely used in the manufacturing of other chemicals and in petroleum refining. It is also contained in cigarette smoke. Although cigarettes emit an insignificant amount of benzene compared to the amount emitted by industry, cigarette smoking is the major source of benzene exposure because smokers directly breathe in this pollutant. In this example, two separate entities, one a behavior (smoking cigarettes) and one an environmental hazard (working in a polluted environment) combine to compound the impact of benzene on the individual.

The good news is that air quality, overall, is getting better. Since the implementation of the Clean Air Act of 1970, controls over concentrations and emissions of pollutants, especially automobile-related pollutants, have successfully reduced the level of criteria pollutants. Total emissions of the six principal air pollutants have fallen 29 percent since 1970, but millions of Americans still live in areas with unhealthy air.

benzene A chemical that can cause leukemia in humans.

carbon monoxide A colorless, odorless, poisonous gas that is produced by the incomplete burning of carbon in fuels.

Principal Air Pollutants

Carbon monoxide is a colorless, odorless, poisonous gas produced by the incomplete burning of carbon in fuels. Carbon monoxide is emitted by internal combustion engines, most of which are gas-powered motor vehicles, including automobiles, trucks, and buses. Carbon monoxide is by far the most plentiful air pollutant. Fortunately, this deadly gas usually does not stay in the environment for long. It tends to convert, by natural processes, into harmless carbon dioxide fast enough to prevent any general buildup. However, it can reach dangerous levels in areas where there is heavy auto traffic and little wind. When breathed, carbon monoxide replaces oxygen in the blood. Because a lack of oxygen affects the brain, one of the first symptoms of carbon monoxide poisoning is impaired perception and thinking. Severe carbon monoxide poisoning can cause heart failure and loss of consciousness (asphyxiation).

Sulfur oxides (the most common of which is SO_2, sulfur dioxide) are acrid poisonous gases produced when fuel containing sulfur is burned. Electrical utilities and industrial plants, particularly those using coal, are the principal producers of sulfur oxides. Although industry is working to reduce the levels of sulfur oxide emissions by switching to low-sulfur fuels or removing sulfur from fuels entirely, sulfur oxides are still a major pollutant. As the level of sulfur oxides in the air increases, breathing becomes more difficult. Respiratory diseases associated with sulfur oxides include chronic coughs and colds, asthma, bronchitis, and emphysema.

Sulfur oxides can also combine with moisture in the air to form sulfuric acids. **Sulfuric acid** dissolves in water droplets in the atmosphere and falls to earth as **acid rain.** This precipitation has a higher level of acid than normal. For example, a fog in southern California was measured and found to have the same acidity level as a hydrochloric acid solution used to clean toilets. As you can imagine, acid rain can be particularly harmful to trees and aquatic life, especially to species that can only live in a narrow range of acidity. In addition, acid rain can also corrode buildings and impair visibility.

Gasoline, which is a mixture of many kinds of **hydrocarbons,** is the major source of hydrocarbon emissions. Hydrocarbon pollution is due in part to gasoline vapors that evaporate from the tank or escape from the tail pipe of a car or truck. Other sources are gasoline stations and industries that use solvents, paint, and dry-cleaning fluids. At the levels usually found in the air, hydrocarbons rarely have an effect on health. In a confined space, however, they can cause asphyxiation. A major problem associated with hydrocarbons is their role in forming smog. **Smog** is a noxious mixture of smoke and fog that develops when hydrocarbons, nitrogen oxides, and other gases are trapped under a layer of warm air.

Particulates are solid particles or liquid droplets so small that they can be transported great distances by the winds and can remain in the air for a long time. They range in size from large pieces of soot to particles too small to detect without a special microscope. Particulates are produced primarily by coal plants and industrial processes as well as by natural sources such as forest fires. The smaller the particulates are, the more likely they are to reach the innermost parts of the lungs and clog the **alveoli,** or lung sacs. Diseases associated with particulates include black lung disease, found among coal miners who inhale coal dust, and brown lung disease, found among textile workers who inhale cotton fibers.

Lead enters the air from automobile exhaust and from industries that smelt or process metal. It is absorbed into the body and accumulates in soft tissues and bones, especially affecting the nervous system and kidneys. Lead exposure causes high blood pressure and increases heart disease, especially in men. Children are highly susceptible to lead poisoning from air pollutants and other environmental sources (see the discussion about lead-based paint on page 269). Although most of the gasoline sold today is lead-free, many gasoline engines and vehicles, including lawn mowers and farm tractors, still use leaded gas.

Nitrogen oxides are poisonous gases produced when fuel is burned at very high temperatures, as in electrical power plants, industrial boilers, and transportation vehicles. At high levels, nitrogen oxides can be fatal. At lower levels, they can irritate the lungs, cause bronchitis and pneumonia, and lower resistance to respiratory infections such as influenza. The principal harm does not come from nitrogen oxides directly but from the photochemical oxidants they form to make ozone and other ingredients of smog.

Ozone is a poisonous form of oxygen and is the principal component of smog. Ozone is not emitted directly into the air but is formed by chemical reactions between two other pollutants—hydrocarbons and nitrogen oxides in the presence of sunlight. Smog irritates the mucous membranes of the respiratory system and can cause coughing, choking, and impaired lung function. It also aggravates chronic respiratory diseases such as

sulfur oxides Acrid poisonous gases that are produced when fuel containing sulfur is burned.

sulfuric acid A corrosive substance produced in the manufacturing process of fertilizers, chemicals, dyes, and petroleum products; when combined with droplets of water in the air it becomes the active component in acid rain.

acid rain Precipitation having a higher than normal level of acid due to the combination of sulfur oxides and moisture in the air.

hydrocarbons A chemical compound made up of hydrogen and carbon; the major chemical ingredient of many fuels.

smog A brownish haze that forms when hydrocarbons react with nitric acid in the presence of sunlight.

particulates Tiny pollutants in the air such as pieces of dust and soot and mold spores.

alveoli The balloon-like air sacs at the end of the bronchioles of the lung.

lead A metal found in exhausts, emissions, and paint.

nitrogen oxides Poisonous gases that are produced when fuel is burned at very high temperatures.

ozone A poisonous form of oxygen that chemically reacts with a variety of substances.

asthma and bronchitis, which is why people who have these conditions are warned to stay inside during periods of high smog levels. Ozone can also irritate the eyes.

Ozone in the air you breathe is not the same as the ozone layer in the stratosphere, which filters out ultraviolet rays from the sun and serves as protection against the sun's radiation—and against skin cancer. There is much scientific debate about how depleted the **ozone layer** is, but it is clearly being threatened to a measurable degree. The major contributors to the destruction of the ozone layer are **chlorofluorocarbons (CFCs),** which had been used as aerosol spray propellants and refrigerants and are present in the exhaust of high-flying jet planes. As of 1996, CFCs can no longer be produced in or imported into the United States. Existing stock can be reused and recycled, so CFC products are not totally eliminated yet. Indeed, over the past two decades, levels of protective ozone in the United States have fallen 10 percent below normal. A thinning area of the ozone layer is commonly referred to as a "hole." The biggest hole in the ozone layer is over the Antarctic, where ozone levels can fall as low as 70 percent below normal.

Many of the air pollutants we have discussed combine to cause what is called the **greenhouse effect,** which many scientists believe is causing **global warming.** It is estimated that global warming will raise the earth's average temperature 1.8° to 6.3° Fahrenheit by the end of the twenty-first century. Although this change may appear small, it could produce extreme weather events such as droughts and floods, threaten coastal resources and wetlands by raising the sea level, and increase the risk for certain diseases by producing new breeding sites for pests and pathogens. (There is a natural greenhouse effect as well, caused by the reflection of the sun's energy from earth back to space. Without this, scientists say that the earth's average temperature would be much colder and the planet would be covered by ice.)

ozone layer A region of the stratosphere, which filters out ultraviolet rays from the sun.

chlorofluorocarbons (CFCs) Compounds used as aerosol spray propellants and refrigerants that contribute to the depletion of the ozone layer.

greenhouse effect The rise in temperature that the earth experiences because certain gases in the atmosphere (e.g., water vapor, carbon dioxide, nitrous oxide, and methane) trap energy from the sun.

global warming The gradual rise in the average temperature of the earth.

point source pollutant A source of pollution that enters a body of water at a specific point.

nonpoint source pollutant A source of pollution that enters a body of water as runoff or seepage.

The Water You Drink

When you are thirsty, you turn on the water faucet and expect to get good, clean water to drink. This is true for most people living in the United States, but there are places where the water supply is contaminated. Toxic chemicals continue to pass through municipal wastewater treatment plants, and it is estimated that about one quarter of waterborne illnesses can be attributed to bacteria or viruses from untreated or inadequately disinfected or filtered wastewater.

Chemicals are added to the water supply to kill microorganisms, and close to 80 percent of U.S. drinking water has chlorine added to it to prevent outbreaks of cholera, typhoid, dysentery, and other waterborne illnesses that were once endemic. While the number of outbreaks of waterborne illnesses is declining in the United States, large outbreaks do take place. In Milwaukee in 1993, for example, four hundred thousand people became ill and fifty died because of a waterborne protozoan, *Cryptosporidium,* in the water supply. This waterborne parasite, which is not killed by chlorine, is excreted by cattle and other animals. Rainwater washes it into rivers, lakes, and reservoirs, where it can get into our water supply. It can also come from overflows from sewage treatment plants.

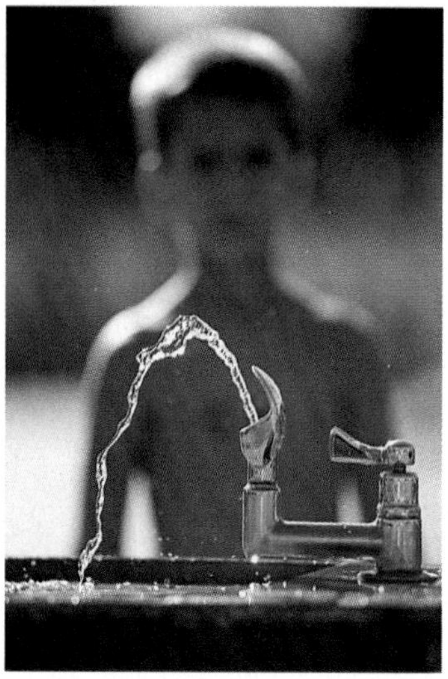

Water continues to be one of our greatest yet most threatened, natural resources.

Sources of Water Pollution

There are numerous sources of water pollution, but the major ones are industrial, municipal, and agricultural. The EPA refers to water pollution sources as point and nonpoint sources. **Point source pollutants** enter a body of water at a specific point—for example, at an industrial plant or a sewage facility. **Nonpoint source pollutants** enter a body of water as runoff or seepage.

Industrial pollutants. Discharges from industry can be both point and nonpoint source pollutants. Discharges may be dumped directly into bodies of water and also carried there indirectly by rainfall. For example, when mercury and arsenic particles are released into the air from factories, they often attach themselves to water droplets and return to earth as rain, thereby contaminating a stream or lake—or further contaminating an already polluted one. Oil spills, as well as other industrial accidents, also contribute to the problem of water pollution.

Toxic chemical compounds in use today find their way into both drinking and recreational waters. Organic chemicals, many of which are suspected of causing cancer, are also found in drinking water. For example, **perchloroethylene (PCE),** a chemical used by the dry-cleaning industry, and **trichloroethylene (TCE),** a chemical used as a degreaser by machine shops, have contaminated large quantities of drinking water because they have leaked into the soil from the waste dumps where they were discarded.

Municipal pollutants. Municipal sources of pollution include urban storm water runoff, septic systems leaking, bacteria, and landfill seepage contaminating the water table.

Agricultural pollutants. Agricultural sources of pollution include large drainage areas (usually resulting when land has been plowed but is not yet held in place by vegetation) and runoff of sediment, agricultural nutrients, and pesticides. Agricultural nutrients, such as fertilizer, can deplete a body of water's oxygen supply by overstimulating plant and algae growth. Billions of pounds of pesticides are applied yearly to U.S. crops. Many believe that the run-off of such pesticides make surface waters unsafe for fishing and swimming because laboratory studies connect pesticides with health problems such as birth defects, nerve damage, and cancer, as well as other effects that might occur over a long period of time. In spite of this, fertilizer and pesticide use continues.

Why Dirty Water Is Unhealthy

The Great Lakes basin provides a good illustration of how water becomes unhealthy. According to a Coast Guard study, the Great Lakes are contaminated by hundreds of oil and chemical spills every month. Spills in estuaries often make fish unsuitable for eating. When oil in water is ingested by organisms in the food chain, highly destructive pollutants can spread throughout the population.

The main health threat from water pollution, however, comes not from oil spills but from toxic wastes dumped into the water. Toxic wastes can cause cancer, food and chemical poisoning, and even an increase in cardiovascular disease when fertilizers with high sodium levels run off into surface and groundwaters. Toxic chemicals move up the food chain from aquatic life to human consumption. Over time, it is anticipated that these contaminants will lead to a variety of problems in humans, including premature births and impaired cognitive and motor development.

As with most pollutants, the effects of water pollution are, for the most part, unknown. But evidence suggests that the cumulative effect of water pollution will result in problems ranging from higher cancer rates to increases in neurological problems.

Solid Waste: The Art of Throwing Things Away

America is sometimes called the throw-away society. We have disposable containers for our fast foods, and convenient trash pickup at our front door. As a result of some of our consumer preferences, our **landfills** are bulging to the point of overflow. In some major cities, solid waste is shipped overland or by barge to other parts of the country simply because there is no longer enough room for the waste. In 2000, the amount of solid waste generated per person per day was estimated to be near 4.5 pounds.

Solid waste is made up of everything from paper and metal cans to old tires, plastic containers, food, yard wastes, and motor oil. Most of it—nearly three quarters—goes into landfills, so it is not surprising that our present landfills will soon need to be replaced (see Figure 15.1).

Consider just one product on the trash heap: disposable diapers. They do not degrade—at least not for hundreds of years—so every disposable diaper ever buried is still there, taking up in total between 1 and 2 percent of all landfill space. A baby uses 4,000 to 5,000 diapers before he or she is toilet trained. (It should be noted that cloth diapers can affect the environment, too. Washing them requires using a lot of hot water, and, the phosphates in detergent add to the burden of water pollution.)

Common household waste can contribute to health problems resulting from the creation of breeding grounds for rats, flies, and mosquitoes as well as from

perchloroethylene (PCE) A suspected carcinogen used in dry cleaning.

trichloroethylene (TCE) A suspected carcinogen used as a degreaser in machine shops.

landfills An area where trash and other wastes are deposited and covered with soil.

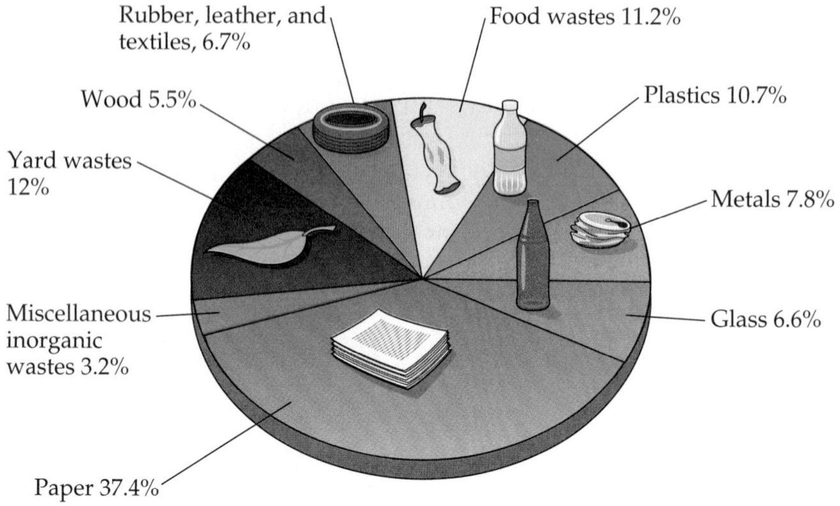

Figure 15.1 **What's in Your Garbage?**
Every person generates about 4.5 pounds of solid waste a day, and most of it goes into a landfill in your community. Paper accounts for most of the solid wastes by weight.
(*Source:* U.S. Environmental Protection Agency)

the emission of noxious smoke from burning trash. Rainwater seeping through buried wastes percolates down through the soil and contaminates groundwater. Other organic wastes, such as garbage and paper products, decompose and can form explosive methane gas. Methane absorbs heat from sunlight and may contribute to global warming.

Precycling and Recycling Options

Reducing the amount of solid waste in the environment is dependent upon two practices, precycling and recycling. **Precycling** is a concept that refers to eliminating solid waste before it is created. This might be considered primary prevention of solid waste.

Precycling is dependent on wise consumer choices. For example, when given the option of buying a product that is highly packaged (e.g., in a Styrofoam box with a molded-plastic cover) or one that is only minimally packaged (e.g., in a paper box that can be recycled), a wise and healthy consumer choice would be the latter. The same concept can be applied to grocery shopping, snack buying, and other consumer purchases. Precycling also involves using packaging for other purposes, and buying products that are made from recycled materials or packaged in containers that can later be reused and recycled locally.

Recycling is a more familiar concept, and refers to the process of collecting and reusing newspapers, plastics, aluminum cans, glass bottles, and many other solid wastes. Recycling can greatly reduce the landfill problem—and save money, natural resources, and energy. It is estimated that recycling a single press run of the Sunday *New York Times,* for example, would save some seventy-five thousand trees. Read the Developing Health Skills box to test your general knowledge about recycling.

Currently, close to 30 percent of the nation's solid waste is recycled. Communities across the country—from major cities like Los Angeles to small towns—have curbside pickup of recyclables. Where curbside pickup is not available, communities may have drop-off centers. In addition, supermarkets across the country are taking back the empty plastic and paper bags that their customers used to carry home foods and other products.

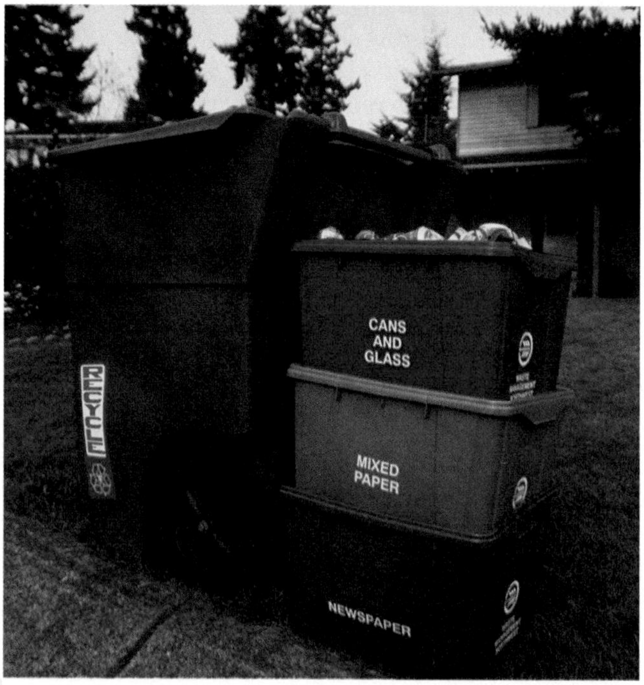

Many communities have curbside pickup so people can recycle newspapers, cans, bottles, and plastic containers. Recycling saves money, natural resources, and energy.

precycling The practice of choosing products that have the potential for reuse, using packaging that can be used for other purposes, or choosing packaging that has already been recycled.

recycling The use over and over again of substances such as metal and glass.

Developing Health Skills

Know Your Recycling

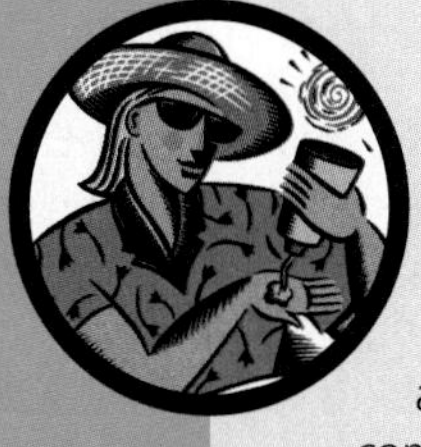

Recycling has been part of the American consciousness long enough for a couple of generations to have ingrained the concepts and philosophy of the movement and adopted the behaviors as a part of daily living. Today, a drive through most communities in the United States will produce signs of recycling bins and compost piles. How well informed are you about recycling and with recycling terms? Answer the following questions to test your knowledge, then check your answers.

1. Which of the following are effective in reducing the amount of waste generated from households?
   a. backyard composting
   b. recycling
   c. Pay As You Throw (PAYT) waste collection and disposal services
   d. collection of yard waste for composting
   e. all of the above
2. What is cullet?
   a. part of a bird's gizzard
   b. glass sorted and crushed for recycling
   c. a drain pipe for storm water
   d. bundled newspapers
3. What material is most commonly collected by curbside recycling programs? (Hint: It is consistently valuable.)
4. Which one of the following should you not put into your compost bin?
   a. shrub trimmings
   b. grass clippings
   c. coffee grounds
   d. meat scraps
   e. egg shells
5. What is a mobius (as related to recycling)?
6. What recycled material is used in toothpaste?
7. This common household recyclable is used to make stuffing for sleeping bags and winter jackets. This stuffing has good insulating qualities.

Answers

1. All of these are effective means of reducing the generation of waste from households. In "Pay As You Throw" (PAYT) communities homeowners pay based on the amount of waste they discard, encouraging participation in other waste reduction practices.
2. Cullet is glass which has been sorted and crushed for recycling. The glass should not be broken at home, because then it cannot be sorted and freed from contaminants. Only glass containers should be put out for recycling. Do not recycle lightbulbs, drinking glasses, ceramics, baking dishes, window glass, or mirrors. Any metal caps or rings should be removed.
3. Aluminum.
4. Meat scraps should not be put into a compost bin because they attract pests and create odors.
5. A mobius is the chasing arrow recycling logo.
6. Tin used to make stannous fluoride is made from detinning old steel cans. The body of the can is made from steel but has a tin coating. The resulting tin is very pure and is ideal for use in toothpaste.
7. PET (polyethylene terephthalate) soft drink bottles are used to make polyethylene fibers for insulation as well as carpets, fabrics, strapping, and engineered resins for the automotive industry.

Source: Adapted from the Pennsylvania Department of Environmental Protection

Health Hazards from Toxic Waste

The word *waste* indicates something not wanted that is to be thrown away. When dealing with toxic materials, how that waste is thrown away carries serious health implications. Some **hazardous wastes** can be disposed of safely by burying them in steel containers. However, too often, toxic wastes are disposed of incorrectly or may otherwise leak into the environment in the form of fumes. Even steel drums rust and corrode over time, allowing toxic wastes to leak out into our environment.

Chlorinated dioxins are hazardous wastes that are emitted by certain chemical processes, including the burning of plastics in high-temperature incinerators. People are exposed to chlorinated dioxins in a variety of ways, but the most common way is through air pollution. They are either exposed to dioxins directly by breathing them in, or indirectly through contaminated water, crops, animals, or fish. Some dioxins accumulate in the body over time and become highly concentrated in human fatty tissue and breast milk.

Toxic chemicals, such as chlorinated dioxins, are chemicals that can have both acute (immediate) and

hazardous waste Waste that is flammable, explosive, corrosive, or toxic.

chlorinated dioxins Hazardous waste emitted by the burning of plastics.

toxic chemical A chemical that is poisonous.

chronic (long-term) poisonous and behavioral effects. Acute reactions are those that are easy to observe—from watery eyes and irritated skin to more serious reactions involving unconsciousness and in some cases, death. It sometimes takes years before chronic effects—such as lung disease and neurological symptoms including blurred vision, muscle weakness, and difficulties in balance—become apparent. The behavioral effects of toxic poisoning are even subtler than chronic effects and can include anxiety, depression, and hyperactivity.

Cancer and birth defects due to toxic wastes usually develop over a long period of time. In many cases, so much time passes that it is often difficult to identify the point of exposure. Love Canal is an example of a toxic waste dump that was associated with a high incidence of miscarriages, stillbirths, urinary and nervous system disorders, and skin disease. More than 15,000 tons of chemicals were buried on this site in upstate New York in the early 1950s. However, it wasn't until the late 1970s that health problems associated with Love Canal became apparent and people were evacuated.

Landfills are another potential source of toxic waste. One housing development in Savannah, Georgia, was built on a former landfill, and when methane gas began escaping from it, residents had to be evacuated.

Even when a toxic material is banned, it can continue to harm the environment for decades. Polychlorinated biphenyls (PCBs), which were produced primarily as electrical insulation, have been banned in the United States since 1977. Although PCBs haven't been produced for more than twenty-five years, these chemicals are still found in older appliances, landfills, and the fatty tissues of fish and other animals—including the fat and breast milk of people who eat those animals.

Radiation Exposure—and Overexposure

The presence of radiation in our environment presents a growing health concern. **Radiation** is energy that travels in waves or particles—some at an extremely low frequency (e.g., energy emitted by power lines) and some at very high frequencies (e.g., energy emitted in tanning booths or medical X rays). Of the different types of radiation, **ionizing radiation** is of greatest concern because it can break chemical bonds and damage DNA.

radiation Energy that travels in waves or particles.

ionizing radiation Radiation such as ultraviolet radiation, X rays, and gamma rays, which is capable of breaking chemical bonds.

radiation absorbed doses (rads) The unit of measurement of radiation exposure.

Radiation is widespread in our environment. It is used to generate electric power, to kill cancer cells, and is a part of many manufacturing processes. When you use a microwave oven, talk on a cell phone, or are out in the sun, you are exposing yourself to radiation. Some naturally occurring elements, such as uranium, also emit radiation.

No one can escape exposure to radiation, but *overexposure* can lead to serious health problems and in some cases, death. Exposure to radiation is measured in **radiation absorbed doses (rads).** Exposure to doses of radiation as low as 100 to 200 rads can cause radiation sickness, such as diarrhea, fatigue, hair loss, and nausea. At 350 to 500 rads, symptoms become more severe, and death becomes a possibility. Long-term exposure to radiation can cause lung cancer, leukemia, skin cancer, bone cancer, and skeletal deformities. Dosages above 600 rads are usually fatal.

Caution is the best advice concerning radiation. Monitor your exposure to the sun, and stay away from tanning booths. Consistent evidence connects sun exposure (and tanning booth exposure) with skin cancer (see Chapter 10). With all medical treatments, particularly X rays, be sure that your physician knows your medical history.

Dangers from Noise

If someone were talking, could you tell whether he or she had said the word *right* or *light?* Normally, you might be able to, but at a live rock concert, where the noise level is over 110 decibels (60 decibels is usually rated as "comfortable"), you might not even realize that someone is talking to you.

Noise is one of the great threats to the quality of life in modern society, but is accepted by many as a necessary evil. Cars, subways, motorcycles, planes, televisions, video games, stereos, power tools, as well as a multitude of other gadgets, have left us in a very noisy world. Sound levels above 85 decibels—roughly equivalent to that produced by a power leaf blower, lawn mower, or food blender—are potentially hazardous. Most Americans live in near-dangerous noise environments, typically experiencing chronic average noise levels of 70 decibels (see Table 15.2).

Who Is at Risk?

Workers especially vulnerable to hearing loss due to high noise levels are firefighters, police officers, musicians, farmers, truck drivers, and construction, airport,

Table 15.2 It's a Noisy World: Noise Levels and Human Response

Common sounds	Decibels	Effects
Normal breathing	10	Just audible
Whisper	30	Very quiet
Normal conversation	50–55	Comfortable under 60 decibels
Vacuum cleaner	70	Intrusive, interferes with telephone
Garbage disposal	80	Annoying, interferes with conversation; Constant exposure may cause damage
Television	70–90	Very annoying; 85 decibels is the noise level at which hearing damage begins after eight hours exposure
Snowmobile	105	Regular exposure of more than one minute risks permanent loss over 100 decibels
Power saw, chain saw	110	
Thunderclap, boom box	120	Threshold of sensation is 120 decibels
Stereos (over 120 watts)	110–125	
Jet takeoff	130	Beyond threshold of pain—125 decibels
Shotgun firing	130	
Rock concerts	110–140	

Source: National Institute on Deafness and Other Communication Disorders

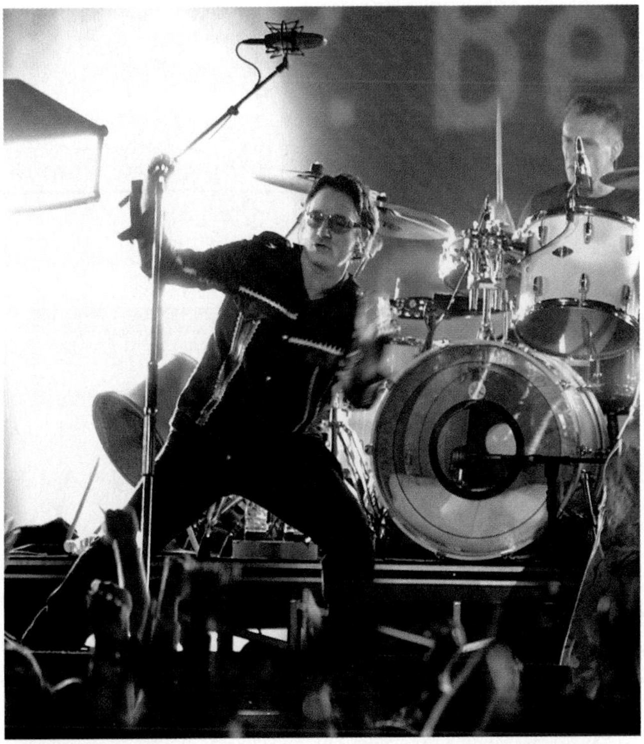

How much is having fun at a rock concert worth to you? Sound levels at rock concerts are in the 110- to 140-decibel range, but anything above 85 decibels is potentially hazardous.

and factory workers. There are regulations designed to protect workers from hazardous noise levels, including those mandating the wearing of protective earplugs, but compliance is inconsistent.

Leisure-related threats—those that can occur in your everyday life—include live or recorded high-volume music, some household appliances, woodworking tools, lawn care equipment, and recreational vehicles such as snowmobiles and trail motorbikes. One important feature of noise-induced hearing loss is that it is preventable in all but certain cases of accidental exposure (see the Developing Health Skills box).

Physical Damage Caused by Noise

A sudden loud noise can leave you temporarily deafened, and you may experience a ringing in the ears, but normal hearing usually returns within a few hours at most. This type of temporary hearing loss is called a **temporary threshold shift (TTS).**

Over time, repeated exposure to loud noise can result in partial or total hearing loss. This is caused by destruction of the cilia in the **cochlea** (inner ear) and their auditory nerve connections. Any time you are exposed to a loud noise, some of your cilia are destroyed. Prolonged or repeated exposure to noises above 85 decibels can cause a total collapse of this sensitive portion of the body.

Noise has other effects on the body, even at levels that do not produce hearing loss. Researchers have found that following a sudden, loud, or unexpected

temporary threshold shift (TTS) Temporary hearing loss usually caused by a sudden loud noise.

cochlea The inner ear.

noise, blood pressure and heart rate increase. In addition, noise also causes the peripheral vessels in the eyes and brain to dilate, which implicates noise as one of the many possible causes of headaches.

Indoor Pollution: Sick Buildings, Sick People

As if there aren't enough dangers resulting from breathing polluted air outside, the air you breathe inside your dorm, home, or office can cause adverse health effects. According to EPA, people may be exposed to greater pollution threats indoors than outdoors because that is where people typically spend 90 percent of their time. The length of exposure multiplies the risk.

In large part, the problem stems from the energy crisis of the early 1970s, when building engineers found that they could save money on energy bills by better insulating offices, schools, and other institutional buildings and recirculating air within the building. During this time, private homes, too, became better insulated. Energy costs fell, but the indoor air became unhealthy as a result of "**sick building syndrome" (SBS)**—unhealthy indoor air quality due to lack of circulation. Office workers and students began complaining about eye and skin irritation, dry throat, fatigue, dizziness, nausea, and respiratory discomfort, including shortness of breath (see Figure 15.2 and Table 15.3).

Millions of private homes also have a problem with **radon.** Radon is a naturally occurring odorless, colorless, radioactive gas that comes from deposits of uranium in soil, rock, and water. It can seep into the home through basements, openings for utility pipes, floor drains, joints between

sick building syndrome (SBS) Characterized by unhealthy indoor air that results from a lack of circulating air or a lack of ventilation.

radon An extremely toxic, colorless gas derived from the radioactive decay of radium; usually arising from uranium in the soil, water, and rock.

Developing Health Skills

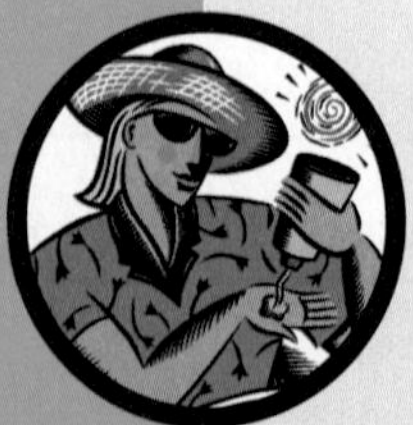

More than Music to Your Ears: Hearing Hazards of Personal Stereo Systems

What do students, joggers, commuters, factory workers, and office workers have in common? They all are likely to listen to music on a personal stereo system with headphones. These systems can be hazardous to your hearing health because they can produce sounds as loud as 120 decibels (sounds above 85 decibels can harm your hearing over time).

Here are some steps to take to protect your hearing while listening to your favorite singers:

- Look for a personal stereo system with an automatic volume limiter, which limits the output to safe levels.
- Set your system at a comfortable level in a quiet room. DO NOT turn it up when you are in a noisy setting to block out the noise. This will only add to the noise and increase the risk to your hearing.
- Limit the amount of time you use it.
- If you are wearing headphones and cannot hear other people talking or if other people have to shout to you to be heard at three feet away, your system is too loud and could be damaging to your hearing.
- If you notice any ringing in your ears, or that speech sounds are muffled after wearing a personal stereo system, discontinue its use and have your hearing checked by a qualified audiologist.

Source: League for the Hard of Hearing

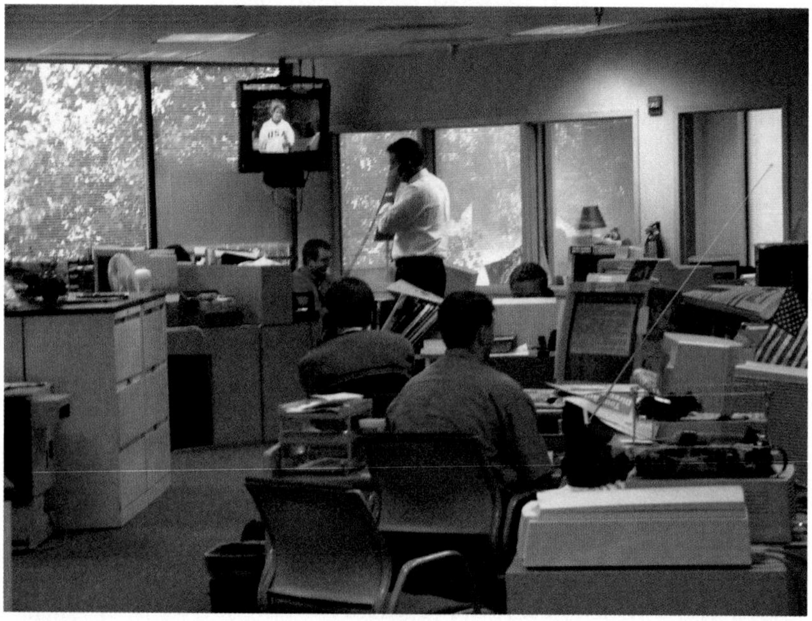

The view may be great, but sealed windows and poor ventilation can result in an unhealthy work environment. Indoor air pollution is invisible and can cause dizziness, nausea, and shortness of breath.

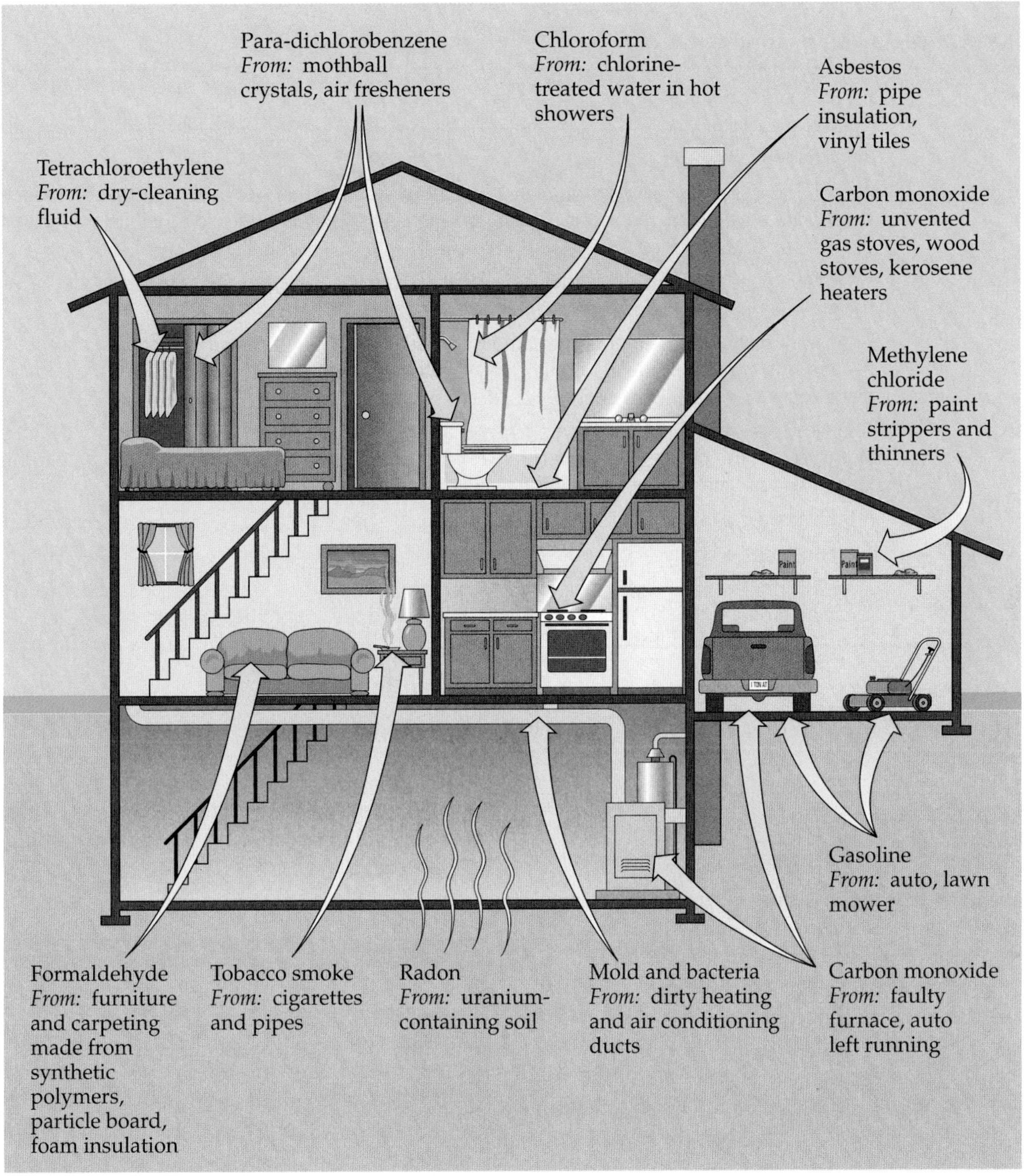

Figure 15.2 Sources of Indoor Air Pollution
How many of these pollutants might be in your home or dorm? People who are sensitive to outdoor air pollution are also likely to be sensitive to indoor air pollution.

walls and floors, and cracks in foundations. Some reports indicate that there is an association between radon in the home and lung cancer; others do not. The good news about radon is that homes built after 1990 have radon-resistant features. In addition, once radon is detected, it is possible to mitigate the problem.

Lead-based paints, which were often used in homes built before 1950, are another environmental problem in the home. They are particularly harmful to inner-city children, who tend to live in older houses and may eat the sweet-tasting paint chips. Children are more vulnerable than adults to lead poisoning because their body mass is small and their nervous systems are still developing. According to the American Academy of Pediatrics, lead is more dangerous to children than the asbestos found in building materials in older schools. In an attempt to remove lead from our indoor environments, the manufacture and sale of leaded paint has been banned.

Table 15.3 Indoor Air Pollutants

Pollutant	Effects on the body
Asbestos fibers	Fibers widely used in insulation and other building materials that can cause lung disease, including lung cancer
Carbon monoxide	An odorless gas produced by incomplete combustion, such as that occurring in tobacco products, gas stoves, and unvented or improperly functioning heating equipment; interferes with the supply of oxygen to the body's tissues
Formaldehyde	An irritating and probably carcinogenic gas emitted from several types of consumer products, including particle board, plywood, insulation, cigarettes, and fabrics
Nitrogen dioxide	The by-product of high-temperature combustion, such as that occurring in gas stoves, unvented space heaters, and tobacco products; a principal respiratory irritant that may interfere with the body's defense against respiratory infections
Pesticides	Chemicals used in the home to control insects and pests that have been associated with health problems such as birth defects, nerve damage, and cancer, as well as other effects that might occur over a long period of time; used in approximately 84 percent of U.S. homes
Radon	A radioactive gas in the earth's crust that can seep into homes; increases the risk of lung cancer
Tobacco smoke	More than 3,800 chemical compounds, most of which are toxic and 60 of which are known carcinogens; a cause of lung cancer and heart disease
Solvents	Cleaning products that contain some chemicals that can cause birth defects

Source: U.S. Environmental Protection Agency

What Are the Risks of Indoor Pollution?

People who are sensitive to outdoor air pollution are also likely to be sensitive to **indoor pollution.** Infants and young children, pregnant women, the elderly, and those who have preexisting chronic illnesses, such as lung or heart disease, are especially sensitive to indoor pollution.

You can do some basic, common-sense things to protect yourself from indoor air pollution at school and at home or at work.

- Ventilate your room with fresh outdoor air or recirculated filtered air.
- Remove the source of the irritant (e.g., tobacco smoke).
- Properly use and store cleaning solvents, paints, and pesticides.
- Repair or remove faulty home heaters.
- Follow manufacturer's specifications for room size and fuel when using kerosene heaters.
- Use an air purifier to reduce odors, tobacco smoke, dust, pollen, and some toxic gases, and change the filter regularly.

indoor pollution The contamination of indoor air by waste products or natural pollutants.

Environmental Ethics

Although environmental awareness is becoming more common in this country, opinions differ greatly on how we should treat the environment. Some people believe that the future of human existence is dependent upon sustaining a healthy environment. Others believe that it is morally appropriate for us to use nature to meet our resource needs without limit. Some suggest that our actions today directly influence the health of our children and grandchildren, while others believe that the impact of environmental degradation affects our personal health today. A study published in the *Journal of Environmental Education* suggests that there are five different "environmental ethics" which form a continuum. These include:

- *Aggressive antienvironmentalism.* Nature needs to be tamed or controlled to prevent human harm.
- *Benign indifference.* Nature is a useful storehouse of raw materials, so we have unlimited use of natural resources.

- *Utilitarian conservation.* The goods and services found in nature are limited, so we have to exercise caution in their use.
- *Stewardship.* Nature is important to future generations so we have a responsibility to take care of it.
- *Radical environmentalism.* Humans have a moral responsibility to protect all living things, and animals should not suffer needless pain.

The researchers found that most people subscribe to a practice of stewardship and utilitarian conservation and acknowledge the limits of natural resources. They recognize that human beings are dependent on nature for a variety of health-enhancing and life-sustaining benefits and are likely to feel a moral obligation to take care of nonhuman elements of the environment.

It is not necessary to be an environmentalist to feel an obligation to protect the environment and to take appropriate actions. One does not have to participate in a political rally supporting an environmental issue or write letters to political leaders to demonstrate personal convictions. Regardless of your philosophical or political position, the day-to-day actions that you take hold the potential of positively or negatively influencing your environment. Perhaps environmental health comes down to thinking globally and acting locally.

CASE STUDY 15: Living in a Healthy Environment

Angela had never been on a hike, but her roommate Lynn really wanted to join the Outdoor Recreation Club on a five-mile hike in the woods on Sunday. Lynn convinced Angela to go on the hike by telling her that it would be fun and a change of pace from studying in the stuffy library all day. In the end, Angela agreed to join Lynn on the hike. It turned out to be a pretty hot day that Sunday and Angela quickly drank the one bottle of water she had brought with her. Soon after, Angela got tired of carrying the empty water bottle and left it on the side of the path. Later, she stopped and drank some water from a beautiful, clear stream that ran through the woods. The next day Angela didn't feel so well. She had an upset stomach, which in two days developed into a serious case of diarrhea. At the student health department, Angela got medication to help her condition, and found out that she had gotten sick in what she thought would be a "squeaky clean" environment: the stream she had drunk water from in the woods was polluted with *Giardia,* an infectious agent.

Karim also went on the Outdoor Recreation Club hike, but in contrast to Angela, he packed several bottles of water in his backpack, knowing that it was a hot day and he would need to drink plenty of water. When he goes on longer camping trips, Karim takes along iodine tablets, and when he is thirsty, he fills his cup with water from a stream and puts in an iodine tablet to purify the water. He also adds a pinch of lemonade mix to make it taste better. Unlike Angela, Karim was careful not to leave any trash behind on the trail. He followed the rule of the outdoors: the only thing, he left behind were his footprints.

In Your Opinion

Although the world around you seems so natural, there are many steps you can take to protect the environment and at the same time protect yourself from it.

- What could Angela have done to better prepare for her hike with the Outdoor Recreation Club?
- What lessons had Karim learned that he followed instinctively?
- When you have been hiking or otherwise spent time outdoors, how have you contributed to keeping the environment sound and your body healthy?
- What more could Angela and Karim do to contribute to the preservation of the environment?

KEY CONCEPTS

1. Many people feel that an "acceptable risk" is one where, although exposure to a specific chemical or other hazardous material might be capable of causing disease, the likelihood of actually getting sick from it is very small.
2. Toxic gases occur naturally in the environment, and under normal circumstances, the body's filtering system ensures that we breathe in safe, naturally filtered air.

3. Air pollution taxes the body's filtering system so that we breathe in noxious particles and gases. The automobile is the most pervasive source of air pollution.
4. The sources of water pollution are numerous, but the major ones are industrial, municipal, and agricultural.
5. The main health threat from water pollution is not from oil spills, but toxic wastes, which can cause cancer, food and chemical poisoning, and an increase in cardiovascular disease.
6. It is estimated that every person generates 4.5 pounds of solid waste a day, with nearly three quarters of it going into landfills.
7. Precycling refers to the reduction of household garbage by making environmentally sensitive consumer choices.
8. Recycling newspapers, plastics, aluminum cans, and glass bottles could greatly reduce the landfill problem and can save money, natural resources, and energy.
9. Sound levels above 85 decibels—roughly equivalent to the level of noise produced by a power leaf blower, lawn mower, or food blender—are potentially hazardous.
10. People may be exposed to a greater pollution threat from chemicals emitted inside a building than outdoors because that is where they typically spend 90 percent of their time and because the length of exposure multiplies the risk.

REVIEW QUESTIONS

1. Differentiate between serious environmental threats and those that are perceived to be serious but that actually present little risk to the global environment.
2. Cite three reasons why measuring environmental health threats is difficult.
3. Explain the differences between carcinogens, teratogens, and mutagens and give an example of each in the environment.
4. List the major pollutants found in the air. Identify a specific disease or health concern associated with each.
5. List the major pollutants found in water. Identify a specific disease or health concern associated with each.
6. Differentiate between the practices of precycling and recycling. Explain how each can contribute to the reduction of solid waste.
7. Explain why toxic wastes pose a threat to health and identify an example of the impact of improper disposal of hazardous waste on human health.
8. Describe the physical damage caused by noise.
9. Estimate the cost of environmental cleanup. What would be the benefits of such activity?
10. Identify five points of view concerning the environment and explain how each is represented in an environmentally related action.

CRITICAL THINKING QUESTIONS

1. Many environmental threats are difficult to quantify. For example, it is difficult to know the impact of air pollution when so many individuals smoke cigarettes. Given our limited ability to measure environmental health, do you think health officials and scientists could be overreacting to environmental health threats? Do you believe there is an acceptable level of risk?
2. The *Healthy People 2010* objectives include the following: "Reduce the proportion of persons exposed to air that does not meet the U.S. Environmental Protection Agency's health-based standards for harmful air pollutants." What is the best way to reach this objective? Should stricter air quality controls be established and enforced? Or should the public be educated on ways to avoid environmental air pollution?
3. Radiation plays an important role in our lives, and we would be hard pressed to attempt to avoid all radiation. For example, we are exposed to low levels of radiation from electrical power lines, cellular phones, and even sunshine. If you were asked to develop a list of guidelines for limiting radiation exposure, what would your list contain?
4. The *Healthy People 2010* objectives include the following two objectives: "Increase the proportion of persons who live in homes tested for radon concentrations" and "increase the number of new homes constructed to be radon resistant." These are two objectives that call for individual action by occupants of homes. Have the national objectives overstepped their boundaries by invading the privacy of the home? What compelling public health issues might justify these objectives?

JOURNAL ACTIVITIES

1. For a period of one day, make a list of all the activities you do that contribute to or harm the environment. For example, driving five blocks instead of walking or riding your bike may be wasting energy resources. Can you think of ways to change some of your habits?
2. Listen for noises around you—jackhammers, loud music, lawn mowers, heavy traffic. Write how you feel about these noises. Don't forget to include noises that might make you feel good, such as the

gentle noise of a spring rain or the laughter of children. Can you describe the difference between noises that make you feel edgy and noises that relax you? Which noises in the environment can affect your hearing?

3. Write a statement about the impact of a particular activity on the environment. For example, consider the implications of placing a sidewalk (or a larger sidewalk) in front of your home or apartment. What would be the impact on your environment? Would you lose a tree or shrub? What pollutants would be produced during construction? Would the environment be improved, or would it deteriorate?
4. Join a clean-up crew picking up bottles and cans from the side of the highway, or help out at a recycling center. Write about your experience. Ask some of the other people working with you why they volunteered for this activity. Does anyone make the connection between a healthy environment and members of the community having good health? Do you think this is a valid connection? Why (or why not)?

SELECTED BIBLIOGRAPHY

Brower, M. *Consumer's Guide to Effective Environmental Choices: Practical Advice from the Union of Concerned Scientists.* New York: Crown Publishing Group, 1999.

EPA Journal. Washington, DC: U.S. Environmental Protection Agency (published bimonthly).

Harte, J., et al. *Toxics A to Z: A Guide to Everyday Pollution Hazards.* Berkeley, CA: University of California Press, 1991.

Healthy Buildings, Healthy People: A Vision for the 21st Century. U.S. Environmental Protection Agency, Office of Air and Radiation (EPA402-K-01-003), July 1997.

Lomborg, B. *The Sceptical Environmentalist: Measuring the Real State of the World.* Cambridge, UK: Cambridge University Press, 2001.

McNeill, J. R. *Something New Under the Sun: An Environmental History of the Twentieth-Century World.* New York: W.W. Norton Co., 2000.

Municipal Solid Waste in the United States: 2000 Facts and Figures Executive Summary. U.S. Environmental Protection Agency, Office of Solid Waste and Emergency Response (EPA530-S-02-001), June 2002.

National Air Quality and Emissions Trend Report. Washington, DC: Environmental Protection Agency (published annually).

National Water Quality Inventory. Washington, DC: Environmental Protection Agency (published biennially).

Water on Tap: A Consumer's Guide to the Nation's Drinking Water. U.S. Environmental Protection Agency, Office of Water (EPA815-K-97-002), July 1997.

The Worldwatch Institute. *Vital Signs 2002: The Trends That Are Shaping Our Future.* New York: W.W. Norton Co., 2002.

HEALTHLINKS

Websites for Living in a Healthy Environment

You can access better health as it relates to this chapter by checking out some of the following sites on the Internet. These sites can be accessed directly from the *Decisions for Healthy Living* Website located at www.aw.com/pruitt.

Ecologia

Ecologia is a nonprofit organization dedicated to environmental issues of public concern. The site provides policy and technical information about environmental health issues.

Environmental Protection Agency (EPA)

The government agency that oversees all environmental issues. This site provides a wealth of information as well as links to other environmental and safety resources.

National Center for Environmental Health

The National Center for Environmental Health collaborates with numerous state and local public and private groups to promote health and quality of life by preventing and controlling disease, birth defects, disability, and death resulting from interactions between people and their environment.

National Institute of Environmental Health Sciences

A division of the National Institute of Health, the National Institute of Environmental Health Sciences provides basic research on environment-related diseases. The site includes press releases about scientific discoveries such as the health effects of urban pollution, a monthly journal with cutting-edge research articles and news of the environment, and access to the NIEHS Clearinghouse.

National Toxicology Program

The National Toxicology Program (NTP) coordinates toxicology research and testing activities and provides information about potentially toxic chemicals to regulatory and research agencies and the public.

HEALTH HOTLINES

Living in a Healthy Environment

Indoor Air Quality Information Clearinghouse
(800) 438-4318
U.S. Environmental Protection Agency
Indoor Environments Division
1200 Pennsylvania Avenue, NW
Mail Code 6609J
Washington, DC 20460

National Institute of Environmental Health Sciences
(919) 541-3345
P.O. Box 12233, Mail Drop B2-05
Research Triangle Park, NC 27709

National Lead Information Center
(800) 424-LEAD (424-5323)
801 Roeder Road, Suite 600
Silver Spring, MD 20910

National Pesticide Information Center
(800) 858-7378
NPIC
Oregon State University
333 Weniger
Corvallis, OR 97331

Occupational Hearing Service
Dial A Hearing Screen Test
(800) 622-3277
P.O. Box 1880
Media, PA 19063

Safe Drinking Water Hotline
(800) 426-4791
U.S. Environmental Protection Agency, Mail Stop 4604
Office of Water (4101M)
1200 Pennsylvania Avenue, NW
Washington, DC 20460

TEST YOUR KNOWLEDGE ANSWERS

1. True. Family size is declining but because the number of children born continues to be greater than the number of parents, the world's population continues to grow, resulting in a strain on the world's limited natural resources.
2. False. Smog is a combination of smoke and fog arising from the burning of hydrocarbons (from automobile exhaust), nitrogen oxides (a form of industrial waste), and other gases trapped under a layer of warm air.
3. True. The ozone layer is located in the stratosphere, but is thinning in recent years due to human-caused factors such as chlorofluorocarbons.
4. False. Disposable diapers are not biodegradable. By some estimates, disposable diapers now constitute up to 1–2 percent of landfills.
5. False. Nonionizing radiation such as radio waves and microwaves are less hazardous than ionizing radiation which can break chemical bonds. Ultraviolet rays are a form of ionizing radiation.

CHAPTER 16

Making Health Care Decisions

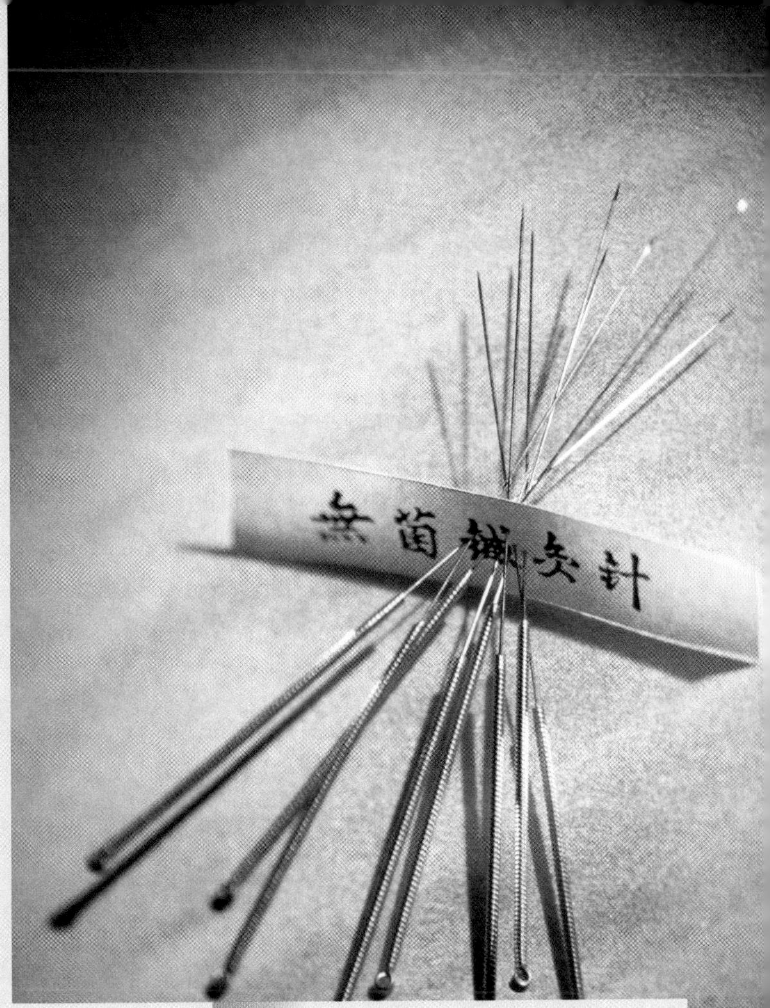

OBJECTIVES

When you finish reading this chapter, you will be able to:

1. Describe the role of information in making consumer decisions about health care.
2. Identify high-quality sources of health information, including reputable hotlines and Internet sites.
3. Describe five advertising techniques used to promote health products and services.
4. Recognize quackery and health fraud and cite examples of each.
5. Learn how to employ several strategies when selecting a physician.
6. Identify a range of alternative and complementary health care providers.
7. Recognize the difference between primary, secondary, and tertiary care and acknowledge your own and your physician's responsibilities in regard to each form of health care.
8. Understand the advantages and disadvantages of traditional indemnity plans, health maintenance organizations, and preferred provider organizations.
9. Differentiate between prescription and over-the-counter drugs and briefly describe how each should be taken.
10. Understand the steps to take before taking a natural product as medicine.

TEST YOUR KNOWLEDGE

1. Most Americans avoid methods of health care that they know little or nothing about to treat medical problems. True or False?
2. Because physicians distrust alternative medicine, most do not refer patients to such practitioners. True or False?
3. The three most commonly performed surgeries today are childbirth by cesarean section, gallbladder removal, and hysterectomy. True or False?
4. Medicare is a government program designed to serve the uninsured or underinsured citizens of the United States. True or False?
5. Generic drugs have the same active chemical ingredients as their brand name counterparts. True or False?

Answers found at end of chapter.

Imagine a health care supermarket that has one aisle for doctors and others for chiropractors, medications, surgery, hospitals, home remedies, and so on. It is not a real place, of course, but such a supermarket does exist in your mind, and each time you need to make a decision concerning your health—which physician to go to, which medication to take, whether to use **conventional medicine** or try **complementary and alternative medicine**—you walk up and down the aisles searching for the right person, place, or product (see Table 16.1 for the major types of complementary and alternative medicine). To do this, you need to be an educated health care consumer.

Americans spend more money on health care than people of any other country in the world. In 2000, Americans spent approximately $1.3 trillion on health care (see Table 16.2). A quick trip to the emergency room for a minor injury can cost several hundred dollars, and a few days in the hospital can cost up to several thousand dollars. The high price of health care is forcing more Americans to become involved in these decisions than in the past.

Buying Health Care: How Do Consumers Make Decisions?

Whether you are aware of it or not, you make decisions about how to spend your health care dollars virtually every day. Do you go to the physician when you have a cold? There is no treatment for a cold other than symptom relief. Do you buy low-cost generic aspirin or a more expensive brand name, thinking it must be better? Generic drugs can cost between 20 percent and 85 percent less than their brand-name counterparts.

When purchasing any product, you probably look for the best value. In terms of health care, the value is the reasonably priced product or service that will lead to good health and/or the improvement of health status. Sometimes that value is expensive to purchase—as with heart surgery. However, sometimes that value can be gained with little or no expense. In certain cases, the healthiest and most economical decision is the decision not to purchase a product or service but to look for a natural way to improve your health. For example, there are times when an aspirin is the appropriate treatment for relief from a stress headache. There are also times when the proper response to a stress headache is to relax, perhaps by lying down in a dark room or taking a walk in the park.

conventional medicine Standard Western medicine based on the rigorous application of the scientific method and the belief that diseases are caused by identifiable physical factors with definable symptoms.

complementary and alternative medicine Interventions that are not part of conventional or mainstream medicine as taught in most U.S. medical schools and available in U.S. hospitals.

patient package insert An information sheet, required by the FDA that, among other things, warns the consumer of possible contraindications for use of a drug or medical product.

Decision Making and Accurate Health Information

To make good health care decisions, it is necessary to be actively involved with your own health and to have complete and accurate information. What do you know about the drugs you buy, the tests your physician performs, or the diet that promises quick and permanent weight loss? Do you have enough reliable and unbiased information to make informed decisions about your health care choices?

Although a lot of accurate information is available, a lot of inaccurate information is also "out there," and it often is difficult to determine which is which. In part this is because the health field includes many people who claim to be experts. In the field of nutrition, for example, whom would you trust: a registered dietician who recommends a balanced diet or an owner of a health food store where supplemental vitamins and minerals are sold?

In addition to having to sort out who really is an expert, you must also decide what data to trust and how to evaluate risks. Consider the decision to take a prescription for allergy medicine. Each package contains a **patient package insert,** an information sheet required by the Food and Drug Administration (FDA), which includes a list of side effects. The consumer needs to examine the benefits and risks of taking the drug and to decide whether the benefits are worth the risks. You can read about any drug

Table 16.1 Major Types of Complementary and Alternative Medicine

Category	What it is based on
Alternative medical systems	Systems built on theory and practice that evolved in part from the conventional medical approach used in the United States. Examples include homeopathic and naturopathic medicine, traditional Chinese medicine, and Ayurveda.
Mind-body interventions	Uses techniques such as meditation, prayer, mental healing, art, music, and dance to enhance the mind's capacity to affect bodily function and symptoms.
Biologically based therapies	Uses natural substances such as herbs, foods, and vitamins.
Manipulative and body-based methods	Manipulates or moves one or more parts of the body.
Energy therapies	Uses energy fields that purportedly surround and penetrate the human body (e.g., by applying pressure and/or manipulating the body by placing hands in or through these fields). Also uses electromagnetic fields.

Source: National Center for Complementary and Alternative Medicine

Table 16.2 Cost of Health Care in the United States

Year	National health expenditures	Percent of gross domestic product
1970	$73.1 billion	7.0
1980	245.8	8.8
1990	696.0	12.0
2000	1,299.5	13.2

Source: Centers for Medicare and Medicaid Services

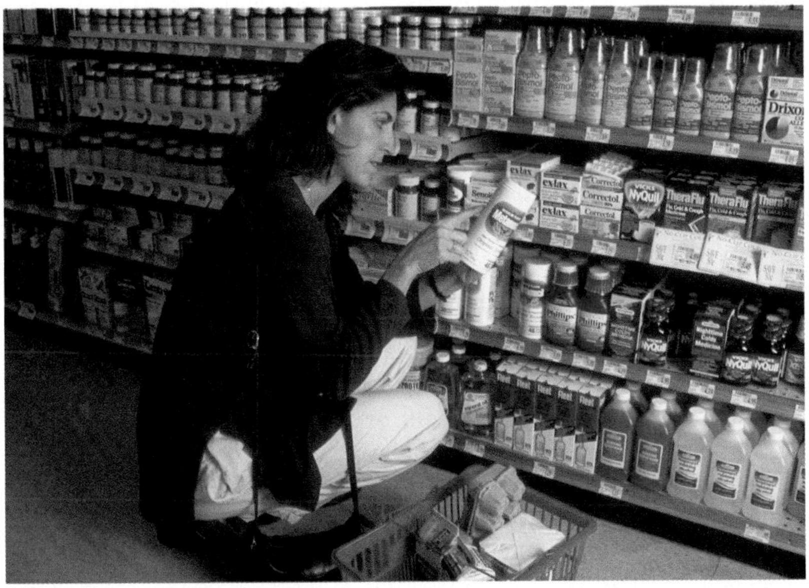

Make good consumer decisions and read about the contraindications (side effects) of over-the-counter medications before you buy them.

sold in the United States in the *Physicians' Desk Reference,* which is available in most libraries and also online.

The Internet can be an excellent source of health information. A good place to begin searching is with the websites listed at the end of each chapter of this textbook. As with any other source of information, be critical of what you read on the Internet. Even the best websites can be biased on occasion (see the Developing Health Skills box).

There also are thousands of toll-free numbers you can call to get free medical information ranging from getting referrals to local physicians to practical information on specific diseases. For example, if you are having a friend with diabetes over for dinner, a call to the American Diabetes Association's 800 number could help you find out what foods you can safely serve. Our Health Hotlines is a compilation of organizations' addresses, telephone numbers, and sites prepared by the National Library of Medicine. You can find selected listings at the end of each chapter of *Decisions for Healthy Living.*

Advertising Health Care

Advertising is the primary way businesses have of informing the public about their products and services. Advertisements for **prescription** and **over-the-counter** (nonprescription) **drugs** appear in magazines, in

prescription drugs Drugs ordered specifically for a person by his or her physician and filled by a registered pharmacist.

over-the-counter drugs Drugs that can be purchased without a prescription.

Developing Health Skills

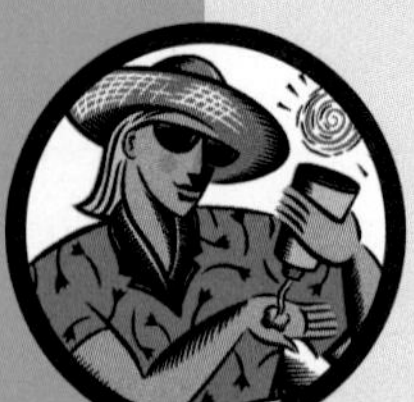

Using the Internet for Health Information

There are more than 100,000 health-related websites on the Internet, and accessing this information is a frequent online activity. Nearly two-thirds of Internet users say they have used it to find health information—more people than those who use it to shop or check sport scores.

Since there is no absolute way to assure that all information found on the Internet is accurate, unbiased, and up-to-date, here are some tips for checking the sources you use:

- *Trust well-known organizations to provide comprehensive information.* For example, the American Cancer Society and the American Lung Association are more likely to provide high-quality information than a site named Bill's Cancer Experience. Federal offices such as the Centers for Disease Control and Prevention (CDC) and the Office of Disease Prevention and Health Promotion in the Department of Health and Human Services are excellent sources of objective information, as are respected medical schools and universities.
- *Always compare sources.* It is not a good idea to look in only one place for information. Even when you find information quickly, compare that information with other sources. The best information found on the Internet is usually cited in or linked to several other sites. Be cautious with information that is not duplicated in trusted sources.
- *Distrust extremes in data.* Good science involves sharing information, so when you find a website that claims to be the only source of a certain "fact," it is probably a good idea to distrust that fact.
- *Check for current information.* How often is the website updated, and who reviews it? Websites should be reviewed and updated on a regular basis. This is particularly important for health-related material.

Keeping these tips in mind when you visit a website will help you evaluate the information you find.

point-of-purchase displays at the drugstore, on the radio, and on television. An educated consumer uses advertisements as a means of finding out what health care products are available. At the same time, the wise consumer seldom depends on advertisements alone as a source of information upon which to base a purchase decision. Advertisements, by their very nature, are biased in favor of the product being promoted.

Advertisers attempt to make a product or service as appealing as possible. They do this through several advertising techniques. *"Scientific studies"* used in many health-related advertisements provide the basis for the statements like the following: "In a doctor-approved research study, brand X relieved headache twice as fast as other brands." However, advertisements do not necessarily provide much data concerning the research design, study population size, or the controls involved in the study.

Another technique used by advertisers is the *bandwagon approach.* In this technique, advertisers claim, "Everyone is using the product," therefore you should use it as well. For example, in a commercial for exercise equipment, an advertiser asserts, "over 8,000 of these devices have been sold." Just because a product is a business success does not mean it is effective.

Some advertisements rely on *testimonials* to sell their product. A famous person—or an attractive model—usually gives the testimonial telling you how well the product worked for him or her. Take notice of the lack of factual data in such advertisements. After reading or hearing the testimonial, the consumer knows little more than that the product exists. The wise consumer does not purchase a product—or ask his or her physician for a prescription for it—without information on the effectiveness, safety, or side effects of the product.

Emotional appeals are used for some products. These advertisements claim that a product is safe or wholesome. Emotional appeals are often used for products designed for children, such as cold remedies. A scene showing a sad and obviously ill child being watched over by a loving mother providing a "soothing" medicine is emotionally touching, but gives the consumer little information.

Finally, some advertisers provide a *comparison to other products* or depend on *price appeal* to sell their products. These approaches are often used with products that are well known to the buying public. Pain relievers, for example, are extremely common, so one way to spur purchase of a particular brand is simply to offer it at a price lower than its competitors'.

Notice that the techniques described here may bend the truth a little or withhold negative information about the product being advertised. Although there are laws that require truth in advertising, consumers should view all promotional material with caution. By recognizing the techniques used by advertisers, you will be better prepared to make wise decisions about health products.

Health Fraud

Some health-related products and services are actually anything but health related. Naive health care consumers in search of the perfect cure for complex health problems seem willing to buy almost anything. In fact, more than 26 percent of Americans surveyed for an FDA poll said that they have used one or more questionable methods of health care to treat medical problems.

Quackery is a health claim made for a product or service that cannot be justified by scientifically derived evidence. It can have serious medical consequences. People have been known to become ill from the product itself or from the failure to get the proper approved and needed therapy when it can be most effective. For example, one quack advertisement stated that 80 percent of women tested got premenstrual relief by taking large doses of vitamin B_6. However, the advertisement neglected to note that the same percentage of women taking a **placebo** (a look-alike pill that has no therapeutic value) thought they got relief, too. More important, the advertisement also failed to mention that the doses of vitamin B_6 they were recommending have been known to cause nerve damage in some individuals.

Cancer and arthritis patients are prone to quackery treatments because many who have these conditions become desperate for "cures." Also, both diseases can go into remission on their own, which allows the quack to claim success. About half of all patients in legitimate cancer therapy also try unproven treatments. Especially popular among cancer patients is metabolic therapy, which includes large doses of vitamins and minerals, a special diet, and detoxification with enemas. Other vulnerable targets for quackery products are people seeking quick weight loss, larger breasts, hair restoration, and removal of wrinkles. If products sound too good to be true, they probably are. Quackery usually depends on sensationalism and false science.

How to Choose Health Care Providers

Suppose you move to a new community and need to find a primary care physician or an alternative practitioner. Who would you choose, and how would you go about making that decision? Similarly, if you had to go to a hospital for an emergency or elective surgery, which one would you choose and why would you make that decision?

The Right Physician for You

There are numerous kinds of medical physicians to choose from. Primary care physicians are most often trained in family practice (and are family practitioners) or in internal medicine (and are internists). Pediatricians provide primary care for children, and obstetrician/gynecologists often provide primary care for women. In general, the type of physician you see is usually not as important as the individual physician. For example, a woman can get her primary care from a family practitioner, an internist, or a gynecologist. No matter which type of physician is chosen, it is important to pick someone you like and feel comfortable talking to.

In most cases, your primary care physician recommends a specialist when you need to see one. For example, if you have allergies, you may be referred to an allergist. If you break a leg, you will need to see an orthopedic surgeon.

There are many kinds of health care practitioners who are not medical doctors (MDs) but are still doctors because they received a doctorate degree and professional training. Examples include psychologists, who are doctors of philosophy (PhDs) or doctors of psychology (PsyDs) and osteopaths, who are doctors of osteopathy (DOs). Psychologists provide therapy as do psychiatrists, but because they are not medical doctors, psychologists cannot prescribe medications. Osteopaths are general practitioners who believe that muscles and bones play a more significant role in most diseases than medical doctors do. They receive training similar to medical doctors but attend schools of osteopathy, not medical schools. Table 16.3 provides examples of some health care professionals and their areas of specialization.

Complementary and Alternative Health Providers

Far from being off beat, many of the complementary and alternative treatments have become mainstream, and licensed practitioners are covered under a growing number of health insurance plans. Some people seek care from alternative health care practitioners, including acupuncturists, herbalists, and massage therapists. In some cases, an acupuncturist is also a

quackery A health claim made for a product or service that cannot be justified by scientifically derived evidence.

placebo A look-alike pill that has no therapeutic value; used in controlled scientific experiments to test the efficacy of another substance.

Table 16.3 Health Care Professionals

Type	Area of Specialty
Acupuncturist	Pain management
Allergist	Allergies
Cardiologist	Heart and blood vessel disorders
Chiropractor	Musculoskeletal structures/body alignment
Dermatologist	Skin disorders
Family practitioner	General practice
Endocrinologist	Glandular disorders
Gastroenterologist	Stomach and intestinal tract disorders
Geneticist	Genetic diseases
Health educator	Health education and health promotion
Hematologist	Blood-related disorders
Naturopath	General practice using natural healing forces within the body
Neurologist	Brain, nervous system, and spinal cord diseases
Neurosurgeon	Brain, nervous system, and spinal cord surgery
Nurse practitioner	Nurse with additional training in a specified area, such as OB/GYN
Obstetrician/gynecologist (OB/GYN)	Female reproductive system
Oncologist	Cancerous growths and tumors
Ophthalmologist	Eye disorders
Orthopedic surgeon	Bone and joint injuries
Osteopath	Musculoskeletal conditions and their relationship to the rest of the body
Otolaryngologist	Ear, nose, and throat disorders
Pediatrician	Well-baby/child care and childhood diseases
Physical therapist	Rehabilitates people after impairment due to injury or disease
Physician assistant	Health care professional trained to assist physicians
Plastic surgeon	Corrective surgery for irregularities of body or facial contours
Psychiatrist	Mental and emotional disorders
Psychologist	Mental and emotional disorders
Pulmonary specialist	Respiratory system disorders
Urologist	Urinary tract

medical doctor. You can read more about this in the Cultural View box.

Naturopaths are sometimes called the general practitioners of the complementary and alternative medical world. As graduates of colleges of naturopathy, they study health sciences for two years, and get hands-on training for two years. They use a variety of alternative treatments, depending on a patient's individual needs. Naturopathy is based on the healing power of nature. These methods can include diet; acupuncture; herbal medicine; water therapy; therapeutic exercise; spinal and soft-tissue manipulation; physical therapies involving electric current, ultrasound, and light therapy; therapeutic counseling; and pharmacology. Just because ingredients are natural, however, doesn't necessarily mean they are safe. In fact, some herbs can cause serious problems, including kidney failure and stroke. A well-trained naturopath will steer you away from risky botanicals. Look for a licensed naturopath in states where that is required.

naturopath A general practitioner of complementary and alternative medicine; uses the natural healing forces within the body.

Selecting a New Health Care Provider

At some point—or at several points in your life, depending on how often you move and your lifestyle circumstances change—you will need a new physician or want to try an alternative therapy. Here are some options you should consider when choosing a new health care practitioner:

- Ask your current physician for a recommendation. Contrary to what you might think, this will not preclude you from getting a recommendation for an alternative practitioner. A national survey found that 60 percent of physicians had at some time referred patients to practitioners of alternative medicine.

Cultural View

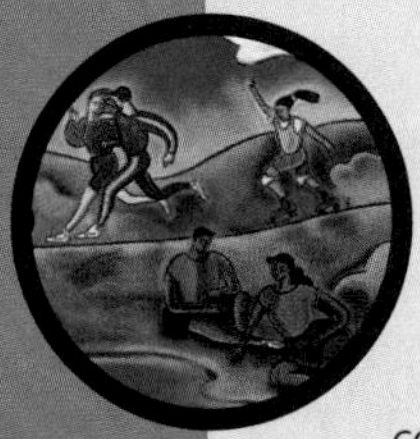

The Chinese Tradition of Acupuncture

Since at least the second century B.C., Chinese doctors have been inserting thin needles into the skin of the ailing. Acupuncture is based on the concept that within the body there are numerous channels called meridians. When energy is blocked along any of the meridians, an excess of energy occurs in some channels and a deficiency occurs in others. Over time, these imbalances can lead to illness. Acupuncture is a way of restoring balance by triggering shifts of energy with hair-thin, disposable needles inserted into the body. These needles are inserted in some of the 361 classical acupuncture points. Typically, acupuncture care involves a series of weekly or twice a week treatments. The needles remain in place between 20 and 30 minutes or longer. Length of treatment can vary, but a course of a dozen treatments is not unusual.

Why acupuncture has the power to heal is a mystery, which is one reason why the U.S. medical establishment has viewed it skeptically—at least until relatively recently. There is a growing contingent of U.S. physicians who swear by it. Frustrated by the limitations of Western medicine, which treats body parts separately, more than 3,000 physicians use acupuncture, which treats the whole body including the mind and the emotions. In addition, there are some 14,000 practicing acupuncturists who are not physicians.

Documented Successes

With findings based on well-conducted studies, National Institutes of Health and other researchers have found that acupuncture is an effective treatment for certain kinds of pain and nausea caused by cancer chemotherapy drugs, surgical anesthesia, or morning sickness during pregnancy. As an example of how successful it can be in reducing pain, patients who received acupuncture before the removal of impacted molars had an average of 17 minutes of post-surgical pain, in contrast to 94 minutes for patients treated with conventional pain drugs. The experts also found evidence—although not as strong—that acupuncture is effective for treating menstrual cramps, drug addiction, strokes, headaches, and even tennis elbow.

Acupuncture is already being used in about one thousand drug addiction treatment facilities, where clinicians have found it has a calming effect on addicts and reduces their craving for drugs. This might be due to a release of endorphins as part of the acupuncture process. Endorphins are pain-relieving substances produced by the body.

Questionable Outcomes

Acupuncture is most commonly used for back pain, headaches/migraines, nerve pain, and osteoarthritis. Yet evidence that it works on these conditions is equivocal or contradictory. In part this is because clinical studies on acupuncture are difficult to design. In a traditional clinical trial, one group receives the real treatment (for example, a certain dose of medicine) while the other receives a placebo or sham treatment (typically a sugar-coated dummy pill). With acupuncture, treatment involves inserting needles at key points in the body. As a result, it is difficult to have a placebo group.

The value of acupuncture remains unproven for a wide variety of other medical conditions, from asthma to smoking cessation.

Increasing Popularity

Whether studies show acupuncture treatment is effective or not, it is gaining popularity with patients. Millions of Americans have tried it at least once, and increasingly health plans are paying for it. Most states have accredited licensure programs for acupuncturists, which require at least 1,750 hours of training. In addition, many states require that physicians practicing acupuncture have 200 to 300 hours of training in the treatment. If you are interested in receiving acupuncture treatment, be sure to inquire about the acupuncturist's training and whether he or she has a license to practice in your state.

Should You Have Acupuncture?

Given that there is not a complete list of when acupuncture should be used, what should you do? One expert says: "What we tell people is that their experience matters. If after a short series of treatments, acupuncture seems to be helping you, then it's worth doing. If not, it's not. You should feel different (after receiving treatments). If you don't, stop it."

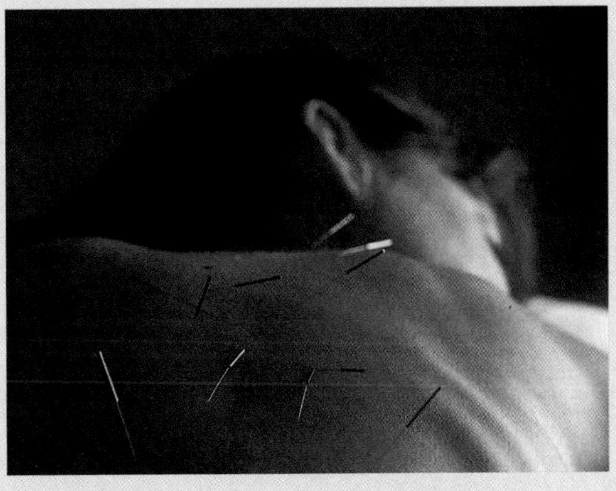

Acupuncturists relieve pain by inserting special needles at key points in the body.

- Ask the student health service or human resources director where you work for the names of physicians whom other students or employees like or dislike.
- If you know a nurse, ask which physicians he or she recommends seeing or avoiding. Nurses know more about good and bad health care practitioners than many other health professionals.
- Get a recommendation from a family member or friend. A solid recommendation is the number one factor influencing people when choosing a doctor.

When You Go to the Hospital

Medical facilities provide a range of care, including primary, secondary, and tertiary care. **Primary care** is provided by a physician in the office or at an emergency room in a hospital or clinic. Examples of this kind of care range from treating cold or flu symptoms to getting a diagnosis and treatment for acute abdominal pain.

Secondary care is usually provided as **inpatient care** in your local community hospital. Uncomplicated surgery is an example of secondary care. The three most commonly performed surgeries today are childbirth by cesarean section, gallbladder removal, and hysterectomy. An alternative to hospitalization for minor procedures is **outpatient care,** or treatment in a special facility within the hospital or in a freestanding facility, where surgery is performed without the patient staying overnight. Examples of the types of surgery where you would not have to stay in the hospital overnight are a bunionectomy and a tonsillectomy.

Tertiary care, which is often provided at hospitals affiliated with medical schools or regional referral centers, includes special procedures, such as open-heart surgery, kidney dialysis, and other sophisticated treatments.

When selecting a hospital for primary emergency care, look for the best one near where you live with good access to secondary care in case additional care is needed (see Figure 16.1). In contrast, you might want to go to a tertiary care facility some distance from your home, perhaps in a different city. For example, some facilities specialize in treating breast cancer, others, lung disease. The selection of a tertiary care hospital is usually made by you in conjunction with your physician.

Unless it is a medical emergency, most health plans have to give advance approval, or **preadmission certification,** before you go to the hospital. Otherwise, the cost of your hospital care may not be covered. Most health plans establish how long you can stay in the hospital for each condition. Many procedures that were once done in the hospital (e.g., tonsillectomy) are now done on an outpatient basis.

Most physicians consider any of the following an emergency and reason to go immediately to the emergency room of the nearest hospital:
abdominal pain (severe) animal bites bleeding (severe, uncontrollable) broken bones bullet or stab wounds burns (severe) chest pains (severe) choking (or difficulty breathing) convulsions diarrhea (prolonged) drug overdose eye injuries or sudden loss of vision head injury heat stroke (dehydration) hypothermia (dangerously low body temperature) inhalation of gaseous fumes or smoke insect stings resulting in shortness of breath poisoning slurred speech (or loss of speech) snake bites temperature over 103° F unconsciousness vomiting (prolonged)

Figure 16.1 What Is Considered an Emergency?
Review the list to see what is considered a medical emergency.

primary care Routine medical care provided by a physician in an office or at an emergency room in a hospital or clinic.

secondary care Care involving surgery and nonroutine medical treatment, usually delivered in a hospital.

inpatient care Health care provided in a hospital.

outpatient care Care provided in a physician's or other health practitioner's office, in an emergency room in a hospital, or in a specialized ambulatory clinic; does not involve hospitalization or overnight stays.

tertiary care Special medical procedures, such as open-heart surgery and transplants, performed mostly at hospitals affiliated with medical schools or at large regional hospitals.

preadmission certification Approval from a health plan of the need for inpatient hospital care prior to the actual admission.

Paying for Health Care

Most people have access to the health care system through their private health insurance plans, which are either provided by their employers, offered through their colleges or through a professional association to which they or their parents belong, or purchased individually. There are also public federal programs that provide insurance and/or access to health care. For example, people over age sixty-five and certain disabled people are covered by **Medicare,** and low-income and disabled persons meeting certain qualifications are covered by **Medicaid.** In addition, there are some people who are **uninsured** (have no health insurance) and some who are **underinsured** (have policies that do not meet their needs or that place them at significant financial risk).

Many employers provide health insurance benefits to workers and their families as part of an employment package. Usually, employers pay most of the cost of the monthly or quarterly premium and employees pay the rest. Full-time students up to age twenty-three or twenty-five (depending on the plan) can be classified as over-age dependents and may remain on their families' insurance plan (see the Developing Health Skills: Consumer Health box).

Shopping for health insurance is complicated because so many different options are available. Choosing a plan can be a costly decision if you select the wrong one. Because your health care needs change, you might want to adjust your health insurance plan over time. For example, having a pregnancy-related benefit is important when you might want to have a family, but it is no longer necessary later in life.

Indemnity (Fee-for-Service) Plans

With an **indemnity plan,** you pay for most of your medical bills and then file a claim to be reimbursed. This is also called **fee-for-service.** This approach gives you the greatest amount of flexibility in choosing physicians, hospitals, and other health-related services. It is also the most costly.

In addition to monthly premiums, indemnity plans have a deductible that you must pay for physician services before the insurer will reimburse your claims. Once that deductible amount is reached, most insurers reimburse only up to a certain amount for legitimate claims. In most plans, insurers pay a larger part of the bill (usually 80 percent) and you pay a smaller part (usually 20 percent).

Fee-for-service plans can also place limits on the extent of coverage for all people insured under a plan, as well as for individual people applying for coverage if they have a **pre-existing condition.** For example, if a person has been seeking medical treatment for a knee injury just prior to joining a plan, the new health insurer can refuse to pay for any treatment for up to twelve months.

Managed Care Plans

Managed care plans have agreements with certain physicians, hospitals, and health care providers to give a range of services to plan members at a reduced cost. This limits your freedom to choose physicians in exchange for lower costs and less paperwork than in a fee-for-service plan. There are three basic types of managed care plans: **health maintenance organizations (HMOs), point-of-service (POS) plans,** and **preferred provider organizations (PPOs).**

Health maintenance organizations HMOs offer a defined set of benefits according to a predetermined monthly premium. Beyond the monthly premium, there are only limited or sometimes no additional costs. A visit to the physician's office, for example, can cost between $10 and $20 a visit, in contrast to between $75 and $100 under a fee-for-service plan.

Medicare A federal program that provides health care coverage to people age sixty-five and older and to some other eligible categories.

Medicaid A federal-state program that provides health care coverage to eligible low-income persons; eligibility can vary by state.

uninsured Having no health insurance.

underinsured Having limited health insurance that compromises one's access to health care services and places one at significant financial risk.

indemnity (fee-for-service) plan Insurance coverage in which a person pays for most of his or her medical bills and then files a claim to be reimbursed.

pre-existing condition A health condition for which a person has been treated prior to joining a health plan; some plans limit coverage for such a condition up to one year after joining the plan.

health maintenance organizations (HMOs) Prepaid plans that offer a defined set of benefits according to a predetermined monthly premium.

point-of-service (POS) plans HMOs having an indemnity-type option that lets members get care from physicians and other providers outside the plan's network.

preferred provider organizations (PPOs) A hybrid form of insurance that merges features of traditional fee-for-service insurance and prepaid plans.

Developing Health Skills

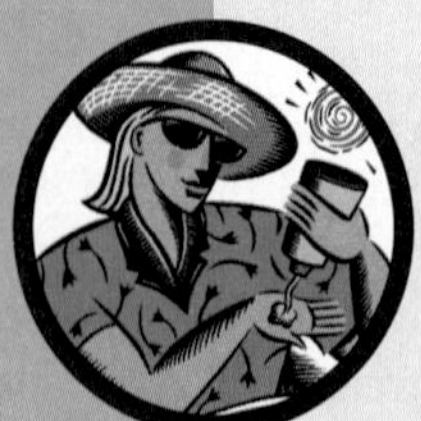

Consumer Health: Covering College Students

Who covers college students for health care when they crash their bikes, twist their knees playing ultimate Frisbee, or come down with a serious illness? In some cases, the answer is no one. More than a quarter of all Americans aged eighteen to twenty-four and a fifth of people aged twenty-five to thirty-four have no insurance.

If you do not have access to health insurance through your parents, there are several affordable options:

- Most colleges and universities offer a student health plan. If you have health insurance through your school, make sure it also covers the summer months.
- If you graduate and do not go directly into a job that provides health insurance, see if your alumni association has a health plan. Often association plans have good rates.
- Some insurance companies provide short-term coverage, from three months up to one year. This is a good option if you think you are likely to be enrolled in an employer's plan soon.

Most colleges and universities also provide some care through the student health service. Typical services include distributing cold medication, treating minor injuries, and providing health education on everything from alcohol abuse and AIDS to hypertension and weight loss. Students should not rely on the college health service for their primary source of care. Most of the services are not set up for this and are not accredited by any national body.

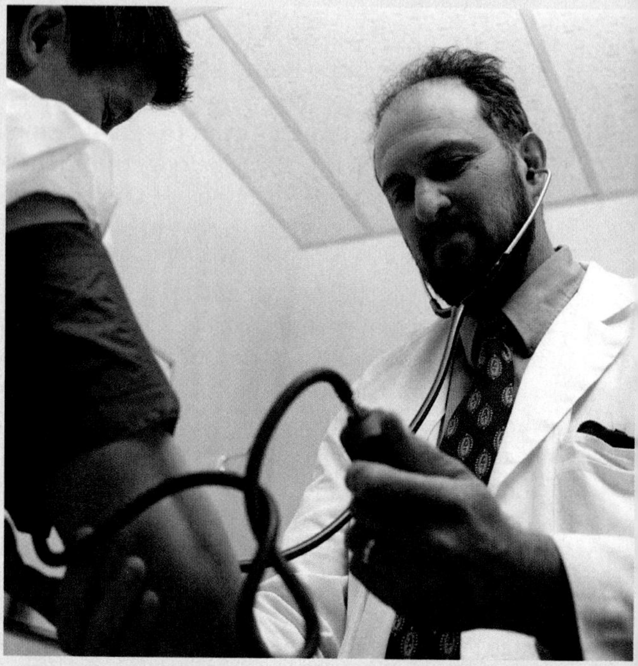

Having a physician who knows you and your health status is important. Your student health center can be a beneficial resource, but you still need a primary care physician.

When you join an HMO, you will be assigned to a family physician or internist who acts as the **gatekeeper** to all of the other health services provided by the HMO. You may be given a choice of several physicians, all contract employees of the HMO. If you want to see a dermatologist or a cardiologist in the HMO, you will first have to see your assigned or chosen gatekeeper, who will determine whether it is necessary for you to see that specialist. This approach holds down costs, but it also severely limits flexibility and choice of physicians and hospitals. Some HMOs allow members to contact certain specialists in the plan without seeing the gatekeeper first. If you choose to see a physician outside the HMO, you may have to pay 100 percent of the cost.

On the plus side, HMOs offer one-stop shopping. Often, you will be able to get all your outpatient medical needs tended to in one treatment center. HMOs are also not permitted to add a waiting period for people who have pre-existing conditions.

Point-of-service plans. These plans are very popular because they offer basic coverage along with an expanded choice of physicians. In a POS plan, members can refer themselves to a physician outside the plan and still get some coverage—although they have to pay additional money for it. A POS option costs more than an HMO but less than fee-for-service.

Preferred provider organizations. Another popular option is a hybrid form of insurance that merges the best features of traditional indemnity insurance and HMOs. Under a PPO, you pay monthly premiums and have deductibles and copayments just as you would in an indemnity plan, but the copayment is lower.

In a PPO, you can choose your own physicians and the services you want as long as they come from a list of preferred physicians and facilities. If you use

gatekeeper The physician in an HMO who refers a patient to specialists or other health services within the HMO.

these preferred providers, your share of the copayment drops to 10 percent. You have to use these preferred providers because they have agreed to treat all participants in the PPO at a discounted rate. This discount contributes to keeping your copayment lower than it would be in a traditional indemnity plan. If you go outside the network, your copayment can rise as high as 50 percent, depending on the type of service provided.

Asking Questions about a Health Plan

Regardless of the type of health insurance you choose, you should ask yourself and others a number of questions before agreeing to join a plan:

- *What type of coverage do you need?* What services are you and/or members of your family most likely to need in the coming years? Will the plan cover them? You may have heard stories about someone who contracted a major illness and then found out that his or her insurance did not provide coverage for it. The only way to avoid such situations is to be informed in advance.
- *How do you feel about having limits placed on your choice of physicians or hospitals?* How important is the cost of services to you? Managed care plans limit your choice. Fee-for-service plans do not place limits but will cost you more money.
- *What is the plan's policy on special areas of coverage* such as maternity, laboratory charges, and prescription fees? Maternity coverage is often incomplete. Some policies offer full coverage if the employee gets pregnant and virtually none if a male employee's wife or dependent child gets pregnant.
- *When does coverage take effect?* This may seem like a simple question, but some employers require that you work for them for three to six months before you can be covered under their plan. Timing can also be critical when pregnancy is concerned, particularly if conception occurs before the insurance takes effect.
- *Does the plan meet your needs?* Are other policyholders satisfied with the extent of coverage? If it is a managed care plan, how long do you have to wait to see a physician? Are there physicians and hospitals in the plan convenient to where you live or work? How much paperwork is involved?

Don't choose an insurance carrier or plan just because it is the cheapest available. As with most consumer decisions, it is usually wise to shop around.

Drugs and Natural Products as Medicine

Each year, Americans spend more than $20 billion on drugs in order to get or stay well. Half of this money is used for prescription drugs, which are ordered specifically for you by your physician and filled by a registered pharmacist. The other half is for over-the-counter drugs, a vast assortment of medicines, ranging from aspirin to wart removers, that you can buy without a prescription. In addition, more than $4 billion is spent on herbal treatments.

What is the difference between these types of drugs? Prescription drugs are defined primarily as those that are unsafe for use except under professional supervision. They can include drugs that are habit forming or unsafe because of their toxicity. Over-the-counter drugs are considered safe for consumers to use if they follow the directions and warnings on the drug's labels. Sometimes, a stronger version of a drug can be obtained by prescription even though a weaker version is available over-the-counter. This is the case with ibuprofen, a popular pain reliever used for headaches, arthritis and joint aches, and soft tissue injuries.

Some drugs are available only under their original brand names. This is especially true of drugs developed by a single pharmaceutical company that are still protected by a seventeen-year, exclusive patent. Most drugs on the market however, are also available as less expensive, generic drugs. **Generic drugs** have the same active chemical ingredients as their brand-name counterparts, but some generic drugs are absorbed at different rates and may not be as effective as their brand-name counterparts.

More than 60 million Americans take herbal remedies and use other natural products, which do not require the same type of rigorous efficacy and safety testing by the FDA as prescription and over-the-counter drugs. Even though they are popular with the public, researchers have found that St. John's wort is ineffective in treating patients with moderate depression and ginkgo supplements do nothing to improve memory in healthy people. Studies are underway on the efficacy and correct doses of other natural products, including echinacea as a treatment to shorten the duration of the common cold and glucosamine and chondroitan to relieve osteoarthritis symptoms.

generic drugs Less expensive drugs that have the same active chemical ingredients as their brand-name counterparts.

If you take herbal supplements or other nontraditional treatments, researchers at the Mayo Clinic recommend the following:

- *Educate yourself.* Before taking a natural product as medicine, check to see if it has side effects, drug-food interactions, and other potential risks associated with your health history.
- *Tell your physician.* Your physician should always know what medications—prescription, over-the-counter, or nontraditional—you take. Studies show that 60 percent of people taking herbal supplements do not tell their physician.
- *Be aware of side effects.* If you have any unusual reactions, stop taking the herb immediately and contact your physician.

The Correct Way to Take Medications

When you have a prescription or buy an over-the-counter drug, do you know when to take it? How many times a day? For how long? To make the most of your health care dollar, use prescription drugs as directed. For example, after a couple of days of taking antibiotics you might feel better, but you still need to take the drug for the full specified period of time to actually cure the illness. The drug needs time to get rid of all of the infectious agent, not just enough of the germ to alleviate the worst symptoms. Similarly, medicines may need to be taken several times throughout the day at specific intervals to maintain the right amount of the drug in your bloodstream at all times. Too much could cause an adverse reaction; too little might not be effective.

Sometimes, a prescription reads "take on an empty stomach—one hour before or two hours after meals." In this case, food in the stomach slows down the absorption of the drug and makes it less effective. Other drugs need to be taken with meals because the food helps the body absorb them better or prevents a feeling of nausea.

The correct time of day to take drugs also varies. It may be best to take a diuretic—a medicine that increases urination—no later than 6 P.M. unless your physician says otherwise, so that you won't have to go to the bathroom several times during the night. But it may be better to take a drug that causes drowsiness, such as an antihistamine, in the evening so that it does not interfere with your daily activities.

Directions for taking drugs are important and you should discuss them with your physician and/or pharmacist. However, most of us don't do this. According to a recent FDA survey, fewer than 4 percent of patients said they asked questions about their prescriptions when they were in their physicians' offices. Although physicians took this as a sign that their patients were clear about how and when to take their medication, the fact is that about half of all prescription drugs are taken improperly. Patients on long-term medications often stop taking them, and each year, more than 230 million prescriptions written by physicians for their patients are not taken at all.

Because of the many problems associated with taking drugs—and with not taking them correctly—it is important to keep your pharmacist informed about which drugs you take. Your pharmacist has a record of all prescribed drugs filled in a particular store (and sometimes in a chain of pharmacies) but does not know which over-the-counter drugs you take unless you inform him or her. With this information, the pharmacist is in a good position to alert you to any possible problems and/or side effects. For this reason, it is recommended that you use the same pharmacy each time you get a prescription drug filled.

The National Council on Patient Information and Education suggests that patients ask these five questions when given a new medication:

1. What is the name of the drug and what is it supposed to do?
2. How and when do I take it, and when do I stop taking it?
3. What food, drinks, other drugs, or activities should I avoid while taking the drug?
4. What are the side effects, and what should I do if they occur?
5. Is there any written information available about the drug?

In addition, the council advises patients to tell their physicians and pharmacists what other medicines they are taking, the names of any drugs they are allergic to, and, for women, whether they are pregnant or plan to become pregnant. Another good tip is to read the patient package inserts for prescription medicines and the new standardized over-the-counter drug label, which tells you what the medicine is supposed to do, who should or should not take it, and how to use it (see Figure 16.2).

Some Concluding Remarks

This book began by presenting the idea that you are responsible for your own health. Nowhere is this truer than in your role as health care consumer. You are the person responsible for the decisions you make, the risks you take, and the products and services you

Drug Facts

Active ingredient (in each tablet)	**Purpose**
Chlorpheniramine maleate 2 mg	Antihistamine

Uses temporarily relieves these symptoms due to hay fever or other upper respiratory allergies:
■ sneezing ■ runny nose ■ itchy, watery eyes ■ itchy throat

Warnings
Ask a doctor before use if you have
■ glaucoma ■ a breathing problem such as emphysema or chronic bronchitis
■ trouble urinating due to an enlarged prostate gland

Ask a doctor or pharmacist before use if you are taking tranquilizers or sedatives

When using this product
■ You may get drowsy ■ avoid alcoholic drinks
■ alcohol, sedatives, and tranquilizers may increase drowsiness
■ be careful when driving a motor vehicle or operating machinery
■ excitability may occur, especially in children

If pregnant or breast-feeding, ask a health professional before use.
Keep out of reach of children. In case of overdose, get medical help or contact a Poison Control Center right away.

Directions

adults and children 12 years and over	take 2 tablets every 4 to 6 hours; not more than 12 tablets in 24 hours
children 6 years to under 12 years	take 1 tablet every 4 to 6 hours; not more than 6 tablets in 24 hours
children under 6 years	ask a doctor

Other information store at 20-25° C (68-77° F) ■ protect from excessive moisture

Inactive ingredients D&C yellow no. 10, lactose, magnesium stearate, microcrystalline cellulose, pregelatinized starch

Figure 16.2 The OTC Drug Label
The FDA requires most over-the-counter drugs to have a label that looks like this one, so the information is in a standardized and easy-to-read format. Use it to compare drug ingredients and to follow dosage instructions and warnings.

use. There is no question that tremendous progress has been made in medical science. There are new surgical procedures that were inconceivable only a few years ago, new drugs to cure illnesses that were once life threatening, and new diagnostic procedures that allow noninvasive inspection of the body and early discovery of disease.

Despite these and other medical advances, your health remains your responsibility, not the responsibility of modern medicine. The good news is that acting responsibly is not very difficult. It involves:

- common sense (sound knowledge about health)
- health skills (patterns of action that develop with practice)
- healthy behaviors (repeated acts that enhance rather than compromise health)

Common sense comes from experience and knowledge. Health skills come from practice. Healthy behaviors come from healthy choices. Now that you are more knowledgeable about your own health and the health of others, and more competent in the application of that health knowledge, you realize that a positive lifestyle offers the best prospect for a healthy, long, happy, and productive life.

CASE STUDY 16: Making Health Care Decisions

Rita was concerned about her sister, Ginger, who had just been diagnosed with chronic fatigue syndrome. Since Rita was adept at online searches for classwork, she logged on to research her sister's health condition. She joined a chat group, learned about other people's experiences, as well as the latest "cure" some people in the chat group swore worked. Instead of checking out the so-called cure in legitimate medical sources, Rita assumed it to be valid because she learned about it on the Internet.

When she called Ginger with the information, Rita was surprised to find that her sister did not want to immediately start the new treatment. In fact, Ginger had a lot of reservations about following medical advice from strangers in a chat room.

Ginger, however, was not against using the Internet to learn more about her illness. She logged onto the National Library of Medicine's Website to find articles from peer-reviewed medical journals about chronic fatigue, so she could become as educated as possible. She also learned some useful information from chat groups about how to deal with the psychosocial aspects of her disease.

In Your Opinion

Both sisters found health information about chronic fatigue syndrome on the Internet. Rita didn't know anything about the source of her information while Ginger did.

- Rita may have encountered incorrect or biased information through her Internet search. What are the risks of giving advice based on misinformation?
- How could Rita check her sources to be sure that the information that she was receiving was correct, complete, and unbiased?
- The Internet is only one source of information related to chronic fatigue syndrome. Where might Ginger and Rita find high-quality information on this illness?

KEY CONCEPTS

1. Americans spend more money on health care than people in any other country. In 2002, $1.3 trillion was spent on health in the United States.
2. Consumers need accurate and unbiased information to make good health care decisions.
3. A vast amount of health information is available on the Internet. This information can be useful in helping consumers make better health care decisions. However, as with all information, it is important to make sure that it is accurate, unbiased, and up to date.
4. Quackery refers to a health claim made for a product or method that cannot be justified by scientifically derived evidence. If a product sounds "too good to be true," it probably is.
5. When selecting a new personal physician, ask your current physician, the student health service or human resources director where you work, a nurse, or a family member for recommendations.
6. Alternative or complementary health providers are becoming more common and, in some cases, the costs are covered under health insurance plans.
7. When you join a health maintenance organization (HMO), you will be assigned to a family physician or internist who will act as the gatekeeper to all other health services provided by the HMO.
8. Go immediately to the emergency room, or nearest hospital, in case of medical emergencies such as severe abdominal pain or prolonged diarrhea or vomiting.
9. About 50 percent of all prescription drugs are taken incorrectly, and more than 230 million prescriptions that are written by physicians for their patients are not taken at all. To get the most out of your health care dollar, use prescription drugs as directed.
10. If you take herbal supplements or other nontraditional treatments, educate yourself on the supplement, keep your physician informed about your practice, and be fully aware of the possible side effects and drug interactions.

REVIEW QUESTIONS

1. Explain the importance of information to wise consumer decision making about health care and describe how information can be incomplete or biased.
2. Explain steps you would take to be sure that your information was accurate. Include in your explanation how you would use hotlines and the Internet.
3. List five advertising techniques used to promote health products and services.
4. Explain the meaning of health fraud.
5. Explain how to go about selecting a physician. Include in your response several approaches to this task.
6. When selecting an alternative or complementary health care provider, how can you be sure about the safety and efficacy of the treatments he or she will provide?
7. When choosing a health insurance plan, what questions should you ask to be sure you select the best policy?
8. Explain the difference between indemnity plans, health maintenance organizations, and preferred provider organizations.
9. Differentiate between prescription and over-the-counter drugs and briefly describe how each should be taken.
10. Herbal remedies and other natural products are not held to the rigorous safety standards like other drugs. What precautions should you take when choosing to use such products?

CRITICAL THINKING QUESTIONS

1. The media is filled with information and advertisements for products making various health claims. Differentiating a true expert from a quack isn't always easy. Do we put too much credence in expertise? Why do you think people are wary of leaving health-related products and services to personal trial and error? What criteria differentiate the true expert from the self-proclaimed expert? What signals alert you to false claims?
2. The *Healthy People 2010* objectives include the following: "Increase the proportion of primary care providers, pharmacists, and other health care professionals who routinely review with their patients aged 65 years and older and patients with chronic illnesses or disabilities all new prescribed and over-the-counter medicines." Is this objective based on the assumption that health care providers are the best source of information? Are there other sources of information that might be more effective?
3. There is concern that some alternative treatments recommend the use of substances for which there is no evidence of effectiveness. What are the possible problems that result from the increased use of such alternatives to traditional medicine? What are the advantages of such treatments? How can you be sure that they won't cause any harm?

4. The *Healthy People 2010* objectives include the following: "Increase the proportion of patients receiving information that meets guidelines for usefulness when their new prescriptions are dispensed." Although prescription drugs are dispensed with patient package inserts, of what use are they to patients who cannot read, do not comprehend the directions, nor recognize the importance of taking prescription medications as directed? Who should be responsible for providing information about prescription drugs? What is the consumer's responsibility?

JOURNAL ACTIVITIES

1. Develop a list of consumer publications or Internet sites that can help you make good, well-informed health decisions. For each publication or Internet site, identify the kind of information you will receive (e.g., pro and con articles, lists of resources to contact, etc.). Be sure to include sources from government agencies such as the Food and Drug Administration.
2. Write down all the medications you currently take—both prescription and over-the-counter. Ask a pharmacist to review this list to make sure you are not at risk for drug interactions. Keep this list up to date. You might want to perform this same activity for your parents or grandparents.
3. Invent your own "quack" product for a health condition or illness. How will you sell this bogus product to the public? What advertising appeals will you use? Write three testimonials praising the product. Do you think they are believable?
4. Go to a local, mail order, or online pharmacy and compare prices of similar products—for example, a name brand and a generic product with the same active ingredients. Do this for several items that you normally buy. What conclusions can you draw from this activity about the value of health products?

SELECTED BIBLIOGRAPHY

Chevallier, A. *Encyclopedia of Herbal Medicine*. New York: DK Publishing Co., 2000.

FDA Consumer. Rockville, MD: Food and Drug Administration (published bimonthly).

Forness, L. M. *Don't Get Duped: A Consumer's Guide to Health and Fitness.* Amherst, NY: Prometheus Books, 2001.

Health Hotlines. Bethesda, MD: National Library of Medicine, 2000.

Institute for the Future. *Health & Health Care 2010: The Forecast, The Challenge.* San Francisco: Jossey-Bass, 2000.

Kaptchuk, T. J. "Acupuncture: Theory, Efficacy, and Practice." *Annals of Internal Medicine 136,* 5 (2002): 374–383.

Lockie, A., and N. Geddes. *Complete Guide to Homeopathy.* New York: DK Publishing Co., 2000.

Physicians' Desk Reference. Montvale, NJ: Medical Economics Company, Inc., 2002.

HEALTHLINKS

Websites for Understanding Health Care

You can access better health as it relates to this chapter by checking out some of the following sites on the Internet. These sites can be accessed directly from the *Decisions for Healthy Living* Website located at www.aw.com/pruitt.

Consumer Product Safety Commission

CPSC is an independent federal regulatory agency that focuses on reducing the risk of injury or death from consumer products, from automatic-drip coffee makers to toys to lawn mowers. Visitors can also use the website to report unsafe products.

Go Ask Alice

An interactive question-and-answer line provided by Columbia University Health Services. "Alice" is available to answer questions each week about any health-related issues, including relationships, nutrition and diet, exercise, drugs, sex, alcohol, and stress.

Institute of Medicine

The Institute of Medicine, a part of the National Academy of Sciences, provides objective, timely, and authoritative information to government, the professions, and the public.

National Center for Complementary and Alternative Medicine Clearinghouse

Managed by the arm of the National Institutes of Health responsible for complementary and alternative medicine, this website provides access to related information and resources.

National Committee for Quality Assurance

The NCQA assesses and reports on the quality of managed care plans such as health maintenance organizations (HMOs).

National Library of Medicine

This site contains every significant program of the National Library of Medicine, from medical history to biotechnology.

HEALTH HOTLINES

Making Health Care Decisions

American Academy of Medical Acupuncture
(800) 521-2262
4929 Wilshire Boulevard, Suite 428
Los Angeles, CA 90010

Department of Health and Human Services, Inspector General's Hotline
(800) HHS-TIPS (447-8477)
Office of Inspector General
Office of Public Affairs
Department of Health and Human Services
Room 5541 Cohen Building
330 Independence Avenue, SW
Washington, DC 20201

National Fraud Information Center
National Consumers League
(800) 876-7060
1701 K. Street, NW, Suite 1200
Washington, DC 20006

National Health Information Center
(800) 336-4797
P.O. Box 1133
Washington, DC 20013-1133

People's Medical Society
(610) 770-1670
P.O. Box 868
Allentown, PA 18105-0868

TEST YOUR KNOWLEDGE ANSWERS

1. False. More than 26 percent of Americans say they have used one or more questionable methods of health care to treat medical problems.
2. False. A national survey found that 60 percent of physicians had at some time referred patients to practitioners of alternative medicine.
3. True. Childbirth by cesarean section, gallbladder removal, and hysterectomy are the three most commonly performed surgeries in hospitals.
4. False. The program for uninsured or underinsured citizens is known as Medicaid. Medicare is designed to aid persons over age 65 and with certain disabilities.
5. True. Some generic drugs, however, are absorbed at a different pace due to the presence of or absence of other ingredients, or, in the case of tablets, due to the shape or size of the tablet.

APPENDIX

Your Sexual Body: A Primer on Reproductive Anatomy and Physiology

Maintaining a healthy life involves making many decisions that relate to diet, exercise, sleep, smoking, and other health-enhancing and health-compromising behaviors. Such health-related decisions generally do not require a full understanding of human anatomy and physiology. For example, you do not need to know the cell structure of skin to know that ultraviolet rays from the sun can cause damage and may result in cancer.

Decisions related to sex and sexuality, however, do require an understanding of human anatomy and physiology. When you want to avoid pregnancy or sexually transmitted infections, it pays to understand the reproductive system. Likewise, when you want to have a baby, it is important to know the mechanics of the reproductive system in order to improve your chances of becoming pregnant.

This special primer examines sex and sexuality from an anatomical and physiological perspective so you can better understand the biological functions of the male and female reproductive systems. The reproductive system is a collective term for the tissue and organs responsible for the production of egg or sperm cells and the secretion of sex hormones. The structures of the reproductive systems of the male and female are also designed to facilitate fertilization of an egg and gestation and delivery of a baby.

In this primer, male reproductive anatomy and physiology are described first, then female anatomy and physiology, followed by a brief introduction to the menstrual cycle.

Male Reproductive Anatomy and Physiology

One of the primary male reproductive functions is to produce sex cells called sperm. Sperm are only visible through a microscope yet contain the genetic information necessary for reproduction. The male reproductive system is designed to facilitate the movement of sperm from the sites of production (the testicles) and storage (the epididymis and vas deferens) into the vagina of a female to allow possible union of sperm and egg. Sperm are deposited through a process called ejaculation, the expulsion of the semen, including sperm, that usually takes place at the peak of sexual excitement, or orgasm. Semen is a whitish fluid containing a variety of substances, mostly water and bicarbonate buffers, that assure the viability of sperm.

A second function of the male reproductive system is to produce androgens, a family of masculinizing hormones. Androgens account for the development of primary male characteristics, including the sex organs, as well as secondary sex characteristics, such as facial hair, deep voice, and muscular build. Testosterone is the major androgen produced by the male reproductive system.

A third male reproductive function relates to sexual response. The external surfaces of the male genitalia have nerve endings responsive to touch and are thus important during sexual interaction. The external organs of the male include the scrotum and the penis. The internal organs include the testes, epididymis, vas deferens, seminal vesicle, prostate gland, and Cowper's gland.

External Organs of the Male Reproductive System

The scrotum is a muscular sac located between the penis and the rectum (see Figure 1). It forms a pouch for holding the testicles. The word scrotum comes from the Latin word meaning "bag," which is an appropriate description of this organ. The testicles are oval-shaped organs and reside inside the scrotum. Sperm are produced in the testicles at a temperature that is three to five degrees below normal body temperature. The muscle of the scrotum, the cremaster muscle, serves as a temperature regulator, and plays a critical role in fertility. When the temperature of the testicles is perceived to be too high, the muscle relaxes, allowing the testicles to hang away from the body, thus lowering their temperature. When the temperature of the testicles is perceived to be too low, the muscle contracts, pulling the testicles up close to the body to provide warmth. It is not uncommon for fertility problems to arise from factors such as tight-fitting underwear, excessive time spent in hot tubs, or continual long-distance driving. In each case, the work of the scrotum is compromised, leading to reduced sperm production. The cremaster muscle may also respond to emotional stress. Thus, some fertility problems may result from continuous contraction of the cremaster muscle due to stress and tension.

The male organ responsible for the transportation of sperm to a female is the penis. The size of the penis varies from man to man and also varies during the stages of sexual excitement. The size of a penis is not associated with virility or fertility.

The penis is an extremely sensitive and responsive organ that becomes hard and erect during sexual excitement. This process is called erection and is necessary for insertion of the penis into a woman's vagina in order to deposit sperm. In an unexcited state, the penis is a limp, tubular organ. In an excited state, the penis is firm, elongated, and capable of penetrating the vagina. The penis is made up of three cylinders of tissue that, upon sexual excitement, fill with blood, making the penis erect. After excitement subsides, each cylinder of tissue releases the blood, and the penis returns to a normal, flaccid state. Running through the penis is the urethra, the outlet of the bladder allowing elimination of urine. Actually, the release of semen and the release of urine take place through the same opening of the penis.

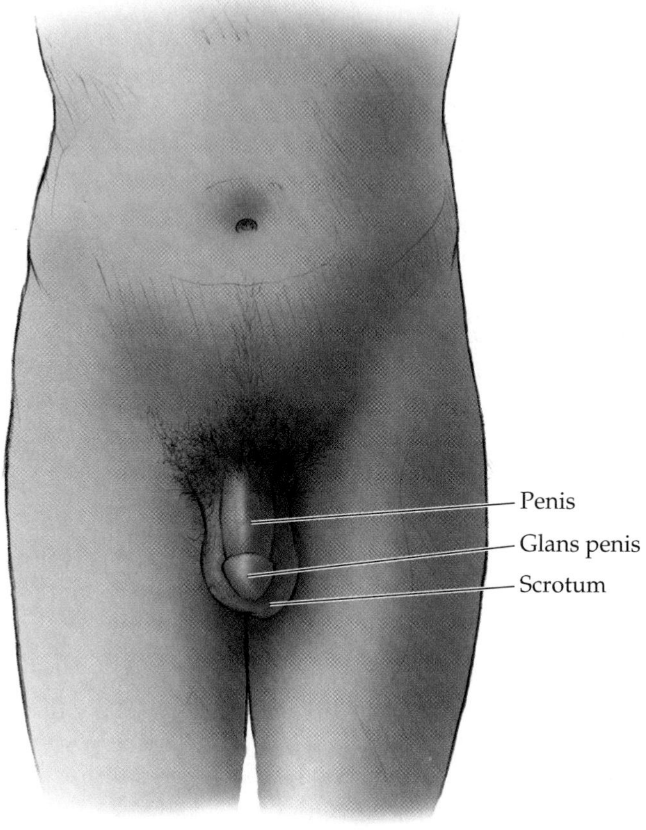

Figure 1 **External Male Reproductive Anatomy**

At the tip of the penis is the head, or glans penis, a highly sensitive area particularly responsive to tactile stimulation. The head is covered with a prepuce, a layer of tissue that is sometimes removed in a surgical procedure called circumcision. The prepuce is also called the foreskin. Some evidence suggests that circumcision may be an effective means of promoting good hygiene and avoiding not only infection but also perhaps some cancers. This surgical procedure is also done for religious reasons. In total, approximately 65 percent of U.S. males are circumcised.

Internal Organs of the Male Reproductive System

The organs of a man's body responsible for the production of both sperm and male hormones are the testes. During fetal development, the testes usually descend through the inguinal canal and into the scrotum, where they will reside. This migration of the testes from within the abdominal cavity to a location outside the abdominal cavity is necessary to produce the lower

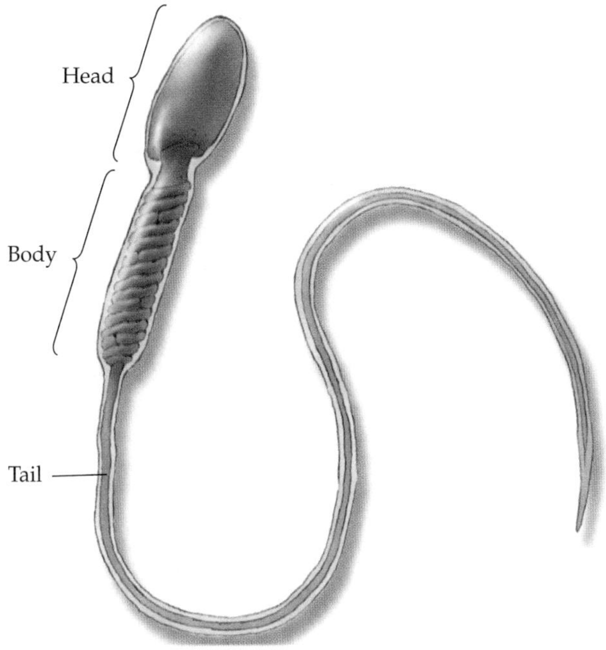

Figure 2 **A Single Sperm**

form sperm. The process of sperm production takes approximately seventy days and continues nonstop from puberty through adulthood.

A normal sperm is microscopic and shaped like a tadpole (see Figure 2). The head contains the genetic material necessary for union with an egg, while the tail is responsible for moving the sperm once it is deposited at the cervical opening to the uterus of a woman. Covering the head are enzymes necessary to penetrate the wall of an egg cell should the sperm come in contact with one.

Sperm produced in the seminiferous tubules migrate to the epididymis, where they reside for two to four weeks before reaching maturity. The epididymis is a coiled organ that functions to transport sperm from the testicle to the vas deferens for eventual ejaculation (see Figure 3). In the epididymis sperm are surrounded by a nourishing fluid that contains proteins necessary for sperm mobility. The time spent in the epididymis is critical to fertility because immature sperm, or sperm that have not been exposed to proteins necessary for the activity of the tail, do not function effectively once deposited into the vagina of a female, and therefore may not be able to find the egg cell.

temperature needed for the production of viable sperm. Failure of testicles to descend is called cryptorchidism. The problem of undescended testicles usually corrects itself during the first few months of a baby's life. It may also be corrected surgically later.

Inside each oval-shaped testicle are numerous seminiferous tubules. This is where sperm develop. Surrounding the seminiferous tubules are the interstitial cells, the site of hormone production. Although the interstitial cells are not the only place where male sex hormones are produced, they are by far the most important source of these hormones, particularly testosterone.

Through the process of meiosis, or reduction division, the cells lining the interior walls of the seminiferous tubules divide and develop into immature spermatids that will eventually break away to

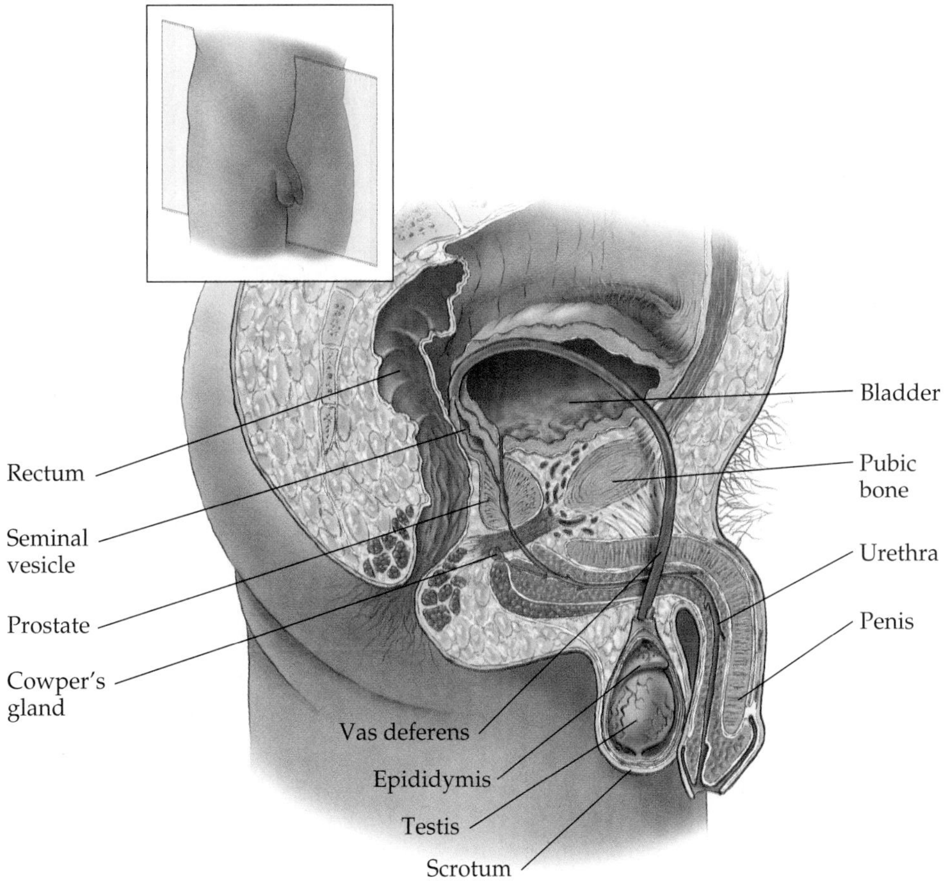

Figure 3 **Internal Male Reproductive Anatomy**

The tube that connects the epididymis to the penis is the vas deferens, which is sometimes called the ejaculatory duct (see Figure 4). This tube is lined with smooth muscle. During ejaculation, the muscle contracts rapidly, moving semen and sperm through and out of the penis. Semen is the fluid that carries sperm during ejaculation. Between 200 million and 400 million sperm are contained in the semen of each ejaculation. Semen is produced in a variety of locations, including the epididymis, the seminal vesicle, and the prostate gland. The seminal vesicle produces about 60 percent of semen. This secretory gland was once thought to be the storage site of sperm, thus the name seminal vesicle, but it is now known as its source. The seminal vesicle secretes water, fructose sugar to be used for energy by the sperm, and coagulators to assure the thickening of semen once it is deposited into the vagina. Thick semen allows sperm to maintain contact with the opening to the uterus from the vagina, thus increasing the chances of successful union of sperm and egg.

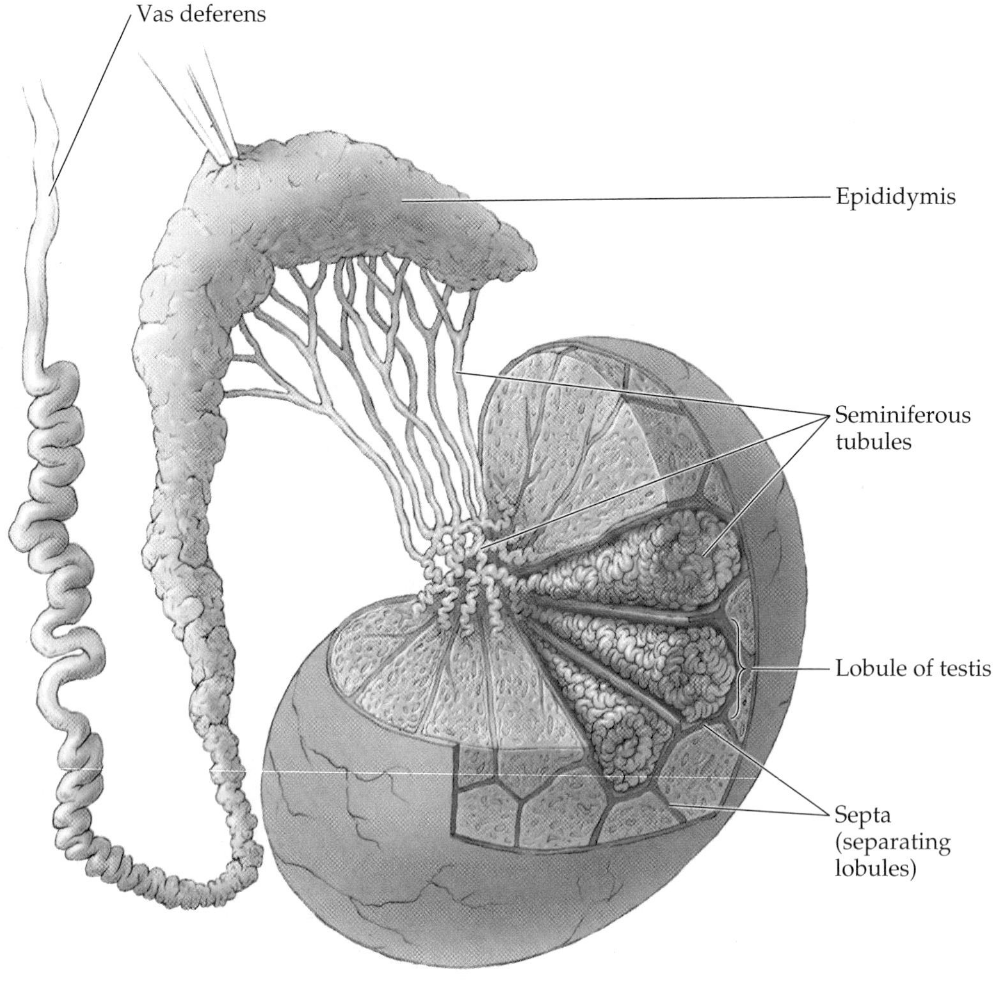

Figure 4 Cross-Section of the Testicle

The vas deferens passes through the prostate gland, where approximately 20 percent of semen is produced. The prostate gland contributes bicarbonate buffers necessary for maintaining a basic environment needed for sperm viability, and more coagulators. Located near the shaft of the penis are the Cowper's glands, two small, pea-like glands that secrete bicarbonate buffers and mucus for lubrication. Secretions from the Cowper's glands occur early in sexual excitement. They counter the acid environment of the pineal portion of the urethra, thus preparing it for ejaculation.

Female Reproductive Anatomy and Physiology

The female reproductive system is designed to carry out several functions, including the production of egg cells and hormones, and the gestation and delivery of a baby.

The primary reproductive function of the ovaries is to produce egg cells, called ova. One ovum (or sometimes two or more) is produced in the ovary approximately every month of a woman's fertile period, which lasts from the onset of menstruation until menopause. The egg is produced in response to hormonal signals, which arise from the ovary and from the pituitary gland in the brain. The production of the hormones estrogen and progesterone is another important function of the ovaries. These hormones account for many female characteristics and contribute to the success of pregnancy.

The structure of the female provides for reception of sperm.

The vagina is a tubular opening leading to the cervix, where sperm must be deposited if pregnancy is to occur. The fallopian tubes provide a place for fertilization and the uterus provides a location for fetal development as well as the musculature necessary to expel a full-term baby. Like the male, the female genitalia play a primary role in sexual responsiveness.

The external organs of the female include the mons veneris, labia majora, labia minora, clitoris, and breasts. The internal organs include the ovaries, fallopian tubes, uterus, cervix, and vagina.

External Organs of the Female Reproductive System

Collectively, most of the external reproductive organs of the female are referred to as the vulva. The vulva includes the mons veneris, labia, clitoris, and hymen (see Figure 5). The breasts, although not a part of the vulva, are also considered external reproductive organs.

The labia majora are the large outer folds of tissue extending from the mons veneris and surrounding the opening of the vagina and urethra. The external sides of these folds of tissue are covered with hair and are pigmented. The internal sides of the folds are smooth and contain numerous sweat glands. During sexual arousal, blood flowing into the pelvic area causes the labia majora to swell in size and separate to some degree. Sweat glands serve to lubricate the area, thus facilitating sexual intercourse.

Inside the labia majora (or outer lips) are the labia minora (or inner lips). The labia minora are a smaller, thinner set of skin folds that also respond to sexual stimulation, secrete lubrication, and become engorged with blood during sexual excitement.

At the point where the folds of the labia minora join, a hood is formed that covers the clitoris, a sensitive organ that is responsive to tactile stimulation. The clitoris apparently has no function other than female sexual gratification. It is composed of erectile tissue and upon sexual excitement becomes engorged with blood. The head of the clitoris, the glans clitoris, is a highly sensitive part of the organ.

In some women, the entrance to the vagina is covered with a partial covering called the hymen. This tissue serves no apparent function, but has become the focus of many myths, particularly those related to virginity. Because the structure of the hymen varies widely, it is not a means of determining whether a woman has had sexual intercourse.

Although not part of the genitalia, the breasts are considered a part of female external sexual anatomy (see Figure 6). The breasts are modified sweat glands that develop during puberty. They are composed of fat cells, glandular tissue, and some fibrous tissue. Combined, these tissues perform an important function—nourishing the newborn. The breasts are mammary, or milk-producing, glands and supply infants with all of their nutritional needs.

The size and shape of breasts vary widely. Breast size is not related to fertility or the ability to breast-feed. The breasts function sexually in two ways. Some women find pleasure from the stimulation of the breasts, particularly the nipple and the areola, the pigmented area surrounding the nipple. Because the nipple is erectile tissue, upon sexual excitement, it engorges with blood and becomes erect.

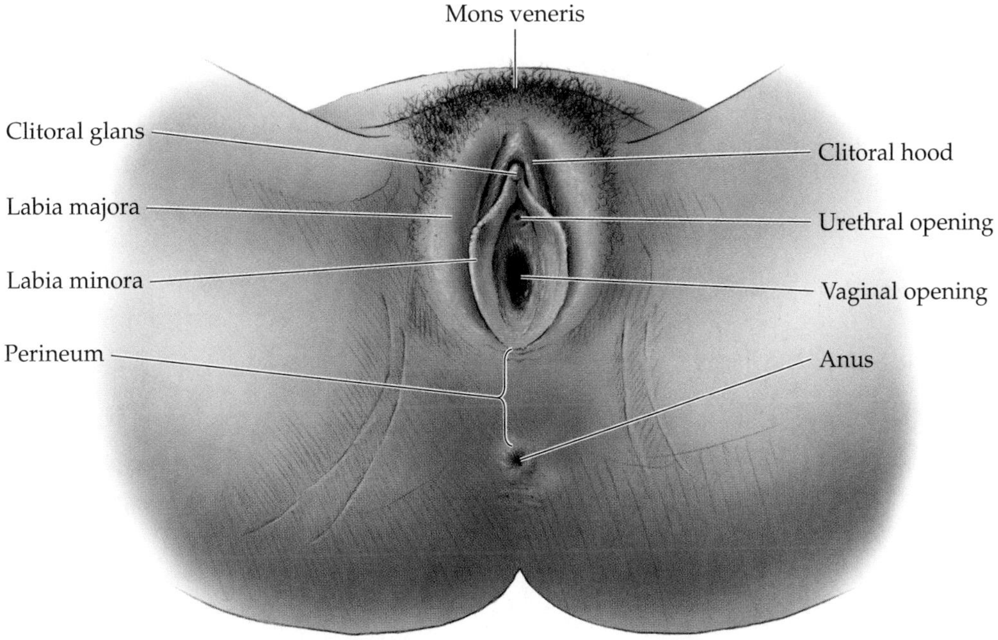

Figure 5 **External Female Reproductive Anatomy**

Internal Organs of the Female Reproductive System

The ovary is the primary sex gland that produces eggs and sex hormones including estrogen, progesterone, and androgens (see

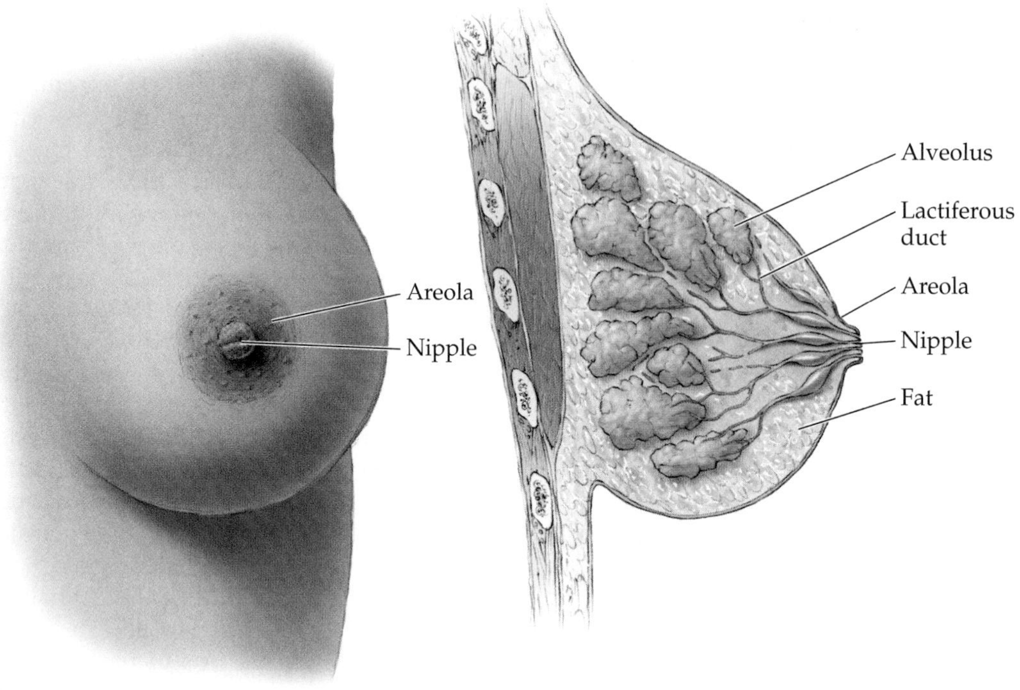

Figure 6 **Frontal View and Cross-Section of the Female Breast**

Figure 7). At birth, a baby girl possesses all of her potential egg cells, which are called follicles. These cells, however, remain in an immature state until they receive hormonal signals from the blood, causing the follicles to begin the maturation process. Many follicles will begin the maturation process each month, but only one (or on rare occasions two or more) will become a fully mature egg and be released into the abdominal cavity to begin its migration to join the sperm. The release of an egg from an ovary is called ovulation.

The fallopian tubes are small tubes extending from the uterus into the abdominal cavity. Named for Gabriele Fallopius, the tubes provide passageways for an egg to move from the abdominal cavity to the uterus. Finger-like structures called fimbriae fan out from one end of each fallopian tube in search of a released egg. The released egg is then carried down

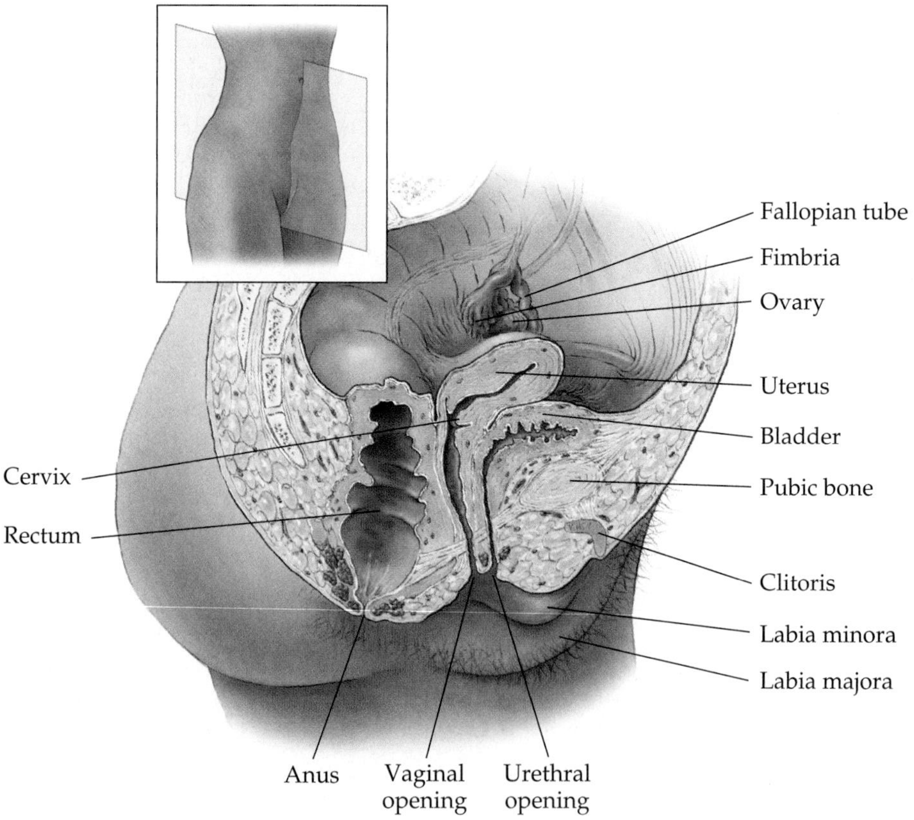

Figure 7 **Internal Female Reproductive Anatomy**

the fallopian tube where fertilization can take place with the sperm that have found their way through the uterus and up the other end of the fallopian tube. The union of sperm and egg takes place in the tube, but implantation and growth of the embryo occurs in the uterus.

The uterus, also called the womb, is a muscular organ shaped like a pear. It is composed of three layers. The perimetrium is the outer thin layer of connective tissue that contains the uterus. The myometrium is a thick middle layer of smooth muscle tissue. This layer is important in that it becomes the muscle that expels a baby at the time of birth. It also provides assistance with menstrual flow by contracting (sometimes cramping). The inner layer, the endometrium, is the mucus membrane where the fertilized egg implants and grows. It provides the nourishment and environment for fetal development.

At the opening of the uterus is the cervix. The actual opening is called the cervical os. It is filled with a plug of mucus that changes characteristics according to the hormonal signals of the body. Sometimes this mucus plug is hostile to sperm. At other times, particularly around the time of ovulation, it is not hostile and in fact serves to aid in the transport of sperm into the uterus and eventually up the fallopian tube.

The vagina is a thin-walled muscular tube that receives the penis during sexual intercourse. This passageway expands at the time of birth to allow movement of a baby from the uterus out of the body.

The Menstrual Cycle

The process of preparing the female body for pregnancy occurs in a cyclic manner beginning at menarche, the first sign of menstrual flow, and ending with menopause, when fertility and regular menstruation cease. Approximately every month, in response to hormonal signals, the uterus develops the capability of supporting a pregnancy. If pregnancy occurs, the uterus provides a location for fetal development over a nine-month period of gestation. If pregnancy does not occur, the uterus discharges the tissue and fluid built up in preparation for sustaining a pregnancy and begins the process of preparing for a possible pregnancy again. This discharge of tissue and fluid is called menstruation.

Although the average menstrual monthly cycle is around twenty-eight days, it varies greatly from woman to woman. It is just as common for a woman to have a twenty-three-, twenty-five-, or twenty-six-day cycle, as it is for a woman to have a thirty-two- or thirty-three-day cycle. Some women seldom have what are considered regular periods beginning at a predictable time. Irregular periods, in which menstrual flow begins at an unpredictable time, are seldom a health problem. Due to the difficulty of predicting the time of ovulation, however, this could become a fertility problem for women attempting to get pregnant—and it can also be a problem for those attempting to avoid pregnancy. Keeping a calendar record of the day when menstrual flow begins is an important health practice for women to follow. This record provides critical information and should be shared with a physician during a woman's annual gynecologic examination.

The easiest way to understand the menstrual cycle is to number the days from the beginning of menstrual flow (day one). Given a twenty-eight-day cycle, several phases can be identified. The first five to seven days are considered the menstrual phase. It is the time of menstrual flow. During this phase, the tissue and fluid from the last month's preparation for pregnancy are sloughed off and passed out of the body. It is also during this phase that the process of developing a new group of follicles for potential ovulation begins. Menstruation is triggered by a drop in the level of both estrogen and progesterone (see Figure 8).

After menstrual flow is well under way, follicle stimulating hormone (FSH) is secreted into the blood by the pituitary gland, thus stimulating the ovary to begin the process of preparing egg cells for possible ovulation. This follicular growth takes several days and occurs somewhere between days six and thirteen in the menstrual cycle. It is influenced by the presence of estrogen levels that rise in response to FSH. This phase of the menstrual cycle is referred to as the follicular phase. The end of the follicular phase is signaled by a sharp rise of another pituitary hormone, luteinizing hormone (LH). The rise in the concentration of LH, sometimes called a spike, causes one (and sometimes more) of the follicles to burst and release its contents, including one egg cell, into the abdominal cavity. The release of the egg from the ovary is called ovulation. In theory, the ovulated egg floats freely in the abdominal cavity. Actually, the finger-like structures at the end of the fallopian tube quickly locate the egg cell and start it on a path down the fallopian tube toward the uterus. It is at this time (around mid-cycle, or day fourteen) that a woman who has sexual intercourse is most apt to become pregnant.

After ovulation, the level of luteinizing hormone remains higher than at other times during the cycle. This causes the tissue that was once the follicle containing an egg cell to alter slightly and to begin secreting higher levels of progesterone. This altered secretory tissue is called the corpus luteum, a term meaning yellow body. The hormone progesterone is critical to the maintenance of pregnancy, and in fact the name progesterone means "for pregnancy." The level of progesterone remains high for several days following ovulation. This phase of the menstrual cycle is called the luteal phase because it is dominated by luteinizing hormone. The luteal phase

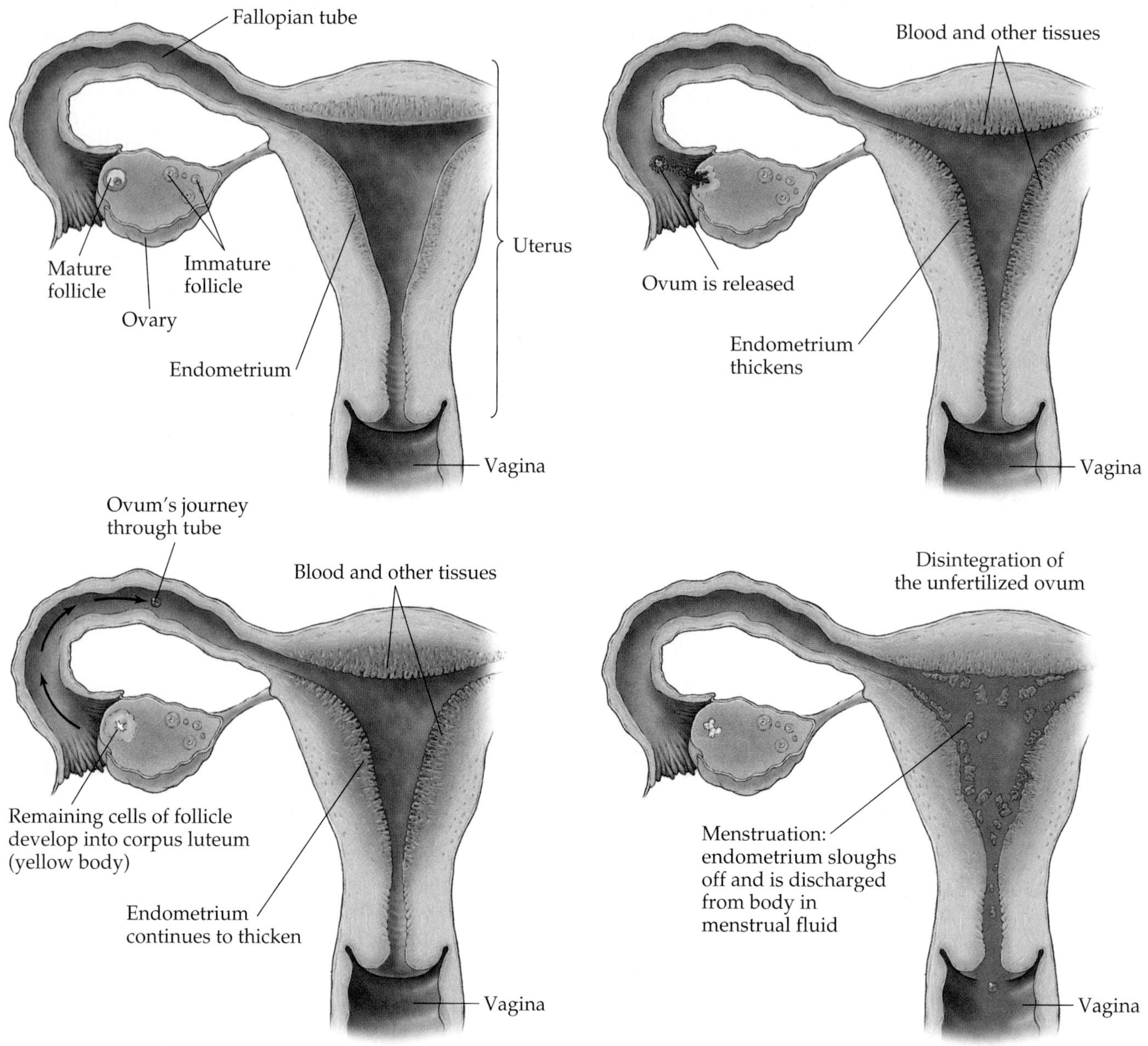

Figure 8 The Menstrual Cycle

usually lasts about fourteen days, even in women who have irregular periods. If pregnancy occurs, signals from the embryonic tissue maintain the level of progesterone and thus delay the onset of menstruation in favor of fetal development. If pregnancy does not occur, however, the level of luteinizing hormone drops, leading to a drop in the level of progesterone, bringing about a breakdown of the endometrium of the uterus. The luteal phase ends with the beginning of menstruation, day one of the next cycle.

TEST YOURSELF

Use the following terms to fill in the blanks below.

breasts	follicular phase	ovulation
cervical os	implantation	testosterone
Cowper's gland	labia majora	seminal vesicle
cremaster muscle	ejaculation	luteal phase
epididymis	menstruation	uterus
erection	semen	vas deferens
fallopian tube	myometrium	

1. _______ is the expulsion of semen, including sperm, that usually takes place at a peak of sexual excitement.
2. ________ is a whitish fluid containing a variety of substances, mostly water and bicarbonate buffers, that assure the viability of sperm.
3. A powerful masculinizing hormone produced in the testicles is _______.
4. As the penis engorges with blood, it becomes hard and erect, a process known as _______.
5. The _______ serves as a temperature regulator for the testicle, a critical role in fertility.
6. The _______ is a coiled organ that functions to move sperm from the testicle to the vas deferens and provides proteins that affect sperm motility.
7. Another name for the ejaculatory duct is the _______.
8. Once thought to be a storage place for sperm, the _______ is actually a secretory gland that produces a portion of the semen.
9. The _______ secretes a substance that prepares the penis for the passage of sperm.
10. The _______ are the large outer folds of tissue extending from the mons pubis and surrounding the opening of the vagina and urethra.
11. Modified sweat glands that develop from puberty into adolescence and eventually may provide nourishment for infants are _______.
12. Fertilization normally occurs in the _______.
13. _______ refers to the release of the egg from the ovary.
14. The muscular layer of the uterus that may cramp during menstruation is the _______.
15. Normally filled with mucus, the _______ provides a passageway for sperm to reach the uterus and eventually the fallopian tubes.
16. Also called the womb, the _______ is a muscular organ shaped like a pear.
17. The sloughing of built-up uterine tissue is ________.
18. The second phase of the menstrual cycle during which estrogen is the dominant hormone is the _______.
19. The final phase of the menstrual cycle during which progesterone is the dominant hormone is the _______.
20. _______ is the burrowing of the embryonic tissue into the wall of the uterus.

Glossary

abortion The termination of pregnancy.

absolute strength The total force that an individual can exert when flexing muscles; usually measured in pounds.

abstinence Deliberately refraining from doing something, e.g., not consuming alcoholic beverages in any form, not having sex before marriage.

acceptable risk A circumstance in which the benefits outweigh the risks; when the likelihood of ill effects is very small.

acceptance The stage of dying in which the person understands that death is inevitable.

acid rain Precipitation having a higher than normal level of acid due to the combination of sulfur oxides and moisture in the air.

acquired immune deficiency syndrome (AIDS) A combination of symptoms caused by the human immunodeficiency virus (HIV).

active immunity The body's development of its own resistance to disease.

acute stage The stage at which symptoms of a disease are fully developed.

addiction Physical or psychological dependence on a drug, often involving tolerance and withdrawal.

adiposity A surplus of body fat.

adrenaline A hormone that speeds up heartbeat and other responses to alarm; also called epinephrine

aerobic To be "with oxygen"; a process of energy production through which carbohydrates, fats, and proteins are used to produce energy and carbon dioxide and water are given off as by-products.

aerobic capacity The largest volume of oxygen that your body can consume in one minute; also called maximal oxygen uptake, or VO_2 max.

affective disorder A condition in which moods or emotions become extreme and interfere with daily life.

air pollution The contamination of air by waste products.

alarm reaction The first stage of the general adaptation syndrome; the body mobilizes its forces to meet a threatening situation.

alcohol addiction Extensive dependence on alcohol; this dependence is so acute that the acquisition and use of alcohol becomes the focus of everyday life.

alcoholic Someone who suffers from alcoholism and who has lost control over his or her drinking.

Alcoholics Anonymous A membership organization of recovering alcoholics who provide social support for avoiding the use of alcohol.

alcoholism A progressive disease related to the uncontrolled use of alcohol that interferes with the drinker's health and social functioning.

allergen A substance that is perceived by the body as an irritant and induces an allergic reaction or hypersensitive state.

alpha-fetoprotein A substance produced by fetal kidneys; high levels could indicate a neural tube defect.

alveoli The balloon-like air sacs at the end of the bronchioles of the lung.

Alzheimer's disease A degenerative disorder that causes dementia in middle to late life.

amino acids A class of organic compounds that are the building blocks of proteins.

amnesia Partial or total loss of memory.

amniocentesis Means of testing amniotic fluid to indicate the presence or absence of certain genetic conditions, such as Down syndrome, in a fetus.

amniotic fluid The fluid in the amniotic sac surrounding the fetus during pregnancy.

anabolic steroid A drug that promotes tissue growth and leads to increased muscle mass and improved strength and power.

anaerobic To be "without oxygen"; the process of energy production in which surges of energy are needed for a brief amount of time.

anger The stage of dying in which the person is angry at almost everything.

angina Chest pain resulting from a lack of blood supply to the heart.

angina pectoris Chest pain; a symptom of a condition in which the heart does not get as much blood as it needs.

anorexia nervosa An eating disorder characterized by starvation behavior brought on by a preoccupation with thinness.

antibiotic A chemical substance that destroys or inhibits the growth of bacteria.

antibodies Specific proteins that are produced principally in the blood in response to foreign substances in the body.

antigens Foreign substances in the body that cause the production of antibodies.

antioxidant A substance that inhibits oxidation; in nutrition, a substance that interferes with LDL cholesterol lipoprotein oxidation.

anxiety A state of apprehension or tension, often accompanied by physiological signs.

arrhythmia An erratic heartbeat.

artificial insemination Introduction of semen into the vagina by artificial means.

assisted reproductive technology (ART) Any procedure in which both eggs and sperm are handled outside the body.

asthma A chronic lung disease characterized by wheezing, shortness of breath, chest tightness, and coughing.

asymptomatic carrier A person who has a disease but no symptoms.

asymptomatic period A period in which a disease exists without outward signs or clinical symptoms.

atherosclerosis Damage to the circulatory system brought about by a buildup of plaque on the inner walls of arteries; sometimes called hardening of the arteries.

auscultation Listening to the sounds made by various body structures.

autopsy An examination and dissection of a dead body to discover the cause of death; usually conducted by a coroner.

bacteria Single-celled microbes that act to produce symptoms of infection.

bacterial pneumonia The main type of pneumonia that follows an attack of influenza.

balanced diet An eating pattern that includes a variety of foods in amounts that result in health enhancement.

bargaining The stage of dying in which the person bargains for more time.

barrier methods Methods of contraception that physically separate the sperm from the egg; include condoms and diaphragms.

basal cell A small, round cell in the lower part (base) of the epidermis.

basal metabolic rate The speed with which the body expends calories on basic functions at a resting state.

behavior modification Therapy designed to change the learned behavior of an individual.

benign tumor A noncancerous tumor that is usually harmless and does not invade other cells or spread to other parts of the body.

benign Not harmful.

benzene A chemical that can cause leukemia in humans.

bereaved Survivors of a recently deceased person who experience a sense of loss and grief.

bereavement The period during which a sense of loss is felt owing to the death of a loved one.

binge drinking Having five drinks in a row for men or four in a row for women on at least one occasion in the past two weeks.

binge eating Eating excessively; consuming much more than the normal amount of food taken in at one sitting.

binge eating disorder An eating disorder characterized by periods of uncontrolled eating.

bioelectrical impedance A test that uses a weak electrical current to measure the body's fat content.

biopsy The removal of bits of living tissue and fluid from the body for diagnostic examination.

bipolar disorder A form of depression characterized by cycles of manic highs and depressive lows; also called manic-depressive illness.

birth control pill A pill, consisting of chemicals similar to hormones normally produced in a woman's body, that prevents pregnancy.

birth control Prevention of pregnancy for the purpose of family planning.

blackout A temporary form of amnesia in which the individual appears to be conscious of what he or she is doing but later cannot remember much, if any, of what happened.

blastocyst The multicellular descendant of the united sperm and egg that will later develop into the embryo then the fetus.

blood alcohol concentration (BAC) A measure of the amount of alcohol in the blood.

body mass index (BMI) A numerical representation of the relationship of height and weight; it correlates positively with measures of body composition such as underwater weighing and the pinch test.

booster A dose of an immunization or vaccination given to renew or maintain the effect of a previous dose.

bradycardia Abnormally slow beating of the heart.

brain dead A state that occurs when there is no longer brain activity.

breast self-examination (BSE) An examination done by a woman to herself to identify abnormal breast tissue; a screening exam for the presence of breast cancer.

breech presentation When the baby's feet or bottom are positioned first in the birth canal.

bulimia An eating disorder characterized by the extreme behavior of binge eating and vomiting.

calcium A mineral important for building strong bones and teeth in growing children and for helping maintain the bones of adults.

calorie A unit measuring the energy produced by food when oxidized in the body.

cannabis Marijuana, hashish, ganga; the dried flowering tops of the hemp plant, *Cannabis sativa.*

carbohydrates Nutrients made of sugars and starches; the body's primary source of energy.

carbon monoxide A colorless, odorless, poisonous gas that is produced by the incomplete burning of carbon in fuels.

carcinogen A cancer-causing agent or factor.

cardiopulmonary resuscitation (CPR) A combination of mouth-to-mouth breathing and chest compression used during cardiac arrest to keep blood flowing to the heart muscle and brain; an emergency procedure.

cardiovascular disease Disease of the heart and blood vessels.

casual drinker A person who drinks an alcoholic beverage every now and then but seldom consumes enough alcohol to become intoxicated.

cataracts Clouding of the lens of the eye.

cerebellum The portion of the brain that contributes to the control of movement.

cerebrum The part of the brain responsible for reasoning and inhibitions.

cervical cap A thimble-shaped contraceptive device that fits snugly onto the cervix.

cervix The opening of the uterus into the vagina.

cesarean section (C-section) Removal of the baby through an incision in the abdominal wall rather than through the birth canal.

chain of infection A metaphor for infectious disease transmission in which each link in the chain represents a single factor necessary for disease to spread.

chancre A painless, round sore with raised edges indicative of syphilis.

chlamydia A common bacterial STI, which, if untreated, can cause serious, painful infections of the urinary tract in men and infection of the reproductive organs in women.

chlorinated dioxins Hazardous waste emitted by the burning of plastics.

chlorofluorocarbons (CFCs) Compounds used as aerosol spray propellants and refrigerants that contribute to the depletion of the ozone layer.

cholesterol A white, crystalline substance found especially in animal fats, blood, nerve tissue, and bile; in excessive amounts, a factor in atherosclerosis.

chorionic villus sampling (CVS) A technique in which the chorionic villi, hair-like projections on a membrane surrounding the interior of the uterus, are tested to determine the presence or absence of certain genetic conditions.

chronic bronchitis A condition in which the bronchial tubes become inflamed as a result of irritation.

chronic fatigue syndrome A group of symptoms that result in a prolonged state of fatigue.

chronic illness An illness marked by gradual onset, long duration, or frequent recurrence.

chronological age A number representing the number of years a person has lived since birth.

cirrhosis of the liver A disease in which scar tissue replaces normal liver tissue and interferes with the liver's ability to function.

club drug A term that refers to a wide variety of dangerous drugs used often in combination with alcohol at all-night dance parties known as *raves,* at dance clubs, and at bars. An example is ecstasy.

cochlea The inner ear.

cohabitation A living arrangement in which two individuals live together in a sexual relationship without being married.

colon cancer Cancer of the large bowel.

colonoscopy A screening procedure in which a physician uses a hollow lighted tube to inspect the entire bowel and some portions of the small intestines.

columbarium A special vault for urns containing ashes of cremated bodies.

complementary and alternative medicine Interventions that are not part of conventional or mainstream medicine as taught in most U.S. medical schools and available in U.S. hospitals.

complementary protein relationship The idea that two foods, neither of which when taken alone would provide a complete protein, can be combined at a meal to provide in a complete protein.

complete protein A protein containing all nine essential amino acids.

complex carbohydrate A basic nutritional component made of long chains of simple sugars that are slowly broken down in the body.

conception The union of sperm and egg.

conditioning period The period of exercise during which a training effect is reached and maintained.

contraception The intentional prevention of conception.

contraimplantation Preventing implantation of the fertilized egg.

controlled substance A chemical that has been identified through legal review as a threat to an individual and/or to society.

convalescence A state characterized by a decline in the severity of disease symptoms.

conventional medicine Standard Western medicine based on the rigorous application of the scientific method and the belief that diseases are caused by identifiable physical factors with definable symptoms.

cool-down period The period of exercise in which the intensity of exercise is reduced to allow the body to recover partially from the conditioning period.

coping Adaptation to stress.

coping skills Strategies used to deal constructively with stressors.

coronary angioplasty A surgical procedure to widen the coronary artery with an inflated balloon catheter.

coronary artery bypass A surgical procedure to reroute blood flow from the blocked part of an artery by using a length of vein taken from another part of the body.

cremation The burning of a dead body into ashes.

crowning The point of labor at which the cervix is completely effaced and dilated to ten centimeters and the baby's head can be seen.

cutaneous anthrax A form of anthrax that results when spores penetrate the skin, usually through of a cut in the skin.

defense mechanisms Coping strategies by which people defend themselves against negative emotions.

dehydration An abnormal loss of water.

delusion A false belief despite obvious truth to the contrary.

dementia A disorder characterized by the general and often slow decline of mental abilities.

denial The stage of dying in which the person does not believe that death is going to happen to him or her.

dental caries Tooth decay.

dental plaque Noncalcified accumulation of microorganisms that attach to the teeth.

dependence A condition in which a person is so physically and/or psychologically attached to a drug that he or she cannot live comfortably without it.

Depo-Provera An injectable method of birth control that lasts for approximately three months.

depressant A drug that slows down the body's functions and movements.

depression A mental disorder marked by sadness, anxiety, fatigue, underactivity, sleeplessness, and reduced ability to function and relate to others; the stage of dying in which anger is replaced with a sense of loss.

dermatitis A skin disorder in which an area of skin may become red, swollen, hot, and itchy.

designer drug A drug that looks like a drug already on the market but has something altered in its molecular structure so that it is a "new" drug. An example is ecstasy.

detection Medical procedures (tests) done on individuals suspected of having a disease, for the purpose of confirming the presence of the disease and, if present, determining the progress of the disease.

detoxification The process of removing all alcohol or drugs from an individual's body.

detoxification program A treatment program that involves a gradual but complete withdrawal from an abused drug.

diagnosis A physician's opinion of the nature or cause of a disease based on observation and laboratory tests.

diaphragm A soft rubber cup that covers the entrance to the uterus.

diastolic pressure The pressure measured in the arteries when the heart relaxes.

dilation Opening of the cervix either for examination or for delivery of a baby.

dilation and evacuation A method of a abortion performed in the second trimester of pregnancy in which the cervix is dilated and medical instruments are used to remove the contents of the uterus through a suction or vacuum procedure.

disordered thinking Disconnected or incoherent thought processes and speech.

distress The type of stress that brings about negative mental or physical responses; also known as bad stress.

diuretic A medication that promotes the excretion of excess body fluids and salt in the urine.

dosage A specified amount of something; in infectious diseases, the amount of pathogens present during disease transmission.

doula A person trained to assist during delivery by providing emotional and physical support; does not deliver the baby.

Down syndrome A birth defect in which the individual has extra genetic material (associated with the number 21 chromosome) that alters the course of development and causes specific physical and mental characteristics associated with the syndrome.

drug A chemical substance that causes a change in the body's functioning, including physiological and psychological activity.

drug abuse The intentional and chronic misuse of a chemical substance.

drug interaction The simultaneous presence of two or more drugs in the body, often having a detrimental effect.

drug misuse The use of a prescribed medication without consulting a physician.

drug use The use of a chemical substance for the purpose intended, to bring about a change in the way the body functions.

dual-career families Families in which both parents work full time.

durable power of attorney for health care A legal document that identifies a representative to speak for a person about his or her health care if the person is unable to do so.

dysfunction The inability to function properly.

dysorganization Pain or difficulty in the process of organization or living.

effacement The thinning of the cervix during the process of childbirth.

elective abortions Abortions that are medically induced.

electrocardiogram (ECG) A screening procedure used to detect heart disease; a graphic record of the heart's action obtained from an instrument that records heart activity.

electroencephalogram (EEG) A device that measures brain activity.

embalming The use of chemicals, internally and externally, to temporarily preserve the body for open-casket viewing and/or transportation.

emphysema A disease of the lungs, particularly of the small air sacs, in which the lungs lose their ability to expand as a result of an accumulation of fluid in the tissue.

empty calories Foods high in calories but with few nutrients; largely made up of sugar.

encephalitis Inflammation of the brain.

endorphin A hormone produced in the brain that helps give a sense of pleasure and satisfaction.

endurance The ability to exercise vigorously at a sustained level for a period of time.

episiotomy The small incision made between the opening of the vagina and the anus to ensure easier passage of the baby's head through the birth canal and to prevent tearing of the tissue.

eradication The removal of a disease by the elimination of all reservoirs of the disease-causing pathogen.

ethyl alcohol The ingredient in alcohol that causes addiction; also called ethanol.

eustress The type of stress that is a healthy part of daily living; it can result in the ability to relax and enjoy a feeling of peacefulness and calm.

euthanasia The hastening of a suffering person's death, also called mercy killing; illegal in the United States.

exercise Bodily movement undertaken to improve or maintain one or more of the components of physical fitness.

exercise duration The length of time a person exercises.

exercise frequency How often an exercise is done.

exercise intensity The degree of energy that is exerted during exercise.

exhaustion The final stage of the general adaptation syndrome; it occurs when the body does not have a chance to restore itself to a state of equilibrium.

extended family Family members connected by blood, marriage, or adoption.

fad diets Diets that are popular for brief periods of time then lose popularity. The loss of popularity usually results when the effectiveness of a fad diet is questioned.

fallopian tube A passageway (tube) that extends from the uterus into the abdominal cavity to a place near the ovary.

family planning A process of establishing the preferred number and spacing of children in one's family and choosing the means by which this is achieved.

fat-soluble vitamins Vitamins that are transported and stored by the body's fat cells; examples are vitamins A, D, E, and K.

female condom Lines the inside of the vagina and covers the cervix; acts to prevent pregnancy and sexually transmitted infections.

fetal alcohol syndrome (FAS) A constellation of birth defects caused by alcohol consumption during pregnancy that is characterized by mental retardation, poor motor coordination, hyperactivity in childhood, facial deformities, and other abnormalities.

fever Above-normal body temperature.

fiber A complex carbohydrate that is indigestible by humans.

fibrillation Irregular convulsive movement of the heart muscle.

fight-or-flight reaction The body's reaction to stress in which it becomes physically ready to resist or fight a stressor or to run from it.

flexibility The range of movement an individual can achieve around a joint or group of joints.

functional age A number representing the ability to function; a tool for comparing actual age with ability to function.

fungal pneumonia Inflammation of the lungs caused by a fungus.

fungi Single-celled or multicelled plant-like organisms that usually grow on the surface of the skin.

gastrointestinal anthrax A form of anthrax acquired by ingesting the spores while eating or drinking.

gatekeeper The physician in an HMO who refers a patient to specialists or other health services within the HMO.

gateway drugs Drugs such as tobacco, alcohol, and marijuana that most users of illicit drugs have tried before their first use of cocaine, heroin, or other illicit drugs.

general adaptation syndrome (GAS) The theory proposed by Hans Selye in which there are three distinct phases to the body's reaction to stress: alarm reaction, resistance, and exhaustion.

generic drugs Less expensive drugs that have the same active chemical ingredients as their brand-name counterparts.

gerontologists Specialists who study the social, biological, behavioral, and psychological aspects of aging.

gingivitis A condition in which the gums are red, tender, and swollen.

global warming The gradual rise in the average temperature of the earth.

gonorrhea A sexually transmitted infection caused by *Niserria gonorrhea,* a bacterium.

greenhouse effect The rise in temperature that the earth experiences because certain gases in the atmosphere (e.g., water vapor, carbon dioxide, nitrous oxide, and methane) trap energy from the sun.

grief A deep sadness caused by a loss.

hallucination The sensation of seeing or hearing things something that is not present.

hallucinogen A drug that causes a great change in perception.

hangover A condition caused by excess alcohol consumption and characterized by nausea, upset stomach, anxiety, and headache.

hazardous waste Waste that is flammable, explosive, corrosive, or toxic.

health attitude A behavioral intention concerning health, usually expressed in positive or negative terms.

health behavior Actions and habits that may lead either to enhancement and protection of a person's health status or to its decline.

health belief A health-related concept thought to be true whether supported by evidence or not.

health history A history of the patient's health as well as of the health of his or her family.

health knowledge The accumulation of factual information that influences health decision making.

health literacy The capacity of an individual to get, interpret, and understand basic health information and services and the competence to use such information and services in ways that are health enhancing.

health maintenance organizations (HMOs) Prepaid plans that offer a defined set of benefits according to a predetermined monthly premium.

health momentum A perception of movement toward or away from good health that results from decisions and health behaviors of the past.

health risk The likelihood of developing a certain disease or health condition.

health skills Abilities that influence health development, health status, and health maintenance.

health style The sum of health knowledge, health skills, and health behavior. Health style is most easily observed in personal health decisions.

health value Something of importance that is related to health.

heart attack (myocardial infarction) A condition that occurs when the blood supply to part of the heart muscle (the myocardium) is severely reduced or stopped. Normally circulating blood brings oxygen and other nutrients to the heart.

heart rate The number of heartbeats per minute.

heart transplant A surgical procedure in which a normally functioning heart from a person who has recently died is implanted into a person with a diseased heart.

helper T-cells White blood cells that are needed by the body's immune system to fight a variety of disease-causing organisms.

hemiplegia The loss of sensory and motor function on one side of the body.

hepatitis An inflammation of the liver, usually caused by a virus.

hepatitis A A form of hepatitis transmitted in human wastes and contaminated food and water.

hepatitis B A form of hepatitis transmitted by blood and sexual contact.

hepatitis C A form of hepatitis, previously known as non-A, non-B hepatitis, that resembles the other forms of hepatitis but cannot be classified as either.

herd immunity The vaccination of a large proportion of a population against a particular disease to significantly reduce the chances of spread of infection.

herpes simplex type 2 A virus usually transmitted by sexual contact and causing open sores on the genitals.

high density lipoproteins (HDLs) A fatty substance that is the type of cholesterol that is considered good and that prevents atherosclerosis.

hospice A specialized health care program, usually for the last weeks or months of life, emphasizing the management of pain and other symptoms associated with terminal illness, in contrast to treatment.

host susceptibility The ease with which a person is exposed to and becomes infected by a pathogen.

human chorionic gonadotropin (HCG) A hormone secreted from placental cells; a pregnancy test looks for the presence of this hormone.

human immunodeficiency virus (HIV) The virus that causes AIDS.

human papilloma virus (HPV) The agent responsible for an STI characterized by warts, usually on the genitalia; also called genital warts.

hydrocarbons A chemical compound made up of hydrogen and carbon; the major chemical ingredient of many fuels.

hypertension High blood pressure; generally means the heart is working harder than normal.

hypoglycemia Low blood sugar.

hypothermia A drop in body temperature to subnormal levels; can result in mental confusion, unconsciousness, and death.

hypothyroidism Not enough thyroid activity.

illicit Illegal.

illness behavior Action taken by a person who has reason to believe that he or she is not well.

immunity The body's ability to destroy pathogens that it has once encountered, before they are able to cause disease.

impact The stage of bereavement in which loved ones react with shock, disbelief, and denial.

in vitro fertilization A procedure in which the sperm and egg from a man and a woman are combined in a glass container, and a fertilized embryo is implanted into the woman.

inappropriate affect Showing emotions that are inconsistent with a person's thoughts.

incomplete protein A protein in which one or more of the essential amino acids is missing.

incontinent Unable to control bowel or bladder function.

incubation The stage during which there are no symptoms of disease and, in most cases, the infected person is not contagious.

indemnity (fee-for-service) plan Insurance coverage in which a person pays for most of his or her medical bills and then files a claim to be reimbursed.

indoor pollution The contamination of indoor air by waste products or natural pollutants.

induction The method of abortion in which labor is artificially induced.

infectious disease A disease caused by pathogens, such as bacteria or viruses, that spread from someone who is infected to someone who is not yet infected; also known as communicable or contagious disease.

infertility The inability of a couple to conceive after one year of intercourse without contraception.

inflammation The body's response to injury; it fights infection and promotes healing.

influenza A severe viral infection involving the respiratory tract; also called the flu.

inhalant A chemical that is inhaled through the nostrils to cause a quick rush to the brain; abused inhalants include airplane glue, paint thinner, and butyl nitrite.

inhalation anthrax A form of anthrax acquired through breathing in anthrax spores.

initiator A carcinogen that starts cell damage that leads to cancer.

inpatient care Health care provided in a hospital.

insulin A substance produced by the pancreas that helps move glucose from the blood into cells; without enough insulin, the body's cells do not function properly.

interferon A chemical substance produced by white blood cells that "interferes" with growth of a virus and also inhibits the virus's ability to infect cells; also made synthetically.

interpersonal skills The techniques involved in relating to other people.

intoxicated Having consumed enough alcohol to experience its effect, usually indicated by a high blood alcohol concentration, delayed muscle coordination, and impaired judgment.

intrauterine device (IUD) A small plastic birth control device that is inserted into the uterus by a physician.

ionizing radiation Radiation such as ultraviolet radiation, x-rays, and gamma rays, which is capable of breaking chemical bonds.

isokinetic exercise An exercise in which there are slow-moving contractions throughout a full range of movement against a constant resistance.

isometric exercise An exercise involving the contraction of muscles performed against an immovable object.

isotonic exercise An exercise involving the contraction of muscles against a movable resistance.

Kaposi's sarcoma A rare, deadly cancer characterized by reddish-purple blotches on the skin; one of the symptoms of AIDS.

keratosis A rough patch or horny growth of the skin.

ketosis An accumulation of chemical compounds called ketones in the blood.

labor The process of childbirth from the initial contractions of the uterus to the delivery of the baby and the placenta.

laboratory tests Procedures that involve the examination of blood, tissue, and other biologic materials for the diagnosis, prevention, or treatment of disease.

lactate A substance formed in the blood when muscles contract.

lactovegetarians Vegetarians whose diet includes dairy products but no other animal products.

landfills An area where trash and other wastes are deposited and covered with soil.

late syphilis A disease characterized by generalized infection that can produce heart failure, blindness, loss of muscle control, brain damage, and death; also called tertiary syphilis.

lead A metal found in exhausts, emissions, and paint.

lesions A localized change in tissue, or sores.

leukoplakia White patches on the oral mucosa that can become malignant.

living-dying interval The time between the diagnosis of a terminal condition and death.

living will A legal document that stipulates which medical treatments are and are not to be used in the final days of life.

low birthweight babies Babies born weighing less than 2,500 grams, or five pounds eight ounces.

low density lipoproteins (LDLs) A fatty substance that is the type of cholesterol that is considered bad and that promotes atherosclerosis.

lumpectomy The surgical removal of only the cancerous lump from the breast.

main effect The desired (intended) physical or mental response of the body to a drug; sometimes called the primary effect.

maintenance program A treatment program that involves providing a less dangerous drug to prevent withdrawal symptoms.

major depression Depression that is extreme, more intense, and longer lasting and that usually interferes with daily life; often characterized as a mood or affective disorder.

male condom A thin rubber sheath for the penis that collects semen ejaculated during sexual intercourse; acts to prevent pregnancy and sexually transmitted infections.

malignant tumor A cancerous tumor that spreads to nearby tissues and organs, crowding out healthy cells and replacing them with cancer cells.

mammography A screening technique used to detect breast cancer.

maximal heart rate The maximum number of heartbeats per minute that should be reached during exercise; usually equal to 220 minus the person's age.

Medicaid A federal-state program that provides health care coverage to eligible low-income persons; eligibility can vary by state.

medical assessment An evaluation conducted by a medical professional that focuses on identification of the presence or absence of a disease.

Medicare A federal program that provides health care coverage to people age sixty-five and older and to some other eligible categories.

medulla The part of the brain that controls breathing.

melanin Brownish-black skin pigment.

melanoma A skin cancer that often starts as a mole-like growth and grows in size and changes color; the most serious of the various types of skin cancer.

meningitis An infectious disease of the fluids and membranes that surround the brain and spinal cord; it can be viral or bacterial.

mental health A state of emotional and social well-being; a state in which an individual is capable of healthy interaction with his or her environment and of enduring the hard times of life, with resilience.

mental illness A disorder or problem of the mind that prevents a person from being productive, adjusting to life, or getting along with other people.

metastasize To spread to other parts of the body through the bloodstream or lymph system.

minor depression An emotional state in which a person's normal feelings of sadness, guilt, and hopelessness are exaggerated.

miscarriage Spontaneous abortion.

MMR vaccine A vaccine that provides immunity to measles, mumps, and rubella.

modified radical mastectomy A selective removal of the breast and surrounding tissue.

mononucleosis A disease caused by the Epstein-Barr virus; symptoms include fever, headache, nausea, extreme fatigue, and swollen spleen and lymph nodes.

monounsaturated fat The type of fat that has one hydrogen available to bond and is liquid at room temperature; usually comes from plant or fish sources.

morning-after pill A form of hormonal contraception used within the first seventy-two hours after unprotected sexual intercourse; generally considered an emergency method of birth control that prevents implantation.

mourning Expressing grief at someone's death.

mucous membranes The moist, protective lining that covers most of the openings to the body and the air passages.

multiple hazards Simultaneous exposure to more than one health threat.

mutagen An agent that causes hereditary changes on the cellular level that may be passed from one generation to another.

mycoplasma A tiny microorganism and causative agent of many diseases of the joints and lungs.

myocardial infarction Damage of heart tissue caused by an interruption of blood supply to the heart that can result in death.

narcotic A drug that reduces pain and induces sleep.

natural childbirth Delivery of a baby "naturally," without the aid of drugs.

naturopath A general practitioner of complementary and alternative medicine; uses the natural healing forces within the body.

neurons The basic cells of the nervous system.

neurotransmitters Chemicals that facilitate the passage of impulses in the brain.

nicotine The ingredient in tobacco smoke that causes addiction.

nicotine addiction The state of being physically and emotionally dependent on nicotine.

nicotine replacement Therapy in which a person who smokes gets nicotine by means other than tobacco.

nitrogen oxides Poisonous gases that are produced when fuel is burned at very high temperatures.

noninfectious disease A disease caused by factors other than infectious microbial agents.

nonpoint source pollutant A source of pollution that enters a body of water as runoff or seepage.

non-REM sleep Sleep during which the eyes are relaxed and not moving; the period of sleep associated with cell regeneration.

nonspecific defense mechanisms The body's various barriers to most disease, as opposed to those defense mechanisms intended to prevent one particular disease.

noradrenaline A hormone that causes blood vessels to constrict and other responses to anger; also called norepinephrine

Norplant A long-lasting method of contraception that consists of hormone-releasing silicon capsules surgically inserted under the skin, usually in a woman's upper arm.

nuclear family The immediate family; parents and/or guardians and their children, usually living together.

nurse-midwife Registered nurse who has completed advanced training in gynecology and obstetrics.

nutrients The basic chemical compounds that make up food.

obesity An excessive amount of body fat relative to body weight.

opportunistic diseases Diseases common to individuals infected with HIV that under normal conditions would be defeated by the body's immune system.

osteoporosis A disorder in which bone density decreases, making the bones more likely to break.

outpatient care Care provided in a physician's or other health practitioner's office, in an emergency room in a hospital, or in a specialized ambulatory clinic; does not involve hospitalization or overnight stays.

overdose A serious reaction to an excessive amount of a drug; it can result in coma or death.

overmedication Consuming a higher drug dosage than prescribed, which can compromise accurate medical care.

over-the-counter drugs Drugs that can be purchased without a prescription.

overweight An excess of body weight relative to a specified standard for height and age.

ovolactovegetarians Vegetarians whose diet includes eggs as well as dairy products.

ovulation-inducing drugs Hormones that bring about ovulation.

ozone A poisonous form of oxygen that chemically reacts with a variety of substances.

ozone layer A region of the stratosphere, which filters out ultraviolet rays from the sun.

palpation Touching body parts with the hands.

Pap test A test for identifying cervical cancer that involves scraping and analyzing cells from the cervix.

parasitic worms Multicelled animals that release toxins inside the body, feed on blood, and compete with the host for food.

partial mastectomy The surgical removal of only the part of the breast containing the cancerous lump.

particulates Tiny pollutants in the air such as pieces of dust and soot and mold spores.

passive immunity Resistance to disease that initially comes from an external source.

passive smoking Inhaling tobacco smoke from the environment, as a result of someone else smoking.

pathogen A microorganism, such as a bacterium, virus, protozoan, parasitic worm, fungus, or rickettsia, that causes disease.

patient package insert An information sheet, required by the FDA that, among other things, warns the consumer of possible contraindications for use of a drug or medical product.

pelvic inflammatory disease (PID) An infection in the pelvic area usually involving the uterus, fallopian tubes, and/or ovaries; half the cases are caused by chlamydia.

perchloroethylene (PCE) A suspected carcinogen used in dry cleaning.

periodontal disease Gum disease.

periodontitis Degeneration of the gum tissue that holds the teeth in place; also called pyorrhea.

personality hardiness A state of resilience due to clear self-concept.

phagocytes White blood cells that attack and consume foreign cells.

phobia An unreasonable fear of some object or situation.

physical examination An examination by a physician that involves inspection, auscultation, and palpation of the body.

physical fitness How efficiently the body works as measured by strength, flexibility, and endurance.

physician-assisted suicide A death that occurs when a physician supplies the means, usually a prescription for a lethal dose of medication, which a competent, terminally ill individual can use to end his or her life; also called physician-hastened death.

pinch test A test that uses special skinfold calipers to pinch layers of fat at specific body sites; a measure of body fat.

placebo A look-alike pill that has not therapeutic value; used in controlled scientific experiments to test the efficacy of another substance.

placenta The structure that develops from the wall of the uterus and serves as an organ of interchange between the mother and the fetus.

plaque A buildup of cholesterol in the arteries, which over time can restrict blood flow.

pneumocystis pneumonia A rare form of pneumonia that is often present in persons living with AIDS.

pneumonia An inflammation of the lung tissue.

point source pollutant A source of pollution that enters a body of water at a specific point.

point-of-service (POS) plans HMOs having an indemnity-type option that lets members get care from physicians and other providers outside the plan's network.

polyunsaturated fat The type of fat that has several hydrogens available to bind and is soft at room temperature; usually comes from plant or fish sources.

portal of exit The means by which the pathogen moves out of the source into a new host.

post-traumatic stress disorder A psychological condition affecting rape victims, combat veterans, and other trauma survivors.

preadmission certification Approval from a health plan of the need for inpatient hospital care prior to the actual admission.

preconception care A health-promoting action taken prior to conception for the purpose of reducing health risks to mother and child.

precycling The practice of choosing products that have the potential for reuse, using packaging that can be used for other purposes, or choosing packaging that has already been recycled.

pre-existing condition A health condition for which a person has been treated prior to joining a health plan; some plans limit coverage for such a condition up to one year after joining the plan.

preferred provider organization (PPOs) A hybrid form of insurance that merges features of traditional fee-for-service insurance and prepaid plans.

premenstrual dysphoric disorder A form of depression occurring just prior to menstruation and characterized by fatigue, irritability, mood swings, and physical symptoms such as abdominal bloating, swollen hands or feet, headaches, and tender breasts; a severe form of premenstrual syndrome.

premenstrual syndrome A combination of emotional and physical features which occur before menstruation; characterized by mood changes, discomfort, swelling and tenderness in the breasts, a bloated feeling, headache, and fatigue.

prenatal care A health-promoting action taken by the mother-to-be after conception and before birth for the purpose of reducing health risks to mother and child; medical care during pregnancy.

presbyopia A difficulty in reading materials at close range; common in older people.

prescription drugs Drugs ordered specifically for a person by his or her physician and filled by a registered pharmacist.

prevention Taking health-promoting action to reduce the risk of disease or injury.

preventive behavior Action taken by a person who is essentially healthy in order to remain healthy.

primary care Routine medical care provided by a physician in an office or at an emergency room in a hospital or clinic.

primary stressor Something that initiates the stress response.

primary syphilis A disease characterized by painless sores, called chancres, at the site of the infection.

prion A mutated, three-dimensional protein that changes the shape of surrounding prions, causing pockets of diseased and dying brain cells.

problem drinker A person who uses alcohol in a manner that causes physical, psychological, or social harm to the drinker and/or others.

pro-choice A political position that supports the idea that a woman has the right to choose whether or not she wishes to continue a pregnancy.

prodromal stage A highly contagious period in a disease in which some symptoms may be apparent but the infected person does not feel ill.

pro-life A political position that supports the idea that a pregnant woman must carry the pregnancy to term because the developing fetus is a human being and has a right to live.

promoter A carcinogen that helps cancer to grow.

proof Two times the percentage of pure alcohol in a beverage.

prostate-specific antigen (PSA) test A blood test that can identify signs of prostate cancer.

protein A group of complex compounds containing amino acids that are essential for growth and repair of tissue.

protozoa Single-celled parasites that produce toxins and release enzymes that interrupt the body's ability to function normally.

protozoal vaginitis A condition transmitted sexually and characterized by a foul or fishy odor, accompanied by itching, burning sensations and pain in the vaginal area.

psychoactive Affecting the mind or behavior.

psychological age A number representing a perceived age (how old you feel).

psychoneuroimmunology A mind–body approach to treatment. It involves the mind and emotions (psycho), the brain and central nervous system (neuro), and the body's natural defense system (immunology).

psychosis A mental disorder that can result in losing touch with reality.

pulse The palpable flow of blood in the arteries caused by the regular contraction of the heart.

purging Self-induced vomiting and/or otherwise ridding the body of excessive food; often done after binges by a bulimic person.

pyrogen A chemical that signals the brain to raise body temperature.

quackery A health claim made for a product or service that cannot be justified by scientifically derived evidence.

quickening Fetal movements felt by the mother.

radiation Energy that travels in waves or particles

radiation absorbed doses (rads) The unit of measurement of radiation exposure.

radical mastectomy The complete surgical removal of the breast and surrounding tissue, particularly the lymph nodes.

radon An extremely toxic, colorless gas derived from the radioactive decay of radium; usually arising from uranium in the soil, water, and rock.

receptor site The location in the body at which a drug triggers a response.

recoil The stage of bereavement in which the bereaved superficially carry on and try to return to normal.

recovery A period in which infection is successfully defeated and the body returns to its healthy state; also the stage of bereavement in which the bereaved begin to show signs of returning to a more normal life.

recycling The use over and over again of substances such as metal and glass.

relative strength A measure of strength determined by dividing absolute strength by body weight.

REM (rapid eye movement) sleep Sleep during which the eyes flicker back and forth behind closed eyelids; the period of sleep associated with dreaming.

reservoir of the pathogen A place (either a human or an animal) where a pathogen resides.

resistance The capacity of the immune system to fight the invasion of an organism; also the second stages of the general adaptation syndrome; the body relaxes and returns to its normal state after the immediate threat has disappeared.

resting heart rate The number of heart beats per minute in a resting state.

rhythm method The method of contraception that relies on knowing when a woman ovulates and then calculating when her fertile and infertile periods occur.

rickettsia A rod-shaped microorganism that is transmitted by vectors and causes a variety of diseases, such as typhus.

risk factor A condition or habit that puts a person in danger of negative health occurrences.

RU-486 A drug that is taken after implantation to induce miscarriage; also called a medical abortion.

runner's high The feeling of euphoria due to an increase in the production of the hormone endorphin during or following exercise.

saturated fat The type of fat that has all hydrogen sites occupied and is usually solid at room temperature; usually comes from animal sources and is thought to encourage plaque build-up.

schizophrenia A complex mental illness in which an individual has a distorted view of reality.

screening Analysis of risk factors done on a person thought to be well, for the purpose of preventing disease or making an early diagnosis.

seasonal affective disorder A form of depression brought on by lack of sufficient daylight.

secondary care Care involving surgery and nonroutine medical treatment, usually delivered in a hospital.

secondary infection An infection that occurs in conjunction with, or as a result of, another infection but which arises from a different pathogen.

secondary stressor An additional stressor that continues the stress response.

secondary syphilis A disease characterized by a general rash on the body, sore throat, fever, and pains in the joints and muscles.

self-actualization The ability to seek the highest and most idealistic state that can lead to a person's fullest possible development.

self-assessment An evaluation of health status based on data collected on oneself by oneself.

self-concept A person's view of himself or herself gained through an assessment of strengths and weaknesses.

self-efficacy A person's belief that he or she is capable of accomplishing a task or series of tasks under certain conditions.

self-esteem How a person values himself or herself.

set point A particular weight at which a person's body functions normally.

sexually transmitted infections (STIs) Infectious diseases and syndromes that are spread primarily through sexual activity.

sick building syndrome (SBS) Characterized by unhealthy indoor air that results from a lack of circulating air or a lack of ventilation.

sick-role behavior Action taken by a person who has been diagnosed as sick.

side effect An unwanted or even dangerous physical or mental effect caused by a drug or medicine.

sidestream smoke The smoke originating from the burning end of the cigarette between puffs, which adversely affects the health of individuals nearby.

sigmoidoscopy A screening procedure in which a physician uses a hollow lighted tube to inspect the rectum and lower colon.

simple carbohydrate A basic nutritional compound made of short chains of simple sugars that are broken down quickly in the body.

single-parent family A family in which only one parent lives in the home and takes care of the children.

smog A brownish haze that forms when hydrocarbons react with nitric acid in the presence of sunlight.

smokeless tobacco Tobacco products that are chewed, placed in the mouth, and/or sniffed through the nose.

smoking cessation The process of breaking a smoking habit stopping the use of tobacco.

social drinker A person who drinks regularly in social settings but seldom consumes enough alcohol to become intoxicated.

sonogram A diagnostic tool that allows a physician to indirectly see the developing fetus and its individual organ systems.

spermicide An acidic substance that kills sperm.

spina bifida A birth defect in which the spinal cord or its covering is incomplete.

squamous cell A flat cell that makes up most of the epidermis.

staging The use of drugs in a predictable progression beginning with gateway drugs, such as tobacco and alcohol, and progressing to hard drugs, such as crack, cocaine and heroin.

starches White, tasteless substances found in potatoes, rice, corn, wheat, and other vegetable products.

sterilization A form of birth control in which steps are taken to permanently end fertility.

stimulant A drug that speeds up the body's functions and movements.

strength The extent to which an individual is capable of exerting force in one effort, as needed.

stress A reaction of the body and mind to the mental and emotional strain place on them.

stress response A series of events, caused by stressors, within the body that involve chemicals, hormones, and neural impulses.

stressor A specific event that disrupts equilibrium and initiates complex biochemical responses.

stressor identification Recognizing stress in order to begin effective management.

stroke A clot or break in a blood vessel in the brain that disrupts blood flow to the brain.

substance abuse Patterns of increasing levels of use of tobacco, alcohol, and other drugs that result in health consequences or impairment in social, psychological, and/or occupational functioning.

suction curettage A method of abortion performed in the first trimester, involving dilation of the cervix and removal of the contents of the uterus by suction; also called vacuum aspiration.

suicidologist A person who studies suicide.

sulfur oxides Acrid poisonous gases that are produced when fuel containing sulfur is burned.

sulfuric acid A corrosive substance produced in the manufacturing process of fertilizers, chemicals, dyes, and petroleum products; when combined with droplets of water in the air it becomes the active component in acid rain.

symptomatic period A period during the course of a disease in which symptoms appear.

synergistic effect When simultaneous actions of two separate entities together have a greater total effect than would be expected from the sum of the individual effects.

syphilis A bacterial STI that spreads through the bloodstream and causes a systemic infection.

systemic infection An infection affecting the body as a whole.

systolic pressure The pressure measured in the arteries when the heart contracts.

tachycardia Excessively rapid beating of the heart.

tar The most carcinogenic substance in cigarettes; the gummy mixture left over from burning.

target heart rate range Heart activity high enough to bring about a training effect and low enough to be safe.

temporary threshold shift (TTS) Temporary hearing loss usually caused by a sudden loud noise.

teratogen An agent that causes birth defects.

tertiary care Special medical procedures, such as open-heart surgery and transplants, performed mostly at hospitals affiliated with medical schools or at large regional hospitals.

testicular self-examination An examination done by a man to himself to identify abnormal testicular tissue; a screening exam for the presence of testicular cancer.

thalamus The part of the brain that plays a part in controlling the senses.

thanatology The study of death and the psychological and social problems associated with it.

therapeutic community A residential treatment center where people who abuse drugs can live and learn to adjust to drug-free lives.

tissue plasminogen activator A natural enzyme that prevents blood from clotting.

tolerance The progressive change in the body's reaction to tobacco, alcohol, or another drug, causing an individual to need more and more of the drug to achieve the same effect.

toxic chemical A chemical that is poisonous.

toxin A poisonous substance produced by a microorganism; can cause certain infectious diseases.

trace minerals Minerals that are essential for proper growth and functioning but are needed in very small amounts.

training effect Health benefits, most notably increased heart efficiency, produced by exercising for a sufficient duration and intensity.

trans fatty acids Fatty acids formed as a part of the hydrogenation process when making margarine that increase LDLs (bad cholesterol) and decrease HDLs (good cholesterol).

transdermal nicotine patch A form of nicotine replacement that, when applied to the skin, releases nicotine into the system at a constant rate.

transient ischemic attack (TIA) A stroke that causes minimal damage but signals the possibility of a more severe stroke.

trichloroethylene (TCE) A suspected carcinogen used as a degreaser in machine shops.

trichomoniasis A protozoal vaginitis transmitted primarily through sexual means.

tubal ligation A surgical procedure in which the fallopian tubes are cut and tied in order to prevent the passage of the egg and the subsequent union of sperm and egg.

tuberculosis An airborne bacterial disease spread by inhaling germs called tubercle bacilli; symptoms include fever, wasting, and cheesy formations in the lungs.

tumor A mass of tissue that accumulates in the body.

type 2 diabetes The most common form of diabetes; also called adult-onset diabetes.

Type A personality Competitive, aggressive, driven, and impatient.

Type B personality Less competitive and more relaxed and patient than Type A personality.

underinsured Having limited health insurance that compromises one's access to health care services and places one at significant financial risk.

undermedication Consuming a lower drug dosage than prescribed, which can compromise accurate medical care.

underwater weighing A test of body fat that weighs a person underwater to determine body composition.

underweight Less body weight relative to a specified standard for height and age.

uniform donor card A card signed by a person age eighteen or older that shows he or she has agreed to donate all or specified parts of his or her body upon death.

uninsured Having no health insurance.

urinary tract infection (UTI) An infection that occurs when bacteria get into the urinary system.

uterus A hollow, pear-shaped muscular organ that functions to house the developing fetus.

vacuum aspiration A method of abortion performed in the first trimester, involving dilation of the cervix and removal of the contents of the uterus by suction; also called suction curettage.

vaginal canal The passage in females leading from the vulva (external orifice) to the uterus.

vaginal ring A soft, flexible, transparent plastic that contains the hormones found in many birth control pills (oral contraceptives). The hormones are released slowly over 3 weeks in order to prevent ovulation.

vaginitis A vaginal infection usually caused by yeast or protozoa.

vagus nerve The nerve that runs between the posterior part of the brain stem and the stomach and gives your brain the message that you are full.

vas deferens A tube that carries mature sperm from the testes to the ejaculatory ducts.

vasectomy Surgically cutting and tying the vas deferens of the man, thus preventing the passage of sperm.

vectors Insects or animals that carry disease.

vegans Vegetarians who do not eat any food of animal origin.

vegetarian A person who follows a diet consisting of no meat, chicken, or fish; all nutrition is obtained from vegetables, fruits, and grains. Some vegetarians eat dairy products.

virulence The strength of pathogens present during disease transmission.

virus A chain of nucleic acid surrounded by a protein coat that invades cells and uses the cells' reproductive capabilities.

warm-up period The period of exercise in which the body becomes prepared for exertion.

water-soluble vitamins Vitamins that are not stored in the body, (and excesses are excreted in the urine); examples are B-complex vitamins and vitamin C.

wellness A description of health that includes the human potential for a high level of well-being while taking into consideration environmental and personal limitations.

Wernicke-Kosakoff syndrome A form of alcohol-related amnesia and personality disorder associated with central nervous system impairment; usually not reversible.

will A legal declaration of a person's wishes about how to dispose of his or her body and personal property after death and other personal issues surrounding death.

withdrawal The symptoms ranging from mild discomfort to very traumatic events when a person stops taking a drug; also the method of contraception in which the man withdraws his penis from the vagina before ejaculation.

yeast infection A condition characterized by itching; burning during urination; a white, thick, odorless discharge; painful intercourse; and general discomfort; caused by *Candida*.

yo-yo dieting Going on and off diets.

Index

Boldface page numbers indicate locations of definitions.

Photo Credits

Chapter 1
Page 1, Jim Cummins/CORBIS; page 2, Kaz Mori/The Image Bank; page 7, Steve Dunwell/The Image Bank; page 9, Eyewire; page 11, Bruce Ayres/Stone; page 13, Digital Stock/CORBIS.

Chapter 2
Page 20, Digital Stock/CORBIS; page 21L, Ed Bailey/AP Photo; page 21R, Darren Huckerby/Topham/The Image Works; page 23, Navaswan/FPG International; page 24, Digital Stock/CORBIS; page 28, Owen Franken/CORBIS; page 30, Jon Bradley/Stone.

Chapter 3
Page 35, David Stoecklein/CORBIS; page 37TL, Duomo/CORBIS; page 37TR, James A. Sugar/ CORBIS; page 37BL, Eyewire; page 37BR, Bob Daemmrich/The Image Works; page 40, Don Spiro/Stone; page 41T, Wartenberg/Picture Press/CORBIS; page 41B, Strauss/Curtis/CORBIS; page 44, Dorling Kindersley.

Chapter 4
Page 48, Phil Schofield/Stone; page 50, Dorling Kindersley; page 52, T. Shumsky/The Image Works; page 57, Bob Torrez/Stone.

Chapter 5
Page 64, Brian Bailey/Stone; page 65, Jeff Greenberg/The Image Works; page 66, Reuters/Fred Prouser/Archive Photos; page 69, Dennie Cody/FPG International; page 70, Tony Freeman; page 73, Jim Cummins/CORBIS; page 74, Yves Forestier/CORBIS SYGMA.

Chapter 6
Page 79, CORBIS; page 81, Tim Pannell/CORBIS; page 83L, Rob Gage/Taxi; page 83R, Nathan Benn/CORBIS; page 84, Gregg Adams/Stone; page 85T, David Ash/CORBIS; page 85B, Steve Chenn/CORBIS; page 86, Lori Adamski Peek/Stone.

Chapter 7
Page 95, Don Tremain/Getty Images; page 96, Peter Vandermark/Stock, Boston; page 97, Peter Poulides/Stone; page 99, Martin M. Rotker. Focus on Careers, Elena Dorfman/Addison Wesley Longman; page 103, Michael Newman/Photo Edit; page 104, Ed Taylor Studio/FPG International; page 108, Terry Quing/FPG International.

Chapter 8
Page 114, Frank Siteman/Stock, Boston; page 116, Ron Chapple/FPG International; page 117, Steve Mason/Getty Images, Inc.; page 120, Mark M. Lawrence/CORBIS.

Chapter 9
Page 131, T. Shumsky/The Image Works; page 132, Mark E. Gibson/CORBIS; page 135, Dorling Kindersley; page 136, Kevin Fleming/CORBIS; page 139, Charles Gupton/CORBIS; page 142, Roy McMahon/CORBIS; page 143, Jose Luis Pelaez, Inc./CORBIS.

Chapter 10
Page 149, Ronnie Kaufman/CORBIS; page 152, Ralph Pleasant/FPG International; page 155, Geoff Tompkinson/SPL/Photo Researchers, Inc.; page 157, David Stoecklein/CORBIS; page 160, Courtesy of the Skin Cancer Foundation, NY; page 161, Mike McGill/CORBIS; page 162, Jeff Kaufman/FPG International; page 166, James Darell/Getty Images.

Chapter 11
Page 172, Tom & Dee Ann McCarthy/CORBIS; page 174, Brendan Beirne/Stone; page 177, Steve Dunwell/Image Bank; page 178, AP Photo/Matt York; page 184, Barry Yee/Getty Images; page 190, Sondra Dawes/The Image Works.

Chapter 12
Page 198, Denis Boissavy/Taxi; page 201L, Andy Sacks/Stone; page 201R, Ken Chernus/Getty Images; page 202, Bruce Ayres/Stone; page 204, Stock, Boston; page 206, Stone.

Chapter 13
Page 214, Christopher Wilhelm/Getty Images; page 215, Will Hart; page 216, Arlene Collins/The Image Works; page 220, Penny Gentieu/Stone; page 223, Sean Cayton/The Image Works; page 233, Joe Marquette/AP Wide World.

Chapter 14
Page 237, Vicky Kasala Productions/Getty Images; page 241, Ken Chernus/FPG International; page 243, Sarto/Lund/Stone; page 248, Al Campanie/Syracuse Newspapers/ The Image Works; page 249, Paul Chiasson/AP Wide World.

Chapter 15
Page 256, Dugald Bremner/Stone; page 262, Frank Pedrick/The Image Works; page 264, Philip James Corwin/CORBIS; page 267, AP/Wide World Photos; page 268, Tom Carter/PhotoEdit.

Chapter 16
Page 275, Andy Whale/Stone; page 277, Michael Newman/PhotoEdit; page 280, Kindra Clineff/Stone; page 284, Kim Steele/Getty Images

CHAPTER 1 HEALTH: YOUR PERSONAL RESPONSIBILITY

Multiple Choice

1. According to Halbert Dunn, an individual's level of wellness depends on:
   a. the individual.
   b. direction and progress.
   c. how the individual functions.
   d. all of the above.
2. The process of becoming healthy is most influenced by which combination of factors?
   a. knowledge, skills, and behaviors
   b. parents, friends, and community
   c. resources, facilities, and opportunity
   d. culture, religion, and politics
3. According to the National Health Education Standards, health literacy means:
   a. adjusting to changes and challenges in a rapidly changing world.
   b. ways of communicating with others about health.
   c. making healthy lifestyle choices.
   d. interpreting, understanding, and using basic health information in ways that enhance the health of self and others.
4. Actions that promote health literacy, maintain and improve health, prevent disease, and reduce health related risk behavior are:
   a. protective factors.
   b. health skills.
   c. resistance skills.
   d. resiliency factors.
5. A heroin addict given methadone through a local treatment program is an example of:
   a. wellness behavior.
   b. sick–role behavior.
   c. illness behavior.
   d. preventive behavior.
6. Getting immunized against a disease such as polio is an example of:
   a. preventive behavior.
   b. illness behavior.
   c. sick–role behavior.
   d. health promotion.
7. Attending a smoking cessation program in an effort to quit the habit of smoking is an example of:
   a. preventive behavior.
   b. illness behavior.
   c. sick–role behavior.
   d. health promotion.
8. An individual's health style (lifestyle) is influenced by personal attitudes, beliefs, values, and:
   a. health momentum.
   b. age.
   c. genes.
   d. gender.
9. The process by which we seek to reduce the risk of disease and injury is called:
   a. wellness.
   b. prevention.
   c. epidemiology.
   d. health promotion.

10. Which of the following risk factors is NOT considered modifiable?
    a. alcohol and/or tobacco use
    b. exposure to environmental pollution
    c. physical activity level
    d. blood pressure

True/False

T F 1. The World Health Organization defines health as hygiene.

T F 2. A medical assessment and self-assessment are synonymous terms for the diagnosis of a disease or medical condition.

T F 3. Changes in one's body temperature and/or weight are measures of a change in health conditions.

T F 4. A health risk refers to the likelihood of having a certain health condition.

T F 5. Health style is best described as the sum total of one's knowledge.

T F 6. If you have every intention to quit smoking within the next month, you are considered to have a positive health attitude.

T F 7. When one positive health behavior influences another positive behavior, this is referred to as prevention.

T F 8. Dietary factors have been linked to heart disease and cancer of the colon.

T F 9. According to the National Center for Health Statistics, the leading causes of death in 2000 were heart disease, accidental injuries, and HIV/AIDS.

T F 10. Physical inactivity has been identified as the most avoidable cause of death in the United States.

ANSWERS:

Multiple Choice: 1. d (p. 3), 2. a (p. 3), 3. d (p. 4), 4. b (p. 5), 5. b (p. 6), 6. a (p. 5), 7. b (p. 6), 8. a (p. 12), 9. b (p. 13), 10. b (p. 10).

True/False: 1. F (p. 2), 2. F (p. 6), 3. T (p. 6), 4. T (p. 9), 5. F (p. 11), 6. T (p. 11), 7. F (p. 13), 8. T (p. 15), 9. F (p. 13), 10. F (p. 15).

Name ______________________________ Date ____________ Section ____________

MARTIN'S INDEX OF HEALTH BEHAVIOR

1. How many days per week do you eat breakfast?

    _____ a. 6–7 _____ b. 4–5 _____ c. 2–3 _____ d. 0–1

2. Which choice most closely describes your daily eating pattern?

    _____ a. eating snack foods (potato chips, soda pop, etc.) whenever I am hungry
    _____ b. eating one balanced meal per day and eating snack foods at other times during the day
    _____ c. eating two balanced meals a day and eating snack foods at other times of the day
    _____ d. eating three balanced meals a day and eating snack foods at other times of the day
    _____ e. eating three balanced meals per day and not snacking

3. How many days/week do you eat a balanced diet that includes the minimum servings from the food groups listed: 2 servings meat/protein substitutes; 2 servings dairy products; 4 servings breads/cereals; 4 servings fruits/vegetables?

    _____ a. 6–7 _____ b. 4–5 _____ c. 2–3 _____ d. 0–1

4. How many servings per day of concentrated sources of sugar (soda pop, candy, cookies, etc.) do you eat?

    _____ a. less than 1 _____ b. 1–2 _____ c. 3–4 _____ d. 5 or more

5. Considering your height and body build, how many pounds within your ideal weight do you fall?

    _____ a. within 10 pounds _____ c. within 30 pounds
    _____ b. within 20 pounds _____ d. more than 30 pounds from ideal

6. Which choice most closely describes your dieting behavior?

    _____ a. never being overweight, so never dieting
    _____ b. being more than 10 pounds overweight, but not dieting
    _____ c. when overweight, going on a fad diet to lose weight quickly
    _____ d. when overweight, attempting to lose weight gradually by increasing exercise *or* decreasing food
    _____ e. when overweight, attempting to lose weight gradually by increasing exercise *and* decreasing food

7. What is the average number of hours per night that you sleep?

    _____ a. more than 10 _____ b. 9–10 _____ c. 7–8 _____ d. 5–6 _____ e. 0–4

8. How often do you use seat belts while driving or riding in a car?

    _____ a. always _____ c. sometimes in town and sometimes on the highway
    _____ b. never in town and always on the highway _____ d. never

9. How often do you drive or ride with someone under the influence of alcohol or drugs?

    _____ a. more than once a week _____ c. a few times per year
    _____ b. once per week _____ d. never

10. Which choice best describes your consumption of alcoholic beverages?

    _____ a. not drinking
    _____ b. drinking one drink or less per day
    _____ c. drinking two drinks or less per day
    _____ d. drinking two drinks or less on weekdays, more than two drinks per day on weekends
    _____ e. drinking more than two drinks per day on most days

11. Which choice best describes your drug use pattern (over-the-counter, prescription, and recreational drugs)?

    _____ a. using the drugs I want whenever I want
    _____ b. using the drugs I feel I need while following common sense
    _____ c. using only medically required drugs exactly as directed
    _____ d. rarely using drugs of any kind

12. How many cups of caffeinated beverages (coffee, tea, cola, etc.) do you drink per day?

    _____ a. none or less than 1 _____ b. 1–3 _____ c. 4–6 _____ d. 7 or more

13. Which choice best describes your cigarette smoking behavior?
    _____ a. not smoking _____ c. smoking 1–2 packs per day
    _____ b. smoking less than one pack per day _____ d. smoking more than 2 packs per day
14. How many times per week do you exercise aerobically (biking, jogging, swimming, aerobics, etc.)?
    _____ a. less than 1 _____ b. 1 _____ c. 2 _____ d. 3–4 _____ e. 5 or more
15. How many times per week do you do other types of exercise (weight lifting, tennis, calisthenics, racquetball, basketball, etc.) besides aerobic activities?
    _____ a. less than 1 _____ b. 1 _____ c. 2 _____ d. 3–4 _____ e. 5 or more
16. How often do you brush your teeth?
    _____ a. after every meal _____ c. once per day
    _____ b. twice per day _____ d. less than once per day
17. How often do you have a dental checkup?
    _____ a. never or only when something is wrong _____ c. every year
    _____ b. every 2–3 years _____ d. every 6 months
18. How often do you have a medical checkup?
    _____ a. never or only when something is wrong _____ c. every 3–5 years
    _____ b. only for Pap tests or other checks _____ d. at least every 2 years
19. How often do you read the labels of foods and over-the-counter drugs before purchasing them?
    _____ a. always _____ b. usually _____ c. sometimes _____ d. rarely
20. How many times per week do you make a conscientious effort to manage your stress by utilizing relaxation, exercise, religion, music, or other stress–reduction techniques?
    _____ a. 6–7 _____ b. 4–5 _____ c. 2–3 _____ d. 0–1
21. Which choice most correctly describes your closest interpersonal relationship?
    _____ a. not having a friend
    _____ b. having a friend, but I am not able to share my real feelings with the person
    _____ c. having a friendship where I can sometimes share my real feelings, but sometimes can't
    _____ d. having a friendship where I can always share my real feelings
22. How many servings/day of foods high in saturated fats or cholesterol (whole milk, eggs, red meat, etc.) do you eat?
    _____ a. 0 _____ b. 1–2 _____ c. 3–4 _____ d. 5 or more
23. How often do you limit your consumption of salt by doing things like not salting your foods at the table, using salt sparingly when preparing foods, and limiting your intake of salty foods?
    _____ a. always _____ b. usually _____ c. sometimes _____ d. rarely
24. How often do you practice breast self-examination (female) or testicular self-examination (male)?
    _____ a. every month _____ c. less frequently than every 6 months
    _____ b. every 2–6 months _____ d. never
25. Which choice best describes your contraceptive use?
    _____ a. not sexually active, so don't use contraceptives
    _____ b. attempting to get pregnant or am pregnant, so don't use contraceptives
    _____ c. sexually active and always use contraceptives
    _____ d. sexually active and usually use contraceptives
    _____ e. sexually active and sometimes use contraceptives
    _____ f. sexually active and rarely use contraceptives

Scoring: For Items: 1, 3, 4, 5, 8, 12, 13, 16, 19, 20, 22, 23, 24 a=3, b=2, c=1, d=0; For Items: 2, 9, 11, 17, 18, 21 a=0, b=1, c=2, d=3; For Item: 6 a=3, b=1, c=0, d=2, e=3; For Item: 7 a=1, b=2, c=3, d=2, e=0; For Item: 10 a=3, b=3, c=2, d=1, e=0; For Items: 14 and 15 a=0, b=1, c=2, d=3, e=3; For Item: 25 a=3, b=3, c=3, d=2, e=1, f=0. Total scores can range from 0–75. Health behavior is generally *poor* if the total score is below 25; *average but needing change* if between 25 and 50; and *good* if over 50.

Source: Joan Peterson Martin, *The Relationship of Self Concept to Health Behavior in Community College Students* (unpublished thesis). University of Chicago, December 1985.

CHAPTER 2 MANAGING YOUR MENTAL HEALTH

Multiple Choice

1. The definition of mental health is:
   a. mental illness.
   b. socio-status health.
   c. a state of emotional and social well-being.
   d. psychoenvironmental health.
2. A mentally healthy person has:
   a. an accurate self-concept.
   b. positive self-esteem.
   c. a good sense of self-efficacy.
   d. all of the above.
3. One's sense of self-respect or self-confidence refers to:
   a. self-esteem.
   b. social support.
   c. self-efficacy.
   d. self-actualization.
4. A person's belief about whether he or she can successfully engage in and execute a specific behavior refers to:
   a. self-esteem.
   b. self-concept.
   c. self-actualization.
   d. self-efficacy.
5. According to Maslow, self-actualization is:
   a. how you value yourself.
   b. how you see yourself.
   c. how well you execute a specific behavior.
   d. the achievement of self-fulfillment.
6. Americans experience this disorder more than any other mental health problem:
   a. psychosis.
   b. anxiety.
   c. mood swings.
   d. suicide.
7. Seasonal affective disorder is associated with:
   a. malfunction of the pituitary gland.
   b. lack of a strong social support network.
   c. reduced exposure to sunlight.
   d. lack of exercise and poor diet.
8. Alterations of the senses and radical changes in emotions, movements, and behaviors are characteristic of what mental disorder?
   a. schizophrenia
   b. anxiety attacks
   c. bipolar disorder
   d. clinical depression
9. Treatment for schizophrenia includes a combination of:
   a. diet, exercise, and rest.
   b. hospitalization, medication, and psychotherapy.
   c. light therapy, electrolysis, and massage therapy.
   d. chiropractic therapy, medication, and exercise.

10. This health issue is the third leading cause of death, following unintentional injuries and homicide, among youth between 15–24 years of age:
    a. cancer.
    b. heart disease.
    c. suicide.
    d. HIV.

True/False

T F 1. Mental health is usually defined according to normal behavior.

T F 2. A mental disorder is evident when the mind prevents a person from getting along with other people.

T F 3. A mentally well person is often referred to as a well-adjusted individual.

T F 4. It is not mentally healthy to express emotions.

T F 5. REM sleep is the time when the body repairs itself.

T F 6. Drinking coffee is recommended for helping to overcome insomnia.

T F 7. A phobia is characterized by an unreasonable fear of a particular object or situation.

T F 8. Most suicidal individuals are depressed.

T F 9. The actual rates of suicide may be much higher due to difficulty in determining the causes of suspicious deaths.

T F 10. Schizophrenia is curable with therapy and drug treatment.

ANSWERS:

Multiple Choice: 1. c (p. 21), 2. d (p. 22), 3. a (p. 24), 4. d (p. 24), 5. d (p. 25), 6. b (p. 26), 7. c (p. 27), 8. a (p. 28), 9. b (p. 28), 10. c (p. 30).
True/False: 1. T (p. 21), 2. T (p. 21), 3. T (p. 22), 4. F (p. 21), 5. F (p. 23), 6. F (p. 24), 7. T (p. 26), 8. T (p. 30), 9. T (p. 30), 10. F (p. 29).

Name ______________________ Date ____________ Section ____________

DOES THIS SOUND LIKE YOU?

Many times people think their feelings are unique, the product of their own lives and experiences. Read these brief descriptions of anxiety disorders. See if they sound like you. Many people share these patterns.

Directions: Check the statements that you feel best describe you.

_____ 1. You are always worried about things, even when there are no signs of trouble.

_____ 2. You have frequent aches and pains that can't be traced to physical illness or injury.

_____ 3. You get tired easily, yet you have trouble sleeping.

_____ 4. Your body is constantly tense.

_____ 5. Out of the blue, your heart starts pounding.

_____ 6. You feel dizzy.

_____ 7. You can't breathe.

_____ 8. You feel like you're about to die.

_____ 9. You've had these symptoms over and over again.

_____ 10. Ever since an assault, you have nightmares almost every night.

_____ 11. The war is over, but the terrifying flashbacks continue.

_____ 12. You avoid places that remind you of the accident.

_____ 13. You feel like you can't trust anyone.

_____ 14. You are so afraid of germs that you wash your hands repeatedly until they're raw and sore.

_____ 15. You can't leave the house until you check the locks on every window and door over and over again.

_____ 16. You are terrified you will harm someone you care about.

_____ 17. You just can't get these thoughts out of your head.

_____ 18. Every day, you fear you will do something very embarrassing.

_____ 19. You've stopped going to parties, because you're afraid to meet new people.

_____ 20. When other people look at you, you break out in a sweat and shake uncontrollably.

_____ 21. You stay home from work, because you're terrified of being called on in a staff meeting.

Assessment: The descriptions within statements 1–4 are symptoms of general anxiety disorder; statements 5–9 are symptoms of panic disorder; statements 10–13 are symptoms of post–traumatic stress disorder (PTSD); statements 14–17 are symptoms of obsessive–compulsive disorder; and statements 18–21 are symptoms of social phobia.
If any of these descriptions sound like you, you may have an anxiety disorder. Anxiety disorders are treatable illnesses. Take a first step to feeling better. Talk to your doctor.

For more information about anxiety disorders, contact NIMH; toll free 1-888-ANXIETY; FAX Back System; 301-443-5158; *www.nimh.nih.gov/anxiety*

Source: www.nimh.nih.gov/soundlikeyou.htm, National Institutes of Mental Health, National Institute of Health, posted October 16, 2000.

CHAPTER 3 COPING WITH STRESS

Multiple Choice

1. The mental and physical response of our bodies to any type of change is called:
   a. eustress.
   b. distress.
   c. stressor.
   d. stress.
2. Which of the following statements is true about stress?
   a. Stress means different things to different people.
   b. Stress is highly addictive.
   c. Stress is genetically predetermined.
   d. It is possible to have a stress-free life.
3. Any event or condition that causes our bodies to have to adjust to a specific situation is known as:
   a. eustress.
   b. distress.
   c. stressor.
   d. stress.
4. In which phase of the general adaptation syndrome does the body attempt to return to its normal state?
   a. alarm reaction.
   b. resistance.
   c. fatigue.
   d. exhaustion.
5. In which phase of the general adaptation syndrome is one susceptible to illness and disease as a result of the physical and psychological energies used to fight stressors have been depleted?
   a. alarm phase
   b. resistance phase
   c. fatigue phase
   d. exhaustion phase
6. Good (positive) stress is defined by Selye as:
   a. strain.
   b. stress.
   c. distress.
   d. eustress.
7. Bad (unpleasant) stress, such as the loss of a job, is defined by Selye as:
   a. strain.
   b. stress.
   c. distress.
   d. eustress.
8. All of the following are examples of events that cause eustress EXCEPT:
   a. burnout at work.
   b. the excitement of a vacation.
   c. the accomplishment of an outstanding personal achievement.
   d. the stimulus of an exciting classroom.
9. All of the following symptoms are typical of stress-related disorders with the exception of:
   a. migraine headaches and irritability.
   b. stomach aches and skin rashes.
   c. insomnia and heart palpitations.
   d. hot flashes and sore throat.

10. Adaptation to stress is referred to as:
    a. coping.
    b. adjusting.
    c. hardiness.
    d. quieting.

True/False

T F 1. Abraham Maslow developed the theoretical basis for the stress response in what he called the general adaptation syndrome (GAS).

T F 2. Epinephrine is a hormone released in the first stage of the GAS, causing the heart to speed up and constrict blood vessels.

T F 3. Sexual harassment and public speaking are examples of psychologic stressors.

T F 4. Eustress is considered an important aspect of healthy living.

T F 5. Taking your driver's test is an example of eustress.

T F 6. There is scientific evidence suggesting a connection between too much stress and the incidence of disease.

T F 7. Recent studies have found that stress can cause a weakening of the immune system.

T F 8. Building a network of personal support that can be used to manage the stress in one's life involves interpersonal skills.

T F 9. There is evidence that exercise functions as a stress reducer.

T F 10. Exercise can reduce stress levels by raising levels of epinephrine in the body.

ANSWERS:

Multiple Choice: 1. d (p. 36), 2. a (p. 36), 3. c (p. 36), 4. b (p. 36), 5. d (p. 37),
6. d (p. 39), 7. c (p. 39), 8. a (p. 39), 9. d (p. 40), 10. a (p. 42).
True/False: 1. F (p. 36), 2. F (p. 36), 3. F (p. 37), 4. T (p. 39), 5. F (p. 39), 6. T (p. 40),
7. T (p. 40), 8. T (p. 44), 9. T (p. 45), 10. F (p. 45).

Name ________________________ Date ____________ Section ____________

AM I A MENTALLY WELL-ADJUSTED PERSON?

Directions: Circle the answer that best applies to you.

	Never		Sometimes		Always
1. I have a positive self-image and good self-esteem.	1	2	3	4	5
2. I experience appropriate and stable moods.	1	2	3	4	5
3. I maintain control of my emotions.	1	2	3	4	5
4. I have the ability to love, feel guilt, and accept remorse.	1	2	3	4	5
5. I demonstrate flexibility and adaptability in social situations.	1	2	3	4	5
6. I acknowledge personal strengths and accept personal limitations.	1	2	3	4	5
7. I tolerate ambiguity and understand that conflict is normal.	1	2	3	4	5
8. I do not distort reality, consciously or unconsciously.	1	2	3	4	5
9. I know how to obtain reliable mental health–related information, products, and services.	1	2	3	4	5

Assessment: Add up your score. The maximum score is 45. The higher the score, the more "mentally well-adjusted" you are.

1. Which area(s) did you score the highest (4 or 5 points)? ____________________

2. Which area(s) did you score the lowest (1 or 2 points)? ____________________

3. What is one change you could make to improve your mental health? ____________________

Source: Rohmer, J.L. and Wanberg, R. *Personalizing Health Action Plans: A Student Resource Manual,* Copyright 1999. Allyn and Bacon.

Multiple Choice

1. Calories are:
   a. one of the three basic nutrient groups.
   b. essential minerals.
   c. a group of nutrients in food sources.
   d. units of measure of energy produced from food.
2. The basic chemical compounds in food that are required for growth are:
   a. nutrients.
   b. amino acids.
   c. dietology.
   d. cellulose.
3. The body's primary source of energy comes from:
   a. carbohydrates.
   b. vitamins.
   c. proteins.
   d. minerals.
4. Carbohydrates that are primarily found in whole grains, fruits, and vegetables are called:
   a. simple carbohydrates.
   b. complex carbohydrates.
   c. sucrose.
   d. glucose.
5. A diet high in fiber may reduce the risk of:
   a. heart disease.
   b. colon cancer.
   c. metabolic disorders.
   d. impetigo.
6. Fats that generally come from animal products such as meat, eggs, milk, and dairy products are called:
   a. unsaturated fats.
   b. saturated fats.
   c. polyunsaturated fats.
   d. monounsaturated fats.
7. The accumulation of _____ fat is a contributing factor to diseases of the cardiovascular system such as high blood pressure and heart attacks.
   a. unsaturated
   b. saturated
   c. polyunsaturated
   d. monounsaturated
8. High levels of _____ cholesterol appear to reduce the risk of heart disease.
   a. LDL
   b. HDL
   c. CDL
   d. MDL
9. The buildup of cholesterol in the walls of the arteries is also called:
   a. plaque.
   b. glycerols.
   c. triglyceride.
   d. fiber.

10. A disorder in which bone density decreases and bones are more likely to break is called:
    a. arthritis.
    b. atherosclerosis.
    c. osteoporosis.
    d. osteoarthritis.

True/False

T F 1. Starches are a source of vitamins and minerals.

T F 2. Sucrose and dextrose are examples of complex carbohydrates.

T F 3. Fiber is any food that is digested by enzymes in the small intestines.

T F 4. Proteins do not need to be consumed in one's daily diet because they are stored in the body.

T F 5. Unsaturated fats can lower body cholesterol.

T F 6. Cholesterol is a fat-like substance that is manufactured by the spleen.

T F 7. Water-soluble vitamins are stored by the body and therefore do not need to be consumed daily.

T F 8. Antioxidants are vitamins that interfere with the oxidation process of LDLs and therefore reduce the risk of atherosclerosis.

T F 9. Minerals form healthy bones and help nerves and muscles react normally.

T F 10. Dehydration is the result of an abnormal loss of water from the body.

ANSWERS:

Multiple Choice: 1. d (p. 49), 2. a (p. 49), 3. a (p. 49), 4. b (p. 49), 5. b (p. 50), 6. b (p. 51), 7. b (p. 51), 8. b (p. 52), 9. a (p. 52), 10. c (p. 54).

True/False: 1. T (p. 50), 2. F (p. 49), 3. F (p. 49), 4. F (p. 50), 5. T (p. 51), 6. F (p. 51), 7. F (p. 52), 8. T (p. 52), 9. T (p. 53), 10. T (p. 55).

Name ______________________ Date ____________ Section ____________

RATE YOUR PLATE

Take a closer look at yourself—your current food decisions and your lifestyle. Think about your typical eating pattern and food decisions.

Do you...

	Usually	Sometimes	Never
Consider nutrition when you make food choices?	2	1	0
Try to eat regular meals (including breakfast), rather than skip or skimp on some?	2	1	0
Choose nutritious snacks?	2	1	0
Try to eat a variety of foods?	2	1	0
Include new-to-you foods in meals and snacks?	2	1	0
Try to balance your energy (calorie) intake with your physical activity?	2	1	0

Now for the details. Do you:

Eat at least 6 servings of grain products daily?	2	1	0
Eat at least 3 servings of vegetables daily?	2	1	0
Eat at least 2 servings of fruits daily?	2	1	0
Consume at least 2 servings of milk, yogurt, or cheese daily?	2	1	0
Go easy on higher-fat foods?	2	1	0
Go easy on sweets?	2	1	0
Drink 8 or more cups of fluids daily?	2	1	0
Limit alcoholic beverages (no more than 1 daily for a woman or 2 for a man)?	2	1	0

Assessment: Add up your score. If you scored:

24 or more points—Healthful eating seems to be your fitness habit already. Still, look for ways to stick to a healthful eating plan—and to make a "good thing" even better.

16 to 23 points—You're on track. A few easy changes could help you make your overall eating plan healthier.

9 to 15 points—Sometimes you eat smart—but not often enough to be your "fitness best."

0 to 8 points—For your good health, you're wise to rethink your overall eating style. Take it gradually—step by step!

Whatever your score, make moves for healthful eating. Gradually turn your "nevers" into "sometimes" and your "sometimes" into "usually."

Source: Adapted from *The American Dietetic Association's Monthly Nutrition Companion: 31 Days to a Healthier Lifestyle,* Chronimed Publishing, 1997.

CHAPTER 5 MAINTAINING PROPER WEIGHT

Multiple Choice

1. Accumulation of fat beyond 30 percent for women and 25 percent for men is called:
   a. body composition. c. overweight.
   b. obesity. d. body fat.
2. Obese people are more likely than their nonobese peers to suffer from all BUT which of the following health problems?
   a. elevated blood cholesterol levels
   b. cardiovascular diseases
   c. adult–onset diabetes
   d. arthritis
3 An eating disorder characterized by binge eating followed by inappropriate compensating measures taken to prevent weight gain is called:
   a. anorexia nervosa c. compulsive eating disorder
   b. bulimia nervosa d. acidosis
4. An acute form of self-starvation motivated by a fear of gaining weight and a severe disturbance in the perception of one's body is called:
   a. anorexia nervosa. c. compulsive eating disorder.
   b. bulimia nervosa. d. acidosis.
5. A drug that promotes the secretion of excess body fluids is called:
   a. a laxative. c. inhalants.
   b. dopamine. d. a diuretic.
6. A body mass index assesses the:
   a. essential fat to storage fat ratio.
   b. relationship of strength to power.
   c. relationship of body weight to height.
   d. fat to muscle ratio.
7. The pinch test measuring technique:
   a. is used to measure muscle mass.
   b. measures subcutaneous fat in various places on the body.
   c. is a more accurate way to measure percent of body fat than other techniques.
   d. is used to measure essential fat stores.
8. The technique of body fat assessment that utilizes electrical currents that pass through fat and lean tissue is called:
   a. body mass index.
   b. pinch test.
   c. bioelectrical impedance.
   d. underwater weighing.
9. The set point theory suggests that the body knows when it:
   a. cannot lose more weight.
   b. is nearest its best height.
   c. is nearest its best weight.
   d. requires more food intake.
10. A unit of energy produced by food and used by the body is called:
    a. metabolism. c. calorie.
    b. body mass. d. appetite.

True/False

T F 1. Obesity is synonymous with being overweight.

T F 2. Weight, by itself, is a valid indicator of obesity.

T F 3. Basal metabolic rate is usually stable throughout life.

T F 4. Women have a higher rate of eating disorders than men.

T F 5. The most common treatments for bulimia include medical intervention and psychotherapy.

T F 6. When the body needs more energy than the amount provided by food, it uses the energy stored in fat tissue.

T F 7. Fats contain more calories per gram than carbohydrates and/or proteins.

T F 8. The number of fat cells and the size of fat cells are both factors related to obesity.

T F 9. Generally, men have higher caloric needs than women because they have a greater amount of muscle tissue.

T F 10. Ketosis is a condition that occurs when the body adapts to prolonged fasting by converting body fat to proteins.

ANSWERS:

Multiple Choice: 1. b (p. 65), 2. d (p. 65), 3. b (p. 66), 4. a (p. 66), 5. d (p. 67), 6. c (p. 67), 7. b (p. 69), 8. c (p. 69), 9. c (p. 70), 10. c (p. 71).

True/False: 1. F (p. 65), 2. F (p. 65), 3. F (p. 73), 4. T (p. 66), 5. T (p. 67), 6. T (p. 73), 7. T (p. 71), 8. T (p. 72), 9. T (p. 73), 10. F (p. 75).

Name ______________________ Date ____________ Section ____________

AM I MAINTAINING MY PROPER WEIGHT?

Directions: Circle the answer that best applies to you.

	Never		Sometimes		Always
1. My body mass index is in the healthy zone.	1	2	3	4	5
2. My body fat ratio is within a healthy range.	1	2	3	4	5
3. When I look in the mirror, I look overweight.	5	4	3	2	1
4. I feel overweight.	5	4	3	2	1
5. Obesity and overweight is in my genetic background.	5	4	3	2	1
6. My family traditions support healthy eating.	1	2	3	4	5
7. My cultural influences support healthy eating.	1	2	3	4	5
8. I am "in tune" with my hunger.	1	2	3	4	5
9 I am preoccupied with "thinness."	5	4	3	2	1
10. I often go on crash diets.	5	4	3	2	1
11. I know how to obtain reliable weight-related information, products, and services.	1	2	3	4	5

Assessment: Add up your score. The maximum score is 55. The higher the score, the more "proper weight" literate you are.

1. Which area(s) did you score the highest (4 or 5 points)? ______________________
2. Which area(s) did you score the lowest (1 or 2 points)? ______________________
3. What is one change you could make to maintain/improve your proper weight? ______________

Source: Rohwer, J.L. and Wandberg, R. *Personalizing Health Action Plans: A Student Resource Manual,* Copyright 1999. Allyn and Bacon.

CHAPTER 6 KEEPING FIT

Multiple Choice

1. According to the U.S. Surgeon General, which of the following is NOT one of the health-related benefits of regular exercise?
   a. reduces the risk of heart disease
   b. reduces the risk of high blood pressure
   c. increases longevity
   d. reduces the risk of colon cancer
2. The bone disease characterized by low bone mass and increased fracture risk is called:
   a. osteoporosis. c. rheumatoid arthritis.
   b. atherosclerosis. d. osteoarthritis.
3. Which type of blood cholesterol is raised due to physical activity?
   a. HDL c. monosaccharide
   b. LDL d. triglycerides
4. The so-called runner's high or feeling of euphoria when exercising is due to the effect of this hormone.
   a. adrenaline c. endorphin
   b. nonadrenaline d. serotonin
5. Strength development exercises in which a weight is moved through a full range of motion are called:
   a. isokinetic. c. isometric.
   b. isotonic. d. isobionic.
6. The volume of oxygen that the body can consume in one minute of exercise is referred to as:
   a. strength. c. muscular endurance.
   b. anaerobic capacity. d. aerobic capacity.
7. Anaerobic literally means:
   a. less anxious. c. with oxygen.
   b. isotonic. d. without oxygen.
8. The improvement in one's heart from regular exercise is known as the:
   a. training effect. c. aerobic effect.
   b. intensity effect. d. target heart rate.
9. Heart activity high enough to bring about a training effect and low enough to be safe is referred to as:
   a. maximal heart rate. c. aerobic capacity rate.
   b. submaximal heart rate. d. target heart rate.
10. Exercise intensity refers to:
    a. how long a person exercises. c. how often one exercises.
    b. how hard one exercises. d. all of the above.

True/False

T F 1. Exercise and physical fitness are synonymous terms.

T F 2. An exercise's intensity can be measured by evaluating blood level.

T F 3. Flexibility is the measure of the range of motion in a particular joint.

T F 4. Aerobic exercise is represented when the body's demand for oxygen is greater than the amount of oxygen available during exertion.

T F 5. An exercise using special machines that provide weight resistance through a full range of motion is known as an isometric exercise.

T F 6. Weight-lifting is an example of an isotonic exercise.

T F 7. A cool-down period following exercise allows blood flow to be redirected back to the heart and brain.

T F 8. Target heart rate denotes the highest number of heart beats per minute that may safely be achieved during an exercise period.

T F 9. The conditioning period varies greatly from individual to individual.

T F 10. Hypothermia is a loss of body temperature that can result from exercising in cold weather while wearing inappropriate attire.

ANSWERS:

Multiple Choice: 1. c (p. 81), 2. a (p. 83), 3. a (p. 83), 4. c (p. 84), 5. a (p. 84), 6. d (p. 85), 7. d (p. 86), 8. a (p. 87), 9. d (p. 87), 10. b (p. 86).

True/False: 1. F (p. 84), 2. F (p. 86), 3. T (p. 84), 4. F (p. 85), 5. F (p. 85), 6. T (p. 85), 7. T (p. 88), 8. F (p. 87), 9. T (p. 88), 10. T (p. 90).

Name ______________________ Date ____________ Section ____________

MOVEMENT AND EXERCISE

Directions: Make a written agreement with yourself about exercise. Set specific goals in Section 1 for increasing your energy and specific goals in Section 2 for increasing activity. Start slowly.

Remember to motivate yourself through a reward system in Section 3. List specific daily and weekly rewards for meeting your exercise goals. Self-payments may range from eating special foods to treating yourself to a night out.

1. Physical activity goals for increasing my energy use during occupational time:
   a. I will park my car or leave public transportation and walk _____ additional minutes per day.
   b. I will spend _____ minutes daily standing instead of sitting while I work.
   c. I will walk up _____ flights of stairs each work day.
   d. I will walk around my work area _____ minutes per day.
   e. I will spend _____ minutes during each coffee break standing instead of sitting.
   f. I will spend _____ minutes during each lunch break walking outside in the open air.
2. Physical activity goals for increasing my energy use during recreational time:
   a. I will spend _____ minutes daily doing stretching activities to increase my flexibility.
   b. I will spend _____ minutes at least three times per week doing aerobic activities to improve my endurance.
   c. I will spend _____ minutes at least three times per week doing strength activities.
   d. I will spend _____ minutes Saturday and Sunday in active recreational activities.
3. My rewards and consequences:
   a. I will reward myself daily with one of the following pleasures when I achieve my daily goals in increased activity.

      1. ______________ 4. ______________
      2. ______________ 5. ______________
      3. ______________ 6. ______________

   b. When I do not make my daily goals I agree to do the following:

      1. ______________ 2. ______________

   c. I will reward myself every week with one of the following pleasures when I achieve my weekly exercise goals:

      1. ______________ 4. ______________
      2. ______________ 5. ______________
      3. ______________ 6. ______________

   d. When I do not make my weekly goals I agree to do the following:

      1. ______________ 2. ______________

Source: Jerrold S. Greenberg/George B. Dintiman, *Exploring Health.* Englewood Cliffs, NJ: Prentice Hall, 1994, p. 225.

CHAPTER 7 THE HEALTH EFFECTS OF SMOKING AND DRINKING

Multiple Choice

1. Which of the following makes a person smoke their first cigarette and continue to smoke?
   a. parents who smoke c. friends who smoke
   b. the allure of advertisements d. all of the above
2. The substance in tobacco responsible for the addictive behavior of tobacco smokers is:
   a. tar. c. hydrocarbon.
   b. nicotine. d. carbon monoxide.
3. All of the negative effects that carbon monoxide produces on the body are related to:
   a. hypertension. c. arthritis.
   b. osteoporosis. d. oxygen deprivation.
4. Two major components of smoke that contribute to heart disease are:
   a. carbon monoxide and carbon dioxide.
   b. carbon monoxide and nicotine.
   c. nicotine and tar.
   d. ash and hydrocarbons.
5. What two respiratory diseases are associated with smoking?
   a. chronic bronchitis and emphysema
   b. pneumonia and strokes
   c. lung cancer and pneumonia
   d. lobar pneumonia and double pneumonia
6. A condition characterized by white patches on the inside of the mouth that are caused by the carcinogens in smokeless tobacco is called:
   a. gingivitis. c. oral cancer.
   b. leukoplakia. d. periodontal disease.
7. Alcohol is processed (metabolized) in the:
   a. stomach. c. skin.
   b. kidneys. d. liver.
8. A condition in which the liver swells due to alcohol is called:
   a. a hangover. c. pancreatitis.
   b. cirrhosis. d. alcohol dementia.
9. Fetal alcohol syndrome can cause the following birth defect(s):
   a. mental retardation.
   b. a small head.
   c. abnormalities of the face, limbs, and heart.
   d. all of the above.
10. Repeated use of alcohol despite the negative effects on the body, mind, and relationships is called:
    a. dependence. c. tolerance.
    b. alcohol dementia. d. problem drinker.

True/False

T F 1. Smoke from the burning end of a cigarette is called sidestream smoke.

T F 2. The nicotine in tobacco causes blood pressure to increase.

T F 3. Tar is the addictive agent in tobacco because it causes physical dependence.

T F 4. An individual with bronchitis has enlarged air sacs that make it harder to take in air but easier to expel it.

T F 5. The inhalation of air polluted by another person's tobacco smoke is called passive smoking.

T F 6. A recurrent drinking episode is called binge drinking.

T F 7. The hangover that follows intoxication is characterized by nausea, upset stomach, anxiety, and a headache.

T F 8. A blackout is an episode of temporary amnesia in which the drinker continues to function but later cannot remember what happened.

T F 9. Researchers have located a genetic link to alcoholism.

T F 10. The treatment process of removing all alcohol from a person's body is called detoxification.

ANSWERS:

Multiple Choice: 1. d (p. 97), 2. b (p. 97), 3. d (p. 98), 4. b (p. 99), 5. a (p. 99),
6. b (p. 101), 7. d (p. 105), 8. b (p. 105), 9. d (p. 106), 10. a (p. 104).
True/False: 1. T (p. 97), 2. T (p. 97), 3. F (p. 97), 4. F (p. 99), 5. T (p. 101),
6. T (p. 103), 7. T (p. 105), 8. T (p. 105), 9. F (p. 107), 10. T (p. 108).

Name ______________________________ Date ____________ Section ____________

WHAT ARE THE SIGNS OF ALCOHOLISM?

Directions: Respond to the following questions by answering yes or no.

_____ 1. Do you occasionally drink heavily after a disappointment, a quarrel, or when the boss gives you a hard time?

_____ 2. When you have trouble or feel under pressure, do you drink more heavily than usual?

_____ 3. Have you noticed that you are able to handle more liquor than you did when you were first drinking?

_____ 4. Did you ever wake up on the "morning after" and discover that you could not remember part of the evening before, even though your friends tell you that you did not pass out?

_____ 5. When drinking with other people, do you try to have a few extra drinks when others will not know it?

_____ 6. Are there certain occasions when you feel uncomfortable if alcohol is not available?

_____ 7. Have you recently noticed that when you begin drinking you are in more of a hurry to get the first drink than you used to be?

_____ 8. Do you sometimes feel a little guilty about your drinking?

_____ 9. Are you secretly irritated when your family or friends discuss your drinking?

_____ 10. Have you recently noticed an increase in the frequency of your memory blackouts?

_____ 11. Do you often find that you wish to continue drinking after your friends say that they have had enough?

_____ 12. Do you have a reason for the occasions when you drink heavily?

_____ 13. When you are sober, do you often regret things you did or said while drinking?

_____ 14. Have you tried switching brands or following different plans for controlling your drinking?

_____ 15. Have you often failed to keep the promises you have made to yourself about controlling or cutting down your drinking?

_____ 16. Have you ever tried to control your drinking by making a change in jobs, or moving to a new location?

_____ 17. Do you try to avoid family or close friends while you are drinking?

_____ 18. Are you having an increasing number of financial and work problems?

_____ 19. Do more people seem to be treating you unfairly without good reason?

_____ 20. Do you eat very little or irregularly when you are drinking?

_____ 21. Do you sometimes have "the shakes" in the morning and find that it helps to have a little drink?

_____ 22. Do you sometimes stay drunk for several days at a time?

_____ 23. Do you sometimes feel very depressed and wonder whether life is worth living?

_____ 24. Sometimes after periods of drinking, do you see or hear things that aren't there?

_____ 25. Do you get terribly frightened after you have been drinking heavily?

Interpretation: If you answered "yes" to two or more of these questions, you may wish to evaluate your drinking behavior in terms of consistency and frequency. Use the following guide to score yourself on questions related to the various stages of alcoholism.

Questions 1 through 8 represent the early stage of alcoholism. If you checked one or more of these, it would be wise to watch your drinking behaviors carefully. Although many people stay at this stage throughout their lives, many others miss the chance to control their drinking before it progresses.

Questions 9 through 21 represent the middle stage of alcoholism. If you checked one or more of these, your dependence on alcohol is probably well established. Outside counseling might be helpful at this stage.

Questions 22 through 25 represent the final stage of alcoholism. If your answers indicate that you are in this stage, you should seek medical help.

CHAPTER 8 UNDERSTANDING THE DANGERS OF DRUG USE

Multiple Choice

1. The intentional misuse of a drug or chemical is called:
   a. addiction. c. drug misuse.
   b. withdrawal. d. drug abuse.
2. Physical dependence is another name for:
   a. tolerance. c. addiction.
   b. psychic dependence. d. withdrawal.
3. Taking one of your friend's prescription pain killers for your own headache is an example of:
   a. drug abuse. c. drug misuse.
   b. drug use. d. a drug reaction.
4. Marijuana and cocaine are examples of:
   a. OTCs. c. controlled substances.
   b. prescription drugs. d. barbiturates.
5. Pain relievers such as ibuprofen and aspirin are examples of:
   a. OTCs. c. controlled substances.
   b. prescription drugs. d. barbiturates.
6. Researchers have identified several risk factors for drug abuse among older teenagers and young adults, the most consistent and powerful predictor being:
   a. families. c. psychological variables.
   b. peer pressure. d. school problems and issues.
7. When two drugs are present in the system at one time but the effect of one reduces or blocks the effect of the other, the effects are referred to as:
   a. additive. c. synergistic.
   b. inhibitory. d. pronounced.
8. A term often used to describe the undesired effects of taking a large amount of a single drug is:
   a. overuse. c. misuse.
   b. overdose. d. dosage effect.
9. What do Librium, Valium, and Xanax have in common?
   a. They are all opiates. c. They are all stimulants.
   b. They are all amphetamines. d. They are all tranquilizers.
10. _____ are either made from or chemically similar to opium.
    a. Stimulants c. Narcotics
    b. Depressants d. Hallucinogens

True/False

T F 1. Habituation is a physical adaptation to a substance that causes it to become less effective with repeated use.

T F 2. The term "additive effect" refers to a drug interaction in which two drugs have a more powerful effect when taken together than they would have if taken separately.

T F 3. Drugs that activate the central nervous system are called stimulants.

T F 4 Cocaine abusers can sniff the drug into their noses, inject it into their bloodstream, or smoke it.

T F 5. Marijuana can be a stimulant, depressant, narcotic, or hallucinogen.

T F 6. The psychoactive drug in marijuana is hashish.

T F 7. While cocaine is highly addictive, tolerance develops slowly.

MULTIPLE CHOICE/TRUE FALSE—*continued*

T F 8. Ecstasy and Rohypnol are examples of club drugs.

T F 9. Anabolic steroids occur naturally in the body.

T F 10. Maintenance programs involve substituting a more socially acceptable and less dangerous drug for the drug of choice.

ANSWERS:

Multiple Choice: 1. d (p. 115), 2. c (p. 116), 3. c (p. 115), 4. c (p. 117), 5. a (p. 116), 6. b (p. 118), 7. b (p. 119), 8. b (p. 120), 9. d (p. 122), 10. c (p. 122).

True/False: 1. F (p. 115), 2. F (p. 119), 3. T (p. 120), 4. T (p. 122), 5. T (p. 122), 6. F (p. 122), 7. F (p. 122), 8. T (p. 123), 9. T (p. 123), 10. T (p. 124).

Name ______________________________ Date ____________ Section ______________

DO YOU HAVE A DRUG PROBLEM?

Directions: Answer the following questions by placing a check next to the appropriate boxes. Base your response on your behavior(s) over the last ten (10) years.

1. Which of the following have you tried more than once outside the direct care of a physician? (Score 2 points for each one checked.)

_____ caffeine

_____ cannabis (hashish, marijuana)

_____ cocaine powder

_____ crack

_____ PCP (angel dust)

_____ heroin, methadone, morphine

_____ LSD

_____ amphetamines

_____ barbiturates

_____ benzodiazapines (Valium and Librium)

2. How often do you use some form of psychoactive drug (exclude caffeine)?

_____ daily or almost daily (16 points)

_____ more often than once a week but less than daily (8 points)

_____ about once a week (4 points)

_____ about once a month (2 points)

_____ rarely if ever (1 point)

3. How would you feel if you did not use any psychoactive drug for more than three days?

_____ I would be very nervous and upset and have an uncontrollable urge to find a drug to use. (16 points)

_____ I would want to use a drug very much but could definitely control myself. (8 points)

_____ I would think quite a bit about using a drug. (4 points)

_____ I would think a little about using a drug. (2 points)

_____ I wouldn't notice that I hadn't used it. (1 point)

4. Which of the following have you recently experienced that accompanied your use of drugs? (Score 3 points for each one checked.)

   _____ missing work or school

   _____ fighting with family or friends

   _____ becoming belligerent, insulting, or fighting

   _____ chest pains

   _____ difficulty breathing

   _____ feelings of dizziness, nausea, or vertigo

5. Which of the following have you experienced recently? (Score 2 points for each one checked.)

   _____ withdrawal symptoms when drug use has been delayed

   _____ an ability to take increased doses of a drug

   _____ a need to take an increased dose of a drug to get a desired effect

   _____ no effect from a drug that used to get you high

   _____ the use of a drug at the same time every day

   _____ losing track of how many times you have used a drug or how much you have taken

   _____ using more than one drug during the same time period

Assessment: Total the points as indicated with each question. Look at the chart below to assess your relationship with drugs.

Score	Label	Danger Rating
2–5	Nonuser	–
6–19	Experimenter	X
20–35	Moderate user	XX
36–50	Heavy user	XXX
51–90	Problem user	XXXX–see a counselor **NOW**

Source: Modified from Joan Luckman's *Your Health!* Englewood Cliffs, NJ: Prentice Hall, 1990.

Multiple Choice

1. Which of the following statements is true regarding unintentional injuries?
   a. Many injuries may be caused by risk-taking behaviors.
   b. Many injuries are caused by hazards in the environment.
   c. Injuries may result from psychological factors.
   d. All of the above are true.
2. The leading cause of death in the United States among 15–24-year-olds is:
   a. homicides. c. unintentional injuries.
   b. suicides. d. cancer.
3. Studies show that motor vehicle accidents in which alcohol plays a role are:
   a. the number one cause of preventable traffic fatalities.
   b. less severe than other crashes.
   c. less fatal than other crashes.
   d. the fifth leading cause of death for all population groups.
4. Which of the following population groups accounts for the largest percentage of unintentional injuries?
   a. men of all ages
   b. teenagers between the ages of 13 and 19
   c. women of all ages
   d. elderly citizens over 65 years of age
5. Motor vehicles account for what percent of all unintentional injuries in the United States?
   a. 25% c. 50%
   b. 33% d. 67%
6. Injuries caused by interpersonal violence such as homicide and assault are sometimes termed:
   a. nonviolent injuries. c. accidental injuries.
   b. natural disasters. d. intentional injuries.
7. Which of the following factors has been linked to violent behavior in the United States?
   a. influence of drugs c. viewing violence on TV
   b. availability of handguns d. all of the above
8. Most acts of violence are committed by:
   a. men. c. people between the ages of 15 and 24.
   b. women. d. the elderly over 65 years of age.
9. A form of verbal battery requiring the abused person to perform demanding, demeaning, and unreasonable tasks is called:
   a. physical abuse. c. social abuse.
   b. psychological abuse. d. sexual abuse.
10. Sexual harassment is a criminal offense involving:
    a. the abuse of power.
    b. personal problems of inadequacy.
    c. a person who is sexually unfulfilled.
    d. a person who feels the need for being dominated.

True/False

T F 1. Deaths from unintentional injuries are more prevalent in urban areas.

T F 2. Falls are the primary reason for on-the-job fatalities.

T F 3. It is illegal in every state to sell alcoholic beverages to anyone under the age of 21.

T F 4. All states have mandatory seat belt use laws.

MULTIPLE CHOICE/TRUE FALSE—*continued*

T F 5. The primary cause of drowning among young adult men is alcohol use in conjunction with water activities.

T F 6. Violence is defined as the use of force with the intent to harm oneself or another person.

T F 7. Wealthy people are more likely to be robbed, raped, or assaulted than poorer people.

T F 8. Homicides are the third leading external cause of death after unintentional injuries and suicide in the United States.

T F 9. Women are more likely to be victims of domestic abuse than men.

T F 10. Forced sexual intercourse between individuals who know each other is termed stranger rape.

ANSWERS:

Multiple Choice: 1. d (p. 132, 133), 2. c (p. 132), 3. a (p. 132), 4. a (p. 133),
5. c (p. 133), 6. d (p. 132), 7. d (p. 138), 8. a (p. 138), 9. b (p. 142), 10. a (p. 142).
True/False: 1. F (p. 133), 2. F (p. 133), 3. T (p. 133), 4. F (p. 133), 5. T (p. 135),
6. T (p. 138), 7. F (p. 138), 8. T (p. 139), 9. T (p. 142), 10. F (p. 144).

Name ____________________ Date ____________ Section ____________

CHARACTERISTICS OF PERPETRATORS OF WORKPLACE VIOLENCE

Directions: Indicate whether or not you work with someone who exhibits the following characteristics.

Yes No Prior verbal threats: If the employee engages in threatening conduct toward other employees or supervisors, this threat should be taken seriously and the employer should respond in an appropriate manner.

Yes No Intimidating behavior: The employee may exhibit any of the following behaviors: repeated phone calls to the victim, following the victim, and/or leaving messages for the victim.

Yes No Mental health problems: Depression, fantasies, irrational/violent thoughts, paranoid delusions, and extreme mood swings all may indicate a potential for workplace violence.

Yes No Obsessions: The employee may be preoccupied with weapons and/or the military, or hurting a specific person. He or she may believe a romantic attachment exists with a co-worker.

Yes No Decline in performance: Recent excessive and unexplained absences from the job, concentration problems, increased signs of poor health or hygiene and the inability to accept responsibility for errors.

Yes No Stress: Increased stress in the employee's personal life including financial problems, problems in his or her marriage or other relationships, inappropriate display of emotions on the job such as uncontrolled anger or excessive crying.

Yes No Substance abuse: Some drugs increase paranoia and others can cause aggressive behavior. Alcohol is present in many violent situations. While there is no scientific evidence to substantiate that substance abuse causes violence, it is present in many of the reported cases of violent behavior.

Interpretation: For every "Yes" you circled, you have identified a common characteristic of those who commit violence in the workplace. These characteristics should give you reason to be more suspicious or careful in any given situation. However, law enforcement personnel still do not have the ability to predict violent behavior in certain specific situations. No definite profile has been accepted by the professionals in this area.

Source: Workplace Violence: Its Nature and Extent, Office for Victims of Crime, Office of Justice Programs, U.S. Department of Justice

CHAPTER 10 REDUCING THE RISK FOR CHRONIC DISEASE

Multiple Choice

1. The leading cause of death in the United States is:
   a. chronic disease.
   b. communicable disease.
   c. suicide.
   d. homicide.
2. Chronic illnesses have all BUT which of the following common characteristics/traits?
   a. They involve some form of permanence.
   b. They result in some form of disability.
   c. They are progressive in nature.
   d. They require short periods of care.
3. Which of the following is NOT considered a chronic disease?
   a. cancer
   b. pneumonia
   c. asthma
   d. diabetes
4. Risk factors for cardiovascular disease that are not related to lifestyle include all BUT which of the following?
   a. family history of the disease
   b. smoking
   c. age
   d. sex (gender)
5. Severe chest pain occurring as a result of reduced blood supply to the heart is called:
   a. myocardial infarction.
   b. angina pectoris.
   c. arrhythmia.
   d. transient ischemia.
6. An irregularity in heartbeat is called:
   a. fibrillation.
   b. tachycardia.
   c. bradycardia.
   d. arrhythmia.
7. Benign tumors:
   a. do not spread by metastatic growth.
   b. eventually change into cancerous tumors.
   c. can do no physical damage.
   d. appear only in the heart muscle.
8. Carcinogens are:
   a. cancer-blocking agents.
   b. cancer-causing substances.
   c. cancer-causing genes.
   d. antigens located in the bloodstream.
9. The process by which cancer spreads from one area to different areas of the body is called:
   a. promoter.
   b. initiator.
   c. metastasis.
   d. mutation.
10. The most common site of cancer for both men and women is the:
    a. lung.
    b. skin.
    c. colon or rectum.
    d. bladder.

True/False

T F 1. The term asymptomatic refers to a period in which a disease exists without any outward signs or clinical symptoms.

T F 2. Alcohol consumption is the single most important factor associated with heart disease.

T F 3. An electrocardiogram is an instrument that records nerve activity.

T F 4. Atherosclerosis is also known as arteriosclerosis.

T F 5. Myocardial infarctions are the number one killer in the United States.

MULTIPLE CHOICE/TRUE FALSE—*continued*

T F 6. A stroke is also known as a myocardial infarction.

T F 7. Cancer is the leading cause of death in the United States.

T F 8. The single behavior that most often results in death from cancer is alcohol consumption.

T F 9. Studies suggest that taking estrogen by post–menopausal women can contribute to cancer of the uterus.

T F 10. A mammography is a screening technique used to detect breast cancer.

ANSWERS:

Multiple Choice: 1. a (p. 150), 2. d (p. 151), 3. b (p. 150), 4. b (p. 152), 5. b (p. 155),
6. d (p. 155), 7. a (p. 157), 8. b (p. 157), 9. c (p. 158), 10. a (p. 159).
True/False: 1. T (p. 151), 2. F (p. 152), 3. F (p. 154), 4. T (p. 155), 5. T (p. 155),
6. F (p. 156), 7. F (p. 157), 8. F (p. 158), 9. T (p. 159), 10. T (p. 162).

Name ______________________ Date ____________ Section ____________

CHECK YOUR HEALTHY HEART I.Q.

Directions: Answer "true" or "false" to the following questions to test your knowledge of heart disease and its risk factors.

_____ 1. The risk factors for heart disease that you can do something about are: high blood pressure, high blood cholesterol, smoking, obesity, and physical inactivity.

_____ 2. A stroke is often the first symptom of high blood pressure, and a heart attack is often the first symptom of high blood cholesterol.

_____ 3. A blood pressure greater than or equal to 140/90 mm Hg is generally considered to be high.

_____ 4. High blood pressure affects the same number of blacks as it does whites.

_____ 5. The best ways to treat and control high blood pressure are to control your weight, exercise, eat less salt (sodium), restrict your intake of alcohol, and take your blood pressure medication, if prescribed by your doctor.

_____ 6. A blood cholesterol of 240 mg/dL is desirable for adults.

_____ 7. The most effective dietary way to lower the level of your blood cholesterol is to eat foods low in cholesterol.

_____ 8. Lowering blood cholesterol levels can help people who have already had a heart attack.

_____ 9. Only children from families at high risk of heart disease need to have their blood cholesterol levels checked.

_____ 10. Smoking is a major risk factor for four of the five leading causes of death including heart attack, stroke, cancer, and lung diseases such as emphysema and bronchitis.

_____ 11. If you have had a heart attack, quitting smoking can help reduce your chances of having a second attack.

_____ 12. Someone who has smoked for 30 to 40 years probably will not be able to quit smoking.

_____ 13. The best way to lose weight is to increase physical activity and eat fewer calories.

_____ 14. Heart disease is the leading killer of men and women in the United States.

Scoring: Compare your responses with the correct quiz answers and explanations that follow:

1. True. High blood pressure, smoking, and high blood cholesterol are the three most important risk factors for heart disease. On the average, each one doubles your chance of developing heart disease. So, a person who has all three of the risk factors is 8 times more likely to develop heart disease than someone who has none. Obesity increases the likelihood of developing high blood cholesterol and high blood pressure, which increase your risk of heart disease. Physical inactivity increases your risk for heart attack. Regular exercise and good nutrition are essential to reducing high blood pressure, high blood cholesterol, and overweight.

2. True. A person with high blood pressure or high blood cholesterol may feel fine and look great; there are often no signs that anything is wrong until a stroke or heart attack occurs. To find out if you have high blood pressure or high blood cholesterol, you should be tested by a doctor, nurse, or other health professional.

3. True. A blood pressure of 140/90 mm Hg or greater is generally classified as high blood pressure. However, blood pressures that fall below 140/90 mm Hg can sometimes be a problem. If the diastolic pressure, the second or lower number, is between 85 and 89, a person is at an increased risk for heart disease or stroke and should have

his/her blood pressure checked at least once a year by a health professional. The higher your blood pressure, the greater your risk of developing heart disease or stroke. Controlling high blood pressure reduces your risk.

4. False. High blood pressure is more common in blacks than whites. It affects 29 out of every 100 black adults compared to 26 out of every 100 white adults. Also, with aging, high blood pressure is generally more severe among blacks than among whites, and therefore causes more strokes, heart disease, and kidney failure.

5. True. Recent studies show that lifestyle changes can help keep blood pressure levels normal even into advanced age and are important in treating and preventing high blood pressure. Limit high-salt foods, which include many snack foods such as potato chips, salted pretzels, and salted crackers; processed foods such as canned soups; and condiments such as ketchup and soy sauce. Also, it is extremely important to take blood pressure medication, if prescribed by your doctor, to make sure your blood pressure stays under control.

6. False. A total blood cholesterol of under 200 mg/dL is desirable and usually puts you at a lower risk for heart disease. A blood cholesterol level of 240 mg/dL or above is high and increases your risk of heart disease. If your cholesterol level is high, your doctor will want to check your levels of LDL-cholesterol ("bad" cholesterol) and HDL-cholesterol ("good" cholesterol). A HIGH level of LDL-cholesterol increases your risk for heart disease, as does a LOW level of HDL-cholesterol. All adults 20 years of age or older should have their blood cholesterol level checked at least once every 5 years.

7. False. Reducing the amount of cholesterol in your diet is important; however, eating foods low in saturated fat is the most effective dietary way to lower blood cholesterol levels, along with eating less total fat and cholesterol. Choose foods low in saturated fats, such as grains, fruits, and vegetables; low-fat or skim milk and milk products; lean cuts of meat; fish; and chicken. Reducing overweight will also help lower your level of LDL-cholesterol as well as increase your level of HDL-cholesterol.

8. True. People who have had one heart attack are at a much higher risk for a second attack. Reducing blood cholesterol levels can greatly slow down (and, in some people, even reverse) the buildup of cholesterol and fat in the walls of the arteries and significantly reduce the chances of a second heart attack.

9. True. Children from "high risk" families, in which a parent has high blood cholesterol (240 mg/dL or above) or in which a parent or grandparent has had heart disease at an early age (at 55 years of age or younger), should have their cholesterol levels tested. If a child from such a family has a cholesterol level that is high, it should be lowered under medical supervision, primarily with diet, to reduce the risk of developing heart disease as an adult.

10. True. Heavy smokers are 2 to 4 times more likely to have a heart attack than nonsmokers, and the heart attack death rate among all smokers is 70 percent greater than that of nonsmokers. Older male smokers are also nearly twice as likely to die from stroke than older men who do not smoke, and these odds are nearly as high for older female smokers. Further, the risk of dying from lung cancer is 22 times higher for male smokers than male nonsmokers and 12 times higher for female smokers than female nonsmokers. Finally, 80 percent of all deaths from emphysema and bronchitis are directly due to smoking.

11. True. One year after quitting, ex-smokers cut their extra risk for heart attack by about half or more, and eventually the risk will return to normal in healthy ex-smokers. Even if you have already had a heart attack, you can reduce your chances of a second attack if you quit smoking. Ex-smokers can also reduce their risk of smoke and cancer, improve blood flow and lung function, and help stop diseases like emphysema and bronchitis from getting worse.

12. False. Older smokers are more likely to succeed at quitting smoking than younger smokers. Quitting helps relieve smoking-related symptoms like shortness of breath, coughing, and chest pain. Many quit to avoid further health problems and take control of their lives.

13. True. Weight control is a question of balance. You get calories from the foods you eat. You burn off calories by exercising. Cutting down on calories, especially calories from fat, is key to losing weight. Losing weight, if you are overweight, may also reduce your blood pressure, lower your LDL-cholesterol, and raise your HDL-cholesterol.

14. True. Coronary heart disease is the number one killer in the United States. Approximately 489,000 Americans died of coronary heart disease in 1990, and approximately half of the deaths were women.

Source: U.S. Department of Health and Human Services, Public Health Service, NATIONAL INSTITUTES OF HEALTH. Revised October 1992, Updated August 1996

CHAPTER 11 REDUCING THE RISK FOR INFECTIOUS DISEASE

Multiple Choice

1. A disease-causing agent is called a(n):
   a. pathogen. c. erythrocyte.
   b. leukocyte. d. T–cell.
2. Antibiotics have no effect in treating which infections?
   a. strep throat/pneumonia c. TB/cholera
   b. herpes/AIDS d. gonorrhea/whooping cough
3. Which of the following conditions is associated with whether or not a person will get sick?
   a. the virulence or strength of the causative agent
   b. the dosage of the causative agent
   c. the degree of resistance of the individual to infection
   d. all of the above
4. What two body structures act as the first line of defense against infectious diseases?
   a. the circulatory and respiratory systems
   b. the nervous and muscular systems
   c. the skin and mucous membranes
   d. the phagocytes and monocytes
5. Phagocytes are:
   a. white blood cells that attack foreign invaders.
   b. vaccines.
   c. the parts of a pathogen that link with human cells.
   d. inflammatory agents.
6. During what stage in the course of an infectious disease is the illness easily and unknowingly spread?
   a. the prodromal period c. the incubation period
   b. the acute stage d. convalescence
7. Pneumonia is known to be caused by:
   a. viruses. c. chemical irritants.
   b. bacteria. d. all of the above.
8. The one common factor that all sexually transmitted infections (STIs) share is:
   a. they have an affinity for the moist, warm genital areas.
   b. they are caused by the same pathogen.
   c. they can be treated with the same antibiotic.
   d. cure rates are very low.
9. AIDS is caused by the virus:
   a. herpes simplex. c. human immunodeficiency.
   b. Kaposi's sarcoma. d. human papilloma.
10. A serious complication from chlamydia infection for women is:
    a. pelvic inflammatory disease. c. yeast infection.
    b. vaginitis. d. pubic lice.

True/False

T F 1. Noninfectious diseases are contagious.

T F 2. Rickettsias, which cause diseases like Rocky Mountain spotted fever, are usually transmitted by insects.

T F 3. People who have a high resistance to disease are less likely to get sick.

T F 4. With passive immunity, the body develops a lifelong immunity to the disease.

T F 5. Tuberculosis initially affects the muscles but can settle into the kidneys, brain, heart, liver, and bones.

T F 6. Hepatitis is an inflammation of the kidneys.

T F 7. As with a chlamydia infection, 80 percent of women with gonorrhea have no symptoms in the early stages.

T F 8. At any stage, syphilis can be diagnosed by visual observation and/or confirmed with a blood test.

T F 9. The main treatment for syphilis is penicillin.

T F 10. Another term for pubic lice is warts.

ANSWERS:

Multiple Choice: 1. a (p. 173), 2. b (p. 176), 3. d (p. 177), 4. c (p. 177), 5. a (p. 177), 6. a (p. 180), 7. d (p. 182), 8. a (p. 184), 9. c (p. 187), 10. a (p. 191).

True/False: 1. F (p. 173), 2. T (p. 176), 3. T (p. 177), 4. F (p. 178), 5. F (p. 183), 6. F (p. 187), 7. T (p. 191), 8. T (p. 192), 9. T (p. 192), 10. F (p. 192).

Name ______________________ Date ____________ Section ____________

AM I REDUCING MY RISK OF INFECTIOUS DISEASE?

Directions: Circle the answer that best applies to you.

	Never		Sometimes		Always
1. My immunizations are up to date.	1	2	3	4	5
2. I wash my hands after bathroom visits.	1	2	3	4	5
3. I wash my hands frequently during the winter months.	1	2	3	4	5
4. My genetic background includes immune deficiency diseases.	5	4	3	2	1
5. I am at risk of HIV infection.	5	4	3	2	1
6. I have blood-to-blood contact with others.	5	4	3	2	1
7. I consider food safety when preparing foods.	1	2	3	4	5
8. I have good eating habits.	1	2	3	4	5
9. I have good exercise habits.	1	2	3	4	5
10. I get plenty of rest.	1	2	3	4	5
11. I maintain a positive mental attitude.	1	2	3	4	5
12. I bathe on a regular basis.	1	2	3	4	5
13. I brush my teeth on a regular basis.	1	2	3	4	5
14. I treat all minor infections seriously.	1	2	3	4	5
15. I know how to obtain reliable infectious disease-related information, products, and services.	1	2	3	4	5

Conclusion: Add up your score. The maximum score is 75. The higher the score, the higher your protection against infectious disease.

1. Which area(s) did you score the highest (4 or 5 points)? ______________________
2. Which area(s) did you score the lowest (2 or 3 points)? ______________________
3. What is one change I could make to lower my infectious disease risk? ______________________

Source: Rohwer, J.L. and Wandberg, R., *Personalizing Health Action Plans: A Student Resource Manual.* Copyright 1999. Allyn and Bacon.

CHAPTER 12 SEXUALITY: DEVELOPING HEALTHY RELATIONSHIPS

Multiple Choice

1. Gender identity is apparent through an individual's:
   a. reproductive organs.
   b. sex role behavior.
   c. sexual orientation.
   d. intimacy level.
2. Sexual orientation refers to:
   a. a person's attraction to individuals of a particular gender.
   b. a state of comfort with one's gender and sex role.
   c. an ability to respond to erotic stimulation with pleasure.
   d. an ability to make mature judgments about sexuality.
3. This sexual orientation is based on an attraction to individuals of both sexes:
   a. heterosexual.
   b. homosexual.
   c. bisexual.
   d. polygamy.
4. According to the Triangular Theory of Love, which of the following is NOT a key ingredient of love?
   a. intimacy.
   b. passion.
   c. infatuation.
   d. commitment.
5. The biological urge or appetite for sexual activity is also known as:
   a. sexual orientation.
   b. libido.
   c. sex role identity.
   d. intimacy level.
6. The erogenous zones include the:
   a. genitals and breasts.
   b. genitals only.
   c. brain and body's extremities like the hands and feet.
   d. body's senses, which include smell, taste, and feeling.
7. Coitus is another name for:
   a. fellatio.
   b. intercourse.
   c. entercourse.
   d. foreplay.
8. The inability to achieve and maintain an erection long enough to participate in sexual intercourse is called:
   a. impotence.
   b. erectile dysfunction.
   c. premature ejaculation.
   d. dyspareunia.
9. Dyspareunia is a term associated with:
   a. failure to reach orgasm.
   b. involuntary constriction of the vagina.
   c. painful intercourse.
   d. sexual addiction.
10. Which therapeutic technique teaches couples the nonverbal communication of touch?
    a. rational-emotive therapy
    b. sensate focus therapy
    c. aversion therapy
    d. psychotherapy

True/False

T F 1. The hormones that most directly affect sexuality are androgens for males and estrogens for females.

T F 2. Men who have an androgen deficiency have a decrease in sexual responsiveness and sexual drive.

T F 3. Individuals who have a homosexual orientation are often referred to as gay or lesbian.

T F 4. Sexual abstinence is a behavioral choice to not engage in sexual intercourse.

T F 5. Passion is the cognitive component of the Triangular Theory of Love.

T F 6. Sex drive refers to the pooling of blood in tissues that takes place during sexual excitement.

T F 7. Myotonia refers to the pooling of blood in tissues that takes place during sexual excitement.

T F 8. Breakdowns in relationships usually begin with changes in communication.

T F 9. An inhibited sexual desire is the persistent or recurrent absence of desire for sexual activity.

T F 10. The inability to achieve orgasm by a woman is known as impotence.

ANSWERS:

Multiple Choice: 1. b (p. 199), 2. a (p. 202), 3. c (p. 202), 4. c (p. 203), 5. b (p. 206),
6. a (p. 206), 7. b (p. 206), 8. a (p. 209), 9. c (p. 210), 10. b (p. 210).
True/False: 1. T (p. 201), 2. T (p. 201), 3. T (p. 202), 4. T (p. 203), 5. F (p. 204),
6. F (p. 206), 7. F (p. 207), 8. T (p. 203), 9. T (p. 208), 10. F (p. 210).

Name ______________________ Date ____________ Section ____________

MUEHLENHARD-QUACKENBUSH SEXUAL ATTITUDE SCALE

Directions: Read each of the statements below carefully and respond using the scale provided.

A=Agree Strongly B=Agree Mildly C=Disagree Mildly D=Disagree Strongly

_____ 1. It's worse for a woman to sleep around than a man.

_____ 2. It's best for a guy to lose his virginity before he's out of his teens.

_____ 3. It's okay for a woman to have more than one sexual relationship at a time.

_____ 4. It is just as important for a man to be a virgin when he marries as it is for a woman.

_____ 5. I approve of a 16-year-old girl having sex just as much as a 16-year-old boy having sex.

_____ 6. I kind of admire a girl who has had sex with a lot of guys.

_____ 7. I feel kind of sorry for a 21-year-old woman who is still a virgin.

_____ 8. A woman having casual sex is just as acceptable to me as a man having casual sex.

_____ 9. It's OK for a man to have sex with a woman he's not in love with.

_____ 10. I kind of admire a man who has had sex with a lot of girls.

_____ 11. A woman who initiates sex is too aggressive.

_____ 12. It's OK for a man to have more than one sexual relationship at a time.

_____ 13. I question the character of a woman who has had a lot of sexual partners.

_____ 14. I admire a man who is a virgin when he gets married.

_____ 15. A man should be more sexually experienced than his wife.

_____ 16. A girl who has had sex on the first date is easy.

_____ 17. I kind of feel sorry for a 21-year-old man who is still a virgin.

_____ 18. I question the character of a guy who has had a lot of sexual partners.

_____ 19. Women are naturally more monogamous (inclined to stick to one partner) than are men.

_____ 20. A man should be sexually experienced when he gets married.

_____ 21. A guy who has sex on the first date is easy.

_____ 22. It's OK for a woman to have sex with a man she is not in love with.

_____ 23. A woman should be sexually experienced when she gets married.

_____ 24. It's best for a girl to lose her virginity before she's out of her teens.

_____ 25. I admire a woman who is a virgin when she gets married.

_____ 26. A man who initiates sex is too aggressive.

Scoring: Convert your A's to zeros, your B's to 1s, your C's to 2s, your D's to 3s. Computing your total involves some simple mathematics:

#4 + #5 + #8 + (3 – #1) + (3 – #15) + (3 – #19) + (#24 – #2) + (#3 – #12) + (#6 – #10) + (#7 – #17) + (#22 – #9) + (#26 – #11) + (#18 – #13) + (#14 – #25) + (21 – #16) + (#23 – #20) = Your Total

Interpretation: The actual name of the scale is the Sexual Double Standard Scale. A person having identical sexual standards for women and men should score zero. A score greater than zero reflects more restrictive sexual standards for women than for men; the highest possible score is 48. A score less than zero reflects more restrictive sexual standards for men than for women; the lowest possible score is –30.

From a sample of college students at a large southwestern university, researchers found that a mean score for women to be 11.99 (N=461) and a mean score for men to be 13.15 (N=255).

Source: Charlene L Muehlenhard and Debra M. Quackenbush *The Sexual Double Standard Scale,* Department of Psychology and Women's Studies University of Kansas. Reprinted with permission.

Multiple Choice

1. The _____ family consists of those who are connected by blood, marriage, or adoption.
   a. nuclear
   b. extended
   c. dysfunctional
   d. single-parent
2. The diagnostic tool that allows the physician to see indirectly the developing fetus and its individual organ systems is called a:
   a. chorionic villus sampling.
   b. mammogram.
   c. CAT scan.
   d. sonogram.
3. A test of the mother's blood to evaluate some health-related conditions of the fetus can detect levels of _____ produced by the fetus's kidneys.
   a. alpha-fetoprotein
   b. beta-fetoprotein
   c. amniocentesis
   d. thalidomide
4. Both amniocentesis and chorionic villus sampling involve which of the following risks to the mother and fetus?
   a. spontaneous abortion
   b. infection
   c. missing or underdeveloped appendages
   d. all of the above
5. Pregnancy can be accurately detected soon after conception by the presence of the hormone _____.
   a. estrogen
   b. progesterone
   c. human chorionic gonadotropin
   d. thalidomide
6. During the first stage of labor:
   a. the amniotic sac breaks.
   b. the baby shifts into a head-down position.
   c. the junction of the pubic bones loosens to permit expansion of the pelvic girth.
   d. all of the above occur.
7. During the third stage of labor:
   a. contractions become more rhythmic and painful.
   b. the amniotic sac breaks.
   c. the baby shifts into a head-down position.
   d. the placenta or afterbirth is expelled from the womb.
8. A cesarean section may be performed when:
   a. the labor is progressing incorrectly.
   b. the mother's blood pressure falls rapidly.
   c. the position of the baby is feet first.
   d. any of the above occurs.
9. Depo-Provera is an example of a(n):
   a. male condom.
   b. injectable birth control drug.
   c. spermicide.
   d. diaphragm.

10. A small plastic device that is implanted by a physician in a woman's uterus to prevent conception is called a(n):
    a. cervical cap.
    b. diaphragm.
    c. intrauterine device.
    d. female condom.

True/False

T F 1. A nuclear family consists of parents and their siblings.

T F 2. Statistically, more women than men remarry after divorce.

T F 3. Research supports the notion that one good reason for wanting a child is that it provides stability to a couple's marriage.

T F 4. Smoking during pregnancy is with higher infant mortality and low birthweight babies.

T F 5. An amniocentesis provides physicians with a reliable way to study fetal cells to test for the presence, or absence, of genetic conditions.

T F 6. The Lamaze method of birthing relies on the use of drugs to relieve pain rather than the art of relaxation.

T F 7. Crowning refers to a breech birth.

T F 8. An incision between the opening of the vagina and the anus to allow ease of passage through the birth canal is known as an episiotomy.

T F 9. Sterilization of the male by cutting and tying of the vas deferens is called tubal ligation.

T F 10. Spontaneous abortions are also referred to as miscarriages.

ANSWERS:

Multiple Choice: 1. b (p. 215), 2. d (p. 221), 3. a (p. 221), 4. d (p. 221), 5. c (p. 219), 6. a (p. 223), 7. d (p. 225), 8. d (p. 225), 9. b (p. 226), 10. c (p. 230).
True/False: 1. F (p. 215), 2. F (p. 216), 3. F (p. 218), 4. T (p. 220), 5. T (p. 221), 6. F (p. 223), 7. F (p. 225), 8. T (p. 225), 9. F (p. 230), 10. T (p. 232).

Name ______________________________ Date ____________ Section ______________

ARE YOU READY FOR A HEALTHY PREGNANCY?

Directions: Indicate which behaviors match your (or your female partner's) behaviors by putting a check mark in the appropriate column.

	Done	Will Do	Won't Do
1. Get a physical exam.	____	____	____
2. Reduce your use of tobacco, alcohol, caffeine, and non-prescription drugs.	____	____	____
3. Get to an optimal weight.	____	____	____
4. Establish a well-balanced, nutritious diet that includes plenty of folic acid.	____	____	____
5. Maintain a regular exercise routine.	____	____	____
6. Talk to your health care professional about any chronic medical conditions you might have.	____	____	____
7. Get any necessary vaccinations.	____	____	____
8. If you are using a hormonal contraceptive method, change to another method.	____	____	____
9. If you are a cat owner, make arrangements for someone else to deal with the kitty litter.	____	____	____
10. Avoid any exposure to X rays.	____	____	____
11. Avoid extremes in body temperatures (e.g., hot tubs).	____	____	____

Interpretation: If all your responses were in the "Done" column, you (or your female partner) are in a good position—from a health point of view—to begin attempting to become pregnant. (Remember, however, that this survey does not replace the need for seeing a physician to truly determine your readiness.) Responses in the "Will Do" column indicate that you are contemplating steps to take to ensure a healthy pregnancy. Any responses in the "Won't Do" column indicate that you are failing to take precautions necessary for a healthy pregnancy.

Source: Based on "From Data to Action," CDC's Public Health Surveillance for Women, Infants and Children

Multiple Choice

1. The specialists who study the social, biological, behavioral, and psychological aspects of aging are:
   a. orthopedists.
   b. podiatrists.
   c. gerontologists.
   d. chiropractors.
2. The _____ theory of aging suggests that foreign elements in the blood accumulate over time in the body.
   a. wear and tear
   b. free radicals
   c. biological clock
   d. high density lipoprotein
3. Which of the following is NOT considered a common measure of one's age?
   a. chronological age
   b. functional age
   c. psychological age
   d. social age
4. A common measure for age that best represents the physiological capacity of the body is:
   a. functional age
   b. chronological age
   c. psychological age
   d. social age
5. More people over the age of 65 die of _____ than of any other cause.
   a. heart disease
   b. cancer
   c. chronic respiratory ailment
   d. stroke
6. The _____ is/are the organs most resistant to change due to aging, provided it is/they are cared for.
   a. heart
   b. lungs
   c. kidneys
   d. liver and pancreas
7. A degenerative bone disease characterized by weakened muscles and decreased bone mass is:
   a. osteoporosis.
   b. hyperglycemia.
   c. calcification.
   d. Alzheimer's.
8. The study of death and psychological and social problems associated with it is called:
   a. gerontology.
   b. thanatology.
   c. mortology.
   d. pediatrics.
9. Administering a lethal drug to hasten the death of a suffering, terminally ill patient is called:
   a. euthanasia.
   b. fantasia.
   c. dyathesia.
   d. cryptothesia.

10. The process of preserving a body using chemicals for open casket viewing is called:
    a. cremation.
    b. columbarium.
    c. embalming.
    d. entombment.

True/False

T F 1. The U.S. Census Bureau defines the elderly as people between the ages of 65 and 74.

T F 2. The ways in which people compare to others of similar age is called biological age.

T F 3. Psychological age represents a perceived age (or how old one feels).

T F 4. Women are at a significantly lower risk for osteoporosis after menopause.

T F 5. Heredity is not a risk factor for osteoporosis.

T F 6. Presbyopia is a condition caused by clouding within the lens of the eye.

T F 7. Incontinence affects all people over the age of 75.

T F 8. Brain death is confirmed by an electroencephalogram (EEG).

T F 9. The goal of hospice care is to relieve pain and suffering during the dying process.

T F 10. Bereavement is the process of grieving that occurs as a result of the death of a loved one.

ANSWERS:

Multiple Choice: 1. c (p. 238), 2. b (p. 238), 3. d (p. 239), 4. a (p. 239), 5. a (p. 239), 6. b (p. 239), 7. a (p. 240), 8. b (p. 244), 9. a (p. 245), 10. c (p. 248).
True/False: 1. T (p. 238), 2. F (p. 239), 3. T (p. 239), 4. F (p. 240), 5. F (p. 240), 6. F (p. 240), 7. F (p. 241), 8. T (p. 244), 9. T (p. 247), 10. T (p. 248).

Name ______________________________ Date ____________ Section ____________

WHAT'S YOUR HOSPICE I.Q.?

Directions: Take this quiz by answering each of the questions below "yes" or "no." When you've completed the quiz, see the table below to check your score and your hospice smarts!

Did *you* know that hospice care:	Yes	No
1. Is made up of an entire group of coordinated services especially designed for people with serious, life limiting illnesses?	____	____
2. Is for the whole family, not just the dying patient?	____	____
3. Is offered according to a plan developed with the patient and the family so that the services meet their needs and expectations?	____	____
4. Focuses on quality of life and includes not only medical and nursing care but also bereavement and spiritual support?	____	____
5. Is provided by an entire team of doctors, nurses, social workers, chaplains, nurse aids, and volunteers?	____	____
6. Is provided by hospice doctors and nurses who are experts in controlling pain and other discomforts?	____	____
7. Ensures that nearly all patients get some relief from pain and other uncomfortable symptoms that often accompany the dying process?	____	____
8. Is offered to people with many different kinds of serious, life-limiting conditions such as cancer, pulmonary disease, heart disease, neurological disorders, Alzheimer's disease, and AIDS?	____	____
9. Serves most patients at home in comfortable, familiar surroundings?	____	____
10. Provides all the equipment and the supplies that are needed to care for a family member at home?	____	____
11. Provides staff who make regular visits to care for the patient and to check in with the family about how they are doing?	____	____
12. Provides staff who teach family members how to take care of the patient at home and what to expect at every stage?	____	____
13. Is available 7-days a week, 24-hours a day with staff to answer questions and offer emotional support?	____	____
14. Provides volunteers to help the patients and family with practical chores and offer emotional support?	____	____
15. Can be provided in hospice inpatient facilities, hospitals, or nursing homes when it is not possible to care for a patient at home?	____	____
16. Offers bereavement services to family members for at least a year after the death of the patient?	____	____
17. Is paid for completely by the Medicare hospice benefit for any Medicare beneficiary?	____	____

18. Is covered by Medicaid in 43 states? _____ _____

19. Is covered by most health insurance and managed health care plans? _____ _____

20. Is covered so well that most hospice patients pay little or nothing directly for hospice care, thus saving the family large medical expenses that often accumulate near the end of life? _____ _____

How did you score?

Assessment: Give yourself 5 points for each "yes" answer, and check score and your hospice smarts below!

85–100 —You are a hospice expert and ready to assist a seriously ill family member or friend to obtain this excellent care near the end of life.
60–80 —You know a lot more about the importance of hospice care than most other Americans.
40–55 —You know about hospice, but probably didn't realize some important facts about this special care available to people as they approach the end of life.
20–35 —You may be missing out on a chance to help a seriously ill family member or friend obtain the special services of hospice as they near the end of life.
5–15 —You have heard of hospice care, but haven't heard about its unique, important benefits for people who are dying and for their family.
0 —You're missing out on important knowledge that could help family members and friends enormously.

Source: Reprinted 2003 with permission of Partnership for Caring, Washington, D.C. 1-800-989-9455.

Multiple Choice

1. A type of toxic chemical capable of promoting birth defects is said to be:
   a. carcinogenic.
   b. pharmogenic.
   c. mutagenic.
   d. teratogenic.
2. When a substance is capable of promoting genetic alterations in cells, it is said to be:
   a. carcinogenic.
   b. pharmogenic.
   c. mutagenic.
   d. teratogenic.
3. Today, the single most significant cause of air pollution is:
   a. motor vehicles.
   b. industrial toxins.
   c. natural sources.
   d. manufacturing corporations.
4. What colorless, odorless, and poisonous gas originates primarily from motor vehicle emissions?
   a. carbon monoxide
   b. carbon dioxide
   c. carbon oxide
   d. bicarbonate
5. The primary origin of sulfur oxide is:
   a. motor vehicle emissions.
   b. electrical utilities and industrial plants.
   c. household chimneys.
   d. the dumping of hazardous wastes.
6. The chemical that plays a major role in the formation of smog is:
   a. carbon monoxide.
   b. lead.
   c. sulfur oxide.
   d. hydrocarbons.
7. The ozone layer:
   a. is a colorless, odorless, poisonous gas.
   b. is formed from sulfur oxides.
   c. filters out ultraviolet rays from the sun.
   d. is formed by high levels of nitrogen oxide.
8. Precipitation that has fallen through acidic air pollutants, particularly those containing sulfur dioxides, is known as:
   a. ozone.
   b. smog.
   c. acid rain.
   d. hydrocarbons.
9. Chemicals that contribute to the depletion of the ozone layer are called:
   a. chlorofluorocarbons.
   b. hydrocarbons.
   c. carbon monoxides.
   d. sulfur oxides.

10. All of the following are sensible ways to reduce the amount of solid waste in the environment, EXCEPT:
    a. precycling.
    b. recycling trash.
    c. reducing the amount of product packaging.
    d. using more disposable products.

True/False

T F 1. A carcinogen is any substance that causes cancer.

T F 2. Toxic gases occur naturally in the environment.

T F 3. The primary origin of carbon monoxide is electrical power plants.

T F 4. Cigarette smoke is a source of particulates in the air.

T F 5. A primary origin of nitrogen oxides is in electrical power plants.

T F 6. Hydrocarbons are included in the six major air pollutants of the Clean Air Act.

T F 7. The gradual rise in the average temperature of the earth is known as global warming.

T F 8. Precycling is the practice of choosing products that have the potential for reuse.

T F 9. Benzene is a suspected carcinogen used in dry cleaning.

T F 10. Cochlea is a condition of temporary hearing loss usually created by a sudden loud noise.

ANSWERS:

Multiple Choice: 1. d (p. 257), 2. c (p. 257), 3. a (p. 258), 4. a (p. 260), 5. b (p. 261), 6. d (p. 261), 7. c (p. 262), 8. c (p. 261), 9. a (p. 262), 10. d (p. 264).
True/False: 1. T (p. 257), 2. T (p. 258), 3. F (p. 260), 4. F (p. 260), 5. T (p. 261), 6. F (p. 260), 7. T (p. 262), 8. T (p. 264), 9. F (p. 260), 10. F (p. 267).

Name ______________________________ Date ____________ Section ______________

THINGS I DO TO PRESERVE THE ENVIRONMENT

Directions: Check the following statements that apply to you.

_____ Whenever I can, I try to walk or ride my bicycle rather than take a car.

_____ I try to carpool to school or work with others.

_____ I have my car tuned up and inspected every year.

_____ When I have the oil changed, I make sure it does not get poured on the ground.

_____ I try to save fuel by not using the air conditioner.

_____ I turn off the lights when a room is not being used.

_____ I take a shower rather than a bath most of the time.

_____ I make sure faucets and toilets do not leak.

_____ I make sure that the washing machine is full before I wash a load of clothes.

_____ I try to purchase biodegradable soaps and detergents.

_____ I try to use biodegradable trash bags.

_____ At home, I use dishes and silverware rather than Styrofoam or plastic.

_____ I try not to subscribe to newspapers and magazines when I can view them online.

_____ I try not to use a hair dryer.

_____ I recycle plastic bags that I get when I bring something home from the store.

_____ I don't run water continuously when washing the dishes, shaving, or brushing my teeth.

_____ I prefer to use unbleached or recycled paper.

_____ If I have items I do not want to use anymore, I donate them to charity so someone else can use them.

_____ I try not to buy drinks in cans with plastic rings attached to them.

_____ I clean up after myself while enjoying the outdoors (picnic, camping, etc.).

For further thought: Review the items you did not check from the list above. Consider whether you might want to adopt some of these behaviors. List other behaviors that are not on the list and share them with class members.

Source: Hilgenkamp, K. and Blesz-Vestal, L., *Take Charge of Your Health! Self-Assessment Workbook,* Copyright 2003 Pearson Education, Inc., Publishing as Benjamin Cummings.

CHAPTER 16 MAKING HEALTH CARE DECISIONS

Multiple Choice

1. The primary purpose of advertising is to:
   a. provide accurate information.
   b. assist customers in making wise choices.
   c. reduce the amount of product packaging.
   d. sell products or services.
2. When advertisers sell a product by claiming that "everyone is using the product," they are using the ____.
   a. emotional appeal
   b. testimonials
   c. bandwagon approach
   d. scientific studies
3. A health claim made by a product or service that cannot be justified by scientific evidence is called:
   a. hijacking.
   b. homeopathy.
   c. quackery.
   d. truth-telling.
4. Treatments used in ____ include acupuncture and herbal medicine.
   a. osteopathy
   b. chiropractic medicine
   c. podiatry
   d. naturopathy
5. Medical care provided in hospitals that specialize in open-heart surgery and organ transplants is an example of:
   a. primary care.
   b. secondary care.
   c. inpatient care.
   d. tertiary care.
6. Outpatient care by a physician in the office is an example of:
   a. primary care.
   b. secondary care.
   c. tertiary care.
   d. extraordinary care.
7. Which traditional method of obtaining health insurance coverage allows you to pay for most of your medical bills and then file a claim to be reimbursed?
   a. cost-sharing
   b. fee-for-service
   c. copayment
   d. deductible
8. Cost-control procedures used by health insurers to coordinate treatment is/are called:
   a. copayments.
   b. managed care.
   c. deductibles.
   d. fee-for-service.
9. A ____ is a type of managed care plan that assigns you to a family physician or internist who acts as the gatekeeper to all other health services provided by the organization.
   a. prepaid group practice (PGP)
   b. health maintenance organization (HMO)
   c. point-of-service plan (POS)
   d. preferred provider organization (PPO)

10. One advantage HMOs have over other managed health care plans is that HMOs:
    a. tend to offer one-stop shopping.
    b. offer more services.
    c. have lower copayments.
    d. offer patients a wider choice of physicians.

True/False

T F 1. Over-the-counter drugs are also known as nonprescription drugs.

T F 2. Primary care physicians are most often trained in family practice or in internal medicine.

T F 3. Health care practitioners may or may not be medical doctors.

T F 4. Medicaid is the federal health insurance program that is only for people over 65 years of age.

T F 5. An indemnity plan for paying health care costs is also called fee-for-service.

T F 6. Inpatient care refers to health care provided in a hospital.

T F 7. A cesarean section is an example of tertiary care.

T F 8. Fee-for-service plans can place a limit on the extent of coverage for all people insured.

T F 9. One advantage of point-of-service plans is that the insured can get all outpatient medical needs tended to in one treatment center.

T F 10. Generic drugs do not have the same active chemical ingredients as their brand-name counterparts.

ANSWERS:

Multiple Choice: 1.d (p.277), 2.c (p.278), 3.c (p.279), 4.d (p.280), 5.d (p.282), 6.b (p.282), 7.b (p.283), 8.b (p.283), 9.b (p.284), 10.a (p.284).

True/False: 1.T (p.277), 2.T (p.279), 3.T (p.279), 4.F (p.283), 5.T (p.283), 6.T (p.282), 7.F (p.282), 8.T (p.283), 9.F (p.284), 10.F (p.285).

Name ______________________ Date ____________ Section ____________

AM I ABLE TO MAKE GOOD HEALTH CARE DECISIONS?

Directions: Circle the answer that best applies to you.

	Never		Sometimes		Always
1. I am actively involved in my own health care decisions.	1	2	3	4	5
2. I have complete information concerning my health.	1	2	3	4	5
3. I understand all of the tests that physicians and other health care workers perform on me.	1	2	3	4	5
4. I understand the variables associated with the purchase of prescription drugs.	1	2	3	4	5
5. I understand the variables associated with the purchase of over-the-counter drugs.	1	2	3	4	5
6. I have the information and knowledge to make reliable and unbiased health care choices.	1	2	3	4	5
7. I am able to analyze health care advertising.	1	2	3	4	5
8. I know how to file a health care consumer complaint.	1	2	3	4	5
9. I know how to choose a health care provider.	1	2	3	4	5
10. I know how to choose health insurance.	1	2	3	4	5
11. I know how to obtain reliable health care-related information, products, and services.	1	2	3	4	5

Assessment: Add up your score. The maximum score is 55. The higher the score, the more "health care" literate you are.

1. Which area(s) did you score the highest (4 or 5 points)? ______________________

____

2. Which area(s) did you score the lowest (1 or 2 points)? ______________________

____

3. What is one change I could make to improve my health care literacy? ______________________

____

Source: Rohwer, J.L. and Wanberg, Robert, *Personalizing Health Action Plans: A Student Resource Manual,* Copyright 1999. Allyn and Bacon.